Basic Science IN Obstetrics AND Gynaecology

Basic Science IN Obstetrics AND Gynaecology

A TEXTBOOK FOR MRCOG PART I

FIFTH EDITION

Edited by

Phillip Bennett, BSc, PhD, MD, FRCOG, FMedSci
Professor of Obstetrics and Gynaecology

David MacIntyre, BSc, PhD
Professor of Reproductive Systems Medicine

Lynne Sykes, BSc, MBBS, PhD, MRCOG
Clinical Senior Lecturer in Obstetrics
Imperial College & Imperial College Healthcare NHS Trust
London, UK

AND

Peter H. Dixon, BSc, PhD
Research Fellow in Women and Children's Health

Catherine Williamson, BSc, MD, FRCP, FMedSci
Professor of Obstetric Medicine
King's College London
London, UK

For additional online content visit eBooks+.com.

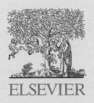

ELSEVIER

First edition 1986
Second edition 1992
Third edition 2002
Fourth edition 2010

ISBN: 978-0-7020-7422-6

Notices

Practitioners and researchers must always rely on their own experience and knowledge in evaluating and using any information, methods, compounds or experiments described herein. Because of rapid advances in the medical sciences, in particular, independent verification of diagnoses and drug dosages should be made. To the fullest extent of the law, no responsibility is assumed by Elsevier, authors, editors or contributors for any injury and/or damage to persons or property as a matter of products liability, negligence or otherwise, or from any use or operation of any methods, products, instructions, or ideas contained in the material herein.

Content Strategist: Alexandra Mortimer
Content Project Manager: Fariha Nadeem
Cover Design: Amy Buxton
Illustration Manager: Nijantha Priyadharshini
Marketing Manager: Deborah Watkins

Printed in India

Last digit is the print number: 9 8 7 6 5 4 3 2 1

Contents

16 *Self-Assessment* *278*
CHARITY KHOO AND ERNA BAYAR

Preface

Training the next generation of obstetricians and gynaecologists requires the provision of a strong foundation in the understanding of the basic science that underpins clinical practice. The MRCOG Part 1 examination has evolved to assess active participation of trainees in acquiring this fundamental scientific knowledge. The updated 2019 MRCOG syllabus and core curriculum acts as a Scientific Platform for Clinical Practice, examining 15 core knowledge areas in four domains of understanding: Cell Function, Human Structure, Measurement and Manipulation and Understating Illness. Assessment has also been reformed to the format of single best answer (SBA) questions.

This new edition has been updated with these adaptations to the MRCOG Part 1 examination in mind. We have brought in new editors and several new authors to update chapters. We have introduced a new chapter with self-assessment questions and answers, to reflect the revised examination format. We include 11 SBA questions per book chapter (17 for the anatomy chapter), and three mock exam papers. Included in this edition is a digital format to the book, to provide more flexibility in learning technique. We are grateful to the previous authors whose work formed the foundation of the current edition.

We hope that this text will continue to help future obstetricians and gynaecologists by providing a solid foundation in the science that underpins the desired high quality clinical practice.

Phillip Bennett, David MacIntyre,
Lynne Sykes, Peter H. Dixon and
Catherine Williamson

London 2022

Contributors

Amanda Ali, MRCPI, MRCOG
Consultant Obstetrician & Gynaecologist
Maternal Medicine Specialist
Kingston Hospital NHS Foundation Trust, UK
Drugs and Drug Therapy

Erna Bayar, BSc, MBBS, MSc, FHEA
Clinical Research Fellow
Queen Charlottes and Chelsea Hospital
Imperial College, London, UK
Self-Assessment

Tom Bourne, PhD, FRCOG, FAIUM (Hons)
Chair in Gynaecology
Tommy's National Centre for Miscarriage Research
Queen Charlottes and Chelsea Hospital
Imperial College, London, UK
Embryology

Annette Briley, SRN, RM, MSc, PhD, FRCOG
Professor of Women's Health and Midwifery Research
Caring Futures Institute, Flinders University and North
    Adelaide Local Health Network
Adelaide, South Australia
Clinical Research Methodology

Louise C. Brown, PhD, MSc, BEng
Professor of Medical Statistics and Clinical Trials
MRC Clinical Trials Unit
University College London
London, UK
Statistics and Evidence-Based Healthcare

Nick Dibb, PhD
Reader
Institute of Research and Developmental Biology
Hammersmith Campus
Imperial College London, UK
Biochemistry

Peter H. Dixon, PhD, BSc
Research Fellow
Department of Women and Children's Health
King's College London
London, UK
Structure and Function of the Genome

Mariane Silva Edge, MRCOG
Senior Specialist Doctor in Obstetrics and Gynaecology
Centre for Reproductive Immunology and Pregnancy
Bramshott House, 137/139 High Street, Epsom, UK
Drugs and Drug Therapy

Andrew J.T. George, MBE, MA, PhD, DSc, FRCPath, FHEA, FRSA, FRSB
Emeritus Professor
Department of Surgery and Cancer
Imperial College London
Hammersmith Hospital
London, UK
Immunology

Bethan Goulden, MBBS, iBSc
Obstetric Medicine and Rheumatology Registrar
Elizabeth Garrett Anderson Wing
University College London Hospital
London, UK
Physiology

Emily J. Greenlay, MSc, CStat
Lead Statistician, The Royal Marsden NHS Foundation
    Trust
And Visiting Lecturer, King's College London, UK
Statistics and Evidence-Based Healthcare

Sheba Jarvis, MBBS, BSc, PhD, MRCP
Honorary Consultant in Endocrinology, Diabetes, Obstetric
    Medicine and Imperial Post CCT Fellow
Imperial College London
Hammersmith hospital
London, UK
Endocrinology

Mark R. Johnson, PhD, MRCP, MRCOG
Professor of Obstetrics
Department of Maternal and Fetal Medicine
Imperial College School of Medicine
Chelsea and Westminster Hospital
London, UK
Endocrinology

Charity Khoo, MRCOG
Training Programme Director for Northwest London
Queen Charlotte's and Chelsea Hospital
Imperial College Healthcare NHS Trust
London, UK
Self-Assessment

Uday Kishore, PhD, FHEA, FRSB
Brunel University London
Kingston Lane
Uxbridge, UK
Immunology

Fiona Lyall, BSc, PhD, FRCPath, MBA
(Formerly) Professor of Maternal and Fetal Health
Maternal and Fetal Medicine Section
Institute of Medical Genetics
University of Glasgow
Glasgow, UK
Biochemistry

Julian R. Marchesi, PhD
Chair of Digestive Health
Department of Metabolism, Digestion and Reproduction,
   St Mary's Hospital, Imperial College, South Wharf
   Road, London, UK
Microbiology and Virology

Sara Paterson-Brown, FRCS, FRCOG
Consultant in Obstetrics and Gynaecology
Queen Charlotte's and Chelsea Hospital
London, UK
Applied Anatomy

Geoffrey L. Ridgway, MD, BSc, FRCP, FRCPath
(Formerly) Consultant Clinical Microbiologist and
   Honorary Senior Lecturer
University College London Hospitals NHS Trust
London, UK
Microbiology and Virology

Srdjan Saso, BSc, MRCS, MRCOG, PhD
Consultant in Gynaecology and Gynaecological
   Oncological Surgery
Honorary Clinical Senior Lecturer, Institute of
   Reproductive and Developmental Biology
Imperial College NHS Trust and Imperial College
   London, UK
Physics in Obstetrics and Gynaecology

Niamh Sayers, BSc, PhD
PhD Molecular Pharmacology
Department of Metabolism, Digestion and Reproduction
Faculty of Medicine
Imperial College London
London, UK
Biochemistry

Neil J. Sebire, MBBS, BClinSci, MD, DRCOG, FRCPath
Consultant in Paediatric Pathology
Department of Histopathology
Camelia Botnar Laboratories
Great Ormond Street Hospital
London, UK
Pathology

Harsha Shah, MA, MBBS
Obstetrics and Gynaecology Specialist Trainee and PhD
   Research Fellow
Queen Charlotte's and Chelsea Hospital
Imperial College London, UK
Embryology

Caroline J. Shaw, MBBS, PhD, MRCOG
Clinical Lecturer
Queen Charlotte's and Chelsea Hospital
Imperial College London, UK
Fetal and Placental Physiology

Hassan Shehata, FRCOG, FRCPI
Obstetric Lead, South West London Maternal Medicine
   Network, London
Consultant Obstetrician and Maternal Medicine Specialist,
   Epsom & St Helier University Hospitals NHS Trust, UK
Drugs and Drug Therapy

Andrew Shennan, MBBS, MD, FRCOG
Professor of Obstetrics
Maternal and Fetal Research Unit
King's College London
St Thomas' Hospital
London, UK
Clinical Research Methodology

Jennifer Summers, PhD, AKC, DHMSA, PGDPH, PGCAP, BSc, CStat, FHEA, MRSNZ
Senior Research Fellow
The Health, Environment & Infection Research Unit
   (HEIRU)
Department of Public Health | Te Tari Hauora Tūmataniui
University of Otago, Wellington | Te Whare Wānanga o
   Otāgo ki Te Whanga-Nui-a-Tara
And
Affiliate of King's College London, London, UK
Statistics and Evidence-Based Healthcare

Paul Taylor
(Formerly) Department of Microbiology & Virology
Royal Brompton and Harefield NHS Trust
Royal Brompton Hospital
London, UK
Microbiology and Virology

Ruth Wheeler, PhD
Clinical Scientist
Molecular Haemostasis Laboratory
Viapath Analytics
St Thomas' Hospital
London, UK
Clinical Genetics

David Williams, MBBS, PhD, FRCP, FRCOG
Professor of Professor of Reproductive Systems Medicine
UCL EGA Institute for Women's Health
University College London Hospital
London, UK
Physiology

Acknowledgements

The editors thank the previous editors, Geoffrey Chamberlain, Michael de Swiet and the late Sir John Dewhurst, the past and present contributors, Emily Sapsed for assisting in proofreading and the production and editorial team at Elsevier.

1 Structure and Function of the Genome

PETER H. DIXON

This chapter will provide a basic introduction to the human genome and some of the tools used to analyse it. Genomics and molecular biology have developed rapidly during the last few decades, and this chapter will highlight some of these advances, in particular with respect to the impact on our knowledge of the structure and function of the genome. The basic science described in this chapter is fundamental to the understanding of the field of clinical genetics, which is described in the following chapter.

Chromosomes

Inheritance is determined by genes, carried on chromosomes in the nuclei of all cells. Each adult cell contains 46 chromosomes, which exist as 23 pairs, one member of each pair having been inherited from each parent. Twenty-two pairs are homologous and are called *autosomes*. The 23rd pair is the sex chromosomes, X and Y in the male, X and X in the female.

Each cell in the body contains two pairs of autosomes plus the sex chromosomes for a total of 46, known as the diploid number (symbol N). Chromosomes are numbered sequentially with the largest first, with the X being almost as large as chromosome 1 and the Y chromosome being the smallest. This means that each cell (except gametes) has two copies of each piece of genetic information. In females, where there are two X chromosomes, one copy is silent (inactive) (i.e. genes on that chromosome are not being transcribed (see later)).

Each individual inherits one chromosome of each pair from the mother and one from the father following fertilisation of the haploid egg (containing one of each autosome and one X chromosome) by the haploid sperm (containing one of each autosome and either an X or a Y chromosome). The sex of the individual is therefore dependent on the sex chromosome in the sperm: an X will lead to a female (with the X chromosome from the egg) and a Y chromosome will lead to a male (with an X from the egg).

Chromosomes are classified by their shape. During metaphase in cell division, chromosomes are constricted and have a distinct recognisable 'H' shape with two chromatids joined by an area of constriction called the centromere. For 'metacentric' chromosomes the centromere is close to the middle of the chromosome, and for 'acrocentric' chromosomes it is near to the end of the chromosome. The area or 'arm' of the chromosome above the centromere is known as the 'p arm', and the area below is the 'q arm'. For acrocentric chromosomes, the p arm is very small, consisting of tiny structures called 'satellites'. Within the two arms, regions are numbered from the centromere outwards to give a specific 'address' for each chromosome region (Fig. 1.1). The ends of the chromosomes are called telomeres. Chromosomes only take on the characteristic 'H' shape during a metaphase when they are undergoing division (hence giving the two chromatids).

Chromosomes are recognised by their banding patterns following staining with various compounds in the cytogenetic laboratory. The most commonly used stain is the Giemsa stain (G-banding), which gives a characteristic black and white banding pattern for each chromosome.

In the cell, the chromosomes are folded many hundreds of times around histone proteins and are usually only visible under a microscope during mitosis and meiosis. DNA is composed of a deoxyribose backbone, the 3-position (3′) of each deoxyribose being linked to the 5-position (5′)

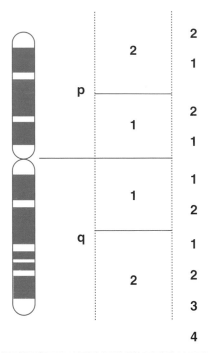

Fig. 1.1 Diagrammatic representation of the X chromosome. Note that the short arm (referred to as *p*) and the long arm (referred to as *q*) are each divided into two main segments labelled 1 and 2, within which the individual bands are also labelled 1, 2, 3, etc. (Courtesy of Dorothy Trump.)

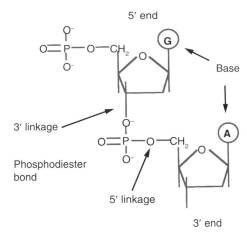

Fig. 1.2 The sugar phosphate backbone of DNA.

Table 1.1   The Genetic Code

1st Position	2nd Position				3rd Position
	T	**C**	**A**	**G**	
T	Phe	Ser	Tyr	Cys	T
	Phe	Ser	Tyr	Cys	C
	Leu	Ser	STOP	STOP	A
	Leu	Ser	STOP	Tyr	G
C	Leu	Pro	His	Arg	T
	Leu	Pro	His	Arg	C
	Leu	Pro	Gln	Arg	A
	Leu	Pro	Gln	Arg	G
A	Ile	Thr	Asn	Ser	T
	Ile	Thr	Asn	Ser	C
	Ile	Thr	Lys	Arg	A
	Met	Thr	Lys	Arg	G
G	Val	Ala	Asp	Gly	T
	Val	Ala	Asp	Gly	C
	Val	Ala	Glu	Gly	A
	Val	Ala	Glu	Gly	G

Note that in RNA thymidine *(T)* is replaced by uracil *(U)*.

of the next by a phosphodiester bond. At the 2-position each deoxyribose is linked to one of four nucleic acids, the purines (adenine or guanine) or the pyrimidines (thymine or cytosine). Each DNA molecule is made up of two such strands in a double helix with the nucleic acid bases on the inside. This is the famous double helix structure that was first proposed by James Watson and Francis Crick in 1953, based upon the x-ray diffraction work of Rosalind Franklin and colleagues. The bases pair by hydrogen bonding, adenine (A) with thymine (T), and cytosine (C) with guanine (G). DNA is replicated by separation of the two strands and synthesis by DNA polymerases of new complementary strands. With one notable exception, the reverse transcriptase produced by viruses, DNA polymerases always add new bases at the 3′ end of the molecule. RNA has a structure similar to that of DNA but is single stranded. The backbone consists of ribose, and uracil (U) is used in place of thymine (Fig. 1.2).

Gene Structure and Function

DNA is organised into discrete functional units known as genes. Genes contain the information for the assembly of every protein in an organism via the translation of the DNA code into a chain of amino acids to form proteins. DNA that encodes a single amino acid consists of three bases, or letters. With four letters and three positions in each 'word', there are 64 possible combinations of DNA, but in fact only 20 amino acids are coded for (Table 1.1). Therefore the third base of a codon is often not crucial to determining the amino acid – a phenomenon known as wobble.

A diagram of a typical gene structure is shown (Fig. 1.3). Each gene gives rise to a messenger RNA (mRNA), which can be interpreted by the cellular machinery to make the protein that the gene encodes.

Genes are split into exons, which contain the coding information, and introns, which are between the coding regions and may contain regulatory sequences that control when and where a gene is expressed. Promoters (which control basal and inducible activity) are usually upstream of the gene, whereas enhancers (which usually regulate inducible activity only) can be found throughout the genomic sequence of a gene. The two base pair sequences at the boundary of introns and exons (the splice acceptor and donor sites), identical in more than 99% of genes, are known as the splice junction (see Fig. 1.3); they signal cellular splicing machinery to cut and paste exonic sequences

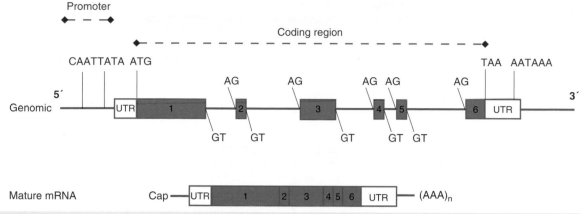

Fig. 1.3 Schematic representation of generalised gene structure. The upper panel shows the genomic organisation of a typical gene (with a variety of key features indicated) and the lower panel the messenger RNA (mRNA) resulting from the transcription of this gene. Key features indicated include the consensus splice sites GT (donor) and AG (acceptor), the initiation codon (ATG), the stop codon (TAA) and polyadenylation signal (AATAAA). Typical promoter motifs are indicated (CAAT and TATA) together with 5′ and 3′ untranslated regions (UTR). Mature mRNAs have a protective 5′ cap (a guanosine nucleotide connected to the mRNA by means of a 5′ to 5′ triphosphate linkage).

together at this point. The first residue of each gene is almost always methionine, encoded by the codon ATG.

Recent estimates based on the genome sequence put the number of genes at less than 23,000, a considerable reduction from earlier estimates. This means that the vast majority of human DNA does not contain a coding sequence (i.e. exons) but is rather an intronic sequence: structural motifs and regulatory regions such as promoters and enhancers. This is distinct from lower organisms (e.g. bacteria), where more than 95% of the DNA is a coding sequence. Just exactly why so much noncoding DNA is present remains somewhat enigmatic but is believed to be linked to the complex layers of gene regulation through interacting regulatory regions. The other key implication of this finding is that the huge complexity of humans compared with other organisms with similar numbers of genes must arise from more subtle regulation of gene expression, rather than greater numbers of different genes.

The Central Dogma of Molecular Biology

The central dogma of molecular biology concerns the information flow pathway in cells and can be simply summarised as: 'DNA makes RNA makes protein, which in turn can facilitate the two prior steps'. These steps are now explained in more detail.

TRANSCRIPTION

'Transcription' is the process of the information encoded in DNA being transferred into a strand of mRNA. During transcription the RNA polymerase, which constructs the complementary mRNA, reads from the DNA strand complementary to the RNA molecule. This is known as the antisense strand, while the opposite strand, which has the same base pair composition as the RNA molecule (with thymidine (T) in place of uracil (U) as mentioned previously), is the sense strand. Gene sequences are expressed

as the sequence of the sense strand of DNA, although it is in fact the antisense strand which is read (Fig. 1.4). The vast majority of genes consist of a 5′ untranslated region (UTR) containing response elements to which proteins may bind that influence transcription. The 5′ regions of genes are frequently characterised by elements such as the TATA and CAAT boxes (see Fig. 1.3) and are often richer in GC pairs than elsewhere in the genome. This is frequently the case around the 5′ ends of 'housekeeping' genes that are constitutively expressed in the majority of tissues. There then follows the transcribed sequence. The expressed coding parts of the gene are known as the exons, while the intervening sequences are known as introns. The coding portion of the gene is often interrupted by one or more noncoding intervening sequences, although numerous examples of single exon genes exist. Initially, the RNA molecule transcribes both introns and exons and is known as heavy nuclear RNA (hnRNA). The exons are perfectly spliced out (as marked by the splice boundary sequences) and a protective cap added before the now mature mRNA exits the nucleus. Hence cytoplasmic mRNA consists only of coding regions flanked by UTRs at the two ends. A polyadenine (poly A) tail is added to most mRNA molecules at their 3′ end, facilitated by the polyadenylation signal found past the stop codon in the coding sequence. This tail, found on the great majority of expressed mRNAs, serves to protect the RNA from degradation prior to translation by the ribosome (see later).

TRANSLATION

The term 'translation' describes the process whereby the cellular machinery reads the mRNA code and creates a chain of polypeptides (i.e. a protein). Once in the cytoplasm, the mRNA message is translated into protein by a ribosome. Ribosomes, consisting of a complex bundle of proteins and ribosomal RNA, attach to mRNA at the 5′ end. Protein synthesis begins at the amino terminal, and amino acids are sequentially added at the freshly made carboxyl end. Amino acids are brought into the reaction by specific transfer RNA

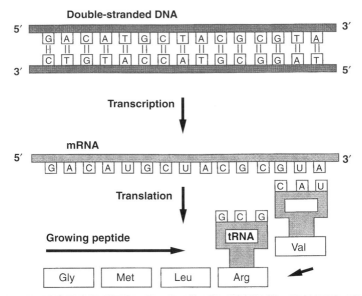

Fig. 1.4 Transcription and translation. Double-stranded DNA is transcribed forming a complementary single-stranded molecule of RNA. The mRNA is translated by transfer RNA *(tRNA)* to form the peptide chain.

(tRNA) molecules. Each tRNA is a single-stranded molecule which folds in a way that allows complementary base pairing between parts of the same strand. The specific configuration allows the tRNA molecule to bind to its specific amino acid. There remains, unpaired, at one end of the molecule, three bases which are complementary to the codon coding for the amino acid. This anticodon binds to the codon of the mRNA and places the amino acid in the correct sequence of the protein (see Fig. 1.4). Usually, several ribosomes translate a single mRNA molecule at any one time.

REPLICATION

'Replication' is the process whereby DNA is copied or replicated to permit transmission of genetic information to offspring. DNA replication is performed prior to cell division, when an identical copy must be made for each daughter cell resulting from division. Replication occurs before mitosis, the normal form of cellular division where resulting cells have identical DNA to the original. Meiosis, the second form of cellular division, occurs during gametogenesis and results in haploid cells (i.e. cells with half the usual complement of DNA). In meiosis the resulting cells (gametes) are haploid (i.e. carry only a single copy of the genomic sequence).

It is important to note that since this dogma was first established in 1958 by Crick, a number of exceptions have been identified. For example, retroviruses (e.g. human immunodeficiency virus (HIV)-1) can cause information to flow from RNA to DNA by integrating their genome (carried as RNA) into that of the host. A second example is ribozymes, which are functional enzymes composed solely of RNA and hence have no need to be translated into protein.

REGULATION OF GENE EXPRESSION

When a gene is actively being transcribed into mRNA and then translated into a protein, it is said to be 'expressed'. Gene expression can be controlled at several levels. Transcription of DNA into mRNA is generally regulated by the binding of specific proteins, known as transcription factors, to the region of DNA just upstream, or 5′, of the coding sequence itself. Other proteins can bind enhancer sequences that may be within the gene or a long way upstream or downstream.

The promoter contains specific DNA sequence motifs which bind transcription factors. In general, transcription factors become active when the cells receive some form of signal and then translocate to the nucleus, where they bind to specific sequences in the promoters of specific genes and activate transcription. Other genes, often known as housekeeping genes, have a constant level of expression and are not induced in this way.

Many different types of transcription factor exist with different modes of action. Typical examples of two types will be considered here, namely intracellular nuclear hormone receptors (which are transcription factors) and cell surface receptors, which are capable of activating transcription factors.

Members of the nuclear hormone receptor superfamily, such as the progesterone receptor and the thyroid hormone receptor, are present mainly in the cytoplasm of the cell. When a steroid hormone crosses the lipid bilayer of the cell membrane, it binds to the receptor which is usually dimerised to form pairs of receptor molecules. The receptor/hormone dimer complex then translocates to the nucleus and binds to response elements in the promoters of target genes, where it activates (or indeed represses) transcription. This process also involves the recruitment of many other cofactors to the dimer complex which are also involved in regulation of the expression of the target gene.

Cell surface receptors, subsequent to binding of ligands, can activate pathways leading to the formation of active transcription factors. For example, activation of tyrosine kinase–linked receptors on the cell surface may lead to a series of phosphorylation events within the cell, culminating in the phosphorylation of the protein Jun. Jun will then combine with the protein Fos to form a dimer transcription factor called AP-1, which can bind to specific AP-1 binding sites in the promoters of responsive genes.

In another example of cell surface receptor action, the 'inflammatory' transcription factor NF-κB exists in the cytoplasm of cells as dimers bound to an inhibitory protein IκB. Mediators of inflammation, such as the inflammatory cytokine interleukin-1β, bind to cell surface receptors and activate a chain of biochemical events that result in the phosphorylation and subsequent breakdown of IκB. Uninhibited NF-κB dimers then translocate to the nucleus to activate genes whose promoters contain NF-κB DNA-binding motifs.

Gene expression can also be controlled by regulation of the stability of the transcript. Most mRNA molecules are protected from degradation by the presence of their poly-A tail. Degradation of mRNA is controlled by specific destabilising elements within the sequence of the molecule. One type of destabilising element has been well characterised. The Shaw–Kayman or AU-rich sequence (ARE) is a region of RNA, usually within the 3′ UTR, in which the motif AUUUA is repeated several times. Rapid response genes, whose expression is rapidly switched on and then off again in response to some signal, often contain an ARE within their 3′ UTR. Binding of specific proteins to the ARE leads to removal of the mRNA's poly-A tails and then to degradation of the molecule.

Epigenetics

The field of epigenetics is concerned with modifications of DNA and chromatin that do not affect the underlying DNA sequence. In recent years, the importance of these modifications has come to light, and this is now a very active area of research.

EPIGENETIC MODIFICATION OF DNA

The principal epigenetic modification of DNA is methylation, whereby a methyl group ($-CH_3$) is added to a cytosine, converting it to 5-methylcytosine. This can only occur where a cytosine is next to a guanine (i.e. joined by a phosphate linkage) and is usually described as CpG to distinguish it from a cytosine base-paired to a guanine via hydrogen bonds across the double helix.

Methylation, particularly in the 5′ promoter regions of genes that are often GC rich, is associated with silencing. Humans have at least three DNA methyltransferases, and the process is critical to imprinting (parent of origin-dependent gene expression) and X inactivation. Abnormal DNA methylation leading to changes in gene expression is being increasingly recognised as playing a role in cancer cell development.

EPIGENETIC MODIFICATION OF HISTONES

Histone proteins are associated with DNA to form nucleosomes, which make up chromatin. Two of each histone protein (2A, 2B, 3 and 4) form the octameric core of the nucleosome, with H1 histone attached and linking nucleosomes to form the 'beads on a string' structure. Chromatin structure plays an important role in regulation of gene expression, and this structure is heavily influenced by modifications of the histone proteins. These modifications usually occur on the tail region of the protein and include methylation (distinct from methylation of DNA itself), acetylation, phosphorylation and ubiquitination. Combinations of modifications are considered to constitute a code (the so-called histone code), which, it is hypothesised, controls DNA–chromatin interaction. A comprehensive understanding of these mechanisms has not yet been elucidated; however, some functions have been worked out in detail. For example, deacetylation allows for tight bunching of chromatin, preventing gene expression.

Mitochondrial DNA

In addition to the genomic DNA present within cells, another type of DNA is present – mitochondrial DNA (mtDNA). The mitochondria are small organelles within cells that have a unique double-layered membrane and are the energy source for cellular activity and metabolism via production of adenosine triphosphate (ATP). They have their own genome (mtDNA), consisting of a single circular piece of DNA of 16,568 base pairs and encoding 37 genes. Mitochondria are only ever inherited maternally because all the mitochondria in a zygote come from the ovum and none from the sperm. mtDNA can be used for confirming family relatedness through analysis of the maternal lineage. In addition, mtDNA has been successfully and reproducibly extracted from ancient DNA samples, largely due to the high copy number compared with nuclear DNA. Mutations in mtDNA are responsible for a number of human diseases (see Chapter 2).

Studying DNA

The vast majority of DNA samples used for genetic analysis originate from a peripheral blood sample, usually collected in a 10-mL tube containing an anticoagulant (e.g. EDTA (ethyelediaminetetraacetic acid)). From this sample, large quantities of DNA are easily extracted from the leucocytes, using one of the many commercial kits available. This has replaced the older method of phenol/chloroform extraction. Alternatively, if only a small amount of DNA is required, buccal swabs can be used to collect DNA or saliva samples collected. Because these are noninvasive, they have considerable advantage (e.g. where patients are needle-phobic, or where DNA is required from small children). It is also possible to extract usable quantities of DNA from very small amounts of tissue or blood from archive samples such as formalin-fixed paraffin-embedded sections. DNA can also be extracted successfully from ancient samples such as teeth and bone.

MENDELIAN GENETICS AND LINKAGE STUDIES

The majority of advances in recent years in disease gene identification have come from the field of mendelian disease. This refers to diseases (e.g. cystic fibrosis or muscular dystrophy) where the inheritance pattern follows classical mendelian principles (i.e. those established by Gregor Mendel at the end of the 19th century). His work, long before the existence of DNA was known, established simple rules for inheritance of characteristics (phenotypes).

That is, a disease can be dominant (requiring only one mutant allele to have the disease), recessive (requires two) or X-linked (one mutant allele on the X chromosome and hence much more common in males). Since the first gene was identified by linkage/positional cloning in 1986, well over 4000 mendelian disease genes have been identified, initially by the use of linkage studies.

Linkage studies rely on the use of large, phenotypically well-characterised families. Typically, 12 or more affected family members are required for tracing autosomal dominant diseases, but far smaller families with as few as three affected individuals can be used for recessive diseases. Family members are typed for polymorphic markers throughout the genome to detect which regions the affected individuals share and hence are more likely to contain the disease gene. The marker of choice for these studies is usually short tandem repeats (STRs), which are more commonly known as microsatellites. These markers are repeat sequences that most commonly consist of dinucleotide base repeats (e.g. $(CA)_n$), but they may also comprise trinucleotide or tetranucleotide repeats. These markers exhibit length polymorphism, such that they are different lengths in different individuals, and can be heterozygous. For example, an individual may carry at one marker position one repeat of five units and one of seven. These different repeat lengths are easily detectable by common molecular biology techniques. If a disease gene is close to a particular marker (i.e. linked), it will almost always be inherited with it. Thus, if affected individuals all show the same length repeat at a particular marker, the disease gene may be close by. Statistical analysis is used to formalise the results and give likelihood ratios, the logarithm of the odds (LOD) score or the location of a disease locus.

In the recent past, linkage studies were followed by positional cloning to identify a disease gene. This method of gene identification is so called because genes are identified primarily on the basis of their position in the genome, with no underlying assumptions about the protein they encode. After the linkage of a disease had been achieved, a physical map of the linked region was constructed. This was done using large-scale cloning vectors such as YACs (yeast artificial chromosomes) or BACs (bacterial artificial chromosomes), which contain inserts of up to a megabase (1,000,000 base pairs) of the human genome. Libraries of the whole genome were screened with the microsatellite markers used that had been linked to the disease and a series of overlapping clones, or contig, of the linked region constructed. Once this had been established, these clones would be searched for genes which, when identified, would be screened for mutations in affected patients. This search would have used a variety of methods such as direct library hybridisation or exon trapping to identify genes within the contig. However, much of this work is now unnecessary due to the greatest advance in the field of human genetics in the past 20 years – the completion of the sequence of the human genome.

THE SEQUENCING OF THE GENOME

The completion of the human genome sequencing project has transformed the field of genetics. In brief, BAC (see earlier) libraries were constructed from the DNA of a handful of anonymous donors and arranged in order around the genome using genetic markers with established positions. Each BAC was then sequenced, and, by the use of high-powered computers, the sequence was assembled, first into the original BAC and then, by matching overlaps, to build up a sequence for the entire genome. The genome centres involved in this project used vast numbers of sequencing machines and a production-line environment to achieve the throughput required. In addition to the publicly funded consortium, a private company also produced a complete human genome sequence using a slightly different methodology.

Individual labs and researchers now have access to the entire genome dataset from the publicly funded project freely available on the internet. This information is an invaluable resource and has greatly accelerated research into the molecular aetiology of genetic disease. Once the position of a disease gene has been confirmed (linkage), scientists can now use an in silico (i.e. computer-based) approach to identifying the disease gene. Practically, this involves searching databases for all the identified genes in a region and then sequencing them in affected individuals to look for mutations. These 'positional candidates' are often prioritised using other sources of information such as tissue expression pattern or predicted function. Once mutations have been identified, functional studies of mutant forms of the protein to determine the exact nature of the molecular aetiology of the disease in question are often pursued.

Completion of this project has enabled genome centres to focus on two other areas: that of whole-genome sequencing of other organisms for comparative purposes, and so-called deep resequencing to identify the spectrum of genetic variation in human populations. With the rapid advances in scale and development of new technology, modern sequencing methods (so-called next-generation sequencing) enable complete human genomes to be determined in a few days.

ANALYSIS OF COMPLEX TRAITS

The vast majority of so-called genetic disease does not fall into the category of mendelian disease. Rather, it is caused by so-called complex genetic disease or traits, where a number of genetic factors interacting with the environment result in a disease phenotype. It is this area of genetics that much current research is most focused upon, together with continued work on rare diseases and single gene disorders. An example of such a disease in obstetrics is preeclampsia (see later chapters). It is important to note that in this type of genetic disease the mutant gene may only be having a small effect on disease susceptibility, caused by subtle effects of relatively common variation, and for each disease a large number of variants at multiple genes (together with environmental influences) may be playing a role. In these cases, the genetic variation of interest is usually single nucleotide polymorphisms (SNPs) or short insertion/deletion polymorphisms (indels). Often the underlying functional effect of the variation is not known but can be investigated with in silico and wet lab approaches.

Methods of analysis of complex traits can be broadly divided into two areas: family-based studies and case–control studies. Family-based studies are usually based upon microsatellite typing approaches (see earlier) or SNP analysis, whereas association studies (otherwise known as case–control studies) generally use another kind of genetic marker, SNPs. SNPs are much more frequent throughout the genome (every 1000 bases or so) and, although they have a lower information content than microsatellites, can be used for much finer mapping studies, thanks to their more frequent occurrence.

Family-based studies rely on large collections of nuclear families, parent–offspring trios and/or affected or discordant sibling (sib) pairs. The term discordant refers to disease status (i.e. a discordant sib pair comprises one affected and one unaffected individual). Unaffected family members act as controls.

The dissection of complex traits using these approaches has been problematic for many years for a variety of reasons. These include insufficient sample size (i.e. underpowered studies), inappropriate controls (in association studies) and a lack of knowledge about the underlying structure of the genome (i.e. the patterns of linkage disequilibrium, or the underlying nonrandom association of markers). In addition, very little was known on a genome-wide scale about the pattern of naturally occurring human variation. However, with a more complete understanding of the structure of the genome, and ever-larger sample resources, significant and reproducible associations of genetic variation with common human disease are emerging. Technology has played a role too, with it now being possible to type many hundreds of thousands of SNPs in a single experiment using DNA array technologies, microbead platforms and current massively parallel sequencing approaches (see later). Much genomic research is now performed at a genome-wide scale such that genome-wide association studies of common diseases are relatively frequent. Large-scale combined analyses of these studies (meta-analysis) in different populations are providing new insights into these common diseases such as heart disease, diabetes and cancer susceptibility. However, this approach is as yet still relatively uncommon in the fields of obstetrics and gynaecology, as the huge cohorts of patients needed have not yet been collected.

Molecular Biology Techniques

The manipulation of DNA, RNA and proteins at a molecular level is collectively referred to as molecular biology. This term encompasses a huge range of techniques, some of which are outlined here. All of these techniques are in routine use in clinical and research labs around the world.

RESTRICTION ENDONUCLEASES

One of the key tools used to manipulate DNA is restriction endonucleases. These enzymes, which have been isolated from a wide range of bacteria, cut or restrict DNA at a certain site determined by the base sequence. The reaction occurs under certain conditions (i.e. at the correct temperature and in the correct buffer (usually supplied by the manufacturer)). These known recognition sites can be used to manipulate DNA for cloning, blotting, etc. The enzymes have usually been isolated from microorganisms, and their name reflects the organism from which they have been isolated. For example, the common restriction enzyme EcoRI,

which cuts or restricts DNA at the sequence GAATTC, was isolated from *Escherichia coli* RY13. *Note*: the recognition of the restriction site depends upon double-stranded DNA, and the cleavage can result in an overhang of a few bases ('sticky ends') or a straight cut across both strands ('blunt ends').

THE POLYMERASE CHAIN REACTION

The polymerase chain reaction (PCR) is the bedrock of molecular biology and refers to a procedure whereby a known sequence of DNA (the target sequence) can be amplified many millions of times to generate enough copies to visualise, clone, sequence or manipulate in many other ways. A known DNA sequence is amplified first by using a uniquely designed pair of primers at the start (5′) and end (3′; on the reverse strand) of the sequence to be amplified. The primers are thus small pieces of DNA, known as oligonucleotides (oligos), and are usually synthesised by commercial companies for relatively minimal cost. The primers are used in combination with a buffer, a source of deoxyribose nucleotide triphosphate (dNTP) building blocks, the target DNA and Taq polymerase. This polymerase, first isolated from *Thermophilus aquaticus*, is able to replicate DNA at high temperatures. Once prepared, the reaction is placed into a thermal cycler. The reaction proceeds through a number of repeated cycles where the DNA template is denatured, the primers anneal and the polymerase extends the products. Cycling of these three temperatures (one for each of the aforementioned steps) results in an exponential amplification of the target sequence. Following amplification, products can be visualised by agarose gel electrophoresis (see later).

Many other commonly used applications are based around the principles of PCR. For example, reverse transcription PCR (RT-PCR), which can be applied to RNA analysis. This technique uses reverse transcriptase enzymes isolated from retroviruses to generate DNA copies of template RNA to detect expression of a particular gene. This approach is further enhanced by quantitative RT-PCR, where relative or absolute expression levels of a particular message can be measured.

Another development of PCR is whole genome amplification, which relies on the use of specialist polymerases to amplify the entire genome in a single reaction, a very useful tool when the amount of sample available is limited.

ELECTROPHORESIS

DNA molecules are slightly negatively charged and hence, under the right conditions, will migrate towards a positive charge. This phenomenon can be exploited to visualise DNA. For example, the results of a PCR reaction (see earlier) can be assessed in this way, or a sample of genomic DNA digested with a restriction enzyme can be separated. DNA samples are loaded onto an agarose gel (a sieving mixture of seaweed extract) in the range of 0.5% to 4% (depending on the size range of DNA to be separated) in a tank containing running buffer (commonly Tris/borate/EDTA). Under an electric current the DNA will migrate at a rate proportional to its size. The samples can then be visualised under an ultraviolet (UV) light box after the addition of ethidium bromide, or one of the newer less toxic alternatives (e.g. Sybersafe). Larger DNA molecules and RNA samples can also be visualised by electrophoresis. Slightly different conditions are used to protect the RNA, which is inherently more unstable than DNA, and specialised running equipment is needed to separate DNA molecules larger than 10 kb in size.

BLOTTING

DNA (in the case of Southern blotting), RNA (Northern) and protein (Western) can be fixed to nylon membranes for further analysis (e.g. for screening with a radioactively labelled probe (DNA/RNA) or with an antibody raised to an epitope of interest (proteins)). This is a fairly straightforward and routine procedure, which enables a range of downstream experiments to be carried out. For example, a genomic DNA digest can be screened with a radiolabelled or biotinylated probe for a gene sequence of interest, or an antibody raised against a particular protein can be used to screen for that protein in cellular extracts.

SEQUENCING

DNA sequencing is now a rapid and straightforward process. The sequence of an amplified fragment of DNA is determined using a variation of the PCR method incorporating fluorescently labelled bases which can be read by a laser detection system. In this application, a PCR cycle is performed using only one primer, either forward or reverse, and the labelled nucleotides (initially radioactive, subsequently with fluorescent dyes). This results in linear amplification of product with consecutive lengths of sequence with a fluorescent tag corresponding to the final base of the fragment. When run on a slab gel or capillary and read by a laser, the sequence is determined by the sequential reading of each base. Recent advances in the use of capillary-based machines with multiple channels have resulted in a huge increase in throughput and capacity and facilitated the rapid acceleration in efforts to sequence the entire human genome. This type of sequencing, called 'Sanger' sequencing after its inventor, Fredrick Sanger, remains the gold standard for DNA sequencing in clinical genetics (see next chapter). However, in the research setting, and very soon across the majority of clinical genetics, next-generation sequencing has become the norm. This describes a range of platforms in current use (from companies such as Illumina and PacBio) that use massively parallel sequencing of millions of strands of DNA concurrently, with subsequent bioinformatic pipelines to map these sequence reads back to the reference human genome. Initially, amplification and pulldown methods were commonplace (generating gene panel screening or whole-exome analysis (WES)), but more recently cost reduction and technologic advances mean that whole-genome sequencing (WGS) is being used more frequently.

CLONING VECTORS AND cDNA ANALYSIS

As outlined earlier, the human genome sequence now makes it unnecessary to clone genes from a candidate region before mutation analysis. However, cloning is still a critical part of the analysis of gene function subsequent to mutation detection. For example, using some of the techniques outlined earlier in the molecular biology section, the expression pattern of a gene can be studied, factors that induce transcription can be identified and so on. Many of these techniques rely on the use of copy DNA (cDNA) clones. These are vectors of much smaller size than YACs and are carried and propagated in bacteria as plasmids or phage. They may also be introduced into cell lines by transfection. The vectors contain an insert of DNA, which corresponds to the full-length mRNA of the gene in question; this is known as cDNA and contains only the exonic material of the gene. Clones may be screened from libraries or in many cases purchased from commercial sources. Isolation and propagation of these clones in a suitable host strain of bacteria allow detailed analysis of gene function.

EXPRESSION STUDIES

A detailed explanation of protein analysis is beyond the scope of this chapter. Key concepts to understand are that proteins can be expressed in mammalian and bacterial systems, their interactions studied and function analysed. A recent approach gaining popularity is to use short interfering RNA (siRNA) to 'knock down' genes of interest in both in vitro and in vivo systems. In this approach, a vector is introduced which expresses short pieces of carefully designed RNA. These RNA molecules interact with cellular machinery and interfere with endogenously expressed mRNA by targeting it for degradation. This results in the reduction, or knocking down, of the expression of the target gene by up to 80% of the original expression level.

IN SILICO ANALYSIS

The free availability of the human genome sequence via the internet has greatly enhanced the use of computer analysis for molecular biology. This has led to an enormous rise in the discipline of 'bioinformatics', which can be simply defined as deriving knowledge from computer analysis of biological data.

A variety of molecular biology databases, also freely available over the web, provide a large amount of useful information. In addition to the human genome sequence already discussed, a huge range of structural and functional databases, together with organism- and disease-specific databases, polymorphism databases and enzyme databases, can be used to aid research (for a few examples, see Table 1.2).

The 'Postgenomic' Era

Following the completion of the sequencing of the human genome, and the ongoing projects to completely sequence the genome of a range of other organisms, focus has shifted into a broad range of fields that consider and analyse cells or whole organisms in their entirety, the so-called postgenomic era. This approach is sometimes referred to as systems biology; broadly it encompasses a range of methodologies to analyse whole systems (be it cells, tissues or whole

Table 1.2 Examples of Online Databases Used by Molecular Biologists

	URL	Description
Genomes	http://genome.ucsc.edu/	Gateways to whole genome sequences including human with huge range of annotation tracks and linked datasets
	https://www.ensembl.org/index.html	
	https://www.ncbi.nlm.nih.gov/genome/gdv/	
RNA	http://www.h-invitational.jp/h-dbas/	Alternative splicing database
	http://www.mirbase.org	MicroRNA database
	http://crdd.osdd.net/servers/virsirnadb/	Human short interfering RNA database
Protein	https://www.ebi.ac.uk/uniprot/	Annotated and curated protein sequence database
	https://gpcrdb.org	Database of G protein–coupled receptors

organisms). The range of techniques used in this field is collectively known as the 'omics' topics. Some of these are as follows:

Proteomics (the large-scale study of proteins). The total protein make-up of a biologic sample can be determined using, for example, automated gas chromatography/mass spectrophotometry (GC/MS) systems. These systems, which combine separation methods (GC) and identification methods (MS), are enhanced through automation and pattern-matching techniques to facilitate rapid and accurate identification of protein content.

Transcriptomics (high-throughput analysis of total mRNA populations). The total mRNA population (or transcriptome) of two groups can be compared by isolating RNA and hybridising it to a chip which has oligos for every identified gene arrayed on its surface. The output of these experiments can, for example, determine changes in gene expression under different conditions or can be used to analyse changes in gene expression during carcinogenesis. Modern sequencing platforms are now often used in place of arrays and can be scaled to a single cell level such that a read of every transcript present in a cell can be performed.

Metabolomics (the analysis of all metabolites in a cellular system). This discipline is concerned with quantitative changes in small molecule metabolites (i.e. molecules changing during the process of normal or abnormal metabolism). This may be analysed using proteomic methodology and nuclear magnetic resonance (NMR) spectroscopy methods.

The Molecular Basis of Inherited Disease – DNA Mutations

DNA mutations occur during cellular replication and division and can result in a range of alterations from large-scale chromosomal abnormalities (which are considered in more detail in Chapter 2) down to single base changes, also called

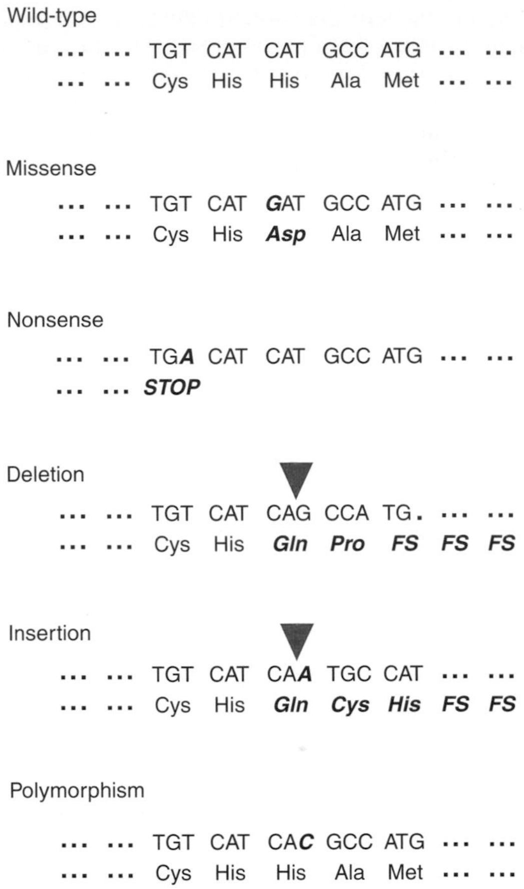

Fig. 1.5 Examples of mutations in DNA sequence and their effect upon the protein. In each case, the result of a base change in the DNA sequence *(upper strand)* is shown on the protein sequence *(lower strand)*. FS, Frameshift.

'point mutations' (which will be considered in general terms here and in more detail in Chapter 2). An important distinction to make is between somatic and germline mutations. Somatic mutations occur in subpopulations of cells and are not inherited. Examples of such somatic mutations are those seen in a variety of cancer cell populations, where cancerous cells accumulate a number of somatic mutations as they develop into tumours. Germline mutations, as the name implies, are present in the germline (i.e. sperm and oocytes) and are inherited down generations. In the rest of this section, only germline mutations will be considered.

Variation in genomic DNA sequence arises from errors in DNA replication. This variation is often repaired by cellular machinery or occurs in noncoding regions of the genome. However, when variations, or polymorphisms, occur within genes and affect protein function, they are considered mutations. A variety of small-scale mutation types are illustrated (Fig. 1.5). This figure illustrates a variety of effects that are possible on encoded proteins by small changes in the DNA sequence. It is important to remember that common variation occurs throughout the human population; for example, SNPs occur every few hundred bases (on average). This causes individuals to be polymorphic (i.e. carry different alleles at the same loci).

The severity of a mutation (i.e. the degree of effect on protein function) often, but not always, correlates with the extent of changes to the protein caused by the change in DNA sequence. For example, a missense mutation will alter only one amino acid, whereas a nonsense mutation will cause a premature truncation of the protein. In some cases, the missense amino acid will not have a great effect.

Due to the degenerative nature of the DNA code (see Table 1.1), some changes occur within coding regions that do not result in an amino acid change. These changes are deemed polymorphisms (see Fig. 1.5).

The application of this knowledge leads to the related clinical specialty, that of the clinical genetics field, which is considered in more detail in Chapter 2.

2 Clinical Genetics

RUTH WHEELER

Clinical genetics is the specialty concerned with the diagnosis and investigation of disorders which are thought to have a genetic basis. The clinical genetics team is multidisciplinary and consists of consultants and specialist registrars working closely with genetic counsellors and laboratory-based diagnostic genetic scientists and cytogeneticists. Genetic risk assessment and non-directive counselling are an important part of the clinical workload and may involve both the proband (the first person to be tested) and also other family members.

Genetic disorders can be broadly classified into the following areas:

1. Chromosomal abnormalities
2. Single gene disorders
3. Familial cancer and cancer-predisposing syndromes
4. Multifactorial disorders

This chapter will deal with each of these types of disorders, with the exception of familial cancer and cancer-predisposing syndromes, and will also cover more unusual mechanisms of disease inheritance, including genetic imprinting and mitochondrial disorders. Diagnostic techniques and interpretation of results will be summarised.

Chromosome Abnormalities

Chromosome abnormalities can be numerical or structural, and it is estimated that they are detected in 50% to 70% of miscarriages. As detailed in Chapter 1, a normal diploid human cell contains 46 chromosomes (22 pairs of autosomes and 1 pair of sex chromosomes) (Fig. 2.1), and any deviation from this is likely to have consequences.

CHROMOSOME NOMENCLATURE

Chromosome abnormalities are described according to an agreed format which forms the basis of cytogenetic reports. The total number of chromosomes is given first, followed by the sex chromosomes (46,XX). Any structural changes, such as translocations, deletions or duplications, are then indicated by the letter 't' (translocation), del (deletion) or dup (duplication), followed by the number of chromosomes concerned in parentheses, with 'p' or 'q' relating to the involvement of long or short arms. The regions of the chromosomes involved are indicated by their numerical address. Fig. 2.2 shows a reciprocal translocation described as 46,XY, t(2;3) (p21;q29), indicating an exchange of genetic material between chromosome 2p21 and chromosome 3q29.

Patient A.C.

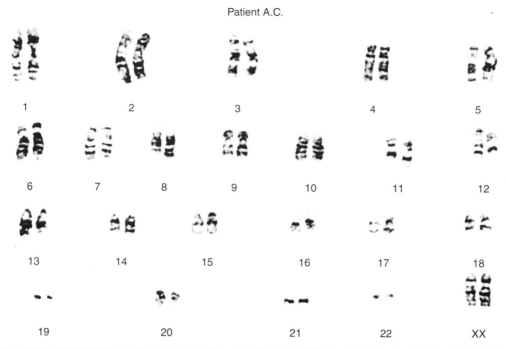

1   2   3   4   5

6   7   8   9   10   11   12

13   14   15   16   17   18

19   20   21   22   XX

Fig. 2.1 A normal female 46,XX G-banded karyotype illustrating the banding patterns which permit identification of each individual chromosome.

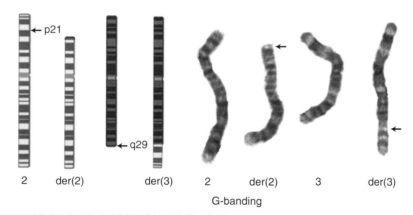

← p21

← q29

2   der(2)   der(3)   2   der(2)   3   der(3)

G-banding

Fig. 2.2 Reciprocal translocation between chromosomes 2 and 3. A portion of the short arm of chromosome 2 has been exchanged with a small portion of the long arm of chromosome 3. The panel on the left shows this in diagrammatic form. The middle panel is the result of G-banding. The right panel shows chromosome painting. This is a balanced translocation. (Figure provided by Dr L. Willett, East Anglian Genetics Service, Cytogenetics Laboratory.)

NUMERICAL DISORDERS

Three types of numerical disorder have been described: aneuploidy, polyploidy and mixoploidy.

Aneuploidy

Aneuploidy is defined as an abnormal number of chromosomes and includes trisomy, monosomy and the presence of additional, structurally abnormal (marker) chromosomes (Table 2.1). It is the most common chromosome anomaly. It can involve any chromosome, but abnormal numbers of sex chromosomes are usually considered a separate group (Table 2.2 and below).

Trisomy. Trisomy is the presence of a single extra chromosome. This occurs when homologous chromosomes fail to separate at meiosis, a process known as non-disjunction, which results in a germ cell containing 24 chromosomes rather than the normal 23. Trisomy of any chromosome can occur, but, with the exception of trisomies 13, 18, 21, X and Y, all are lethal in utero.

Trisomy 21, also known as Down syndrome, is the most common of the viable trisomies and affects around 1 in every 650 live births in the absence of prenatal screening. The clinical features are summarised in Table 2.1. The risk of having a child with Down syndrome increases with maternal age, with a live-born risk of under 1 in 1000 in a 25-year-old woman rising to 1 in 100 at a maternal age of 40. Screening is offered to all pregnant women in the UK between weeks 10 and 14 of pregnancy. A small number of cases of Down syndrome (~2%) are due to mitotic

Table 2.1   Numerical Abnormalities of Autosomes

Condition	Karyotype	Clinical Picture
Polyploidy	69,XXX or 69,XXY	Usually spontaneous abortion. Occasional live born, die soon after birth. Growth retardation, congenital malformation, mental retardation.
Diandry polyploidy	69,XXX or 69,XXY extra chromosomes from father	Usually spontaneous abortion. Can lead to partial hydatidiform mole.
Trisomy		
Trisomy 21 (Down syndrome)	47,XX + 21 or 47,XY + 21	Characteristic facial dysmorphology, mental retardation, congenital cardiac anomalies, duodenal atresia.
Trisomy 13 (Patau syndrome)	47,XX + 13 or 47,XY + 13	Cleft lip and palate, microcephaly, holoprosencephaly, closely spaced eyes, post-axial polydactyly. Death usually within few weeks of birth.
Trisomy 18 (Edward syndrome)	47,XX + 18 or 47,XY + 18	Low birth weight, small chin, narrow palpebral fissures, overlapping fingers, rocker bottom feet, congenital heart defects, death usually within few weeks of birth.
Monosomy		Monosomy of autosomes not viable.

Table 2.2   Sex Chromosome Anomalies

Condition	Karyotype	Clinical Picture
Triple X syndrome	47,XXX	Slender body habitus, mild learning difficulties, as a group reduction in IQ, individually may not be noticeable.
Tetrasomy X	48,XXXX	Mental retardation more severe than 47,XXX (mean IQ around 60).
Klinefelter syndrome	47,XXY	1 in 1000 newborns but often not diagnosed until much later. Tall, small testes, gynaecomastia, sparse facial hair, infertility, mild reduction in IQ.
XYY syndrome	47,XYY	Often undiagnosed, can cause mild learning difficulty, behavioural problems.
Turner syndrome	45,X	Often causes spontaneous miscarriage, short stature, webbing of neck, congenital heart defect, wide-spaced nipples, gonadal dysgenesis leading to delayed or absent puberty.

non-disjunction, which occurs after zygote formation. In such cases, only a percentage of cells will be trisomy 21, and the baby is said to be a mosaic. There is no correlation between the degree of mosaicism and the severity of symptoms.

Trisomies 13 (Patau syndrome) and 18 (Edward syndrome) are much rarer (1 in 12,000 and 1 in 6000 live births respectively). Both these trisomies cause severe congenital malformations (see Table 2.1) and mental retardation, and affected babies usually die within the first few months of life. Although the risk also increases with

maternal age, it is much lower than for Down syndrome at all ages.

Monosomy. Monosomy, the absence of one of a pair of chromosomes is usually lethal to the embryo and therefore rare in live-born infants. The only exception is monosomy X or Turner syndrome (see Sex Chromosome Anomalies).

Polyploidy

Polyploid cells possess whole extra copies of the haploid genome (i.e. one set of all chromosomes). The most common polyploidies in humans are triploidy, in which 69 chromosomes are present, and tetraploidy (92 chromosomes). Triploidy occurs in 1% to 3% of conceptions and usually results in spontaneous abortion, although there have been occasional reports of live births of affected infants, who present with growth restriction and congenital malformations and die shortly after birth. The extra set of chromosomes can come from either the father (Type 1 triploidy or diandry) or mother (Type 2 triploidy or digyny). Diandry usually arises due to the fertilisation of a single haploid ovum by two sperm or, less frequently, by a single diploid sperm which has arisen due to an error in meiosis during spermatogenesis (see Table 2.1). Digyny is much less common and occurs when a diploid egg or nucleated primary oocyte is fertilised. Diploid ova arise as the result of non-disjunction of all chromosomes during meiosis I or II.

Examples of polyploidy include partial hydatidiform mole and diploid-triploid mosaicism. In both cases some cells have the normal two copies of each chromosome, whilst others have three copies. Partial hydatidiform mole is usually due to fertilisation of an ovum by two sperm and does not result in a viable fetus. Diploid-triploid mosaicism is most frequently due to second polar body incorporation in which the polar body (produced in the ovary at the same time as the egg and containing an extra set of chromosomes) is included in the cells that will become the baby. It is associated with truncal obesity, body/facial asymmetry, hypotonia, growth delay, mild differences in facial features, syndactyly and irregularities in the skin pigmentation. Intellectual impairment may be present but is highly variable, depending on the degree of mosaicism present. Interestingly, triploid cells are not normally present in the blood, so diagnosis relies on the analysis of other cell types, such as skin cells.

Tetraploidy, in which there are four copies of each chromosome per cell, is extremely rare. It is predominantly associated with miscarriage but infants surviving to term present with a severe phenotype characterised by multiple congenital abnormalities, and/or genital malformations and limb defects.

Mixoploidy

Mixoploidy includes mosaicism and chimerism.

Mosaicism. Mosaicism occurs when an individual has two cell populations, derived from a single zygote, each with a different genotype, such as diploid/triploid mosaicism (see above). Aneuploidy mosaicism is common and is usually caused by non-disjunction during early cleavage of the zygote or the loss of one chromosome due to a failure to travel along the nuclear spindle properly during cell division (anaphase lagging). Turner syndrome is often mosaic and this may explain the occasional reports of fertility in affected women.

Chimerism. In chimerism, an individual has two or more genetically distinct cell lines originating from different zygotes. The exact frequency of chimerism is not known, but there have been reports in association with the rare pigment disorder hypomelanosis of Ito.

SEX CHROMOSOME ANOMALIES

The consequences of aneuploidy involving the sex chromosomes are generally less severe than those observed in autosomal aneuploidy. This is thought to be due to the presence of normal mechanisms which control gene dosage effects. In a normal female cell (46,XX), one randomly selected, complete copy of the X chromosome is switched off in a process known as X-inactivation or lyonisation. This ensures that both males and females express the same number of X-encoded genes. There is no such mechanism for Y chromosomes, but, as this contains very few genes, predominantly concerned with determining maleness, there is no impact of dosage differences. The features of sex chromosome aneuploidies are summarised in Table 2.2. Trisomy of the sex chromosomes is often undetected, particularly in Klinefelter syndrome (47,XXY), unless a karyotype is performed. Monosomy, resulting in Turner syndrome (45,X or 45,X0), is the only viable monosomy and has an incidence of approximately 1 in 2500 in newborn females. The features are summarised in Table 2.2. A much larger number of affected pregnancies miscarry, and monosomy X accounts for about 18% of chromosomal abnormalities seen in spontaneous abortion. Absence of the X chromosome, leaving only the Y chromosome, is incompatible with embryonic development and will always result in early abortion. Tetrasomy (48,XXXX) and pentasomy (49,XXXXX) of sex chromosomes are compatible with normal physical development, but affected individuals usually have some degree of mental retardation. It appears that the greater the number of X chromosomes, the greater the degree of mental impairment. Whatever the number of X chromosomes, the presence of a normal Y chromosome always produces the male phenotype.

STRUCTURAL CHROMOSOME ABNORMALITIES

Structural chromosome abnormalities are very variable and occur when breaks in chromosomes are misrepaired. These breakages occur naturally during cell divisions to allow the exchange of genetic material between sister chromatids. Structural abnormalities are described as balanced, if there is no overall loss or gain of genetic material, or unbalanced, which is characterised by the loss or gain of genetic material. Generally, the loss of chromosomal material is more harmful and, due to the high number of genes expressed, the brain tends to be the most vulnerable organ, with affected individuals usually showing some reduction of mental and/or intellectual function.

Chromosome Deletions

The loss of part of a chromosome leads to monosomy for that particular region of deoxyribonucleic acid (DNA). Any part of either the long or the short arm of a chromosome may be lost. Deletions are described as interstitial, if they occur within chromosome arms, or terminal, if they involve the ends of the chromosome, the telomeres. The consequences of a chromosome deletion depend on the genes deleted. Several rare syndromes are associated with specific chromosome deletions, such as cri du chat or 5p deletion syndrome (5p-), a condition associated with severe intellectual disability and a characteristic cry from birth which is said to sound like a cat, and Wolf Hirschhorn Syndrome (4p-), which is characterised by severe intellectual disability, microcephaly, hypertelorism and a characteristic facial appearance.

Large deletions (≥4 Mb) can be identified by conventional karyotyping, but syndromes are increasingly being identified in which the chromosome deletion is too small to be detected using traditional G-banding. These microdeletion syndromes require specific tests, such as fluorescence *in situ* hybridisation (FISH), for diagnosis (see later). An example of a microdeletion syndrome is 22q- or DiGeorge syndrome, in which affected individuals have heart defects, palate abnormalities, a characteristic facial appearance, learning difficulties and immune problems.

Chromosome Duplications

Duplications (dup on a karyotype report) can involve any chromosomal region and result in one or more copies of a region of DNA. The most common cause of chromosomal duplication is unequal sister chromatid exchange due to chromosomal misalignment during meiosis. The resulting duplicated region can be located immediately adjacent to the normal region, either in the same or opposite orientation to the original (tandem duplication and inverted duplication respectively), elsewhere on the same chromosome or attached to a completely different chromosome. There is usually little or no loss of genetic material, so duplications are more often compatible with life than other chromosomal abnormalities and are therefore found more frequently. Any observed phenotype is due to gene dosage effects and will depend on the region involved and the size of the duplication. Examples of chromosome duplication disorders include chromosome 16p11.2 duplication, a rare disorder associated with developmental delay and behavioural problems, such as attention-deficit/hyperactivity disorder and recurrent seizures, and *MECP2* (Methyl-CpG-Binding Protein 2) duplication disorder, which involves duplication of part of the long arm of the X chromosome. The condition is seen mainly in males, although females can be affected, and is characterised by moderate to severe intellectual disability. Some duplications are known to occur without phenotypic effect and can be classified as polymorphisms.

Chromosome Inversions

An inversion is a chromosomal rearrangement in which a region of DNA is reversed with respect to its normal orientation ('inv' on the karyotype report). It occurs if there are two breaks in a chromosome, followed by rotation of the region through 180 degrees. It can involve a single arm of the chromosome (paracentric inversion) or both arms on either side of the centromere (pericentric inversion). Inversions may not be associated with a phenotype since there is usually neither loss nor gain of chromosomal material, but if the break occurs within a gene or within the controlling region associated with a gene, then a phenotype may be observed.

Translocations

Translocations occur when chromosomes become broken during meiosis and the resulting fragment becomes attached to another chromosome.

Reciprocal translocations: These are the most common type of translocation and usually involve the exchange of material between non-homologous chromosomes. They are described as balanced or unbalanced (see Fig. 2.2). The portions exchanged are known as 'translocated segments' and the rearranged chromosome is called a 'derivative', reported as 'der', and is named according to its centromere. It is estimated that around 1 in 500 individuals carry a reciprocal translocation. Balanced translocations usually result in normal development, unless the break occurs within a gene or separates a gene from its controlling elements, in which case a phenotype may be observed. However, in carriers of balanced translocations, there is an increased risk of recurrent miscarriages or of having a child with congenital abnormalities and/or learning difficulties, as there is a possibility of the fetus inheriting the unbalanced form of the translocation. During meiosis, homologous chromosomes pair. When a reciprocal translocation is present, the four chromosomes (i.e. the two derivatives and two normal chromosomes) come together as a structure known as a 'quadrivalent'. Two of these chromosomes then pass into the gamete. There are four possible outcomes: the gamete contains the two normal chromosomes and will result in a normal karyotype in the offspring; the gamete contains the two derivative chromosomes and will result in offspring with the reciprocal balanced translocation like the parent or one of the two derivatives, and the other normal chromosomes pass into the gamete (or vice versa), resulting in offspring with monosomy for one region of the genome and trisomy for another. This can result in either miscarriage or, if the chromosome segments involved are small, a viable offspring with congenital abnormalities. The phenotype obviously depends on the genes present on the segments of chromosome involved. The risk of giving birth to a live-born infant with an unbalanced translocation is not one in four, but rather is specific to each reciprocal translocation and is difficult to calculate, as it depends on which segments of chromosomes are involved and how large they are. Reciprocal translocations are found in approximately 3% of couples presenting with recurrent miscarriage, and testing is recommended in women who have had three or more miscarriages.

Robertsonian translocations: These are a specific type of translocations involving only the acrocentric chromosomes 13, 14, 15, 21 and 22, which all have a very short p arm. Robertsonian translocations occur following breakages within the short arms of two acrocentric chromosomes and fusion of the long arms to form a single large, derivative chromosome usually described as rob (1stchrq;2ndchrq) (Fig. 2.3). There is usually loss of the short arms but, as these consist mainly of non-coding satellite DNA, this has little or no effect. An individual carrying a Robertsonian translocation has only 45 chromosomes.

Robertsonian translocations are amongst the most common, balanced structural rearrangements, with a frequency of about 1 in 1000 live births. The majority arise spontaneously during gamete formation (usually oogenesis) and are said to be *de novo*. Individuals with Robertsonian translocations are phenotypically normal and are described as healthy carriers. However, they are at risk of having repeated miscarriages or children with abnormalities due to incorrect segregation of the derivative chromosome during meiosis. This can lead to the formation of gametes containing either two copies of the chromosome or none. If both the abnormal, derivative chromosome and the normal homologue are present, the fetus will be trisomic for that chromosome. Translocation involving chromosomes 13 and 21 give rise to (translocation) Patau and Down syndrome, respectively, and account for a small percentage of these disorders. Alternatively, if trisomy or monosomy rescue occurs, uniparental disomy (UPD) can arise, in which both copies of the chromosome are derived from only one parent.

Ring Chromosomes

A ring chromosome is a circular structure formed when a chromosome breaks in two places and the broken ends then fuse. It is denoted by the symbol *r*. Formation is always associated with the loss of some chromosomal material, although identification of which region is missing may be difficult. FISH studies can be helpful in the investigation of this. Ring chromosomes almost always arise during the formation of gametes or during early embryogenesis and are rarely inherited. Ring chromosome disorders are extremely rare and are characterised by intellectual disability and seizures.

Isochromosomes

Isochromosomes are unbalanced structural anomalies consisting of either two long or two short arms. They arise when the centromere divides transversely rather than longitudinally during meiosis (Fig. 2.4) and are abbreviated as

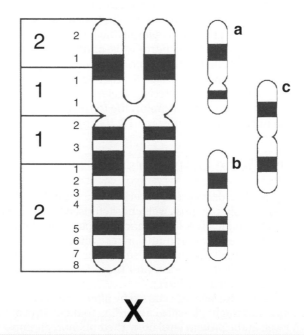

Fig. 2.3 Chromosome deletion and isochromosome formation. The large X chromosome at metaphase is seen on the left; (a, b) deletion of the long arm at different points; (c) isochromosome formation; only the two short arms of the X chromosome are represented here since division has been transverse instead of longitudinal, and the isochromosome for the short arm of the X has been formed.

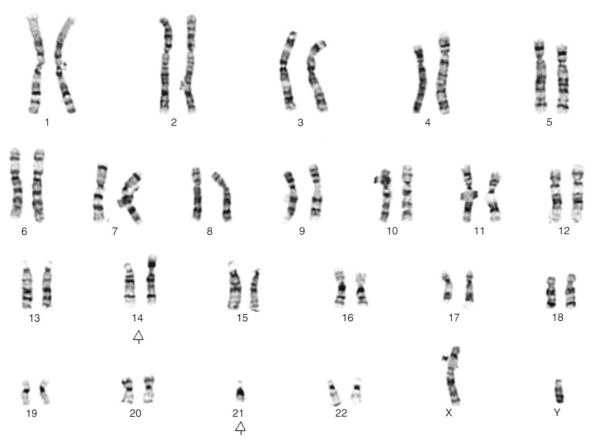

Fig. 2.4 Robertsonian translocation between chromosomes 14 and 21. (Figure provided by Dr L. Gaunt, Manchester Regional Genetics Service, Cytogenetics Laboratory.)

i(chromosome number and arm). Around 15% of Turner syndrome cases are associated with isochromosome X, which is composed of two copies of the long, q arm (i(Xq)). Pallister-Killian mosaic syndrome is another example of a disorder associated with the presence of an isochromosome. It is a rare developmental disorder which is characterised by hypotonia, a characteristic facial appearance, sparse hair and intellectual impairment due to the presence of an extra, abnormal isochromosome 12, i(12p).

Single Gene Disorders

Single gene disorders can be inherited in a number of ways and are probably the most well characterised of all genetic disease. They typically follow Mendelian patterns of inheritance and are either dominant or recessive, autosomal or sex-linked. A small number of disorders are caused by variants in mitochondrial genes, and these follow a maternal inheritance pattern (see later).

Single gene disorders are caused by alterations in the gene sequence and can be classified according to their effect at the DNA level, at the protein level or by their phenotypic impact.

At the DNA level variants include:

- substitutions
- deletions (del)
- duplications (dup)
- insertions (ins)
- deletion-insertions (delins)

Single base pair substitutions are the most common type of variant observed and involve the replacement of one nucleotide by another. They are sometimes referred to as point mutations. Deletions and duplications are less frequent and can involve one or more bases. Insertions involve one or more nucleotides from elsewhere in the genome being inserted into the coding sequence of a gene. More complex types of DNA changes can also occur, such as deletion-insertions, which involves one or more nucleotides being replaced by one or more different nucleotides.

All of these types of changes lead to an alteration of the DNA sequence of a gene which can have an impact at the protein level and result in a phenotype.

At the protein level, variants are described as:

- Missense (non-synonymous)
- Silent (synonymous)
- Nonsense
- Frameshift

Missense, or non-synonymous, variants occur when a single base pair substitution results in an alteration to a codon and leads to a change in the amino acid being coded for. The impact of these variants varies; they may affect key regions of the protein and alter its function or cause misfolding of the protein, which may result in it being degraded, leading to reduced levels and reduced activity. Synonymous variants do not cause a change in the amino acid, and they were often described as silent mutations as they were thought to have no impact on protein function. However, more recently it has been shown that such variants can affect ribonucleic acid (RNA) secondary structure, stability and splicing, which may result in a disease phenotype. To date, over 50 synonymous variants have been described in association with human disease.

Nonsense variants occur when single base pair substitutions cause the generation of a premature stop codon. They can result in the production of either a truncated, nonfunctional protein or no protein at all due to degradation of the aberrant messenger RNA (mRNA) by a quality control process known as nonsense-mediated decay.

Frameshift variants occur when the insertion and/or deletion of nucleotides causes a change to the translational reading frame of a gene, the sequence of consecutive nucleotide triplets which code for the amino acids that make up a protein. This leads to the introduction of a premature termination codon, and the resulting protein is usually absent or nonfunctional.

Variants in non-coding DNA can also cause disease. Those occurring in the upstream, promoter region of a gene can affect when, where and how much of the protein is produced and lead to disease. Variants affecting the DNA sequence at the intron-exon boundary (the splice sites) can disrupt RNA splicing and result in the exon skipping or the inclusion of intronic DNA with the subsequent production of an altered protein.

Phenotypically single gene disorders are due to:

- Haploinsufficiency
- Loss of function
- Gain of function

Haploinsufficiency occurs when one copy of a gene is either deleted or inactivated and the normal function of the protein cannot be maintained by the remaining copy.

Loss of function variants are usually recessive. The DNA variant causes an alteration to the protein product which leads to a loss of function. However, in most cases, the protein produced by the wild type allele still functions normally and a phenotype is not observed in the heterozygous state.

Gain-of-function variants describe variants which lead to an alteration in protein which confer a new function. They are almost always dominant.

AUTOSOMAL DOMINANT DISEASES

In autosomal dominant disorders, a variant in only one of the two gene copies (alleles) is sufficient to cause disease. Therefore, affected individuals have a 50% risk of transmitting the variant to their offspring. Typical features of autosomal dominant inheritance are:

- An equal ratio of affected males and females
- Affected individuals in every generation
- Transmission of the disease from either sex to either sex

In dominant disorders, the presence of the mutant allele causes the disease phenotype. This may simply be due to a lack of the normal level of functioning protein (i.e. a dosage effect or haploinsufficiency). Alternatively, the mutant protein can interfere with the function of the normal protein, the so-called 'dominant negative' effect.

Another feature of autosomal dominant disorders is variable expressivity whereby the phenotype may be more or less severe in different individuals (e.g. neurofibromatosis type 1). On occasion, the phenotype can be so mild that the disease appears to skip a generation (e.g. autosomal dominant deafness). In other disorders there may be rare individuals who carry the mutant allele but exhibit none of the features of the disease. This is called nonpenetrance. If a child is diagnosed with an autosomal dominant condition and there is no family history of the condition, then the variant may have arisen in the child for the first time (de novo). However, because some conditions are known to exhibit variable expressivity and penetrance, it is extremely important to examine both parents for any features of the disease to determine if they do in fact carry the variant allele in order to be able to give accurate figures for the risk of recurrence in another child. If either parent is affected, the risk will be 50%, but if neither has the condition, the risk is very low, although it is not zero, as occasionally germinal mosaicism may be present, with one parent having a small proportion of germ cells which harbour the variant.

Examples of more common autosomal dominant conditions include:

- Achondroplasia
- Myotonic dystrophy
- Huntington disease
- Marfan syndrome
- Neurofibromatosis type 1
- Multiple polyposis of the colon
- Osteogenesis imperfecta
- Autosomal dominant polycystic kidney disease
- Tuberous sclerosis.

AUTOSOMAL RECESSIVE DISEASES

Autosomal recessive disorders occur when both copies of a gene carry a variant. An individual is described as homozygous if both the maternal and paternal alleles carry the same variant. This is often seen in cases of intermarriage or consanguinity where both parents have inherited the same variant from a common ancestor, or if there is a common or founding variant which is present at a high frequency in the population.

If an individual has a different variant on each allele, they are described as being a compound heterozygote. This occurs in diseases such as cystic fibrosis, where many different variants can cause the disease.

Individuals who have only one mutated copy of the gene will be unaffected and usually unaware that they carry the disease. Occasionally, these carriers may exhibit symptoms of disease; for example, individuals who are heterozygous for the sickle cell variant may become symptomatic under extreme conditions, especially if they also carry thalassaemia variants or the haemoglobin C variant. Carriers of autosomal recessive diseases are unlikely to have any family history, and their carrier status is often only detected following the birth of an affected child.

For an individual to be affected with an autosomal recessive disorder, both parents must be carriers. In this case there will be a one in four risk of having an affected child each time they have a child. There will also be a one in two chance of a child being a carrier (and therefore unaffected) and a one in four chance of a child being unaffected and not a carrier. It follows therefore that the *unaffected* sibling of an affected child has a two in three risk of being a carrier.

Examples of autosomal recessive conditions include:

- Cystic fibrosis
- Congenital adrenal hyperplasia
- Usher syndrome
- Galactosaemia
- Spinal muscular atrophy
- Phenylketonuria.

The most frequently encountered autosomal recessive disorders in obstetric practice are (1) cystic fibrosis and (2) the haemoglobinopathies (sickle cell disease and the thalassaemias).

Cystic Fibrosis

Cystic fibrosis (CF) is the most common autosomal recessive disorder in the UK Caucasian population, with a carrier frequency of about 1 in 25 individuals and an incidence of around 1 per 2500 live births. The disease is due to variants in the gene encoding a chloride channel protein called cystic fibrosis conductance transmembrane regulator *(CFTR)*. Variants in this gene lead to the production of thick sticky secretions resulting in lung disease and recurrent bacterial infections, pancreatic insufficiency and male infertility. Patients often present in infancy, with respiratory and gastrointestinal problems and failure to thrive. Life expectancy is reduced but has increased significantly over recent years due to improvements in management of the condition and the availability of lung transplants, and many children born with CF today will live to their mid-20s or 30s. This is an important consideration as many families may have a much more pessimistic understanding of life expectancy based on past experience. In the UK, all babies are screened at or shortly after birth using blood collected by heel prick. If screening suggests the baby has CF, additional tests are performed to confirm the diagnosis. This can involve measuring the concentration of chloride in sweat (the sweat test) as this is abnormally high in CF. Additionally mutation analysis may be offered (see DNA sequencing section).

Prenatal diagnosis (PND) following chorionic villous sampling (CVS) is also possible for couples known to carry CF variants.

Sickle Cell Disease and the Thalassaemias

These disorders are described as haemoglobinopathies. Haemoglobins are the molecules responsible for binding oxygen and transporting it around the body. They are made up of four globin chains which are encoded by several different genes. Adult haemoglobin consists of two alpha and two beta subunits. The two alpha haemoglobin genes, *α1* and *α2*, are located close together on chromosome 16, and the *β* genes are clustered together on chromosome 11.

Sickle Cell Disease. Sickle cell disease is the most common inherited blood disorder and is characterised by a tendency for red cells to deform into a characteristic sickle shape under conditions of low oxygen tension. These sickled erythrocytes are haemolysed prematurely, which can lead to chronic anaemia and jaundice. They also have a tendency to block small capillaries leading to recurrent episodes of lung, spleen and bone infarction and extreme pain (sickle cell crisis). Sickle cell disease is due to a single amino acid change from valine to glutamine in the β-globin molecule, p.(Glu7Val), resulting from a single base-pair substitution in *HBB* (Haemoglobin Beta). The disease is particularly prevalent in individuals with African or Caribbean heritage where natural selection has resulted in the mutant allele being maintained at high frequency, as it is protective against malaria in the heterozygous state. In the UK, screening for sickle cell disease is included in the newborn screening programme. Prenatal diagnosis is also available.

Thalassaemias. The thalassaemias are a group of inherited blood disorders characterised by abnormal haemoglobin production.

Alpha thalassaemia is caused by reduced synthesis of the alpha chain of haemoglobin. Disease severity is determined by the number of functioning *α* genes, and alpha thalassaemia has two clinically distinct phenotypes: Hb Bart hydrops fetalis (Hb Bart) syndrome and haemoglobin H (HbH) disease. Hb Bart syndrome is the most severe form, caused by mutations or deletions affecting all four α globin alleles causing a total lack of production of α haemoglobin. This leads to oedema and intrauterine hypoxia resulting in stillbirth or death in the neonatal period. HbH disease occurs when only one of the four α globin genes is functioning and causes a microcytic hypochromic haemolytic anaemia, hepatosplenomegaly and mild jaundice.

Beta thalassaemia is caused by reduced synthesis of the haemoglobin beta chain which results in microcytic hypochromic anaemia, nucleated red blood cells and reduced haemoglobin A (HbA). Affected individuals (thalassaemia major) have anaemia and hepatosplenomegaly, and without treatment affected children fail to thrive and have a shortened life expectancy. Carriers (thalassaemia minor) are symptom free but have a mild microcytic hypochromic anaemia. There are many different molecular pathologies that cause β-thalassaemia, and disease severity can be affected by modifying factors.

SEX-LINKED INHERITANCE

Unlike the autosomes, females have two X chromosomes whilst males have only one and they are described as hemizygous. In order to ensure that gene dosage is equal in both sexes, a process known as X inactivation occurs, which results in only one allele being active in female cells. X inactivation begins in early embryogenesis and is random, although once an individual cell has set its inactivated X chromosome, all daughter cells will have the same X chromosome switched off. In general, X inactivation is random, so in an adult female the maternal and paternal X chromosomes will each show approximately 50% expression in any particular tissue.

X-Linked Recessive Diseases

Females who inherit a mutant allele carried on the X chromosome will usually be protected from its effects by the presence of the normal homologue on their other X chromosome. They will therefore be unaffected, although, since expression of the 'normal' chromosome will be limited to approximately 50%, it is often possible to detect female carriers of an X-linked disease by measurement of the gene product. For example, female carriers of haemophilia may have reduced circulating factor VIII concentrations. The main characteristics of an X-linked family pedigree include:

- Usually only males are affected (see later).
- Females may be carriers.
- Male-to-male transmission of the disease is not possible.
- The disease is invariable in phenotype.
- There is a 50% risk that the sons of a carrier female will be affected.
- There is a 50% risk that the daughters of a carrier female will be carriers.
- All the daughters of an affected male will be (obligate) carriers.

Occasionally females are affected by X-linked recessive diseases. This can be due to skewed X-inactivation, where by chance the normal allele is disproportionately inactivated resulting in the mutant allele being expressed, if there is homozygosity for a variant (i.e. affected father and carrier mother) in Turner syndrome, if the variant is present on the single X chromosome present, and in X-autosome translocations (part of the X chromosome is translocated to an autosome), which can interfere with random inactivation. Examples of recessive X-linked conditions include:

- Duchenne muscular dystrophy
- Glucose-6-phosphate dehydrogenase deficiency
- Haemophilia A (Factor VIII deficiency)
- Haemophilia B (Factor IX deficiency)

X-Linked Dominant Diseases

X-linked dominant diseases are caused by a variant in a gene on one copy of the X chromosome, which means that both males and females can be affected.

The most frequently observed X-linked dominant disorder is Fragile X. Almost all cases of this disease involve the expansion of a DNA segment in the promoter region of the *FMR1* (Fragile X Messenger Ribonucleoprotein 1) gene, known as a triplet repeat, from the usual 5 to 40 copies to over 200. This expansion effectively switches the gene off and results in the disease which is characterised by developmental delay, learning disability, behavioural problems and autism-spectrum disorder.

X-linked dominant disorders have a similar family pedigree to autosomal dominant diseases, with the exception that a father cannot pass the disease to his son. In addition, the disease tends to be more severe in males, as females are protected to a greater or lesser extent by the presence of the homologous 'normal' chromosome.

Y-Linked Diseases

The main function of the Y chromosome is to direct male sexual development, and there are no known examples of Y-linked disease. Variants in *SRY* (Sex Determining Region , Y), a gene in the so-called 'sex determining region of Y' are known to cause failure of testicular development and result in XY females. XY females are not fertile, and the mutation cannot be further propagated.

MITOCHONDRIAL INHERITANCE

The mitochondrial genome consists of 1.6 kb of double-stranded, circular DNA. It codes for a total of 37 genes, which include 2 ribosomal RNAs, 22 transfer RNAs and 13 polypeptides. The polypeptides are all subunits of enzyme complexes which form the oxidative phosphorylation system. The consequences of variants in genes of the mitochondrial genome are difficult to predict, as it will depend on the degree of heteroplasmy, that is the percentage of mitochondria within the cell that carry the variant. Heteroplasmy arises due to the random distribution of mitochondria to the daughter cells during cell division. This means daughter cells can have a different proportion of mutant mitochondria than the parent cells. Within an individual, there can be great variation in this proportion between tissues and cells, leading to a variable phenotype.

Mitochondrial diseases are rare and have a characteristic inheritance pattern as they are always maternally inherited. The embryo derives all its mitochondria from the egg, that is, the mother. If the mother has a mitochondrial variant, then all maternal offspring are usually affected. Males do not transmit mitochondrial variants. Mitochondrial diseases characteristically affect muscles and the nervous system, and the phenotype is variable. Examples of mitochondrial diseases include:

- Leber hereditary optic neuropathy (LHON)
- Chronic progressive external ophthalmoplegia (CPEO)
- Myoclonic epilepsy with ragged red fibres (MERRF)
- Mitochondrial myopathy, encephalopathy, lactic acidosis with stroke-like episodes (MELAS)

GENOMIC IMPRINTING

An individual carries two copies of every autosomal gene, one inherited from the father and one inherited from the mother, and for the majority of genes both alleles are functional and contribute equally to the phenotype. However, for a small subset of genes, one copy is switched off in a parent-of-origin dependent manner and this is termed imprinting. Genomic imprinting occurs during germ cell production and is thought to involve selective methylation of the genome. Once it has occurred, the differences between the maternally and paternally derived chromosomes appear to remain fixed through successive mitotic divisions but are reset at meiosis.

Only nine chromosomes carry genes which are imprinted, and these are often associated with growth and development, such as the insulin-like growth factor receptor. Imprinted genes play a role in early embryogenesis with paternally derived genes controlling the development of the placental tissues, whilst maternally derived genes play a more important role in development of the embryo.

The most frequently encountered imprinting disorders are Prader–Willi syndrome (PWS), characterised by hypotonia in infancy, developmental delay, obesity and hypogonadism and Angelman syndrome (AS), characterised by developmental delay, ataxic movements, seizures and characteristic behaviour including frequent laughter and being easily excitable. Both conditions involve deletions or variants in the same region of chromosome 15q11–13. Part of this region is maternally imprinted, the PWS region, and part is paternally imprinted, the AS region. In PWS the mutated chromosome is always paternally derived, whereas in AS the variant is maternally derived.

Imprinting has also been observed in some autosomal dominant conditions, with affected individuals showing differences in the expression, severity or age of onset of the disease depending upon which parent they inherited the disorder from. The clearest example of the effects of genomic imprinting on a single gene disease is hereditary glomus tumour. This rare, benign tumour has an autosomal dominant inheritance but is only seen in individuals who have inherited the mutant allele from their father. The gene is presumably imprinted in the female germ cell line so that it is not expressed in the offspring of affected mothers. The disease often appears to skip a generation when inherited by a female, whose sons would not exhibit the disease but whose grandchildren could do so.

UNIPARENTAL DISOMY

Uniparental disomy (UPD) occurs when a child inherits both copies of a chromosome from only one parent. It is due to errors during meiosis, but the exact mechanism is not fully understood. There are two types of UPD: (1) isodisomy, where both copies of the chromosome are identical, and (2) heterodisomy, when two non-identical homologues are present.

As the gene content is normal, UPD is only associated with disease if the chromosome carries imprinted genes. Thus, a small percentage of PWS and AS are associated with UPD. Other disorders associated with UPD are Beckwith-Wiedemann syndrome (parental UPD of chromosome 11) and Russell-Silver syndrome (maternal UPD of chromosome 7).

There are numerous recognised cases of UPD of the sex chromosomes, 47,XXX and 47,XXY, as these are easily identified by cytogenetic studies.

Multifactorial Inheritance

Many common disorders do not have a single genetic cause; rather, they are due to multiple genes (polygenic) interacting with environmental and lifestyle factors. This is termed multifactorial or complex inheritance. Such disorders tend to cluster within a family but do not have clearly defined inheritance pattern. Examples of complex traits include:

- Major neural tube defects (spina bifida and anencephaly)
- Congenital heart disease
- Cleft lip and palate
- Hypertension
- Pre-eclampsia
- Diabetes mellitus
- Atopy

For more information on the analysis of complex traits, see Chapter 1.

Genetic Testing and Interpretation of a Genetic Result

A variety of tests are available to aid in the diagnosis of disorders suspected to be genetic in origin. Tests may be indicated prenatally following an abnormal ultrasound or because of a family history of genetic disease, or postnatally if an infant presents with an abnormal phenotype at birth or if there are unexplained growth or developmental problems and/or learning difficulties. In addition, genetic follow-up is advised for women who have suffered multiple miscarriages. The type of test(s) offered depends on the suspected diagnosis. Cytogenetic techniques including karyotyping, FISH, multiplex ligation-dependent probe amplification (MLPA), quantitative-fluorescence polymerase chain reaction (QF-PCR) and microarray-based comparative genomic hybridisation are useful for detecting chromosomal abnormalities and are often offered in combination, whereas single gene disorders are usually diagnosed by sequence analysis.

A brief outline of the different methodologies used in the Clinical Genetics Laboratory is included to allow an understanding of how the investigations are performed, their interpretation and their limitations.

CYTOGENETICS

Cytogenetics is the study of chromosomes and diseases caused by structural and numerical abnormalities.

Karyotyping

Karyotyping is the analysis of the chromosomal content of a cell and is typically used to detect numerical abnormalities, large imbalances and chromosomal rearrangements. Chromosomes are only visible in actively dividing cells and, although these are difficult to obtain, T-lymphocytes from peripheral blood can be induced to divide by treatment with a lectin such as phytohemagglutinin. Cells are obtained from a blood sample and allowed to divide for 48 to 72 hours. A spindle-disrupting agent such as Colcemid is then added, which causes the cells to pause at the M-phase of the cell cycle. During this phase chromosomes are condensed and easily visible after staining with DNA-specific dyes. The most commonly used dye is Giemsa which, following trypsin digestion, gives rise to characteristic G-banded (black and white) chromosomes (see Fig. 2.1). Although usually performed on a sample of peripheral blood, cells from other tissues can also be used for karyotyping, with fibroblasts from skin biopsies being a common source. For prenatal diagnosis, chorionic villi or fetal cells that are shed into the amniotic fluid can also be used. Cytogeneticists in the laboratory are able to read the karyotype to identify individual chromosomes and determine whether there are any anomalies present.

Although considered the gold standard test for many years following its introduction in the 1970s, karyotyping is not without limitations. In addition to being both time consuming and costly, karyotyping cannot be used to detect deletions or duplications of less than 5 Mb (5 million base pairs). Deletions in this range are seen in microdeletion/duplication syndromes such as velocardiofacial/DiGeorge syndrome (22q11.2 deletion), Williams-Beuren syndrome (7q11.23 deletion) and *MECP2* (Xq28 duplication). These disorders involve the loss or gain of multiple genes and are sometimes referred to as contiguous gene disorders. Although the individual disorders are quite rare, together microdeletions/duplications represent a large subset of human disease. Symptoms vary but frequently include mental retardation, autism, physical dysmorphism and/or organ malformations. The inability of karyotyping to detect this group of disorders prompted the development of alternative technologies, and karyotyping has been largely superseded by higher resolution molecular tests such as FISH and microarrays. Karyotyping is now predominantly offered in cases of unexplained infertility to identify balanced chromosomal rearrangements which may affect fertility by disrupting the formation of germ cells. It is also used in the diagnosis of sex chromosome aneuploidies such as Klinefelter syndrome (47,XXY).

Fluorescence in situ Hybridisation

FISH was introduced as a diagnostic tool in the late 1980s and combines DNA hybridisation with traditional karyotyping to offer targeted analysis. Briefly, a fluorescently labelled DNA probe, specific to the chromosomal region under investigation, is hybridised to denatured DNA from the patient which is fixed onto a microscope slide. The probe binds to its complementary region and the subsequent fluorescent signal is detected, and the copy number can then be calculated. In a normal cell, two signals should be observed for autosomal genes (one from each chromosome), whereas in a cell with a deletion, there will be only one signal. Resolution of detection is about 10 kb, which means that FISH can be used to detect microdeletions and duplications.

A related technique, known as chromosome painting, uses a large probe set across the entire genome to identify unbalanced translocations.

Although still a labour-intensive procedure, an advantage of FISH is that, unlike traditional karyotyping, there is no requirement for dividing cells and the technique is more sensitive.

Multiplex Ligation-Dependent Probe Amplification

MLPA is a PCR-based method which allows the simultaneous analysis of multiple regions of DNA in a single reaction. The procedure is rapid and robust and is routinely used to detect small deletions and duplications, such as the exon 7 and 8 deletion in the *SMN1* gene which causes spinal muscular atrophy 1.

Quantitative-Fluorescence Polymerase Chain Reaction

QF-PCR is another targeted approach used to determine copy number. It involves PCR amplification of repeat sequences at known polymorphic loci across a chromosome using fluorescently labelled primers. Several loci can be analysed simultaneously by multiplexing primers. QF-PCR is a rapid, robust and cost-effective test for the detection of copy number variation, and in many genetic laboratories this is now the first line test for the diagnosis of aneuploidies, such as trisomy 13 and 18, and sex chromosome anomalies. QF-PCR can also be used to detect UPD disorders such as Prader–Willi syndrome, Angelman syndrome and Russell–Silver syndrome.

Chromosomal Microarray

Chromosomal microarray is sometimes referred to as molecular karyotyping and it allows genome-wide detection of submicroscopic chromosome imbalances. Briefly, the technique involves the comparison of patient DNA with control DNA to identify any differences. The procedure is quicker than traditional karyotyping and offers a higher resolution of detection at around 1 Mb. There are two types of chromosomal array, comparative genomic hybridisation (aCGH) and single nucleotide polymorphism (SNP array).

Array CGH is now the first line diagnostic test in most UK laboratories for neonatal, paediatric and adult patients presenting with neurodevelopmental disorders and dysmorphism or multiple congenital anomalies, and for the detection of pathogenic genomic imbalances at prenatal diagnosis or in fetal losses. However, it should be noted that microarray cannot be used to detect balanced translocations.

Deoxyribonucleic Acid (DNA) Sequencing

When a patient presents with a clear phenotype associated with a well-characterised disorder, analysis of only a few or even a single gene by DNA sequencing may be sufficient to provide a definitive diagnosis.

In some cases, a screening approach may be adopted which focuses only on the most common variants associated with a particular disease. A good example of this is in the diagnosis of CF. Although over 1000 different variants have been described in CF, the majority of disease (85% to 90%) is caused by just 30 variants; in the UK the most common variant, present in around 76% of all cases, is a 3 base deletion in the *CFTR* gene which results in the loss of a single amino acid from the protein (c.1521_1523del, p.(Phe508del)). Genetic testing for CF in the UK focuses initially on the detection of known variants, including the c.1521_1523del, with further analysis only in the 10% to 15% of patients who do not carry this variant.

When interpreting a genetic result, it is important to remember that even if no variant has been detected, the original diagnosis may still be correct. This is because of the limitations of the testing. This is particularly true if a screening approach has been used, as only the most common variants will be detected. Laboratory reports usually describe the detection rate of the technique used to allow for informed interpretation of the result.

Following recent technological advances, genetic diagnosis has been transformed, and laboratories are increasingly offering high-throughput sequencing techniques.

High-Throughput Sequence Analysis/Genomic Analysis

A large number of Mendelian disorders are heterogeneous both phenotypically and genetically, and it can be difficult to decide which genes to analyse and in what order to prioritise analysis. As a result, many patients have had to endure a long and painful journey involving years of tests and investigations before receiving a definitive diagnosis, the so called 'diagnostic odyssey'. The development of high-throughput sequencing technology, also known as next generation sequencing, has revolutionised the field of human genetics. Briefly, it involves fragmenting and sequencing short stretches of patient DNA and comparing it to a reference sequence using computer software. Any differences between the two are flagged by the software and can then be interrogated to determine if they are potentially pathogenic and involved in the disorder under investigation.

Next generation sequencing technology is now being offered as a diagnostic test. Depending on the diagnosis, DNA is either analysed against a panel of genes known to be involved in the suspected disorder, or if the aetiology is unknown, whole exome sequencing (WES) may be offered. This looks at all the coding DNA within the genome (only about 1.5% of the total 3000 Mb DNA) and has been shown to be particularly valuable in the diagnosis of disorders where there is a broad differential diagnosis, such as the estimated 2% to 3% of pregnancies that present with ultrasound anomalies. Samples from these pregnancies are usually taken for karyotyping or microarray analysis, but the diagnostic hit rate is low at around 14% to 16%. The use of WES in such cases has been shown to be able to identify causative variants in a further 25% to 30% of cases.

High-throughput sequence analysis is not without its limitations and challenges. In many cases a potential variant will be identified which has not previously been described. Scientists analyse the possible impact of these variants using a variety of techniques but are often unable to say unequivocally that they are the causative variant. Instead, a report will be issued which describes the sequence change seen as 'a variant of unknown significance' (VUS) which obviously poses a challenge as to how to counsel a patient and their family. Whole exome sequencing is also able to identify changes in copy number but cannot be used to detect imprinting errors, UPD, nucleotide repeats or expansion. Alternatively, whole genome sequencing (WGS) may be offered. Again, this is useful if the aetiology of the disease is unknown, and it offers an advantage over WES in that it also allows analysis of non-coding DNA.

High-throughput technologies have revolutionised prenatal testing.

Non-Invasive Prenatal Testing/Diagnosis

The blood of all individuals contains fragmented DNA which is released by dying cells, and in 1997 it was discovered that the blood of pregnant women also contains fragmented DNA derived from the placenta. This cell-free fetal-DNA (cffDNA) accounts for between 10% and 20% of the total cell-free DNA in maternal blood and it can be detected as early as 7 weeks post-conception. The concentration of cffDNA increases with gestational age, but it is rapidly cleared from maternal circulation following delivery. The analysis of maternal and cffDNA using high-throughput sequencing technologies offers a non-invasive screening test for aneuploidies. Tests are typically performed at around 10 weeks, gestation and require only a maternal blood sample. Results are reported as either 'low risk'/'very unlikely to be affected' or 'high risk'/'likely to be affected'. Women with a 'high risk' result are then offered CVS or amniocentesis to obtain a definitive diagnosis. Although not diagnostic, NIPT is a very sensitive screening test with a detection rate for Down syndrome of around 99%.

Non-invasive prenatal diagnosis (NIPD), which does provide a definitive result, is used for fetal sexing where there is a risk of an X-linked disorder, for dominant conditions such as the *FGHFR3*-related disorders achondroplasia and thanotrophic dysplasias and the *FGFR2*-related disorders Apert syndrome and other craniosynostoses. At present it is only offered by a small number of laboratories.

The Future – Genomic Testing

In December 2018 the ground-breaking UK 100,000 Genome Project was completed, with the genomes of approximately 85,000 people with rare disease and cancer being fully sequenced. This project was delivered by a joint partnership between the NHS and Genomics England and showed that it was possible to integrate genomic medicine into routine healthcare. This led to the development of the national genomic medicine service (GMS) which was launched in 2019. This initiative, part of the NHS Long Term Plan, aims to:

- Offer consistent and equitable care to everyone
- Operate to common national standards, specifications and protocols
- Deliver a single national testing directory covering the use of all genomic technologies from single gene testing to whole genome sequencing (replacing the UK Genetic Testing Network directory)
- Give all patients the opportunity to participate in research for their own benefit and to inform future care for other patients
- Build a national genomic knowledge base to provide real world data to inform academic and industrial research and development

The GMS is underpinned by a network of seven regional genomic laboratory hubs (GLHs) each hosted by an acute NHS trust which provides genomic testing.

The tests offered by the GMS are listed in the National Genomic Test Directory (https://www.england.nhs.uk/publication/national-genomic-test-directories/) together with details about the technologies used and which patients are eligible for testing. Tests range from karyotyping to single gene analysis right through to WGS. Genomics England PanelApp (https://panelapp.genomicsengland.co.uk/), a publicly available knowledge base, is used as the platform for achieving consensus on gene panels offered by the GMS. Virtual gene panels related to different genetic disorders have been created in such a way that genes and genomic entities, such as copy number variants, can be added and reviewed by experts from the international scientific community. This ensures that only those genes with sufficient evidence for disease association are included.

There are over 20 different groups of clinical indications as listed below:

- Acutely unwell children
- Cardiology
- Developmental disorders
- Endocrinology
- Eyes
- Fetal (including NIPD)
- Gastrohepatology
- Haematology

- Hearing
- Immunology
- Inherited cancer
- Lipids
- Metabolic
- Mitochondrial
- Mosaic and structural chromosomal disorders
- Musculoskeletal
- Neurology
- Renal
- Respiratory
- Skin
- Ultra-rare and atypical monogenic disorders
- Multipurpose tests

The implementation of this service means that clinicians are now able to order genomic testing without having to refer their patients to a clinical geneticist. However, all referrals will be triaged by the local GLH to ensure the most appropriate test is performed. In instances where testing is requested by the clinical indication, the GLH will review the test request and relevant clinical information and select the most appropriate constituent test(s) to facilitate the request. Testing can be targeted at those patients where a genetic or genomic diagnosis will guide management for them and/or their family.

A separate directory is available for cancer genetics (National Genomic Test Directory for Cancer).

3 Embryology

HARSHA SHAH, TOM BOURNE AND KATE HARDY

Oogenesis and Spermatogenesis

The process of fertilisation involves the union of female and male gametes, the ovum and spermatozoon, respectively. In humans there is a ready supply of spermatozoa constantly available from the normal healthy male after the age of puberty. By contrast, the normal healthy female will bring only one ovum to maturity and ovulation in each 28-day cycle.

OOGENESIS

During fetal life the developing ovaries become populated with primordial germ cells (gamete precursors) which differentiate into oogonia and continue to divide by mitosis until a few weeks before birth. After this time, no new oocytes are produced, and the female is born with all the oocytes she will ever have (approximately 1,000,000), which are not replaced. From early in gestation, fetal oogonia enter meiosis, reaching the first prophase stage, whereupon they become arrested and remain so beyond birth and until just before ovulation. During this arrest, the single diplotene oocyte becomes surrounded with a monolayer of flattened granulosa cells and becomes known as a *primordial follicle*. These primordial follicles are scattered throughout the cortex of the ovaries, surrounded by interstitial connective tissue. The primordial follicles can remain in this arrested state for up to 50 years whilst awaiting signalling to resume development. The majority of ovarian oocytes become atretic by puberty, leaving only approximately 250,000 available in the reproductive phase of life. Of these, only approximately 400 will be ovulated.

In the ovary there is continual recruitment of small numbers of primordial follicles to start folliculogenesis, which is a lengthy process taking 6 months or longer. This recruitment continues until the supply of primordial follicles is exhausted, around the time of the menopause. Folliculogenesis encompasses recruitment of a cohort of primordial follicles from the resting pool, initiation of follicle and oocyte growth; this is followed by final selection and maturation of a single preovulatory follicle, with the remaining follicles being eliminated by atresia. During this time, the oocyte grows from 35 to 120 μm in diameter, undergoes meiosis to produce a haploid gamete, produces large amounts of stable RNA to support early embryonic development and acquires the nuclear and cytoplasmic maturity to undergo fertilisation and embryogenesis.

Following recruitment, the granulosa cells of the primordial follicle become cuboidal in shape and undergo cell division. When the follicle reaches the secondary stage, with two layers of granulosa cells, a layer of theca cells develops around the follicle. The theca and granulosa cells of the follicle, which are epithelial in nature, create a specialised microenvironment for the developing oocyte. At the same time, the granulosa cells secrete a glycoprotein coat around the oocyte, which forms a translucent acellular layer separating the oocyte from the surrounding granulosa cells, known as the *zona pellucida*. Later on, this will provide species-specific sperm receptors at fertilisation and protect the embryo before implantation. Microvilli extend from the granulosa cells through the zona pellucida to the plasma membrane of the oocyte and are intimately involved in the transfer of nutrients and signalling molecules between the two.

When there are several layers of granulosa cells and the oocyte is fully grown, a fluid-filled cavity (the antrum) appears and starts expanding. The oocyte itself becomes suspended in this fluid and is pushed to one side and surrounded by two or three layers of tightly knit granulosa cells, the corona radiata. The oocyte and surrounding corona radiata are attached to the rim of peripheral granulosa cells by a thin 'stalk' of cells. From now until ovulation, follicular development is subject to endocrine control, predominantly by follicle-stimulating hormone (FSH). At the beginning of each menstrual cycle, there is a group of approximately 20 small antral follicles, only one of which will ovulate 2 weeks later. The rest of the group undergo atresia and die by apoptosis.

After antrum formation, the rate of cell division in the granulosa cell population slows down, and these cells differentiate and become steroidogenic, using theca-derived androgen to produce increasing amounts of oestradiol. In the midfollicular phase, a dominant follicle emerges, and its secretion is responsible for approximately 95% of circulating oestradiol levels in the late follicular phase. During the final maturation of the follicle, the corona cells become columnar and less tightly packed. The primary oocyte resumes meiotic maturation in response to the onset of the midcycle surge of luteinising hormone (LH). The germinal vesicle breaks down and the first meiotic division is completed in which half the chromosomes (one of each homologous pair, 23 in total made up of two chromatids) and almost all the cytoplasm go to one cell, which is now known as the secondary oocyte. The remaining chromosomes and a minute amount of cytoplasm are extruded in the first polar body. The oocyte proceeds at this time through the second meiotic division, where it arrests again at metaphase II, and is stimulated to complete meiosis only at fertilisation. The ovarian follicle now undergoes further growth, which culminates in ovulation. As the follicle continues to grow, it begins to bulge from the ovarian surface, and a slightly raised nipple on the thinning follicle wall (known as the stigma) breaks down and allows release of the secondary oocyte from this site. The oocyte oozes out in a sticky envelope of cumulus cells loosely packed around it, with the innermost layer of these cells known as the corona radiata. The collapsed follicle transforms after ovulation into the corpus luteum.

SPERMATOGENESIS

By comparison with the mature ovum, the mature spermatozoon is very small, the headpiece measuring only 4 to 5 μm in length. Maturation of an ovum is a prolonged process starting in fetal life and involving two substantial resting phases before producing the definitive cell in the adult female. By contrast, the spermatozoon is produced in 70 to 80 days in a continuous process of development and maturation, which occurs only after puberty in the male. Spermatozoa develop from the basic germ cells of the male, the spermatogonia, which line the basal lamina of the seminiferous tubules interspersed with Sertoli cells. Spermatogenesis, the process by which spermatozoa are formed, depends on the hormonal drive of two principal gonadotrophins from the pituitary gland: FSH, which provides the impetus for the early development stages, and LH, which provokes the Leydig cells to produce testosterone, thus stimulating spermatogenesis. FSH acts both

independently and in synergy with testosterone, for the proliferation, maturation and function of the supporting Sertoli cells that produce regulatory signals and nutrients for the maintenance of developing germ cells.

At the onset of puberty, spermatogonia are reactivated to constantly divide by mitosis, providing an endless supply of spermatogonial stem cells. From this pool of self-regenerating stem cells, some distinct spermatogonia emerge at intervals, which increase in size and develop into primary spermatocytes, each containing 46 chromosomes. Like the primary oocytes, these primary spermatocytes undergo a reduction division, known as the first meiotic division, in which the two daughter haploid cells receive 23 chromosomes (each consisting of a pair of duplicate chromatids) and are known as secondary spermatocytes. The first meiotic division of the oocyte produces one secondary oocyte and one polar body which is expelled, whereas the same division in the male produces two equal secondary spermatocytes of the same size and cytoplasmic content. Each of the secondary spermatocytes undergoes a further meiotic division to form two equal spermatids, each with 23 chromosomes. As the spermatozoa develop through the phases of primary spermatocyte, secondary spermatocyte and spermatid, they progress towards the lumen of the seminiferous tubule. The various generations of spermatogonia, spermatocytes and spermatids are linked in small groups by cytoplasmic bridges, possibly as an aid to nutrition and also to ensure synchronous development. The occasional occurrence of twinned mature sperm may represent failure of separation of these bridges.

The individual spermatids undergo substantial metamorphosis known as spermiogenesis to produce mature spermatozoa. Until now, the spermatids have been radially symmetric and round but now develop polarity to become elongated. The nuclear material migrates to form the dense sperm head and the cytoplasm is gradually reduced, leaving the head piece almost totally full of nuclear material. The sperm head becomes covered by the acrosomal cap (Fig. 3.1) which is developed from vacuoles in the Golgi apparatus that fuse to form the acrosomal vesicle, which

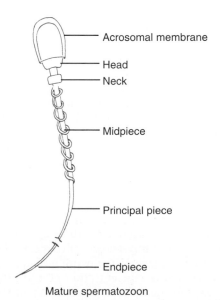

Acrosomal membrane

Head

Neck

Midpiece

Principal piece

Endpiece

Mature spermatozoon

Fig. 3.1 Diagram of a mature spermatozoon showing its principal features.

spreads out over the nucleus. The very important function of the acrosomal contents in penetrating the ovum is considered under the section Fertilisation. Meanwhile, the centriole which lies at the opposite pole of the nuclear membrane divides into two, and it is from here that the axial filament or flagellum develops. Most of the mitochondria form a sheath for the proximal part of the middle piece of the spermatozoon, whereas the tail piece develops a thin fibrous sheath. The centrioles link the midpiece and tail to the headpiece of the spermatozoon. The mature spermatozoon thus consists of a head piece covered by an acrosomal membrane, and a tail divided into four sections; the neck, midpiece, principal piece and endpiece. The DNA is confined to the nucleus in the head piece, and this alone penetrates the ovum at fertilisation. The remainder of the spermatozoon is responsible for its movement.

The ripe spermatozoa are released into the lumen of the seminiferous tubules of the testis and through to the epididymis together with the residual fragments of cytoplasm, mitochondria and Golgi apparatus, which separate from the sperm and eventually degenerate. Taken from this source they are known to have the capacity for fertilisation in vivo and in vitro. During ejaculation the spermatozoa are ejected through the vas deferens and prostatic urethra, where they combine with local secretions to form the seminal fluid.

EARLY EMBRYOGENESIS

Fertilisation

The complicated process of fertilisation implies the union of the mature germ cells, the ovum and spermatozoon. In humans there is a ready supply of spermatozoa constantly available from the normal healthy male after the age of puberty. An average ejaculate will consist of 2 to 5 mL of seminal fluid with an average sperm density of 60×10^6/mL.

By contrast, the normal healthy female will bring only one ovum to maturity and ovulation in each 28-day cycle. Other follicles do develop partially in the same cycle but rarely will more than one reach full maturity. The timing of ovulation is regulated by the cyclical release of gonadotrophins from the pituitary, and, at this time, the fimbrial end of the ipsilateral fallopian tube gently folds over the ovary and comes to rest over the stigma from where the ovum is released so that it can be taken up into the tube directly. Although this is the normal pattern, it is also possible for the ovum to move over the peritoneal surface of the pelvis behind the uterus to reach the fimbrial end of the contralateral tube.

Once inside the tube, the ovum is wafted medially by the rhythmic action of the cilia, which line the lumen. This movement is augmented by the finely tuned muscular activity of the fallopian tube, which by a combination of peristalsis and shunting squeezes the contents towards the uterus. This process is then temporarily halted for up to 38 hours, when the ovum reaches the ampulla of the tube. There appears to be a physiologic valve mechanism which prevents further passage of the ovum and is possibly only released by the rising concentration of the progesterone from the newly formed corpus luteum. When the valve is released, the ovum is moved on once again by the combination of cilial and muscular activity.

This temporary hold-up of the ovum in the ampulla allows additional time for fertilisation and means that sexual intercourse need not coincide precisely with ovulation. Furthermore, spermatozoa have the capacity to retain their potency in the tube for at least 48 hours after ejaculation, with the implication that, providing coitus occurs within 2 days before or after ovulation, fertilisation of the ovum is possible. Because the ovum is temporarily held up at the ampulla, the majority of fertilisations occur at that site. Experimental work in which the fallopian tubes have been cut into sections after insemination have defined the section of the tubes in which most newly fertilised ova are found.

Sexual intercourse occurs at random in humans, although the female may be more responsive at ovulation time, when the cervical glands produce a copious watery secretion which not only serves to lubricate the vagina but also assists the ascent of the spermatozoa. Normal ejaculation will occur into the upper vagina, where the semen forms a coagulum for approximately 20 minutes before liquefying. The coagulum prevents immediate loss of fluid from the vagina after sexual intercourse. The surface cells of the vagina are rich in glycogen, especially when under the influence of oestrogen in the follicular phase of the menstrual cycle. Döderlein bacilli convert glycogen to lactic acid with the result that the vagina becomes weakly acidic and, as such, is hostile to spermatozoa. However, the seminal fluid is alkaline and acts as a buffer for the sperm until they can reach the cervical fluid, which is also alkaline. At midcycle the flow of cervical mucus will increase the pH of the upper vagina and facilitate the activity of the sperm. The early progress of the spermatozoa is dependent on the propulsive effect of the tail piece, which acts as a flagellum; thus poor motility of the sperm in the seminal sample is an important cause of male infertility. In addition, the passage of the spermatozoa is aided by low-grade contractions of the uterus, which produce a slight negative pressure in the cavity serving to draw the sperm upwards. Spermatozoa have the ability to pass through the uterus and fallopian tubes with amazing rapidity. It is possible to aspirate viable sperm from the pouch of Douglas within 30 minutes of artificial insemination in the upper vagina.

To be able to penetrate and fertilise an egg, spermatozoa must undergo physiologic maturation changes in a process known as capacitation. This process occurs during the first 6 hours of the sperm being in the female genital tract, and capacitated sperm are distinguished by the development of hyperactivated motility, a change in their surface properties which allows them to be responsive to signals near the oocyte and the ability to bind to the zona pellucida of the ovum. Following capacitation, when a spermatozoon reaches the cumulus around the ovum, the spermatozoon plasma membrane initially attaches loosely to it and then more firmly to specific sperm receptors on the zona pellucida. Following initial binding a quite definite change occurs in the acrosomal cap and the sperm undergoes an irreversible form of lysosome exocytosis. The outer acrosomal membrane fuses with the spermatozoon plasma membrane and, as they coalesce, fine pores open up to release various lytic enzymes which have the ability to break up the oocyte cumulus cells and corona radiata to penetrate the zona pellucida, through a narrow channel. The first spermatozoon to reach the cell membrane of the ovum fuses with it, and the head piece containing the nucleus passes into the cytoplasm of the oocyte, where it appears as the male pronucleus. It is easily discernible by light microscopy next to the nucleus of the oocyte, which forms the female pronucleus. The tail piece of the spermatozoon is left behind outside the cell membrane of the oocyte.

As soon as the head piece has penetrated the oocyte, cortical granules release their contents into the space between the egg and the zona pellucida, changing the cell membrane and preventing further penetration by any other spermatozoa, thus establishing a block to polyspermy. Although only one spermatozoon out of many millions produced in a single ejaculation is needed for fertilisation, hundreds of spermatozoa will undergo the acrosomal reaction to help degrade the cumulus and zona pellucida, thereby allowing one sperm to reach the cell membrane of the oocyte and fuse with it. Hence low-density semen of less than 20 million/mL is associated with relative infertility. In vitro, however, a much lower sperm density is compatible with fertilisation, providing that the motility and morphology are normal.

In the majority of cases a woman will release a single egg during each ovulation cycle. However, if two ova are released and fertilised independently by two sperm, this leads to two zygotes forming and developing, resulting in dizygotic (nonidentical) twins. Much less commonly, if a single zygote splits into two embryos this results in monozygotic (identical) twins.

Postfertilisation Transportation and Implantation

Following fertilisation, the ovum continues to move towards the uterus aided as before by the muscle activity of the tube and to a lesser extent by the cilia, which are sparser at the medial end of the tubes where the glandular secretory cells are more numerous. The early development of the fertilised ovum depends on the nutrients derived from the secretions from these cells.

The first 4 or 5 days after fertilisation produce the most remarkable series of changes in the oocyte, all of which have now been followed clearly during in vitro experiments. Following fertilisation the second meiotic division of the oocyte is completed, at which time the pairs of chromatids separate, with 23 being retained in the oocyte and 23 being expelled in the second polar body (see Oogenesis earlier). Thereafter a nuclear membrane re-forms around the ovum's set of haploid chromosomes, as well as those from the sperm, resulting in the formation of female and male pronuclei, which each contain 23 chromosomes. The pronuclei migrate towards each other, but it is not until the time of the first cleavage division that the maternally derived and paternally derived chromosomes finally come together on the first mitotic spindle. The resulting diploid zygote now has 23 pairs of chromosomes, with each pair consisting of one chromosome from the mother and one from the father. The genetic features of the offspring are thus ordained with all of the genetic material required for development.

Following fertilisation, the zygote traverses the fallopian tube over the course of 4 days to reach the uterine cavity. Within 30 hours of fertilisation, the first mitotic division occurs, in which the fertilised ovum splits equally into two separate cells (Fig. 3.2). This process is known as 'cleavage'; each of the daughter cells, or blastomeres, contains a nucleus with a full complement of 46 chromosomes. Within 12 hours, a second cleavage occurs when each of the daughter cells divides into two again by mitotic division. Subsequent cleavage of successive generations of cells

follows in quick succession and not always synchronously, so that at any particular time there may be an uneven number of cells. During the preimplantation period there is no growth; blastomeres cleave to form successively smaller daughter cells until, just before implantation, they attain the size of adult somatic cells. During early cleavage the cells are spherical, loosely attached to each other, and totipotent (i.e. able to contribute to any embryonic or extraembryonic lineage). During the first few cleavage divisions the conceptus is solely dependent on maternal stores of RNA laid down during oogenesis because the genetic material brought in by the sperm is not active. Between the 4- and 8-cell stages the 'embryonic' genome is activated.

When the conceptus has between 16 and 32 cells, after the fourth cleavage division, it undergoes a process known as compaction. The cells maximise their intercellular contacts with each other, and flatten onto each other. It becomes impossible to discern the cell outlines, and the embryo becomes known as a morula (Fig. 3.3), Latin for a mulberry, which it resembles. At the morula stage, the embryo moves from the fallopian tube to the uterine cavity, at which stage a fluid-filled cavity (the blastocoele) develops between the cells and a blastocyst is formed (see Fig. 3.22).

After morula formation, the cells differentiate for the first time, when the embryo has approximately 32 cells. The outer cells (adjacent to the zona pellucida) become polarised and epithelial, forming zonular tight junctions with each other to make a watertight seal. Sodium is actively pumped into the interstitial spaces inside the conceptus, which in turn draws in water through the cells by osmosis, with the formation of a blastocoele cavity. This outer epithelial layer is known as the trophectoderm, which gives rise

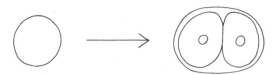

Fig. 3.2 Diagrammatic representation of the first cleavage division.

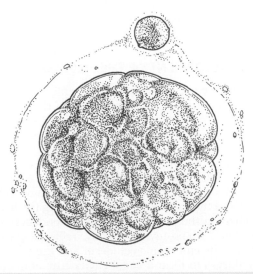

Fig. 3.3 The morula stage of development.

mainly to the extraembryonic membranes and the fetal portion of the placenta. The inner cells remain totipotent and form an eccentrically positioned clump of cells which are fated to become the embryo.

In vitro studies of human preimplantation embryo development have shown that human embryos have variable morphology and developmental potential. Approximately 75% of embryos have varying numbers of cytoplasmic membrane-bound fragments, and blastomeres are frequently uneven in size. Only approximately 50% of embryos cultured in vitro will reach the blastocyst stage, with the remaining embryos arresting development mainly between the 4-cell and morula stages. The reasons for this embryonic arrest are unclear but may reflect a combination of suboptimal culture conditions, chromosomal abnormalities or inadequate oocyte maturation. It is becoming apparent that a large proportion (approximately 20%) of human embryos have gross chromosomal abnormalities, and nearly 70% of embryos have one or more blastomeres with two or more nuclei. These factors, combined with a sensitivity to the environment, may contribute to the low rates of implantation (approximately 25%) following in vitro fertilisation and transfer of embryos at the 2- to 4-cell stage. High levels of embryonic arrest, coupled with low implantation rates, suggest that in the human there are very high levels of embryonic loss during the first 2 weeks following fertilisation.

The blastocyst implants into the secretory endometrium of the uterus approximately 6 days after fertilisation. The trophoblast cells produce a proteolytic enzyme which degrades the zona pellucida, thus allowing the blastocyst to break free in a process known as 'hatching'. At this time, the trophoblast divides and proliferates rapidly, and a more superficial syncytium of cells, the syncytiotrophoblast (ST) (outer layer), is produced along with the basal (inner layer) cytotrophoblast (CT) (see Fig. 3.17). The ST invades the uterine wall and interlocks into the spongy network of the endometrium so that the blastocyst is secured firmly to it, thus establishing the maternal and embryonic interface. By the end of 10 days, the early embryo has burrowed into the endometrium to such an extent that it is completely covered. It extracts nutrients from the endometrial secretions and is already producing human chorionic gonadotropin (hCG), which may be measured in maternal serum or urine. The trophoblast cells go on to form the placenta, which is described later in this chapter.

EARLY DEVELOPMENT OF THE EMBRYO

The cells known as the inner cell mass which give rise to the embryo and contribute to the formation of the yolk sac and amnion start a rapid development from the 10th day following conception. They are heaped up on one wall and thus remain in contact with the CT on the inner aspect of the blastocyst wall. At this time, the inner cell mass arranges itself into a bilaminar disc, the outer, which is in contact with the CT, forming the primitive embryonic ectoderm (epiblast) and the inner layer (i.e. that facing the blastocyst cavity) forming the primitive embryonic endoderm (hypoblast). By the 12th postovulatory day, a slit-like space opens up between the embryonic ectoderm and the adjacent CT, which enlarges to form a small cavity (the amniotic vesicle, later becoming the amniotic sac) the base of which is formed by embryonic ectoderm and the walls and roof of which are formed of CT. At the same time, hypoblast cells migrate out from the deeper layer of the embryonic disc and migrate along the inner surface of the CT to create a cavity in the lower half of the blastocyst, which is called the endocervical vesicle, later becoming the yolk sac (see Fig. 3.23).

Only two layers of cells lie between the two fluid cavities of the amniotic sac and yolk sac – the epiblast and hypoblast. Between the epiblast and hypoblast a third layer of cells grows in the third week of development in a process known as gastrulation. Gastrulation is initiated with the formation of the primitive streak, with epiblast cell migration and invagination, displacing the hypoblast to form two cells layers, the mesoderm (which lies between the epiblast and hypoblast) and endoderm (which displaces much of the hypoblast tissue). The remaining epiblast develops into ectoderm, forming the trilaminar germ disc.

The ectoderm cells adjacent to the amniotic sac are tall columnar cells from which all the ectodermal tissues of the fetus develop (i.e. the skin and all its appendages) and also the neural tube and its derivatives (the brain, spinal cord, nerves, autonomic ganglia and adrenal medulla).

The endodermal cells adjacent to the yolk sac form all the endodermal tissues of the developing fetus (i.e. the lining of the gut and the epithelial cells of the gut derivatives – the thyroid, parathyroid, trachea, lungs, liver and pancreas).

The middle layer forms the intraembryonic mesoderm, and, from it, all the mesodermal tissues of the fetus develop (i.e. the bones, muscles, cartilage and subcutaneous tissues of the skin, heart, blood vessels and kidneys). Extraembryonic mesoderm cells migrate between the CT and yolk sac and amniotic sac largely separating the blastocyst from the trophoblast except at the connecting stalk (primitive body stalk), which is the primordium of the umbilical cord.

ORGANOGENESIS

Development of the Germ Layers

The three layers of ectoderm, mesoderm and endoderm initially take the form of a flat circular sandwich, but later there is a disproportionate growth of the ectoderm at opposite poles so that the embryonic plate elongates into an oval, each end of which curves towards the yolk sac, thus forming a C-shape with a head fold and tail fold. Intraembryonic mesoderm lies between the ectoderm and endoderm except at two locations – the prochordal plate (buccopharyngeal membrane), which breaks down in the fourth week, and the cloacal plate membrane, which breaks down at the seventh week.

On the dorsal or amniotic surface of the ectoderm, specialised neuroectodermal tissue thickens into the neural plate. A groove develops in the middle of the neural plate from the head to the tail of the embryo, and tissues on either side fold upwards into a neural fold. The edges grow over and eventually unite and close to change the groove into a tube – the neural tube – from which the nervous system will develop (Fig. 3.4). Meanwhile, the mesodermal layer, which is now adjacent to the neural tube, is growing laterally, the part nearest the midline becoming the paraxial mesoderm, the part further out becoming the intermediate mesoderm (intermediate cell mass) and the part that is most lateral becoming the lateral plate mesoderm (see Fig. 3.4). The amniotic sac, which was sitting on top of the bilaminar flat embryo, enlarges as the embryo grows and folds until it completely surrounds the developing embryo and yolk sac.

Growth of the endoderm is at first lateral and then ventral, eventually folding round to envelop a portion of the yolk sac and creating a tube, the primitive gut. The gut tube has three distinct sections: foregut, midgut and hindgut. At first, the midgut is in direct continuity with the diminishing yolk sac, but as the lateral folds of the embryo grow round, they constrict the opening to the yolk sac, which eventually becomes separated from the gut altogether and forms a tubular stalk, the vitellointestinal duct. Occasionally, the connection with the gut may persist as Meckel diverticulum.

The lateral plate of the mesoderm divides into the somatopleure, which remains adjacent to the ectoderm, and the splanchnopleure, which grows round the developing gut. The space between the somatopleure and splanchnopleure forms the coelomic cavity (Fig. 3.5), later the pleural and peritoneal cavities.

The paraxial mesoderm becomes segmented into discrete masses of cells, or somites, which appear on either side of the neural tube under the surface of the ectoderm on the dorsal aspect of the embryo progressively along its length from the base of skull to the tail. The paraxial mesoderm somites develop into the vertebrae, dura mater, muscles of

the body wall and part of the dermis of the neck and trunk. The intermediate mesoderm develops in a ventral direction towards the coelomic cavity and forms the origins of the urogenital system. The limb buds develop from the lateral plate mesoderm, pushing out a covering of ectoderm. The nerve supply to the limb buds comes off the neural tube at the level at which they originate.

Much of the early development of the embryo is at the head end, where the coverings of the neural tube develop with the brain. In addition, a condensation of mesoderm occurs at the cranial end of the coelomic cavity, and this forms the pericardial cavity and the primitive heart tubes. A further accumulation of mesoderm caudal to the developing heart is called the septum transversum and is destined to become the centre of the diaphragm.

As the head fold grows more quickly on the dorsal surface than on the ventral surface, it begins to curl round the developing heart and diaphragm (Fig. 3.6). The foregut also curves round behind the pericardium and reaches the surface at the pit between the forebrain and pericardium, known as the stomatodeum (see Fig. 3.6). The thin buccopharyngeal membrane at this point breaks down at the fourth week of embryonic life, leaving a continuous channel between mouth, lined with ectoderm, and foregut or pharynx, lined with endoderm. A small outpouch in the roof of the mouth grows up into the developing brain. This is the Rathke pouch, which develops into the anterior lobe of the pituitary gland.

Central Nervous System

As described earlier, the cells of the central nervous system develop from the dorsal surface of the embryonic plate, which is induced to become neuroectoderm and develops into a neural plate. The neural plate folds along its central axis to form a shallow neural groove which later becomes covered by the neural folds which fuse and pinch off, thus forming the neural tube. As the tube closes, some neural cells are excluded on the dorsal aspect and form the neural crest between the spinal cord and the ectodermal surface. These neural crest cells are pluripotent and will differentiate to form most of the peripheral nervous system. Some of these cells migrate laterally on either side of the midline to become the cell bodies in the autonomic ganglia, including the suprarenal medulla, and the posterior root ganglia (Fig. 3.7).

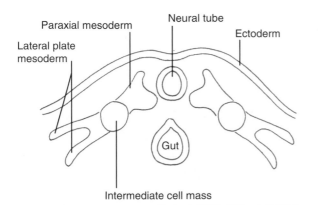

Fig. 3.4 Diagram to indicate the formation of the neural tube, the paraxial mesoderm, intermediate cell mass and lateral plate mesoderm.

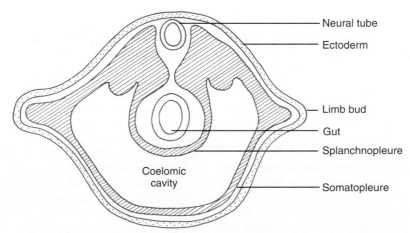

Fig. 3.5 Diagram showing division of the mesoderm into splanchnopleure and somatopleure to form the coelomic cavity.

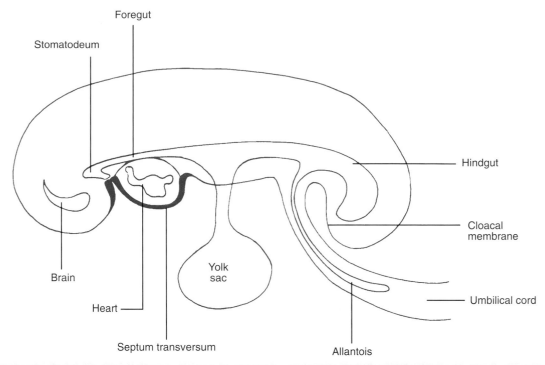

Fig. 3.6 Sagittal section of the early embryo indicating the relationship of the various features referred to in the text.

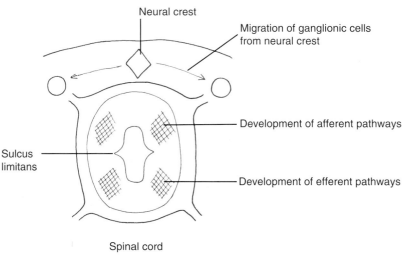

Fig. 3.7 Early development of the spinal cord.

The anterior end of the neural tube forms the forebrain limited by the lamina terminalis. The side walls of the foremost part of the neural tube develop into the hypothalamus, while the two cerebral hemispheres originate as two hollow diverticula, the cerebral vesicles. They grow forwards and laterally from the hypothalamus, and the cavities of the cerebral hemispheres form the lateral ventricles of the mature brain and interconnect through the interventricular foramen.

The midbrain, brain stem and cerebellum develop by further cell proliferation at the cranial end of the neural tube, while the caudal section develops into a spinal cord. When the neural tube closes over, a rapid proliferation of neural cells occurs throughout the length of the brain stem and spinal cord. These cells then undergo functional differentiation, arranging themselves into distinct bundles to become the visceral and somatic, and efferent and afferent pathways.

At the level of the brain stem, the central canal is wider and flatter as it opens up into the fourth ventricle. The distribution of afferent and efferent pathways is similar to that in the cord, but the afferent groups lie more laterally. In addition, special branchial afferent and efferent nerve cell groups appear supplying the pharyngeal arch derivatives as the cranial nerves (Fig. 3.8).

Failure of closure of the neural tube on its dorsal aspect gives rise to the variety of neural tube defect abnormalities, most commonly seen at the caudal end as an open spina bifida.

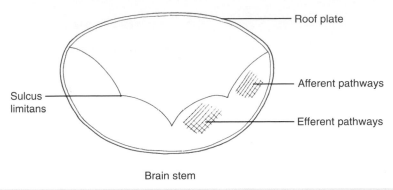

Fig. 3.8 Diagram showing spinal cord development at the level of the brain stem.

Pharyngeal Region

The lower part of the face (mandibles) and the whole of the neck region are developed from condensations of lateral mesoderm into a series of symmetrical arches which grow round the sides of the pharynx and eventually meet ventrally in the midline, thus becoming horseshoe shaped. In fish, these are the gill arches and the spaces between them are the gills, but in humans the condensations of ectoderm and endoderm between the pharyngeal arches remain intact and a very thick layer of mesoderm interleaves between them (Fig. 3.9). In each pharyngeal arch there develops a cartilage bar and surrounding muscle supplied by segmental blood vessels and nerves (derived from neural crest cells). Between the arches, a series of pharyngeal pouches develops. Humans have five arches (1, 2, 3, 4 and 6).

Various structures develop from each of the pharyngeal arches and their adjacent pouches. From the first arch, the upper and lower jaws, the palate, incus, malleus, anterior two-thirds of the tongue and muscles of mastication develop. Served by the fifth (trigeminal) cranial nerve, the first pouch elongates and extends laterally as the eustachian tube and the middle ear.

The second pharyngeal arch structures include part of the hyoid bone, the stylohyoid ligament, the styloid process and stapes, as well as the muscles of facial expression served by the seventh (facial) cranial nerve. The second pouch contributes to the tympanic cavity and forms the tonsil and supratonsillar fossa.

The third pharyngeal arch gives rise to the lower part of the hyoid bone and stylopharyngeus muscle served by the ninth (glossopharyngeal) cranial nerve. The posterior third of the tongue and anterior part of the epiglottis are covered with mucous membranes derived from this arch. In the third pharyngeal pouch, the inferior parathyroids and the thymus gland develop.

The fourth pharyngeal arch gives rise to the thyroid, cricothyroid and laryngeal cartilages, muscles of the soft palate and some muscles of the pharynx supplied by the tenth (vagus) cranial nerve. From the fourth pouch, the superior parathyroid glands are formed.

The fifth arch regresses, and the sixth pharyngeal arch fuses with the fourth and gives rise to the laryngeal cartilages.

Each of the pharyngeal arches has its own blood vessels and nerve supplying the structure derived from it. Each

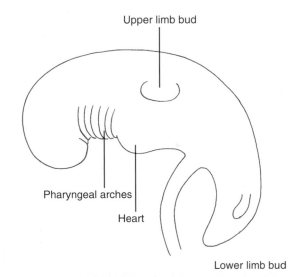

Fig. 3.9 Diagram showing embryonic development at the stage of preliminary pharyngeal arches.

nerve divides into an anterior and posterior division, which in certain situations may supply the adjacent arch structures. Not all the pharyngeal arch arteries survive; the first and second regress apart from the small maxillary and stapedial arteries, and the fifth disappears altogether. The third arch arteries form part of the internal carotid artery, while the right fourth arch artery forms the right subclavian artery and the left fourth arch artery forms the arch of the aorta. The sixth arch arteries form the pulmonary arteries and also the ductus arteriosus on the left side (Fig. 3.10).

From the floor of the pharynx, three important midline structures develop: the tongue, thyroid and respiratory system.

The muscles of the tongue develop from three occipital myotomes, but the connective tissue, lymph glands and mucosa are derived from the first and third pharyngeal arches, supplying the anterior two-thirds and posterior one-third, respectively. Between the two components the thyroglossal duct exists in the fetus but is usually obliterated before birth. The thyroid glands develop as a downwards growth from the floor of the pharynx called the thyroid diverticulum. As it descends down the neck, it remains connected to the tongue via the thyroglossal duct.

At the caudal end of the ventral aspect of the pharynx, a fossa develops, and this gradually grows away from the

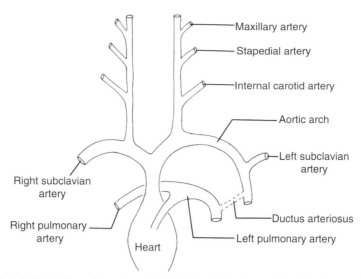

Fig. 3.10 The arterial development from the pharyngeal arch arteries as described in the text.

pharynx as the trachea. From this, the bronchi and primitive lungs are derived. The cartilage of the fourth and sixth arches contributes to the bones of the larynx which border the opening to the trachea.

The development of the pharyngeal region, face and mouth is a complex one, sometimes occurring imperfectly. Among the more common developmental abnormalities that may arise are failure of fusion of the palate or maxillary processes, giving rise to cleft palate or harelip. Failure of occlusion of the second pharyngeal pouch may give rise to a branchial cyst, and failure of regression of the thyroglossal duct may produce thyroglossal cysts.

Cardiovascular System

The heart is one of the earliest differentiating and functioning organs and begins to beat in the fourth week of development, reflecting the increasing size and nutritional requirements of the embryo at this early stage, which cannot be fulfilled by diffusion alone. Angiogenic tissue is recognisable in the very early presomite embryo and will soon develop into the heart and blood vessels of the fetus. The heart is formed as a pair of endocardial heart tubes developing from an accumulation of angiogenic cells (which originated as progenitor heart cells in the epiblast and migrated) in the area of the pericardial mesoderm. These left and right endocardial heart tubes are brought together in the central midline during cephalocaudal bending and lateral folding of the embryo, which causes them to fuse to form a single chamber within the pericardial mesoderm known as the primitive heart tube. The primitive heart tube does not fuse at the caudal-most ends and therefore has an inverted Y shape, with the arms of the Y receiving venous blood from the confluence of the vitelline, umbilical and cardinal veins, which run into the left and right sinus venosus. The cranial end of the heart tube leads into the bulbus cordis and on to the newly formed aorta. The heart tube consists of an outer myocardium and inner endocardium and by day 23 has initiated rhythmic contractions; fetal heart activity can be recognised with ultrasound techniques by the 32nd day of intrauterine life.

The two ends of the heart tube are soon fixed to the pericardium, so that further growth of the bulbus cordis and ventricle causes the tube to bend up on itself and form an S shape. Cardiac looping is the first manifestation of left–right asymmetry within the embryo. The heart tube bends so that the cranial (ventricular) portion bends caudally and right, whilst the caudal (atrial) portion expands cranially and left up creating an S-shaped loop. The atrium expands laterally and the two lateral expansions become the left and right auricles in a process known as ballooning. The atrium now receives blood through an opening on its dorsocaudal part from the sinus venosus. Blood leaves the atrium through an opening on the ventral surface, the atrioventricular canal, which leads to the single ventricle.

Next, extensive remodelling occurs through the formation of septa, which is necessary to produce dual circulation. This occurs at three main levels: the atria, ventricles and the atrioventricular canal. Endocardial cushions appear on the dorsal and ventral surfaces of the atrioventricular canal and eventually fuse, dividing the canal into right and left atrioventricular canals. The division of the atrium into two cavities is brought about by the growth of two septa: the septum primum and septum secundum, which overlap. This creates a valve opening called the foramen ovale, which allows the unidirectional passage of blood from the right to the left atrium. Throughout fetal life, the foramen is patent but closes at birth.

A more complex development of septa occurs in the ventricle and the truncus arteriosus, to form a left and right ventricle, and an aortic and pulmonary artery. Dorsal and ventral ridges arise on the walls of the ventricular cavity, eventually fusing to divide the right and left ventricle as they expand. Failure of fusion leaves a patent interventricular foramen. The final part of septation is that of the truncus arteriosus (forms the proximal aorta and pulmonary artery) and the conus cordis (forms the outflow tracts of both ventricles). The truncus is divided by endocardial cushions which grow inwards to fuse, and spiral around each other to produce an aorticopulmonary septum which has a twist forming the aorta and pulmonary artery, which are intertwined in the adult heart. Failure of this spiral-ling process leads to transposition of the great vessels. The conus divides in a similar manner with the resultant sep-tum being continuous with the membranous ventricular septum inferiorly and the truncus septum superiorly, thus ensuring continuity of the outflow tracts.

Finally, the heart valves are formed from endothelial pro-jections at the atrioventricular orifices and also at the distal end of the cordis at the pulmonary and aortic orifices. The total development from heart tube to completion occurs between the fourth and seventh weeks of intrauterine life.

Fetal Circulation

Prior to birth, the fetus obtains oxygen and nutrients and discards waste products via the umbilical vein and placenta. Oxygenated blood from the placenta returns to the fetus in the umbilical vein which joins the left branch of the por-tal vein. The majority of this blood bypasses the sinusoids of the liver by passing through the ductus venosus shunt directly to the inferior vena cava. Blood entering the infe-rior vena cava is transported to the right atrium, and thence the majority is deflected through the patent foramen ovale to the left atrium and on to the left ventricle, thus bypass-ing the pulmonary circulation. From the left ventricle, the blood flows into the aorta to supply the fetal tissues, in particular the brain, coronary circulation and upper body. Deoxygenated blood returning from the head of the fetus passes through the superior vena cava to the right atrium and straight on to the right ventricle and pulmonary artery. However, only approximately 15% of this blood reaches the pulmonary circulation because most is directed into the descending aorta via the wide-patency ductus arteriosus to supply the lower body and placenta. Aortic blood is carried via the umbilical arteries back to the placenta for reoxygen-ation. At birth, the three short circuits, the ductus venosus, foramen ovale and ductus arteriosus, close, but occasion-ally the ductus arteriosus fails to do so. The ductus venosus is obliterated and becomes the ligamentum venosum, and the distal umbilical vein becomes the ligamentum teres.

Alimentary System, Pulmonary and Peritoneal Cavities

The gut, which develops in continuity with the pharynx, may be subdivided into three sections, each with its own blood supply. The caudal portion of the foregut extends as a tube, the oesophagus, to the stomach, which forms as a sac at the fifth week of intrauterine life. Below the stomach the liver grows out from the ventral aspect of the foregut. At first it is a hollow diverticulum pushing up into the septum transversum, but later it produces two solid buds of cells which form the left and right lobes of the liver. The gall-bladder develops from a ventral outpouching of the hepatic diverticulum. The duodenum arises from the foregut and midgut and gives rise to the pancreas from its endodermal lining. The foregut structures are supplied by blood from the coeliac artery (Fig. 3.11). The spleen, which takes its blood supply from the splenic branch of the coeliac artery, arises from cellular islands in the coelomic epithelium and is not a derivative of the foregut.

The midgut starts at the midpoint of the duodenum at the level of the entry of the bile duct and terminates approx-imately two-thirds of the way along the transverse colon.

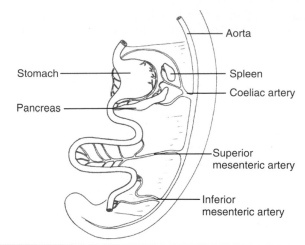

Fig. 3.11 The vascular supply to the developing alimentary system.

The pancreas develops initially at 4 weeks of development as a ventral and dorsal part; the two parts subsequently fuse, and a common opening to the duodenum forms. The midgut rapidly elongates but, because the peritoneal cavity is small at this stage, herniates out into the umbili-cal cord at 6 weeks as a physiological umbilical hernia. This herniated bowel returns to the abdominal cavity at 10 weeks and undergoes rotation. Failure of this process to occur can cause two types of abnormal midgut hernia-tion to persist – omphalocele or gastroschisis. The midgut extends down to the splenic flexure of the colon and is sup-plied with blood from the superior mesenteric artery. This part of the gut grows far more rapidly than the vertebral column and therefore produces a large ventral loop held in place by an extensive dorsal mesentery, through which the blood vessels run. Fixation of folds in the lower part of the loop produces the characteristic position of ascending and transverse colon in the adult, while the ileum retains its mesentery and mobility.

The hindgut forms the distal third of the transverse colon, descending colon and rectum and is supplied by the inferior mesenteric artery, although the anal canal is also supplied by middle and inferior rectal arteries. The hindgut opens into the dorsal part of the cloaca.

Respiratory Organs

In the midline of the ventral surface of the primitive pharynx (part of foregut), the endoderm furrows to form the laryngotracheal groove which grows into the primi-tive mesoderm appears at the fourth week of intrauterine life. Between the fourth pair of pharyngeal pouches, this groove extends ventrally as the laryngotracheal tube, with the proximal portion elongating to form the larynx and trachea, and the distal portion diving into two lung buds which eventually develop into the primary bronchi. The lining of the respiratory passages is endodermal in origin. A tracheooesophageal septum forms posterior to the laryn-gotracheal tube, separating it from the oesophagus. By the fifth week of gestation, the lung buds grow further to fill the pleural coeloms and form the secondary lung buds. These then subdivide into lobules, three on the right and two on the left, which in turn will form the lobes of the mature lungs. Growth of the trachea and lung buds proceeds in a caudal direction so that by full term the bifurcation of the trachea is at the level of the fourth thoracic vertebra. The alveoli do not appear until the sixth month of intrauterine life.

The pleural coeloms fold back on themselves to form the fluid-filled pleural cavities, which are separated from the pericardial cavity by the pleuropericardial membrane and from the peritoneal cavity by the developing diaphragm.

The diaphragm itself develops from the septum transversum, the pleuroperitoneal membrane, the costal margin and the gastrohepatic ligament. There is a very small contribution from the dorsal mesentery behind the oesophagus and from the mesoderm around the aorta.

Skeletal System

The embryonic mesenchyme gives rise to all the bones of the body and is derived from mesodermal cells of the somites, the somatopleuric layer of lateral plate mesoderm and neural crest cells. Some of the bones are preformed in cartilage before undergoing ossification, while others are ossified directly from membranous precursors. The vertebrae are formed from the segmental sclerotomes around the notochord and neural tube. These sclerotomes are derived from the mesodermal somites. Each vertebra is preformed as a cartilaginous ring in which three centres of ossification appear: one for the body and one for each half of the neural arch. The process is complete by the eighth week of intrauterine life. The notochordal remnant eventually disappears in the centre of each vertebral body but persists as the nucleus pulposus of the intervertebral discs.

The ribs are also preformed in cartilage and develop from the costal processes of the primitive vertebral arches. The ribs grow laterally towards the sternum, which forms from two sternal plates which develop to link the central ends of the upper nine ribs on each side. The two plates pass through a cartilaginous phase before undergoing ossification and fusion to form the definitive single sternum.

The skull develops from the mesenchyme that envelops the cerebral vesicles. The vault of the skull and part of the base are ossified directly from membranous bone, while the major part of the base, excluding the orbital part of the frontal bone and the lateral part of the greater wing, is preformed in cartilage.

The limbs appear as small limb buds at the end of the fourth week of intrauterine life (see Fig. 3.9). The upper limb buds develop a little in advance of the lower ones. Each bud is derived from several primitive somites and carries with it the corresponding ventral ramus of the spinal nerve. The central mesenchyme forms the cartilaginous skeleton, which eventually ossifies to form the limb bones. The muscles pertaining to the skeleton are derived from the surrounding mesoderm. The feet and hands appear very similar to start with, as flat extensions of the limb buds. Later, the mesenchyme condenses into distinct digits, and failure of this phase gives rise to webbing of the fingers or toes.

The joints between bones evolve from the residual core of mesenchyme which does not differentiate into membranous bone. This mesenchyme may develop into fibrous tissue as in the fibrous joints between the skull bones, or it may become cartilaginous as in the cartilage joints. Synovial joints occur when the mesenchyme loosens out and a cavity forms in the centre, while some of the cells liquefy to fill the space.

Muscles, Skin and Appendages

It has already been observed that the muscles of the limbs develop from the mesenchyme of the limb buds, and the muscles of the head and neck develop from the mesenchyme of the pharyngeal arches and neural crest mesenchyme. The muscles of the trunk all develop from the dorsolateral part of the somites known as the dermomyotome. Spindle cells proliferate from it to form the muscle plate, while the remainder forms the skin plate. The muscle plate or myotome divides into a dorsal part supplied by the dorsal ramus of the corresponding spinal nerve and a ventral part supplied by the ventral ramus. The dorsal part develops into the muscle groups of the back, and the ventral part forms the muscles of the body wall.

Some of the myotome derivatives degenerate and disappear, while others may fuse and form fibrous aponeuroses, as seen in the anterior abdominal wall. Involuntary muscles of the gut, ureters, bladder and uterus are developed from the splanchnopleuric mesoderm in situ. The skin plate or dermatome develops into the true dermis, while the overlying ectoderm forms the epidermis, hairs, nails, sweat glands and sebaceous glands.

The dermis and subcutaneous areolar tissue develop towards the end of the third month, and the dermal papillae appear in the fourth month. The primary nailfolds are also seen in the third month, and the sweat glands appear approximately 1 month later. The mammary glands develop as a collection of modified sweat glands at the cranial end of the milk ridge or nipple line. Occasionally, supernumerary nipples and even gland tissue may develop caudally in the same line. The epithelial lining of the ducts and glands is derived from the ectoderm, while the connective tissue and fat are developed from the underlying mesenchyme.

Development of the Genital Organs

The genital organs develop in close association with those of the urinary tract because the genital ridges are originally part of the larger, urogenital ridges. The urogenital ridges arise in the intermediate mesoderm on each side of the root of the mesentery beneath the epithelium of the coelom along with the nephrogenic cord (which becomes the urinary apparatus).

The urogenital ridges are composed of a pronephros, mesonephros (the gonad) and metonnephros (the definitive kidney). The pronephroi, a few transient tubules in the cervical region, appear first and quickly degenerate.

The mesonephros develops as a long bulge into the dorsal wall of the coelom in the thoracic and upper lumbar regions. It will later degenerate to a different extent in the two sexes (Fig. 3.12). Two important structures appear on the coelomic surface of the mesonephros: (1) the genital ridge from which the gonad will form and (2) the paramesonephric (müllerian) duct alongside the wolffian duct.

The genital ridge appears as a swelling on the medial aspect of the mesonephros; at first it covers the whole extent of the latter but later contracts to the central part only. The paramesonephric duct forms laterally as an invagination of the coelomic epithelium overlying the mesonephros, which

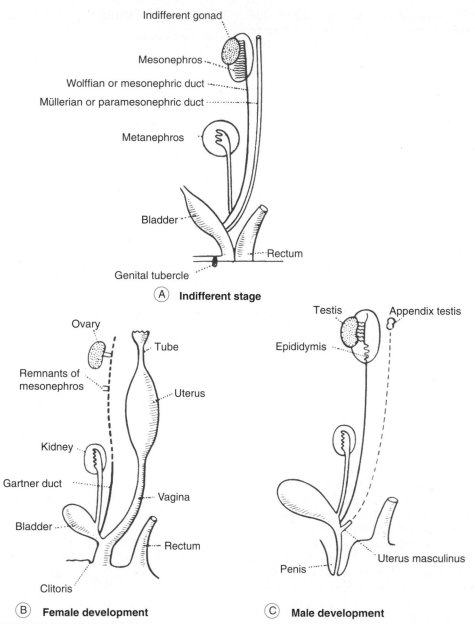

Fig. 3.12 Diagrammatic representation of genital tract development. (A) Indifferent stage. (B) Female development. (C) Male development.

closes to form a tube, or duct. This occurs in embryos of some 10-mm crown–rump length (5 to 6 weeks).

GONADS

The first sign of a primitive gonad may be seen at approximately 5 weeks.

The gonad has a triple origin from:

1. The coelomic epithelium of the genital ridge
2. The underlying mesoderm
3. The primordial germ cells which enter it from an extragonadal source.

We have seen that the gonads begin as bulges on the medial aspect of the mesonephric ridge on either side of the aorta in the upper lumbar region. These two bilateral prominences consist of mesonephric mesenchyme overlain by coelomic epithelium. First, there is proliferation of the coelomic epithelium and then further proliferation of the mesenchyme beneath that epithelium. By 5 to 6 weeks, irregular, finger-like projections of coelomic epithelium can be seen invaginating into the substance of the developing mesenchyme of the gonad below and breaking it into loose strands to form the primitive sex cords. Rapid development of these cords follows, and in the deeper layers they become branched and complex. During these early stages, primordial germ cells (bipotential gamete precursors) can be seen lying between the cords. These germ cells have originated from beneath the epithelium of the yolk sac, from which site they migrate via the hindgut and the dorsal mesentery to enter the genital ridge. They can be seen in the region of the genital ridge at approximately 4 weeks. By 6 to 7 weeks, therefore, the sex cords which have developed from the coelomic epithelium, the primitive mesenchymal tissue and the primordial germ cells all lie together in the developing bipotential gonad, which is at its indifferent stage. At this point the activation or absence of the sex-determining region of the Y chromosome (SRY) gene will determine male or female differentiation, respectively.

In the presence of the SRY gene, gonadal differentiation can first be seen in the testis at approximately 7 weeks. Sertoli cells are the first testis-specific cells to appear and, in conjunction with interstitial gonad cells, form the testis cords, which envelop the germ cells (spermatozoa precursors). The Sertoli cells are also responsible for secreting antimüllerian hormone (AMH), which causes atrophy of the paramesonephric duct. There is rapid development of the sex cords as they continue to grow into the medulla, where they branch out and differentiate to become the straight and convoluted seminiferous tubules. The mesenchymal cells between the testicular cords differentiate to become Leydig cells, which produce testosterone. Thus this stabilises and maintains the mesonephric duct, which opens into the urogenital sinus and persists in males and regressed in females. The ends of the straight seminiferous tubules anastomose into a network of tiny tubules – the rete testis. Efferent ductules form the connection between the rete testis and mesonephric duct, and their cranial portion becomes tightly coiled to form the ductal epididymis. The mesenchymal stroma becomes differentiated into spindle-shaped fibroblasts which subdivide the testes into lobules and ultimately form the tunica albuginea.

The ovary cannot be clearly identified until approximately 10 weeks, and it is possible to distinguish three groups of cells: the larger primordial germ cells, the supporting cells, which may now be called pregranulosa cells, and more spindle-shaped cells which have formed from the mesenchyme of the genital ridge. There is a phase of tremendous growth, and, in particular, the primordial germ cells differentiate into oogonia and increase markedly in number. By 20 weeks, they have almost reached 7 million in number, after which many die by a process known as atresia. The outer cortex remains less differentiated and in a state of more rapid proliferation compared with the inner cortex.

Histological examination of the developing ovary shows that there is a gradient, from the surface of the ovary inwards, of differentiation of oocytes from oogonia, entry of oocytes into meiosis and formation of follicles. Germ cells at the inner cortex–medulla boundary are the first to undergo these processes, so that it is possible simultaneously to see dividing oogonia in the outer cortex and fully formed follicles deeper in the ovary. By 20 to 24 weeks, follicle formation is taking place, whereby oocytes become surrounded by flattened pregranulosa cells. An interesting feature is that those germ cells which do not succeed in surrounding themselves with a protective layer of pregranulosa cells die. This destruction along with atresia of some follicles, which have passed into the early stage of development, results in many germ cells being eliminated, so that perhaps only 1 to 2 million remain at birth.

UTERUS AND TUBES

The paramesonephric (müllerian) and the mesonephric (wolffian) ducts are tubular tissue structures which give rise to the male and female reproductive tracts, respectively, originate from the mesonephros and initially coexist. After an initial indifferent stage during gonad development, in females, in the absence of AMH and testosterone, the paramesonephric (müllerian) ducts continue to develop and the mesonephric (wolffian) ones degenerate; in the male the opposite occurs (see Fig. 3.12). The paramesonephric ducts are formed from a longitudinal invagination of coelomic epithelium, with the cranial end forming a funnel which opens into the peritoneal/coelomic cavity (becomes the future ampulla of the fallopian tube) and the lower end extending caudally to reach the dorsal wall of the urogenital sinus by approximately 9 weeks (Fig. 3.13). As the paramesonephric ducts progress caudally, their lower portions come together in the midline and fuse; during the fourth month (12 to 16 weeks), proliferation of mesoderm around the fused lower parts of the ducts forms the muscular walls of the uterus and cervix.

VAGINA

Vaginal development is more complex (Figs. 3.14 and 3.15). Where the paramesonephric ducts reach the urogenital sinus, endodermal proliferation is induced to form

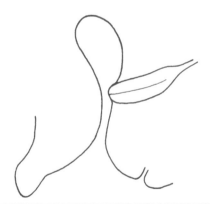

Fig. 3.13 The paramesonephric ducts which have reached the dorsal wall of the urogenital sinus by approximately 9 weeks.

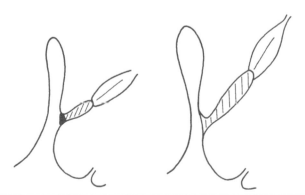

Fig. 3.14 Formation of the vaginal plate. This vaginal plate displaces the lower end of the fused müllerian ducts cranially as indicated by the hatched areas.

the müllerian tubercle, which is an area of thickened tissue. This tissue growth forms the solid vaginal plate (see Fig. 3.14), which is thus composed of sinus epithelium and paramesonephric ducts. The vaginal plate grows rapidly, pushing the remnants of the mesonephric duct, which had also reached the urogenital sinus, cranially. From this vaginal plate, the vagina forms. At first it is a solid organ, but at approximately 16 to 18 weeks the central core canalises to form the vaginal lumen (see Fig. 3.15). Because of the great growth of the plate, it is not possible to be sure how much vagina is developed from the paramesonephric ducts and how much from the urogenital sinus.

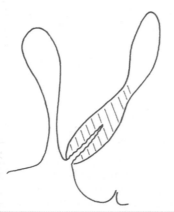

Fig. 3.15 The solid vaginal plate is beginning to break down to form the vaginal lumen at approximately 16 to 18 weeks.

EXTERNAL GENITALIA

The early development of the external genitalia is similar in males and females. At approximately 5 weeks, the primitive cloaca becomes divided by a transverse septum (the urorectal septum) into an anterior primitive urogenital sinus and a posterior rectal portion. From the upper part of the cloaca to approximately the level of the müllerian tubercle, this septum grows downwards; below that, the septum grows inwards from each side. Shortly after division is complete, the urogenital portion of the cloacal membrane breaks down.

Soon afterwards the urogenital sinus is seen to be made up of three parts (Fig. 3.16). In its lower portion there is an expanded urogenital sinus, above which is a narrow pelvic part (the pelvic urethra) which reaches as far cranially as a point where the müllerian ducts reach the sinus wall. The superior portion of the urogenital sinus, above the pelvic urethra, forms the presumptive bladder, which extends superiorly and is continuous with the allantois. On the external surface of the embryo, the genital tubercle can be seen, which is a conical projection encircling the

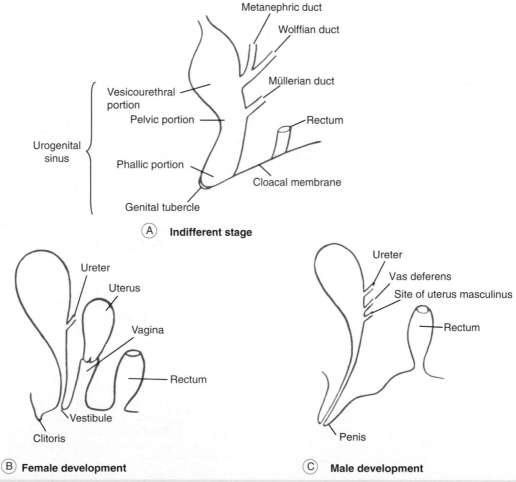

Fig. 3.16 Diagrammatic representation of lower genital tract development. (A) Indifferent stage. (B) Female development. (C) Male development.

anterior part of the cloacal (or urogenital) membrane; the tubercle can be seen before cloacal division is complete (6 weeks). As division of the primitive cloaca (described earlier) reaches completion, the urorectal septum fuses with the cloacal membrane, creating the perineum, which separates the anus from the urogenital region. The urogenital, or cloacal, membrane breaks down, opening the urogenital sinus to the amniotic fluid. Externally, on either side of the urogenital sinus may be seen two pairs of eminences – a medial pair called the genital folds and a lateral pair called the labioscrotal swellings. These are formed by the proliferation of mesoderm around the lower portion of the sinus.

Until approximately 10 weeks, the external appearances of the male and female are similar, and it is not possible to determine the sex of a fetus. Then, differentiation occurs in the presence or absence of steroidal sex hormones. The bladder and urethra are formed from the upper part of the vesicourethral division of the urogenital sinus, while, in the female, the pelvic and inferior portions become shallow and, ultimately, form the vestibule of the vagina (see Fig. 3.16B). In females, the genital tubercle remains small and becomes the clitoris; the genital folds form the labia minora, and the labioscrotal swellings enlarge to become the labia majora. The primitive perineum does not lengthen. In males, the genital tubercle enlarges to become the penis; the genital folds fuse to form the phallic portion of the male urethra, and the labioscrotal swellings enlarge and fuse to form the scrotum.

Finally, proliferating mesoderm spreads ventrally around the lower part of the body wall, uniting with its fellow part from the opposite side to complete the development of the clitoris or penis and the anterior surface of the bladder and anterior abdominal wall below the umbilicus.

Development of the Placenta

Once the ovum is fertilised in the fallopian tube, it enters the uterine cavity as a morula, which rapidly sheds its surrounding zona pellucida and converts into a blastocyst.

The outer cell layer of the blastocyst then proliferates to form the primary trophoblastic cell mass (Fig. 3.17A), from which cells infiltrate between those of the endometrial epithelium. The endometrium then degenerates, and the trophoblast thus comes into direct contact with the endometrial stroma; this process of implantation is complete by the 10th or 11th postovulatory day.

In the 7-day blastocyst, the trophoblast forms a peripheral plaque which rapidly differentiates into two layers, an inner layer of larger clear mononuclear CT cells with well-defined limiting membranes, and an outer layer of multinucleated ST (see Fig. 3.17B), this latter being a true syncytium. The ST is derived from the CT, not only at this early stage but also throughout gestation and is formed by fusion of CT cells. Apoptosis of uterine stromal cells creates spaces through which the blastocyst penetrates further into the endometrium.

Placental development commences when the blastocyst evokes the decidual reaction in the maternal endometrium, which transforms this into an exceedingly well perfused source of nutrition – the basal plate. The placenta is structurally composed of two parts: (1) the chorionic plate, which is of fetal origin, and (2) the basal plate, which has fetal- and maternal-derived parts (from the decidua basalis).

Between the 10th and 13th postovulatory days, a series of intercommunicating clefts, or lacunae, appears in the rapidly enlarging trophoblastic cell mass (Fig. 3.18); these are probably formed as a result of engulfment within the trophoblast of endometrial capillaries. The lacunae soon become partially confluent to form the precursor of the intervillous space, and, as maternal vessels are progressively eroded, they become filled with maternal blood. At this stage, the lacunae are incompletely separated off from each other by trabecular columns of ST which, between the 14th and 21st postovulatory days, tend to become radially orientated and come to possess a central cellular core that is produced by proliferation and invasion of CT cells from the chorionic base. These trabecular columns are not true villi but serve as the framework from which the villous tree will later develop; the placenta at this stage is a labyrinthine

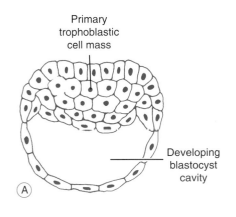
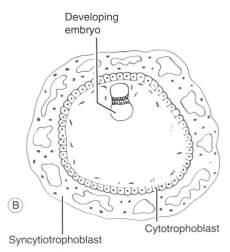

Fig. 3.17 Diagrammatic representation of (A) formation of primary trophoblastic cell mass and (B) the differentiation of this into the cytotrophoblast and syncytiotrophoblast.

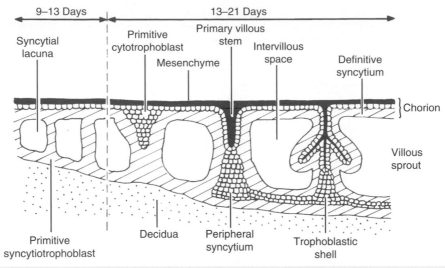

Fig. 3.18 Diagrammatic representation of the development of the placenta during the first 21 days of gestation.

rather than a villous organ, and the trabeculae are therefore best known as primary chorionic villi.

Continued growth of the CT leads to its distal extension into the region of decidual attachment. Concurrently, extraembryonic mesoderm invades the core of the primary chorionic villi, converting them into secondary chorionic villi. Later, the villous stems become vascularised, and in due course, the vessels within the stems establish functional continuity with others differentiating from the embryo body stalk and inner chorionic mesenchyme, and are now known as tertiary villi.

The distal part of the tertiary villous stems is formed almost entirely by CT, which is not invaded by mesenchyme and not vascularised but which is anchored to the decidua of the basal plate and known as anchoring villi. The CT cells of these anchoring villi proliferate and spread laterally to form a continuous CT shell between the ST and the uterine endometrium. This splits the ST into two layers: the definitive syncytium on the fetal aspect of the shell, which persists as the limiting layer of the intervillous space, and the peripheral syncytium between the shell and the decidua, which degenerates and is replaced by a layer of fibrinoid material (Nitabuch layer). The establishment of the trophoblastic shell is a mechanism to allow for rapid circumferential growth of the developing placenta, and this leads to an expansion of the intervillous space into which sprouts extend from the primary villous stems. These offshoots consist initially only of ST, but as they enlarge, they pass through the stages previously seen during the development of the primary villous stems (i.e. intrusion of CT), formation of a mesenchymal core and eventual vascularisation. These sprouts form the primary stem villi, and, because these are true villous structures, the placenta is by the 21st day of gestation a vascularised villous organ. The primary stem villi grow and divide to form secondary and tertiary stem villi, and these latter eventually break up into the terminal villous tree.

During the early weeks of gestation, CT cells from the trophoblastic shell break through the peripheral layer of ST and spread into the underlying decidua. However, groups of CT cells also grow into the lumen of the spiral arteries and extend as far as the deciduomyometrial junction; these cells replace the vessel endothelium and invade the walls of the intradecidual portion of the spiral vessels and appear to destroy the muscular and elastic tissue of the media. Because the walls of the intradecidual portions of the spiral vessels are markedly weakened as a result of this process of trophoblastic invasion, these vessels dilate considerably under the pressure of the maternal blood (Fig. 3.19); this is an important factor in allowing for a greatly augmented blood flow.

Between the 21st postovulatory day and the end of the fourth month of gestation, those villi orientated towards the uterine cavity degenerate and form the chorion laeve, while the thin rim of decidua covering this area gradually disappears to allow the chorion laeve (consisting of extraembryonic mesenchyma and CT) to come into contact with the parietal decidua of the opposite wall of the uterus. This merging causes the uterine cavity to obliterate. The villi on the side of the chorion towards the decidua basalis proliferate and progressively arborise to form the chorion frondosum, which develops into the definitive placenta. During this period, there is some regression of the CT elements in the chorionic plate and in the trophoblastic shell where the CT cell columns degenerate and are largely replaced by fibrinoid material (Rohr layer). Although there is CT regression in the basal plate, during the fourth month of gestation a further proliferation of endovascular CT occurs, a wave of these cells moving in retrograde direction to involve the intramyometrial segments of the spiral vessels. Again, this is where they replace the endothelium, invade and destroy the medial muscular and elastic tissue and lead to deposition of fibrinoid material in the wall; these changes extend almost to the origin of the spiral vessels from the radial arteries and, when complete, result in the transformation of the coiled spiral arteries of the placental bed into dilated, funnel-shaped, flaccid uteroplacental arteries. These arteries can accommodate the progressively increasing blood flow to the placenta (see Fig. 3.19).

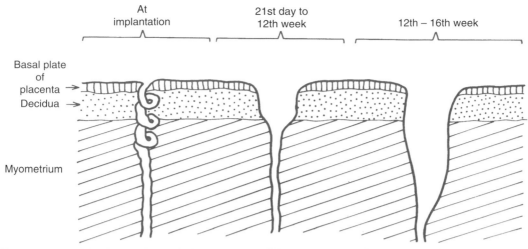

Fig. 3.19 Diagrammatic representation of the conversion of the spiral arteries into uteroplacental arteries.

The placental septa appear during the third month of gestation; they protrude into the intervillous space from the basal plate and divide the maternal surface of the placenta into between 15 and 20 lobes. These septa are simply folds of the basal plate, being formed partly as a result of regional variability in placental growth and partly by the pulling up of basal plate into the intervillous space by anchoring columns which have a poor growth rate. Because the basal plate is formed principally by the remnants of the CT shell embedded in fibrinoid material, it follows that the septa will have a similar composition, although some decidual cells may also be carried up into the folds. The septa are therefore simply an incidental by-product of the architectural refashioning of the placenta and have no physiologic or morphologic importance.

The lobes between the septa are not functional or structural subunits of the fetal placenta; this role is played by the lobules. Each placental lobule is derived from a single secondary stem villus which breaks up into tertiary stem villi, which sweep down towards the basal plate to form a hollow globular structure. The terminal villous tree, derived from the tertiary stem, is mainly in the outer shell of the hollow globule, and the centre of the lobule is relatively empty and villus free. The term cotyledon, if used at all, is best defined as that part of the villous tree which has arisen from a single primary stem villus; such a primary stem villus may give rise to a varying number of secondary stem villi, and hence the number of lobules in a cotyledon varies from two to five.

Each fetal lobule is supplied by a single uteroplacental artery, this being not coincidental but due to the preferential formation of the lobules in relationship to the opening of a maternal vessel. The blood from the uteroplacental artery, driven by the maternal head of pressure, flows up, rather like a fountain, in the central hollow core of the lobule towards the chorionic plate (Fig. 3.20). Towards the apex of the lobule, the driving pressure force becomes dissipated and the blood disperses laterally to flow back towards the basal plate in the outer shell of the lobule. Hence it is only in the outer shell of the lobule that the maternal blood comes into contact with the terminal villi, and only here is there a true physiological intervillous space, which is probably of capillary dimensions throughout.

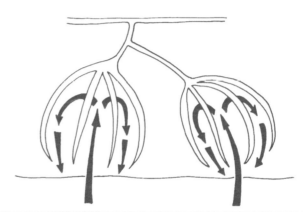

Fig. 3.20 Diagrammatic representation of the flow of maternal blood *(blue arrows)* through the fetal lobule.

By the end of the fourth month of gestation, the placenta has achieved its definitive form and undergoes no further anatomical modification. However, growth continues until term, and this is due principally to continuous arborisation of the villous tree and formation of fresh villi. This continuing growth is accompanied by a progressive alteration in the morphological appearances of the most distal villi of the tree, these being the only villi that are concerned with maternofoetal transfer. In the first trimester, the villi are large and have a regular circumferential mantle of trophoblast which consists of an inner layer of CT cells and an outer layer of ST; the villous stroma is formed of loose mesenchymal tissue in which, towards the end of the first trimester, small centrally placed fetal vessels are present (Fig. 3.21). During the second trimester the villi are smaller, the trophoblastic covering is less regular and the CT cells less numerous; more collagen is present in the stroma, and the fetal vessels are becoming larger in diameter and are beginning to move towards the periphery of the villus. In the third trimester the villi are much smaller in diameter, the trophoblastic layer is irregularly thinned and the CT cells are few and inconspicuous. Much of the trophoblastic irregularity is due to the formation of thinned anuclear areas of ST; these vasculosyncytial membranes are areas

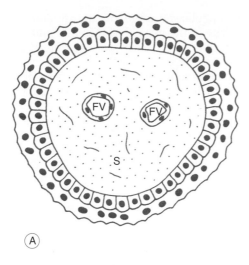

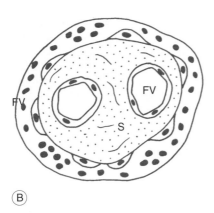

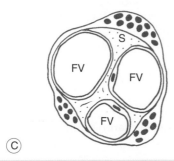

Fig. 3.21 Diagrammatic representation of the histologic appearances of the placental villi in (A) the first trimester, (B) the second trimester and (C) at term. *FV*, fetal vessels; *S*, villous stroma.

- approximate the fetal and maternal circulation
- increase the maternofoetal concentration gradient
- provide optimal conditions for maternofoetal transfer.

PLACENTAL BED

The term placental bed is applied to the decidua and myometrium, which directly underlie the placenta. As previously described, the placental bed is extensively colonised by extravillous CT cells during the early stages of gestation. The intravascular component of this extravillous trophoblastic cell population plays a crucial role in converting the spiral arteries of the placental bed into uteroplacental vessels while the interstitial component intermingles with the basal decidual cells and infiltrates between the myometrial fibres.

The function of the interstitial trophoblastic cells in the placental bed is unknown, but their principal secretory product is, unlike villous trophoblast, human placental lactogen rather than hCG.

The maternal component of the placental bed includes decidualised endometrial stromal cells and two leucocytic populations: macrophages and granular lymphocytes. The macrophages are prominent throughout pregnancy and may well play an immunologic role, whereas the granular lymphocytes are most conspicuous in the early months of gestation and may be of importance in the processes of implantation and placentation.

Residual endometrial glands are present in the placental bed but are usually attenuated or compressed into slits and identifiable only with epithelial markers.

Development of Membranes and Formation of Amniotic Fluid

MEMBRANES

The conversion of the early morula to a blastocyst is accomplished by the formation of a central fluid-filled cavity. This largely separates the primary trophoblastic cell mass, from which the placenta and extraplacental chorion develop, from those cells which give rise to the embryo and contribute to the formation of the yolk sac and amnion; these latter cells form the eccentrically situated inner cell mass which remains in contact with the CT on the inner aspect of the blastocyst wall (Fig. 3.22). During the eighth and ninth postovulatory days, the inner cell mass arranges itself into a bilaminar disc, the inner layer (i.e. that facing the blastocyst cavity) forming the primitive embryonic endoderm and the outer, which is in contact with the CT, forming the primitive embryonic ectoderm. The amniotic cavity first appears as a slit-like space between the embryonic ectoderm and the adjacent CT; this enlarges to form, by the 12th postovulatory day, a small cavity, the base of which is formed by embryonic ectoderm and the walls and roof of which are formed of CT (Fig. 3.23). At the same time, endodermal cells migrate out from the deeper layer of the embryonic disc to line the blastocyst cavity and thus form the primary yolk sac. The extraembryonic mesenchyme subsequently appears (Fig. 3.24), possibly derived from the trophoblast, and separates off the primary yolk sac from the blastocyst wall; the extraembryonic mesenchyme also intrudes between, and largely separates off, the

of trophoblast specially differentiated for gaseous transfer. The fetal villous stromal vessels are sinusoidally dilated and occupy most of the cross-sectional area of the villus; they have moved peripherally and lie in an immediately subtrophoblastic position. These villous changes represent a form of functional maturation and are not an indication of ageing; the net result of these intermediate changes is to:

- increase the surface area of trophoblast in contact with the maternal blood in the intervillous space

roof of the amniotic sac and the trophoblast of the chorion. However, a connection between the two is maintained for a time by the persistence of a column of cells, the amniotic duct, which provides a pathway for the continuing migration

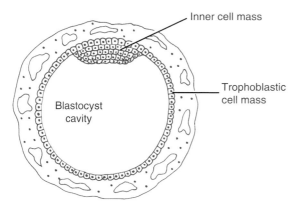

Fig. 3.22 Diagrammatic representation of the blastocyst and inner cell mass.

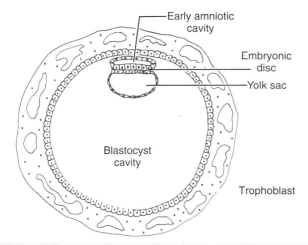

Fig. 3.23 Diagrammatic representation of early stage in the formation of the amniotic cavity and yolk sac.

of cells of trophoblastic origin into the amniotic epithelium. Mitotic activity at the margin of the embryonic ectodermal disc suggests that the ectoderm is also a continuing source of supply of amniotic epithelial cells.

The extraembryonic mesenchyme forms a loose reticulum in which small cystic spaces appear; these gradually enlarge and fuse to form the extraembryonic coelom, which splits the extraembryonic mesenchyme into two layers, one opposed to the trophoblast and also covering the amnion (the parietal extraembryonic mesenchyme) and the other covering the yolk sac (the visceral extraembryonic mesenchyme) (Fig. 3.25). The progressively enlarging extraembryonic coelom also separates the amnion away from the inner aspect of the chorion, except at the caudal end of the embryo, where an attachment of extraembryonic mesenchyme persists to form the body stalk from which the umbilical cord will eventually be derived (Fig. 3.26). Subsequently, the amniotic space enlarges at the expense of the extraembryonic coelom, and the developing embryo bulges into the expanding amniotic cavity.

Meanwhile, the yolk sac becomes partially incorporated into the embryo, where it gives rise to the gut; that part of the yolk sac remaining outside the embryo communicates with the primitive gut. However, this communicating channel gradually becomes elongated and attenuated to form the vitelline duct; the extraembryonic yolk sac becomes progressively removed further away from the embryo, to be eventually incorporated into the lower end of the body stalk.

Further expansion of the amniotic sac leads to more or less complete obliteration of the extraembryonic coelom, with eventual fusion of the extraembryonic mesenchyme covering the amnion with that lining the chorion. At the same time, the extraplacental chorion (the chorion laeve) ceases to produce ST, and the CT component undergoes a partial regression. Hence the single fused amniochorionic membrane is now fully formed and will consist of, from fetal to maternal side, amniotic epithelium, condensed extraembryonic mesenchyme, a loose reticular layer (which possibly represents the vestige of the extraembryonic coelom), extraembryonic mesenchyme and trophoblast.

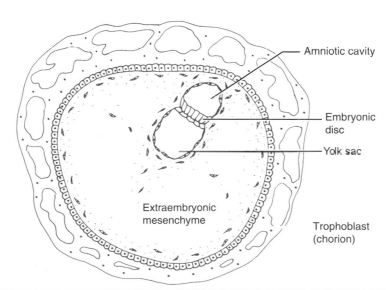

Fig. 3.24 Diagrammatic representation of relationship between developing amniotic cavity and extraembryonic mesenchyme.

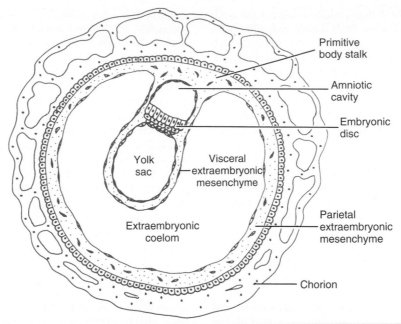

Fig. 3.25 Diagrammatic representation of relationship between developing amniotic cavity, extraembryonic mesenchyme, extraembryonic coelom and primitive body stalk.

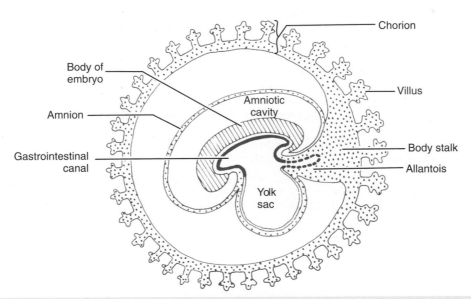

Fig. 3.26 Diagrammatic representation of the relationship between the expanding amniotic cavity and the developing embryo.

AMNIOTIC FLUID

Amniotic fluid is found in the amniotic cavity and, after the fourth week of pregnancy, completely surrounds the embryo. Amniotic fluid volume can be measured by ultrasound; at 12 weeks, it is approximately 50 mL and at 16 weeks, when amniocentesis is often carried out, it is approximately 150 mL. The volume increases to 900 or 1000 mL in late pregnancy, falling again just before term to 800 to 900 mL.

Initially the fluid is formed from the primitive cells around the amniotic vesicle. Later there is a transudate of fetal extracellular fluid, which is passed through the fetal skin and umbilical cord. There is also some diffusion of fluid across that part of the amniotic membrane which covers the placenta. In the second trimester, as the skin becomes keratinised and waterproof, there is an increasing contribution from fetal urine and fetal lung secretions. As the fetus develops an ability to swallow, a circulation of fluid occurs whereby urine excreted from the kidneys is passed through the bladder into the amniotic pool. This fluid is then swallowed, digested and reexcreted. Additional contributions to the amniotic pool continue to come from amniotic membrane secretions. At term there is an exchange of 500 mL/24 h, most of which is swallowed and reexcreted by the fetus, and up to 250 mL is transferred to the mother through the membranes.

A reduced liquor volume is found in conjunction with fetal renal agenesis and also with lower urinary tract obstruction. It also occurs to a lesser extent with growth restriction associated with insufficient placental function. Excessive liquor volumes are found where there is any dysfunction of fetal swallowing and also in cases of open spina bifida lesions, where the spinal fluid may leak out. Polyhydramnios is also found in some cases of twinning, in some diabetic pregnancies and in the rare presence of a haemangioma of the placenta.

Composition of Amniotic Fluid

As a result of its mixed origins, amniotic fluid is heterogeneous in composition. The cells found in amniotic fluid at term are of three main types: fetal epithelial cells, amniotic cells and dermal fibroblasts. The epithelial cells and amniotic cells grow poorly in culture, but the fibroblasts grow well and are used for karyotyping and other analyses. In the presence of renal tube defects, glial cells are also found.

Nitrogenous waste, in the form of urea, creatinine and uric acid, increases in concentration from the end of the first trimester until term and reflects the increasing function of the fetal kidneys. Amino acids are found in approximately the same concentration as in maternal plasma.

Proteins increase in concentration as pregnancy progresses, but the concentrations level off after 30 weeks of gestation. They are mainly albumin and globulins in a ratio of 6:4. There is virtually no fibrinogen or protein-bound lipids. α-Fetoprotein is found in early pregnancy but in a concentration 10 times lower than in fetal blood. Higher levels of α-fetoprotein may indicate an open neural tube defect, whereas abnormally low levels may be associated with Down syndrome.

Lipids in the amniotic fluid increase to a concentration of approximately 400 mg/L at term, half of which is in the form of free fatty acids. There are small amounts of phospholipids, cholesterol and lecithin; the lecithin, which is secreted from the lungs, is used as an indicator of surfactant maturation.

Carbohydrates are present in amniotic fluid in concentrations approximately half those found in maternal serum. Glucose predominates, with only smaller quantities of fructose and sucrose. Concentrations of lactate, citrate, pyruvate and α-ketoglutarate are similar to those in maternal blood.

Various enzymes and hormone assays have been recorded, although in some cases considerable variations have been noted. Oestrogens, mainly oestradiol, are found in their conjugated forms. Progesterone and its metabolite pregnanediol are also present. Cortisone and 17-hydroxycortisone are found in trace amounts only. Insulin levels rise towards term and are much higher in diabetic pregnancies.

Pigment from bilirubin and meconium may stain the amniotic fluid. Bilirubin normally decreases towards term, except in cases of fetal haemolysis. Meconium may be present in late pregnancy, and in labour it is often taken to be an indication of fetal distress, but its presence correlates only with biochemical evidence of fetal hypoxia in approximately 20% of cases.

The partial pressure of oxygen (PO_2) at 2 to 15 mm Hg is lower than that of the maternal arterial blood, whereas the partial pressure of carbon dioxide (PCO_2) at 55 to 60 mm Hg is higher. Compared with blood, the amniotic fluid pH is slightly acidic at 7.0. This fact may be used as a diagnostic test on vaginal fluid when there is doubt about rupture of the membranes and amniotic fluid leakage. The amniotic fluid is thought to have some antibacterial activity, possibly generated by the pH, and also by the presence of lysozyme, peroxidase and α-interferon.

4 Fetal and Placental Physiology

CAROLINE J. SHAW

Introduction

The subject of fetal and placental physiology encompasses a large and complex branch of the reproductive sciences, and any one of the subsections below could form the subject of an entire textbook. The concepts described here should aid the understanding of how fetal and placental physiology influence clinical assessment of fetal wellbeing, as well as diseases of prematurity and the unwell term neonate.

Understanding of the physiology of the fetus and placenta is inextricably linked to the developmental stage of the pregnancy. Unlike the chapters on maternal physiology, where in the absence of maternal disease, complete structural (anatomical) and functional maturation can be assumed, both must be considered in relation to gestational age (GA) of the fetus at birth. Throughout their development, fetal organ systems continue to modify their function to meet the demands of in utero, compared to postnatal life, while also maturing the fetal body for the transition into neonatal life.

Fetal Development and Preparation for Birth

CARDIOVASCULAR

The primitive heart tube is formed during the third week of pregnancy, with a heartbeat detectable from around the third to fourth week. A complex pattern of folding, rotation and remodelling results in the four-chamber heart with multiple arterial and venous connections and which anatomically resembles the adult heart, but contains additional fetal vascular shunts to support the unique requirements of the fetus (Fig. 4.1).

In utero, the source of oxygenated blood is the placenta not the lungs, so oxygen-rich blood is delivered by umbilical vein (UV) to the inferior vena cava (IVC) and right atrium through the first of the fetal shunts, the ductus venosus (DV), instead of the left atrium via the pulmonary vein. The DV allows newly oxygenated blood to bypass the portal sinus supplying the liver significant depletion of its oxygen content, before passing through the second of the fetal shunts, the foramen ovale into the left atrium, then ventricle. Deoxygenated blood from the fetal brain also enters the right atrium via the superior vena cava (SVC) with a downward flow pattern. This angle of entry is different to that of the blood from the IVC, which stays medial and is directed towards the medially placed foramen ovale. This ensures that there is minimal mixing of partially deoxygenated blood from the SVC, which enters the right ventricle, and well-oxygenated blood.

The oxygen-rich blood is pumped by the left ventricle into the ascending aorta and the aortic arch, where it supplies the first four branches of the aorta: the coronary arteries, the brachiocephalic trunk, the left common carotid artery and the left subclavian artery. Partially deoxygenated blood is pumped from the right ventricle through the third of the fetal shunts, the ductus arteriosus (DA), which links the pulmonary artery to the descending aorta: this allows blood to bypass the non-gas-exchanging fetal lungs and high-pressure pulmonary arteries. The DA inserts at the aortic isthmus, just distal to the origin of the subclavian artery, allowing mixing of richly oxygenated blood coming from the aortic arch with partially deoxygenated blood to deliver oxygen to the remainder of the fetal organs via arterial branches of the descending aorta before returning to the placenta via the umbilical arteries, which arise from the internal iliac arteries.

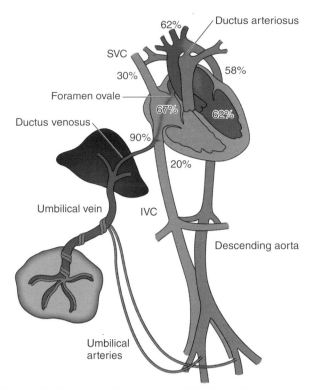

Fig. 4.1 The diagram shows the organisation of the fetal circulation to include the placenta as the source of oxygenation, with the three fetal shunts, the ductus venosus, foramen ovale and ductus arteriosus allowing oxygenated blood to bypass the fetal liver and lungs. Percentage figures relate to the oxygen saturation at that point in the circulation. *IVC*, Inferior vena cava; *SVC*, superior vena cava.

It is important to recognise that the fetal ventricles beat in parallel, with no temporal offset in closure of pulmonary and aortic valve. Additionally, both sides of the heart supply the systemic circulation, unlike in postnatal life. Therefore the convention is to refer to combined cardiac output (CCO) during fetal life rather than to consider left ventricular output equal to cardiac output as in the adult. Fetal ventricular output is unequal, with around 55% of cardiac output coming from the right ventricle and 45% coming from the left in normal conditions, although the balance becomes inverted during fetal compromise. This organisation of the fetal cardiovascular system lends a degree of plasticity to the fetal circulation, allowing it to respond to in utero acute and chronic hypoxic or hypotensive challenges in a different way to postnatal life, when ventilatory responses can also be made, referred to as cardiovascular defence mechanisms or fetal brain sparing.

Cardiovascular Defence Mechanisms

The fetus has several mechanisms to protect itself against acute hypoxia. Firstly, fetal heart rate (FHR) decreases due to parasympathetic nervous system (PNS) activation (causing a deceleration or bradycardia), so reducing myocardial oxygen consumption. CCO is maintained as the longer diastolic filling time increases the stroke volume (SV) and myocardial contractility (Starling's law), which offsets the effect of reduced heart rate (CCO = SV × FHR). Secondly, blood flow is redistributed away from the peripheries to the

central circulation, ensuring adequate oxygenation to brain and heart, known as 'fetal brain sparing'. Hypoxia and the resultant hypercapnia, sensed by peripheral chemoreceptors, trigger peripheral vasoconstriction due to sympathetic nervous system (SNS) activity. Cerebral vasodilation also occurs under paracrine control, and the combination of high peripheral pressure and low central pressure directs blood preferentially into the central circulation. Finally, oxygen consumption is downregulated: fetal movements and breathing movements cease. These mechanisms mature from the second trimester onwards in line with the maturation of the PNS and SNS; immaturity or failure of these processes is associated with adverse pregnancy outcomes.

However, when exposed to chronic hypoxia, as in fetal growth restriction (FGR), only the fetal brain sparing response persists. The FHR returns to normal, even without recovery of normal oxygenation as PNS activity attenuates, and SNS activity converts to an perpetuated endocrine response. Fetal movements and breathing movements recommence and may be perceived as normal. Ongoing reduction in supply of oxygen and nutrients to the peripheral circulation has adverse effects on the development of organs, notably the kidneys, pancreas and intestines, which mature slower than anticipated, and leads to asymmetric growth restriction. Persistent high peripheral resistance causes remodelling of the cardiomyocytes and resetting of arterial baroreflex functions. Prolonged SNS activation causes dysregulation of the fetal autonomic system, with reduction in FHR variability and blunting of bradycardic responses to further episodes of superadded acute hypoxia. Unsurprisingly, such a wide-ranging series of compromises to maintain central oxygenation, while beneficial in utero, persist postnatally, when they present a risk of adult disease (see later).

Heart Rate Variability

The fetal heart shows beat-to-beat differences in rate, which results in variability in the baseline FHR, excluding periods of acceleration and deceleration. This variability can be assessed using cardiotocography (CTG), can be quantified using computerised CTG as short- or long-term variation (STV, LTV), and is understood to be a powerful predictor of fetal wellbeing. FHR fluctuates under the influence of basal sympathetic and parasympathetic tone, different fetal sleep states, and has some intrinsic diurnal variability. The sympathetic tone predominates for much of the third trimester, with parasympathetic tone only increasing near term. FHR variability increases with advancing gestation and is higher in active sleep states (associated with fetal body and eye movements) and lower in quiet sleep states (Fetal rest). FGR has been suggested to impair the expected increases in FHR variability with GA. Chronic reduction in STV particularly has been associated with adverse pregnancy outcomes, although the mechanisms underlying this remains to be understood. Animal models suggest that autonomic system dysregulation, potentially through an action on the fetal brain stem or desensitisation to catecholamines, plays a key role.

Postnatal Cardiovascular Changes

Following delivery, the source of oxygenated blood shifts from the placenta to the lungs, and the circulation needs to divide into systemic (left-sided) and pulmonary (right-sided) aspects. This change relies on closure of the fetal shunts and removal of the umbilical arteries and veins from the circulation. While the umbilical cord is often clamped and cut to achieve this, this is not the evolutionary solution, and anatomical remodelling of the cord remnant is also required regardless. The Wharton's jelly which surrounds the vessels in the umbilical cord vessels swells in response to lower temperatures, promoting vascular closure. The umbilical arteries constrict due to serotonin and thromboxane A_2 release within minutes of delivery, achieving functional closure, before degenerating into the median umbilical ligaments over months. The UV remains open after birth, allowing passive flow of blood from the placenta to the neonate, before it degenerates over days into the ligamentum teres hepatis. Finally, the umbilical cord remanent detaches spontaneously leaving the umbilicus.

The DA closes within hours of birth: its smooth muscle is sensitive to the bradykinins, endothelin, and acetylcholine released as a result of respiration and rising oxygen content in the fetal lungs and blood; the effect can be reversed using a prostaglandin-E infusion if patency of the DA is required in the neonate for clinical reasons (usually in the context of congenital heart disease). Until functional closure is achieved, peripheral saturations in the neonate are interpreted as pre-ductal (higher) or post-ductal (lower), and oxygen saturation in the right hand may be compared to the feet to illustrate this difference. Functional closure is followed by anatomical closure: the DA becomes the ligamentum arteriosum over months. Patent DA causes left-to-right shunting (differences in systolic pressure cause reversal of flow) and may result in pulmonary hypertension and right heart failure if untreated.

Breathing changes the relative pressures of the left and right atria, pushing the atrial septum primum against the septum secundum, functionally closing the foramen ovale. The two septa fuse over weeks (anatomical closure): the resulting tissue becomes the fossa ovalis. Patent foramen ovale (PFO) is common, usually of little clinical significance as left atrial pressures typically remain higher than right atrial pressures, preventing shunting, although PFO may allow paradoxical embolus to occur.

The DV shrinks progressively during fetal life, as hepatic blood supply increases with gestation, and collapses at birth once the UV is obliterated. Over months, it becomes the ligamentum venosum, and prolonged patency leads to a portocaval shunt and liver failure, although this remains rare.

RESPIRATORY

The development of the lung in utero is divided into four stages defined by GA: pseudoglandular, canalicular, terminal sac and alveolar.

In the pseudoglandular stage (5 to 16 weeks GA), the embryonic fetal lung develops into five bronchopulmonary segments with branched airways, lined by respiratory epithelium. The pulmonary vasculature, cartilage, smooth muscle and connective tissue also form by 16 weeks. Progressive branching of the airways is directly proportional to the exposure of the endodermal lung buds to surrounding mesenchymal tissue, but also requires the presence of amniotic fluid to expand the lungs. Hence, processes leading to oligo- or anhydramnios during this period of development represent the most significant risk of pulmonary hypoplasia. The mesenchyme is also required to allow the first differentiation of lung epithelium into cilia in proximal airways and alveolar type II pneumocytes in the bronchi.

In the canalicular stage (16 to 25 weeks GA), the gas-exchanging function of the lung develops. Around 20 weeks GA the respiratory epithelium differentiates into type I pneumocytes and inclusion bodies storing surfactant are found in type II pneumocytes. There is a decrease in interstitial tissue thickness, growth of the capillary network of the lungs, as well as elongation and widening of existing airways. Pulmonary blood vessels are formed from mesenchyme, which are thick walled with high vasomotor tone. This stage of development corresponds to the potential for gaseous transfer, and so ex-utero survival to occur, although the respiratory function of the lungs remains underdeveloped. While amniotic fluid remains important in distending fetal lungs during this period and stimulating normal growth, oligohydramnios from this stage onwards produced less profound pulmonary hypoplasia than when it occurs during the pseudoglandular stage.

From 26 weeks until birth, the lungs enter the terminal sac stage, during which the surface area for gaseous exchange increases and interstitial tissue continues to thin. During this phase of development, sporadic breathing (diaphragmatic) movements begin to occur; the resultant stimulation of mechanoreceptors allows the lungs to continue to grow in physical size, and without these breathing movements, pulmonary hypoplasia can still occur.

Surfactant Production

The terminal branches of the primitive airways do not yet resemble adult alveoli, and remain as primitive saccules. Numbers of type I and II pneumocytes increase, as do numbers of inclusion bodies containing pulmonary surfactant. Surfactant is a monomolecular phospholipid layer which coats the bronchioles and small airways of the lung to reduce the work of breathing by preventing the collapse of alveoli and air spaces. The stability of the lung at birth depends on the number of inclusion bodies present in type II pneumocytes and their activity in producing surfactant; without adequate surfactant respiratory distress syndrome (RDS) results. Surfactant production is developmentally regulated, controlled by several hormones, the best known of which are thyroid hormones and cortisol. As such, exogenous glucocorticoids are used antenatally to stimulate surfactant production when early preterm delivery is anticipated. Surfactant can also be deactivated in the term infant by the presence of meconium in the airways, pulmonary haemorrhage, Fetal hyperinsulinemia, and pulmonary or alveolar oedema. RDS secondary to deficiency can be corrected with the use exogenous surfactant more reliably than RDS secondary to deactivation.

Postnatal Respiratory Function

The alveolar stage of lung development typically occurs postnatally but can occur near term. It is marked by the development of primitive saccules into functioning alveoli, usually completed by 5 weeks after birth, although the number of alveoli present continue to increase into childhood.

The alveolar stage overlaps with the changes that are required in the fetal lung at birth to support ex utero life. Until birth, the fetal lungs are hyperextended with fluid, which is produced within the fetal lungs and removed via the trachea. This maintains high extraluminal pressures and keep pulmonary blood flow low. The pulmonary vasculature has a high resistance and a low blood flow, receiving only around 13% of the CCO at 20 weeks gestation. In preparation for delivery, pulmonary fluid drains from lungs into pulmonary vasculature or lymphatics, under the influence of rising endogenous adrenaline, vasopressin and cortisol, or is mechanically displaced by uterine contractions even preceding vaginal delivery. However, this reduction in extraluminal pressure only increases pulmonary blood flow to around 25% of CCO. Historically, both cord occlusion and removal of facial immersion were thought to be involved in increasing pulmonary blood flow, but neither have been shown in translational models to have an effect.

Pulmonary vascular resistance falls due to activation of pulmonary mechanoreceptors in response to insufflation of the lungs with air, mediated by endothelially derived nitric oxide. The resultant 35% fall in pulmonary vascular resistance with the first breaths causes up to a 400% increase in pulmonary blood flow but does not change pulmonary arterial pressure. Dysfunction of this nitric oxide release from the pulmonary vascular bed leads to persistent pulmonary hypertension of the newborn. Pulmonary arterial pressure is partially reduced by exposure to oxygen, and the vasculature becomes more reactive to hyperoxygenation as gestation increases. Ventilation with an increased inspired fraction of oxygen can result in up to a further 10% fall in pulmonary vascular resistance. At the same time, there is a rapid reorganisation of pulmonary vessel walls after birth, with a reduction in wall thickness, and ongoing vascular remodelling mediated by vasoactive nitric oxide, prostaglandin I_2 and enodothelin-1, leading to a permanent reduction in pulmonary arterial pressure.

RENAL AND AMNIOTIC FLUID

The fetal kidney is functional by around the 12 weeks gestation, although nephrons continue developing until around 36 weeks. Before birth the fetal kidney produces urine but has minimal filtration capacity, relying on the materno-placental interface for removal of waste usually renally excreted. The renal blood flow is around 5% of the CCO of the fetus and the glomerular filtration rate (GFR) at term is around 30% of the adult. The urine produced is isotonic, as is the amniotic fluid in which the fetus is bathed. In animal models, increases in maternal urea, creatinine and haematocrit have been shown to increase the osmolality of amniotic fluid and fetal urine due to increased fetal production of arginine vasopressin, while maintaining a stable amniotic fluid volume.

After birth, the kidney needs to be able to concentrate urine to a greater degree and excrete nitrogenous waste products. Much of the expected 5% to 10% loss in birth weight over the first week of life is due to diuresis from the immature kidney, also resulting in increased sodium excretion. Renal blood flow increases to around 25% of the neonatal cardiac output, which, coupled with increases in surface area and permeability of the glomerular basement membrane, leads to increased blood flow in the kidneys and transfer of plasma into the nephrons. The GFR increases threefold in the first weeks of life, before reaching adult levels around 2 years of age.

Amniotic Fluid Regulation

While the fetal kidney is functional from early second trimester, amniotic fluid volume is not solely dependent on fetal urination and swallowing (Fig. 4.2). During embryogenesis, amniotic fluid generation far exceeds what would be expected related to embryonic size and comes from passage of maternal plasma through the fetal membranes, before becoming proportionate to fetal size in the second trimester. During this phase of development, the amnion, placenta and umbilical cord remain permeable to water and solutes, as does the fetus until keratinisation of the skin at around 20 weeks, allowing diffusion to occur based on hydrostatic and osmotic pressures. After keratinisation of the fetal skin, amniotic fluid is generated by fetal urine (around 300 mL/kg fetal weight/day) and secretion of fluids from the airway due to fetal breathing (around 75 mL/kg fetal weight/day) but removed by fetal swallowing (200 to 250 mL/kg fetal weight/day). While intra-membranous (direct absorption into cord and placenta) and transmembranous transfer of maternal plasma to amniotic fluid still occurs, this accounts for a much smaller proportion of change in amniotic fluid volume than earlier in pregnancy. Amniotic fluid reaches its maximum volume in early third trimester, before declining naturally as the fetus approaches term, despite increasing fetal size. It appears likely that a control mechanism for amniotic fluid volume exists, although this has not been fully elucidated; intra-membranous absorption of amniotic fluid is increased in animal models with oesophageal

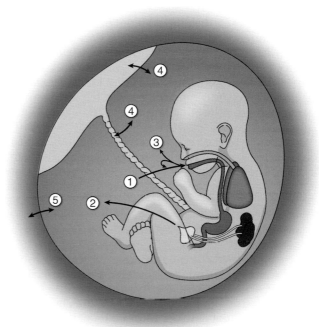

Fig. 4.2 Amniotic fluid is depleted and returned to the fetal circulation by swallowing and absorption from the gut (1), and to a lesser extent by intermembranous absorption into the placenta and umbilical cord (4). The amniotic fluid is replenished by fetal urination (2) and expiration of secretions from the respiratory tract (3), a proportion of which is swallowed from the oropharynx before reaching the amniotic fluid. Amniotic fluid can also be replenished by intermembranous secretion (4) and transmembranous transfer (5) which facilitates transfer between maternal plasma and amniotic fluid, so can also deplete amniotic fluid.

atresia, and only two thirds of fetuses with oesophageal or intestinal atresia show increased amniotic fluid volume.

LIVER

The fetal liver develops from the foregut region of the endoderm, initially as a hepatic diverticulum around the third gestational week, growing rapidly until around 10 weeks of gestation. During fetal life, the liver has two key functions: haematopoiesis and cardiovascular communication.

Haematopoiesis – or the production of blood cells and plasma – occurs in the embryonic period in the yolk sac. At 10 weeks of gestation, haematopoietic progenitor cells migrate to the newly formed fetal liver, thymus and spleen. Erythroid precursors, along with other erythroid cell lines, are predominantly found in the liver compared with the thymus or spleen. At this stage of development, the liver is an environment in which stem cells can proliferate and give rise to mature blood cells, notably erythrocytes (containing haemoglobin F, HbF), macrophages and fibroblasts. The fetal liver remains the main site of erythrocyte production until the third trimester when erythropoiesis shifts to the fetal bone marrow. The transcriptional switch in erythroid precursor cells from forming HbF (2 α-globulin and 2 γ-globulin chains) to haemoglobin A (HbA, 2 α-globulin and 2 β-globulin chains) occurs progressively during the neonatal period, until virtually all HbF is replaced by around 6 to 12 months of age. In the absence of underlying haemoglobinopathy, HbF is expected to form less than 1% of adult haemoglobin.

The fetal liver also contains an important connection between the placental and fetal circulations. Blood flow from the UV enters the fetal abdomen at the umbilicus and travels along the free margin of the falciform ligament of the fetal liver to the inferior surface of the liver, enabling shunting of a varying proportion of this highly oxygenated blood through the DV into the IVC, as described above.

Before birth, hepatic digestive and detoxification functions are heavily replicated by the placenta, while synthetic function is partially preserved. The fetal liver stores amino acids in a similar way to postnatal life and plasma protein synthetic pathways are active, resulting in an albumin level equal to adult normal values at term. Coagulation proteins levels vary: vitamin K-dependent clotting factors (FII, FVII, FIX, FX), contact factors (FXI, FXII), and protein C, S, antithrombin and plasminogen are around 50% of adult levels at birth and reach 100% by 6 months of age. Factor V, VIII, and XIII are normal at birth; despite this apparent functional immaturity of coagulation, clinically significant bleeding events in the term neonate in the absence of co-existing pathology remains rare.

Once the placental supply of glucose is removed, neonatal blood glucose will fall rapidly after birth, but typically stabilises within around 3 hours without enteral intake. This is due to a reduction in neonatal insulin levels and an increase in glucagon levels, which releases glucose from the hepatic glycogen stores lain down in utero; these stores are usually depleted within around 12 hours of life and thereafter enteral intake of glucose or gluconeogenesis is required to maintain blood glucose levels. At birth, the gluconeogenesis capacity is around 10% of adult levels, but the activity of glucose-6-phosphatase, phosphoenolpyruvate carboxykinase and lipolysis (which allows ketogenesis) all increase rapidly over the first 2 to 3 days of life, when the approach near adult levels of activity.

The biotransformative capacity of the liver is the slowest to mature. Phase I reactions (those involving cytochrome P450 enzymes, essential for the metabolism of many medications) are at around 30% of adult activity at birth and take up to a full year to mature. Phase II reactions (conjugation reactions which allow renal excretion of waste products) are more variable: the process of converting ammonia to urea is mature at birth; but conjugation of bilirubin is around 1% of adult activity and takes 1 to 2 weeks to mature to adult levels, underlying the neonatal vulnerability to jaundice.

GUT AND METABOLISM

The fetal gut arises from the endoderm as a flat, pseudostratified intestinal tube present by around the fifth week of gestation. From the eighth week a rapid expansion in the surface area begins due to villi formation, which progresses in a proximal to distal wave, ending in the large bowel. The gut also begins to lengthen from the eighth week by intervillous epithelial proliferation. This rapid expansion leads to physiological herniation of the bowel into the umbilicus, until the abdomen enlarges sufficiently by 12 weeks to allow all the gut return intra-abdominal; failure of this herniation to resolve is termed 'exomphalos'.

While there is no in utero requirement for nutrient absorption, differentiation of stem cells in the intestinal crypts into different epithelial cell types and expression of specialised enzymes for terminal digestion of nutrients and related transporters are completed by around 20 weeks GA. By this time, the gut is also vascularised. The activity of these enzymes and transporters increase with gestation and animal models have linked lower levels of activity with increased risk of necrotising enterocolitis (NEC), a significant complication of prematurity.

Hence, while the structure and cellular differentiation of the gut are in place at birth (even if preterm), adaption to the ex utero environment requires colonisation by commensal microorganisms, which occurs during birth, breast feeding and neonatal oral to skin contact. Disruption in gut bacterial colonisation has been linked to autoimmune and inflammatory diseases and infection risk; however, these commensal bacteria must also be contained. To do so, the gut has mechanical (tight junctions, mucous) and chemical (secreted antimicrobial peptides) host defences. If these are immature, this leads to an increased risk of microbiological invasion, an additional cause of NEC.

The neonatal gut has evolved to accept mammary milk, which contains proteins, lipids, carbohydrates and immunoglobulins (IgA, which provides passive immunity against enteric pathogens), and inflammatory mediators (attenuation of immune response, antigenic tolerance). Enhanced maturation and function of the neonatal gut have been observed in breastfed compared with formula-fed infants.

Meconium Passage

The formation and innervation of smooth muscle layers, which provide structure to the gut and aid in peristalsis, are completed by 26 weeks GA, from when peristalsis can be observed. During this development, the fetus continues to swallow, as discussed earlier: the fluid, electrolytes and cellular debris contained within the amniotic fluid are almost completely reabsorbed, and the residue leads to formation of meconium in distal fetal colon.

Passage of meconium is a developmentally programmed event and typically occurs postnatally. While delay in passing meconium is associated with defects in colonic innervation (e.g. Hirschsprung disease), little is known about the regulation of meconium passage in utero; gut peristalsis alone is not sufficient. Meconium-stained liquor is more common with advancing gestation and uncommon in preterm deliveries, suggested by some to be a sign of post maturity not pathology. Observationally, the coexistence of in utero hypoxia or infection has been noted to increase the passage of meconium, independent of GA. Animal models support that activation of the fetal SNS (i.e. a fetal stress response, not exogenous glucocorticoids alone) can cause meconium passage at term, but has lesser stimulatory effect on the colon in preterm situations.

CENTRAL NERVOUS SYSTEM

The development of the fetal central nervous system (CNS) is an extremely complex process controlled by numerous genetic and environmental factors, with many processes yet to be understood.

Brain development starts around 3 weeks of GA, with neural progenitor cells differentiating into neurons and glia soon after, although development will continue into early adulthood. During pregnancy the brain continues to grow and change in structure; at each stage anatomical appearances are used as a marker to reflect the changes occurring at a cellular level as neurons form chemical and axonal signalling pathways that allow communication between themselves, and glia differentiate into their subspecialised cell types. By term, the brain is formed but needs sensory input to further develop and increase the number of neural connections present in the brain. In utero, direct sensory input is limited and consists largely of materno-fetal biochemical signals, including prenatal maternal stress exposure, although it remains difficult to disentangle the relative effects of pre- and postnatal environmental exposure to stressors, which typically overlap.

One such signal which is prenatal, and increasingly debated, is the effect of exogenous glucocorticoids (as used for fetal lung maturation) on fetal brain development. Glucocorticoids can pass the blood-brain barrier and target receptors throughout the CNS. Animal models suggest that exposure to exogenous glucocorticoids can reduce brain weight, decrease cell proliferation, alter neuron activity and disrupt myelination, predominantly affecting limbic and prefrontal regions. These studies commonly use doses and durations of exposure which are not adjusted for shorter gestational length or smaller fetal weight of animals, so are not equivalent to human fetal exposure. However, while there is limited evidence to support cognitive impairment in fetuses treated with preterm glucocorticoids but born at term, there is some suggestion of neurobehavioural alterations predisposing to mental health conditions.

Perinatal Brain Injury

The most common forms of perinatal brain injury are hypoxic-ischaemic encephalopathy (HIE), intraventricular haemorrhage (IVH) and periventricular leukomalacia (PVL), any of which may result in long-term disability, including cerebral palsy, and neurodevelopmental delay. While their causes are multifactorial, of which the quality of perinatal care is undoubtedly one, the discussion here will focus on underlying physiological mechanisms.

Perinatal brain injury can affect fetuses born at any gestation but is more common in preterm infants, as their cerebral autoregulation pathways and cardiovascular defence mechanisms to hypoxia (see earlier) are less well developed. Cerebral autoregulation describes the ability of the cerebral vasculature to maintain a stable blood flow despite changes in systemic blood pressure and corresponding cerebral perfusion pressure. In brief, a combination of endothelial, metabolic, neurogenic and myogenic responses to changes in cerebral perfusion pressure controls cerebral arterial diameter and vascular resistance. As vessels dilate, so the resistance decreases, and cerebral perfusion increases. Autoregulation is therefore a response to perfusion changes, protecting the brain from under- or over-perfusion, not due to direct sensing of hypoxaemia or hypercapnia. Together, cerebral autoregulation and cardiovascular defence mechanisms allow the fetus to prioritise oxygen supply to the brain during hypoxic insults, meaning that not all such events result in neurological damage.

It is important to understand that the majority of hypoxic insults to the fetal brain are not the result of oxygen unavailability (while it may be reduced, it is rarely absent in the blood while the mother has adequate cardio-respiratory function), but rather a secondary failure of oxygen delivery when cardiovascular defence mechanisms and autoregulation are immature or fail, causing an initial hypoxic insult. During this time, neurons have insufficient oxygen to meet their metabolic demands, leading to death by necrosis or apoptosis. If oxygen supply is restored, a secondary injury occurs with reperfusion. Excitatory amino acids and reactive oxygen species are released and have a toxic effect on the developing brain, causing further cell death and inflammation, leading to a larger degree of cerebral injury than the initial hypoxic insult alone. Fetal infection is also known to dysregulate the cerebral response to hypoxia, rendering the brain more susceptible to hypoxic insults when there is co-existing infection.

These principles can be applied to the understanding of observed forms of perinatal brain injury. The incidence of IVH and PVL has a strong inverse correlation to GA at delivery. IVH, or bleeding from thin-walled capillaries in the subependymal germinal matrix, which ruptures into lateral ventricles, can occur spontaneously, but it is linked to dysregulation of cerebral blood flow. As such, infection, hypoxia and hypotension have been implicated in promoting rupture. Administration of antenatal steroids where preterm delivery is anticipated below 34 weeks is shown to reduce rates, as is delayed cord clamping at birth. However, 'milking' of the umbilical cord, which causes rapid increases in venous return and so CCO and cerebral perfusion in the neonate, is linked with increased rates of IVH. PVL is characterised by white matter injury in characteristic patterns, correlating to the regions of brain tissue with high metabolic requirements for oxygen but at greatest risk of hypoperfusion when cerebral blood flow is reduced. Again, uncompensated changes in cerebral blood flow due to systemic infection, hypoxia and hypotension have been implicated in the pathogenesis of PVL.

HIE is the term for CNS dysfunction secondary to prolonged hypoxia occurring in late preterm or term fetus, either antenatally or intrapartum. Due to the protective mechanisms described previously, it does not occur after all events causing fetal hypoxia or hypotension but is potentiated by fetal infection. One study suggested it affects around 10% of fetuses with a single, prolonged period of hypoxia, and 2.5% of fetuses with non-reassuring CTG monitoring in labour (Martinez-Biarge et al., 2012). Postnatal outcomes are variable and related to severity and type of brain injury. The heterogeneity of effects in survivors emphasise the role of neonatal brain plasticity in recovery from such insults.

Administration of magnesium sulphate to mothers at risk of preterm delivery (32 weeks and below) in the 24 hours before birth has been shown in randomised controlled trials to reduce rates of cerebral palsy in neonates. While the mechanism of action is not fully understood, magnesium sulphate can reduce both reperfusion injury and cytokine medicated injury, and acts as a vasodilator, all of which could reduce the incidence of primary and secondary cerebral insults during episodes of hypoxia or hypotension. However, as hypoxia is estimated to result in only around 20% of cases of cerebral palsy, a different mechanism of mitigating neuronal injury may also be possible.

TEMPERATURE REGULATION

In utero, the fetal temperature is regulated by amniotic fluid. The developing fetus produces excess heat due to the degree of metabolic activity; however the large surface area to volume ratio promotes heat loss from the fetus to the amniotic fluid. The mother regulates the temperature of the amniotic fluid, although the temperature is 0.5 to 1.0°C higher than the maternal temperature. The amniotic fluid temperature is thought to show corresponding increases with maternal basal temperature during pregnancy.

After birth, the neonate is no longer protected from heat loss by the amniotic fluid and is vulnerable to hypothermia. While parental/caregiver behaviour is the primary way in which neonatal temperature is controlled, neonates also have stores of brown adipose tissue which allows non-shivering thermogenesis, under the control of the SNS. The skeletal muscle mass in the newborn is insufficient to maintain body temperature through shivering, so brown adipose is laid down from around 35 weeks to perform this protective function.

Placental Growth and Development

In humans, placentation is invasive, meaning during implantation fetal trophoblast cells invade into the inner third of maternal uterine decidua. The trophoblast divides into three parts: the cytotrophoblast (proliferation), syncytiotrophoblast (exchange and biosynthesis) and extravillous trophoblast (EVT). During the embryonic period, while the placenta is formed, the embryo relies on histotrophic nutrition, protecting the fetus from damage by reactive oxygen species during organogenesis. From the 10th week of gestation, the haemochorial function of the placenta replaces this, in which maternal blood is in direct contact with the chorion and the placenta acts as the interface between the maternal and fetal circulations, meeting the increasing needs of the developing fetus for oxygen and nutrients and waste product elimination. As the placenta increases in size, so the surface area available for exchange increases.

NUTRIENT TRANSFER

The syncytiotrophoblast has both maternal-facing microvillous membrane (MVM) and fetalfacing basal membrane (BM); nutrients must cross both to be supplied to the fetus. This can occur by passive, active or vesicular transport.

Passive transport includes simple diffusion, by which non-polar and fat-soluble molecules move across the placenta following the concentration gradient. This process accounts for the transfer of oxygen (although maximised by the double Bohr effect (see below)), carbon dioxide (Haldane effect), fats and alcohols. Water, a polar molecule, enters the placenta by osmosis using specialised pores known as aquaporins along a concentration gradient, as does glucose, which crosses the placenta by a process of facilitated diffusion reliant on glucose transporter proteins (GLUTs). None of these processes consume energy but are reliant on preserved surface area for exchange and blood flow to continue.

Active transport is required for larger molecules, or where transfer against a concentration gradient is required (sodium, potassium, calcium ions), and requires energy. Where needed, it allows fetal concentrations to exceed maternal for these substrates and ions. Amnio acids are transported across the placenta by a combination of accumulative, facilitated and exchanger transporters expressed by the syncytiotrophoblast; more than 20 different types have been described. The MVM expresses several lipases, which hydrolyse triglycerides in the maternal circulation into fatty acids, which are taken up by the placenta using fatty acid transport proteins, and bound to fatty acid binding proteins, before being delivered to the fetal circulation.

Vesicular transport describes a process whereby the macro-molecules, typically immunoglobulin G (IgG), enter the MVM by endocytosis and leave the BM by exocytosis. This process, which also consumes energy, again allows fetal concentrations of IgG to exceed maternal concentrations. Placental transfer of immunoglobulins is increased greatly in the third trimester, allowing the fetus to acquire passive immunity relative to the pathogens in the maternal environment prior to birth. This is the basis on which maternal vaccination to support neonatal immunity may be offered.

OXYGEN TRANSFER

Well-oxygenated maternal blood from the uterine arteries reaches the maternal side of the chorionic plate; by contrast, deoxygenated fetal blood from the umbilical artery has a much lower partial pressure of oxygen and higher partial pressure of carbon dioxide. Hence, while there is already a concentration gradient which will allow maternal to fetal transfer of oxygen, this is maximised by the double Bohr effect.

Binding to, or release of, oxygen from haemoglobin is controlled by the Bohr effect, whereby an increase in hydrogen ions (i.e. an increase in the partial pressure of carbon dioxide resulting in a decrease in pH of the blood) results in disassociation of oxygen from haemoglobin, and an decrease in hydrogen ions results in uptake of oxygen. Therefore, as fetal carbon dioxide diffuses from the fetal to maternal circulation, it results in an increase in hydrogen ions on the maternal side and decrease on the fetal side. This drives disassociation of oxygen on the maternal side and greater uptake on the fetal side, further widening the concentration gradient increasing the rate of diffusion.

Despite this, the placenta remains an estimated five times less efficient than the lungs at oxygenating blood, and partial pressures of oxygen remain lower in the fetal compared with maternal circulations at all times. Famously, Barcroft coined the phrase 'Mt. Everest in utero' in 1935 to describe the unavailability of oxygen to the fetus. This effect is offset by the greater affinity of fetal HbF for oxygen compared with adult HbA, and the higher fetal haematocrit compared with adult life. As a result, HbF is able to maintain a higher saturation of oxygen at a lower partial pressure than HbA, and in combination with a higher oxygen carrying capacity in the blood, the fetal oxygen content of the blood remains adequate to meet its needs in normal circumstances, despite saturations which would be inadequate in adult life.

ENDOCRINE

Before implantation, maternal hormonal production is reliant on the hypothalamic-pituitary-adrenal (HPA) axis and ovarian function; however, by the end of the first trimester the syncytiotrophoblast is functioning as an endocrine gland. Thereafter, hormonal concentrations are regulated by the HPA axis, placental and fetal adrenal glands. The placental produces an array of steroid, polypeptide, metalloproteinases, dimeric glycoproteins and adipokine hormones that are beyond the scope of this text, so a brief mention of key hormones will be made here.

Steroid biosynthesis is shared between the placenta and fetus, protecting the fetus from excess active steroid hormones (mainly testosterones) while making them available to the maternal circulation. Both the fetus and the placenta synthesise progesterones from cholesterol; however only the fetus can convert this to testosterone precursors, in the sulphated (inactivated) form. Placental sulfatases remove sulphates and allow testosterones to become active, but placental aromatases convert the majority into oestrogens, which are released into the maternal circulation. As such, the placenta is the main producer of progesterone and oestrogen during pregnancy.

Human placental lactogen is a polypeptide hormone which increases with placental mass and regulates maternal lipid and carbohydrate metabolism. Human placental growth hormone is a highly homologous polypeptide hormone which replaces maternal growth hormone and also promotes lipolysis, anabolism and gluconeogenesis.

Together, these hormones increase nutrient availability for transplacental transfer, and contribute to the pathogenesis of insulin resistance (and gestational diabetes in susceptible individuals) during pregnancy.

The placenta also produces human chorionic gonadotrophin (hCG) and pregnancy-associated plasma protein A (PAPP-A), mentioned here as due to their presence in the first trimester combined screening test. Once pregnancy is established, hCG is involved in the growth of the uterus and angiogenesis of vasculature, fetal, placental and umbilical cord growth and development, and quiescence of uterine muscle contractions. The role of PAPP-A is less well understood, but cleaves insulin like growth factor binding protein 4, elevated levels of which have been associated with FGR.

INADEQUATE INVASION

During invasion, EVTs migrate from the body of the placenta through the maternal decidua and can be found in the tunica media of the spiral arteries (terminal branches of the uterine arteries which supply maternal blood to the placental bed). They are involved in remodelling the spiral arteries, a process in which muscular arteries with high resistance become thin-walled capacitance vessels, allowing high-flow, low-resistance supply of maternal blood to the placenta. As such, the placental bed becomes a vascular sink to offset the changes in maternal cardiac output and circulating volume which occur early in pregnancy and underlie healthy maternal adaption to pregnancy. Failure of spiral artery modelling, which is completed by 24 weeks of gestation, is associated with FGR, maternal preeclampsia. Assessment of resistance to flow and waveform characteristics using uterine artery Dopplers in the second trimester is intended to identify pregnancies in which spiral artery remodelling has not occurred, and are at risk of these complications, although the negative predictive power outweighs the positive predictive power.

Fetal Growth and Growth Restriction

Fetal growth is influenced by multiple genetic and environmental factors, which, in this setting, refers to the utero-placental environment. FGR describes the failure of the fetus to achieve its genetic growth potential. Maternal factors (notably maternal height which restricts uterine size) and periconceptional health are understood to have an important role in determining fetal growth potential. Maternal smoking is strongly associated with reduced placental invasion, reduced spiral artery remodelling, FGR and indicators of hypoxia in the third trimester fetus. Maternal alcohol intake is associated with reduced placental weight, but in the absence of fetal alcohol syndrome, not growth restriction. Inadequate periconceptional and first trimester nutrition is strongly associated with FGR; however historical studies suggest that calorie restriction of less than 500 kcal/day is required to produce this effect. Chronic maternal disease, particularly active inflammatory conditions, or conditions resulting in maternal hypoxia, also restrict fetal growth.

However, in the UK, in the absence of underlying fetal chromosomal or genetic abnormality, the majority of FGR results from idiopathic utero-placental dysfunction, and subsequent reduction in supply of oxygen and nutrients to the fetus to support fetal growth.

DEVELOPMENTAL ORIGINS OF ADULT HEALTH AND DISEASE

It is now well recognised that lifelong health is intrinsically linked to in utero conditions, not just events and influences after birth. The original epidemiological observations of Barker that rates of low birth weight influenced rates of adult cardiovascular disease 50 years later have developed into the multidisciplinary field which investigates the developmental origins of health and disease. Multiple avenues of research have linked adverse in utero conditions to a predisposition to develop cardiovascular disease, stroke, obesity, diabetes, metabolic syndrome, reduce cognitive function and mental wellbeing and cause adoption of health-risk behaviours, making clear the implications for public and population health. Studies have linked low birth weight to SNS overactivity and elevated cortisol in adults. Chronic SNS overactivity is associated with the development of hypertension, obesity, insulin resistance, left ventricular hypertrophy and carotid atherosclerosis, all highly predictive of cardiovascular adverse events.

References

Martinez-Biarge M, Madero R, Gonzalez A, et al. 2012. Perinatal morbidity and risk of hypoxic-ischemic encephalopathy associated with intrapartum sentinel events. American Journal of Obstetrics and Gynecology 206:148.e1–7

5

Applied Anatomy

SARA PATERSON-BROWN

Introduction

This chapter will address general anatomical principles as well as cover detailed anatomy relevant to the obstetrician and gynaecologist and the Membership of Royal College of Obstetricians and Gynaecologists (MRCOG) exams. Particular attention is given to how this knowledge should be applied clinically, and readers are advised to refer to more detailed comprehensive anatomy books to supplement this applied anatomy approach.

Body Tissues and Cells

These are composed of four elements:

- Epithelium
- Connective tissue
- Muscle
- Nerve

Epithelium can be simple or stratified:

1. Simple means it is one layer thick and this is seen with absorptive or secretory surfaces:
   Simple squamous – flat cells (e.g. endothelium)
   Simple cuboidal – collecting ducts
   Simple columnar – gut lining/fallopian tubes
2. Stratified means it has multiple layers and this affords protection:
   Stratified squamous – and if this is also keratinised it comprises skin – vagina
   Stratified cuboidal – (2 to 3 cells thick) (e.g. excretory duct)

Stratified transitional – cuboidal cells right up to surface (i.e. surface cells remain large; e.g. urinary epithelium)
Other histology details are addressed in the relevant sections of the text.

The Nervous System

The central nervous system (CNS) comprises the brain and the spinal cord, while the peripheral nervous system includes the cranial and spinal nerves. Both central and peripheral systems have somatic (aware/voluntary) and autonomic (unaware/involuntary) components.

THE SOMATIC NERVOUS SYSTEM

This both transmits sensory information (afferent pathways) and innervates skeletal muscle (efferent pathways). The sensory cells are derived from the neural crest and are bipolar with their cell bodies lying in the dorsal root ganglia (*Note* there is no synapse in dorsal root ganglia), while the motor cells grow out in the ventral root from the neural tube (i.e. single myelinated cells with no synapses before their end organs). Somatic nerves do not cross the midline (Fig. 5.1).

Spinal nerves consist of:

- Posterior primary rami sequentially supplying erector spinae and overlying skin
- Anterior primary rami supply the rest of the body's muscles and skin and are often involved in forming nerve plexuses before branching and joining together for more distal distribution (cervical, brachial, lumbar and sacral plexuses)

Autonomic nerves often 'hitch a ride' on these nerves (as they do on blood vessels).

THE AUTONOMIC NERVOUS SYSTEM

Unlike the somatic nervous system, this is involuntary and regulates the body's internal environment. It has the distinctive feature of comprising two neurones in its motor pathway which synapse outside the CNS: one neurone grows out from the CNS and is myelinated (preganglionic) while the postganglionic neurone (derived from neural crest cells) is unmyelinated. Two components (sympathetic and parasympathetic) form the autonomic system and tend to oppose each other to maintain internal homeostasis. The sympathetic nervous system originates from the thoracolumbar regions and the ganglia form a chain bilaterally down each side of the vertebral column, while the parasympathetic nerves have craniosacral outlets and their ganglia are situated distally near their target organs. These differences together with pharmacological features are illustrated in Fig. 5.2.

In addition to these efferent autonomic motor neurones, there are afferent fibres which are conveyed via the sympathetic and parasympathetic nerves, but they are independent of them and do not relay in the ganglia. Like other sensory fibres, their cell bodies lie in the dorsal root ganglia from where they ascend centrally to the hypothalamus and thence to the orbital and frontal gyri of the cerebral cortex (see Fig. 5.1).

Clinical Application

In normal circumstances, we are unaware of autonomic afferent impulses but if sufficiently strong they can cause the sensation of visceral pain (intestinal colic, uterine pain, etc.) which can also produce referred pain in the dermatome of the relevant segmental supply (e.g. cervix S2 and S3, ovary T10 and T11, body of the uterus, lower thoracic and upper lumbar roots). Dermatomes are shown in Fig. 5.3.

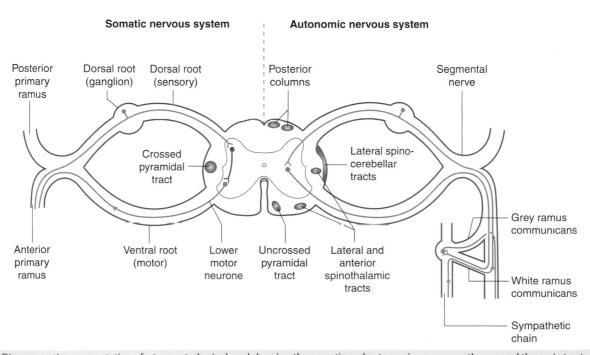

Fig. 5.1 Diagrammatic representation of a transected spinal cord showing the somatic and autonomic neurone pathways and the main tracts running within the cord.

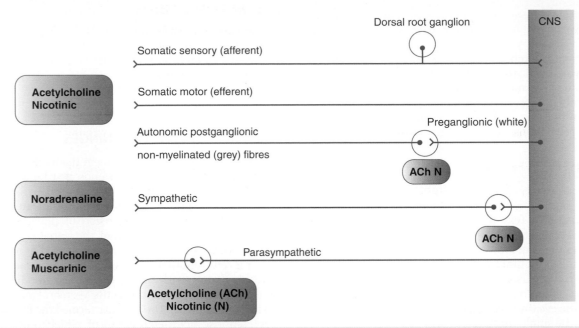

Fig. 5.2 Diagrammatic representation of the neurone arrangements and neurotransmitters of the somatic and autonomic nervous systems. *CNS*, Central nervous system.

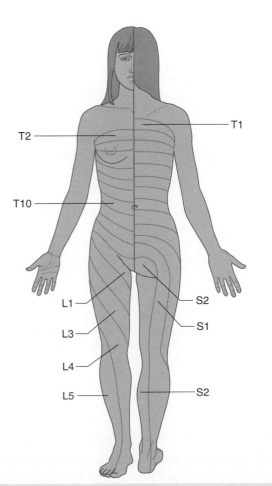

Fig. 5.3 An approximate pattern of anterior and posterior dermatomes.

SYMPATHETIC (THORACOLUMBAR) NERVOUS SYSTEM

These cells are derived from the lateral horn of T1–L2 but the preganglionic fibres travel up and down to form a chain of ganglia extending from the cervical to the coccygeal region (i.e. the root value of the autonomic component may be different from the spinal component with which it emerges). Postganglionic neurones then form sympathetic nerve plexuses, the main ones being:

- Cardiac plexus (below the aortic arch)
- Pulmonary plexus (at the root of the lungs)
- Coeliac plexus (on the coeliac axis and around the origin of the superior mesenteric artery)
- Superior hypogastric plexus (anterior to the aortic bifurcation)
- Inferior hypogastric plexus (lateral to the rectum, cervix and vaginal fornix)

The peripheral distribution of the sympathetic fibres includes branches for somatic distribution which travel with each spinal nerve to supply the corresponding segmental skin, and the visceral distribution which tends to reach its end organ by means of the arterial pathways.

Approximate segmental supplies:

T1–2 head and neck
T1–4 thoracic viscera
T2–5 upper limb
T4–L2 abdominal viscera

T10–L2 pelvic viscera
T11–L2 lower limb

Note: Thoracic, lumbar and sacral splanchnic nerves emerge from the sympathetic plexuses while the *pelvic* splanchnics, in contrast, are parasympathetic (S23 – nervi erigentes). These parasympathetic preganglionic fibres join the sympathetic fibres (from the inferior hypogastric plexus) for distribution within the pelvis and are described in more detail later.

SYMPATHETIC EFFECTS

These are essentially of fight and flight:

- Vasoconstrictor (except to coronary arteries which it dilates)
- Increases the heart rate
- Dilates the bronchial tree
- Relaxes the detrusor muscle
- Contracts smooth muscle sphincters
- Dilates the eye (by relaxing the ciliary muscle)
- Relaxes the small intestine

THE ADRENAL MEDULLA

This is derived from neural crest cells and comprises approximately 10% of the adrenal gland (the remainder being the cortex). The myelinated preganglionic sympathetic fibres from the splanchnic nerves travel via the coeliac plexus and synapse directly with the medullary (chromaffin) cells which secrete catecholamines.

PARASYMPATHETIC (CRANIOSACRAL) NERVOUS SYSTEM

Unlike the sympathetic, the parasympathetic system has no somatic distribution and is purely visceral. Four cranial nerves and two sacral roots are involved.

Cranial: III, VII, IX, X

The vagus is particularly important, travelling widely. It forms a plexus round the oesophagus and the fibres from each side mix and thence continue as anterior and posterior nerves. The vagus contributes to the:

- Cardiac, pulmonary and oesophageal plexuses
- Stomach and liver (via the anterior vagus)
- Small and large intestine as far as the splenic flexure (travelling via the superior mesenteric artery)

Sacral: S2 and S3

Preganglionic cell bodies lie in the lateral horn of the grey matter in the spinal cord from where they pass out as nervi erigentes to intermingle with the inferior hypogastric plexus to supply the:

- Gut beyond the splenic flexure (travel via the inferior mesenteric artery)
- Bladder
- Genital organs
- Pelvic blood vessels

Parasympathetic Effects

- Decreases the heart rate
- Bronchoconstrictor
- Increases glandular secretions
- Increases peristalsis
- Stimulates detrusor contractions
- Relaxes sphincters

THE SPINAL CORD AND MENINGES

This extension of the CNS begins in the medulla oblongata at the foramen magnum and ends at L1/L2. The nerve roots that continue after the spinal cord has terminated at the conus medullaris comprise the cauda equina, while the filum terminale (the extension of pia mater) inserts into the coccyx. As the length of the spinal cord is shorter than the vertebral column, nerve roots arise at increasingly higher levels than their corresponding vertebrae and travel increasingly longer distances within the vertebral column before exiting from their respective vertebral foramina.

The membranes of the cord are termed the meninges and they comprise neuroepithelium of which there are three layers. From outside inwards these are:

1. Dura mater (under which lies the subdural space)
2. Arachnoid mater (under this is the subarachnoid space containing cerebrospinal fluid)
3. Pia mater

Both pia and arachnoid are continued out along the spinal nerve roots, while the dura forms a tough sheath for the cord ending at S2, and it extends out over each nerve root blending with its sheath.

The epidural (extradural) space lies between the dura mater and the spinal canal and is filled with fat and vessels (lymphatic and blood).

The spinal cord has neuronal cell bodies in its grey matter, and its external white matter comprises axonal tracts (see Fig. 5.1).

Afferent neurones include those for:

- Touch and vibration – cell bodies in dorsal root ganglia, tracts in posterior columns
- Pain and temperature – cell bodies in contralateral posterior horn, axons in lateral and anterior spinothalamic tracts
- Proprioception – axons in lateral spinocerebellar tracts

Efferent neurones are motor and pass along the:

- Lateral cerebrospinal (or corticospinal) tract. These neurones originate in the motor cortex but the fibres cross before descending in what is also referred to as the crossed pyramidal tract.
- Anterior cerebrospinal (or direct pyramidal) tract. These neurones are uncrossed.

SPINAL NERVE ROOTS AND THEIR PLEXUSES

Each pair of spinal nerves emerges from the vertebral column as illustrated in Fig. 5.1, and branches proceed to supply the skin in a pattern which can be mapped out diagrammatically (see Fig. 5.3).

Clinical Application

Pain can be referred to the dermatome which is supplied by the same nerve root as the area in question. Some spinal nerves merge and re-divide with other nerve roots before proceeding. This produces nerve plexuses and these occur in the cervical, brachial, lumbar and sacral regions. Although the cervical/brachial plexus can be relevant in situations of obstetric trauma to the neonate (in the clinical situations of shoulder dystocia), detailed knowledge of it is beyond the remit of this chapter. The relevant clinical message is to respect the fetal neck and avoid undue traction on it (which can stretch and damage the nerve roots).

The lumbar and sacral plexuses are described in the relevant regional anatomy sections (pp. 22 and 24).

Anatomy of the Brain

The brain develops from the neural tube and its cavity persists in the three resulting components:

- The forebrain
  - the cerebral hemispheres, each with their lateral ventricle
  - the deeper diencephalon surrounding the third ventricle
- The midbrain
  - connects the forebrain to the hind brain
  - the aqueduct (of Sylvius) runs through it
- The hindbrain
  - pons, medulla oblongata and cerebellum
  - the fourth ventricle
- The midbrain, pons and medulla comprise the brain stem

THE THALAMI

The two thalami lie laterally in the diencephalon forming the lateral walls of the third ventricle. The internal capsule lies laterally, separating them from the basal ganglia. The thalamus is sensory in function and relays impulses on to the cerebral cortex via the internal capsule. It also connects to the hypothalamus.

THE HYPOTHALAMUS

The hypothalamus is also in the diencephalon forming the floor of the third ventricle and is concerned with the autonomic nervous system. It contains many cell types, in particular the supraoptic and paraventricular nuclei whose axons connect it to the posterior lobe of the pituitary via the pituitary stalk. It also connects with the basal nuclei caudally and via long axons to the sympathetic and parasympathetic cells in the lateral horns of the spinal cord.

THE PINEAL GLAND

The pineal gland lies posterior to the thalamus at the posterior end of the third ventricle and is innervated by the sympathetic nervous system. It is most active at night, produces melatonin and tends to have an inhibitory effect on other endocrine glands and gonads. It calcifies with age and may be visible on a skull x-ray after the age of 40 years.

THE PITUITARY GLAND

The pituitary gland is composed of two parts; both are derived from ectodermal tissue but of different origins:

- The small posterior pituitary is derived from a downgrowth of ectodermal neural plate and these neurones have their cell stations in the hypothalamus. These neurosecretory cells produce oxytocin and antidiuretic hormone (adh)
- The larger anterior pituitary (pars tuberalis) forms from Rathke's pouch growing up from the roof of the mouth and consists of glandular cells:
  - chromophobes – account for 50% of the anterior pituitary
  - eosinophilic/acidophilic cells produce growth hormone (GH) and prolactin
  - basophilic cells produce adrenocorticotrophic hormones (ACTH), follicle stimulating hormones (FSH), luteinizing hormones (LH) and thyroid stimulating hormones (TSH)

This gland occupies the pituitary fossa with:

- The diaphragma sellae and optic chiasma above
- The cavernous sinuses laterally
- The body of the sphenoid below

Clinical Application

Pituitary tumours (including prolactinomas) can grow upwards to press on the medial sides of the optic nerves in the lower anterior part of the optic chiasma causing temporal hemianopia (tunnel vision).

The Lymphatic System

LYMPHATIC VESSELS

The extracellular tissues of the body are constantly gaining fluid and debris (from capillary leakage, cell death, etc.) and the function of the lymphatics is to remove this and return it to the venous circulation. The lymphatic capillaries have the same basic structure as vascular capillaries but their distribution is not uniform throughout the body. The lymphatics in the limbs tend to be superficial, while those of the viscera tend to drain via channels on the posterior abdominal and thoracic walls.

The lymphatic vessels return the lymph to the venous system via two main channels:

- *The right lymphatic duct* drains the right thorax, upper limb, head and neck
- *The thoracic duct* drains all lymph from the lower half of the body

The pre- and para-aortic lymphatics drain into the cisterna chyli which is an elongated sac-like vessel that lies over the body of L1 and L2 behind the inferior vena cava (IVC) and between the aorta and the azygous vein. It becomes the thoracic duct as it ascends through the diaphragm at the level of T12. It starts on the right side of the oesophagus, but as it ascends through the thorax the thoracic duct passes behind the oesophagus (at T5) to reach its left side, then superiorly it passes over the left subclavian artery and the dome of the left pleura to drain into the confluence of the left subclavian with the left internal jugular veins.

Lymphatics, like blood vessels (and unlike somatic nerves), can cross the midline, but in contrast they pass to and from lymph nodes (afferent and efferent lymphatics) and they comprise an anastomosing low-pressure system.

LYMPHATIC TISSUE

These comprise concentrations of lymphocytes and occur in mucosal and submucosal collections in the gut (e.g. Peyer's patches in the ileum) as well as in the thymus, the spleen and lymph nodes themselves.

The anatomical clinical importance of this system relates to the drainage patterns of each group of nodes, which is summarised in Table 5.1, but also described for the individual organs in their relevant regional anatomy sections.

The Vascular System

FETAL CIRCULATION AND CHANGES AFTER BIRTH

Oxygenated Blood

- *The ductus venosus* bypasses the liver taking oxygenated blood from the left branch of the portal vein (from the umbilical vein) to the IVC
- This flows into the right atrium and is directed towards the *foramen ovale* passing through into the left atrium and thence out to supply the head and neck.

Deoxygenated Blood

- Flows back from the superior vena cava (SVC) and is directed through the tricuspid valve to the right ventricle
- *The ductus arteriosus* bypasses the lungs taking blood from the left branch of the pulmonary trunk to the aorta distal to its three main primary branches
- The blood in the descending aorta then passes out to the placenta via the umbilical arteries which branch off from the internal iliac arteries

Table 5.1   Lymphatic Drainage Patterns

Lymph Node Group	Location	Tissues/Structures Drained
Superficial inguinal nodes	Longitudinally along the great saphenous vein and horizontally distal to the inguinal ligament	Anterior abdominal wall (below umbilicus)
		Upper part of uterus and round ligament
		Lower third of vagina, vulva, perineum and anus
		Superficial part of leg and buttock
Deep inguinal lymph nodes	Lie medial to the femoral vein	The superficial inguinal nodes
		Deep part of leg
		Clitoris
Deep femoral lymph node of Cloquet	Lies in the femoral canal	Vulva
External iliac nodes	Along the external iliac arteries	Deep inguinal lymph nodes
		Bladder
		Lower uterus and cervix
Internal iliac nodes	Along the internal iliac arteries	Urethra and deep perineum
		Cervix and upper two-thirds of vagina
		Lower rectum
Common iliac nodes	Along the common iliac arteries	Internal and external iliac nodes
		Abdominal part of the ureter
		Fallopian tubes and upper uterus
Obturator nodes	Along the obturator artery	Cervix
Para-aortic nodes	Lie alongside the aorta near the origins of the paired arterial branches	Common iliac nodes
		Posterior abdominal wall
		Lumbar region
		Kidneys and ovaries
Pre-aortic nodes	Anterior to the aorta around the origin of coeliac, superior and inferior mesenteric arteries	Pelvis and abdomen corresponding to ventral aortic arterial branches

Changes at and After Birth

- The pressure changes due to inflation of the lungs and the increased flow through the pulmonary arteries close the foramen ovale
- The ductus arteriosus muscular wall contracts and closes, and is effectively obliterated within 2 months, becoming the ligamentum arteriosum
- The ductus venosus becomes the ligamentum venosum (passing round the caudate lobe of the liver)
- The intra-abdominal umbilical vein becomes the ligamentum teres
- The umbilical arteries become obliterated and form the medial umbilical ligaments (not to be confused with the median umbilical ligament which is the obliterated remains of the urachus)

The Arterial System

THE AORTA

The aorta (Fig. 5.4) enters the abdomen behind the diaphragm between its crura at T12 and descends to divide into the common iliac arteries at L4. It has three ventral branches which give rise to the portal circulation, while the other branches are systemic.

Three Ventral Branches.

- The coeliac artery (axis/trunk) is very short (1 cm long) arising at level L1
- The superior mesenteric artery arises at level L2
- The inferior mesenteric artery arises at level L3

Three Terminal Branches.

- The right and left common iliac arteries arise at level L4
- The median sacral artery continues over L5

Four Pairs of Branches.

- Phrenic arteries
- Suprarenal arteries
- Renal arteries
- Gonadal arteries

Four Lateral Pairs.

- The four lumbar segmental arteries.

The Common Iliac Arteries

The common iliac arteries diverge from in front of the fourth lumbar vertebra and then divide into internal and external iliac arteries in front of the sacroiliac joint.

The external iliac artery is essentially involved in the blood supply to the leg (becoming the femoral artery when it passes behind the inguinal ligament), but it gives two important branches off just above the inguinal ligament: the inferior epigastric and the deep circumflex iliac arteries.

The internal iliac artery divides into anterior and posterior branches to supply the pelvis and buttock, respectively. Details of these vessels are given in the section on the pelvis.

Details of individual vessels and their relations are given in the relevant regional anatomy sections.

The Venous System

This is a relatively low-pressure valved system for draining blood back to the heart. Flow fluctuates with the arterial pulse while muscle pumps further encourage flow in the limbs and inspiration increases flow in the IVC and SVC centrally. Excepting the portal circulation, veins generally follow the pattern and path of arteries and have sympathetic innervation.

THE INFERIOR VENA CAVA

The common iliac veins join to form the IVC (Fig. 5.5) behind the right external iliac artery at L5. The IVC ascends through the abdomen on the right of the aorta piercing the central tendon of the diaphragm at T8. It receives:

- Segmental lumbar veins
- The right gonadal vein (the left gonadal vein drains into left renal vein)
- The renal and suprarenal veins
- The hepatic veins
- The inferior phrenic veins

COLLATERAL VENOUS DRAINAGE PATHWAYS

There is an extensive network of potential collateral circulations which open when thrombosis of the IVC occurs.

Superficial venous channels which can eventually drain to the SVC are:

- Epigastric
- Circumflex iliac
- Superficial epigastric and lateral thoracic (via thoraco-epigastric vein)
- Internal thoracic
- Posterior intercostals

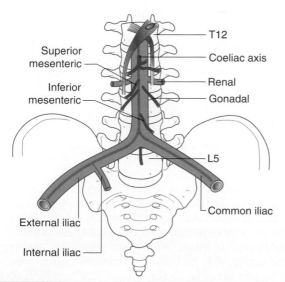

Fig. 5.4 The abdominal aorta and its branches.

Superior mesenteric

Inferior mesenteric

External iliac

Internal iliac

T12

Coeliac axis

Renal

Gonadal

L5

Common iliac

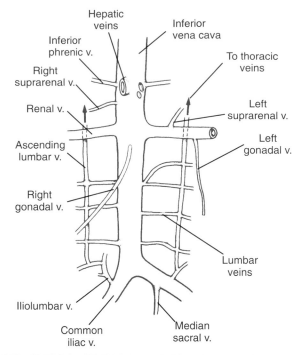

Fig. 5.5 The inferior vena cava and its tributaries.

- External pudendal
- Lumbovertebral

Deep channels which provide deep anastomoses are:

- Azygous
- Hemiazygos
- Lumbar

The vertebral venous plexus also provides effective collateral circulation between IVC and SVC.

Clinical Application

This collateral circulation is so efficient that, even when there is substantial obstruction to venous flow by a large deep vein thrombosis in the iliac vessels, there can be an absence of clinical symptoms or signs.

THE PORTAL VENOUS DRAINAGE AND PORTOSYSTEMIC VENOUS ANASTOMOSES

The portal venous system drains blood to the liver from the abdominal part of the alimentary canal (except the anus), the spleen, pancreas and gall bladder. The superior and inferior mesenteric veins join the splenic vein behind the pancreas to form the portal vein which carries blood to the liver, which in turn is drained by the hepatic veins which pass into the IVC. This pathway may be obstructed causing portal hypertension and then collaterals open up between the portal and the systemic venous systems:

- Lower oesophagus – tributaries of: left gastric with hemiazygos/azygous
- Anal wall – superior rectal with middle and inferior rectal

- Caput medusa – tributary from left branch of portal vein (paraumbilical) with epigastrics
- Retroperitoneal veins of abdominal wall with veins of the ascending colon and the bare area of the liver
- Very rarely a patent ductus venosus

VERTEBRAL COLUMN

Venous drainage from both the internal and the external vertebral plexus drain to regional segmental veins providing potential communication with systems which also drain segmentally. This is a largely valveless system and therefore the spread of malignancy is possible (especially likely from breast, uterus, prostate and thyroid):

- Pelvic viscera via the lateral sacral vessels
- Abdomen via the lumbar veins
- Breast via the posterior intercostals
- Neck via the vertebral vein

The Musculoskeletal System

TYPES OF JOINT

- Fibrous (bone/fibrous tissue/bone) (e.g. skull sutures although these ossify in later life)
- Cartilaginous:
  - primary (bone/hyaline cartilage/bone) (e.g. epiphyses or costochondral junctions)
  - secondary (bone/hyaline cartilage/fibrocartilage/hyaline cartilage/bone) – these only occur in the midline (e.g. pubic symphysis, intervertebral joints)
- Synovial joints that allow movement (e.g. hip joint). The sacroiliac joint is also a synovial joint but atypical in that the movement allowed is extremely limited

THE VERTEBRAL COLUMN

The vertebral column has 33 vertebrae (7 cervical, 12 thoracic, 5 lumbar, 5 sacral and 4 coccygeal). The five sacral vertebrae are fused to form the sacrum, and the coccygeal components can be variably fused.

There are 31 pairs of spinal nerves whose nerve roots travel variable distances within the vertebral column to exit the spine by passing across the disc of the vertebra above (therefore problems with, e.g. L4 disc will affect L5 nerve root).

THE PELVIS

The bony pelvis comprises the sacrum and the os innominatum.

- The sacrum is composed of five fused vertebrae (with four sacral foramina). It articulates with the fifth lumbar vertebra above, the coccyx below and the ilium laterally.
- The os innominatum is made up of three bones: ilium, pubis and ischium, which are joined by cartilage in the young, but by bone in adulthood. They meet in a Y-shaped junction in the acetabulum to which they all contribute.

Clinical Application

Movement at the pelvic joints is minimal in the non-pregnant state, but there is considerable joint relaxation during pregnancy. In some women, instability can occur with sacroiliitis or pubic symphysis dysfunction which can be extremely debilitating. Limiting abduction of the legs in these conditions is crucial in preventing further deterioration or even permanent instability, and pain-free abduction distances should be measured (knee to knee) and recorded prior to labour so that nursing of the woman (when pain-free with an epidural) does not silently cause more damage.

OBSTETRIC PELVIC DEFINITIONS AND DIMENSIONS

The pelvic inlet is oval being widest transversely, the pelvic mid-cavity is circular, while the outlet is oval being widest anteroposteriorly. Normally, the fetal head enters the pelvis transversely due to the shape of the inlet and subsequent rotation of the fetal head during the descent through the pelvis in labour takes advantage of the bony dimensions, but the rotation itself is caused by the muscular pelvic gutter (Table 5.2).

The Pelvic Inlet

The pelvic inlet is oval shaped and is widest from side to side. It divides the bony pelvis into the false pelvis above (made up mainly of the ala of the ilium on each side which forms the lower lateral portion of the abdomen), and the true pelvis below (the pelvic cavity). The boundaries of the pelvic inlet include:

- The promontory of the sacrum
- The arcuate line of the ilium
- The iliopubic eminence
- The pectineal line
- The pubic crest
- The symphysis pubis

The Pelvic Outlet

The pelvic outlet is widest from front to back and lies between:

- The lower border of the symphysis pubis anteriorly
- The ischial tuberosities laterally
- The tip of the last sacral vertebra posteriorly

The true obstetric conjugate extends from the sacral promontory to the upper border of the pubic symphysis. The diagonal conjugate extends from the sacral promontory to the lower border of the pubic symphysis. The important landmarks of the pelvis are indicated in Figs. 5.6 and 5.7.

The Male and Female Pelvis

General differences in structure between the male and female pelvis relate to the heavier thick-set skeleton of the male, with more obvious and well-marked muscle attachments and larger joint surfaces compared with the female, but there are also notable sex differences (Table 5.3).

Variations in Pelvic Shape (Fig. 5.8)

- Gynaecoid – normal female
- Android – normal male
- Anthropoid – the pelvic brim is longer anteroposteriorly than transversely
- Platypelloid – the pelvic brim is much wider transversely and foreshortened anteroposteriorly
- Rachitic pelvis – typical of rickets and the result of vitamin D deficiency. The sacral promontory projects forwards reducing the anteroposterior diameter
- The contracted pelvis – can be symmetrical associated with a small stature, or asymmetrical due to a variety of disease processes
- A narrow (gothic) subpubic arch foreshortens the effective pelvic outlet because the narrow anterior triangle (the waste space of Morrison) cannot accommodate the fetal head. In such circumstances, more space is required posteriorly to enable vaginal delivery (Fig. 5.9).

Table 5.2 Approximate Pelvic Obstetric Dimensions (cm)

	Transverse	Oblique	Anteroposterior
Inlet	13	11	11
Mid-pelvis	12	12	12
Outlet	10.5	11.5	12.5

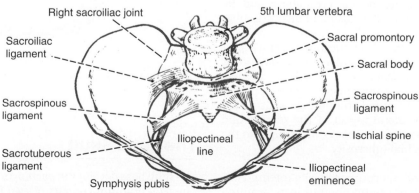

Fig. 5.6 Important landmarks of the pelvis.

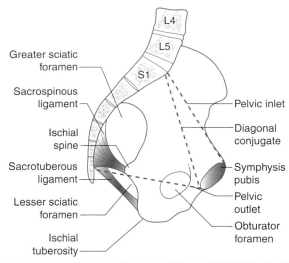

Fig. 5.7 Lateral view of the pelvis showing the obstetric conjugates.

Table 5.3   Differences Between the Male and Female Pelvis

Sex Differences	Female	Male
Sacral curve	Short, wide and flat	Long and narrow
	Curved in the lower part	General curve
Articular surfaces of the sacrum	Laterally with two sacral bodies	Laterally with three sacral bodies
	Superiorly with L5: oval and occupies one-third of alar surface	Superiorly with L5 and occupies half of the alar surface
Pelvic inlet	Oval	Heart shaped
Pelvic canal	Short and almost cylindrical	Long and tapered
Pelvic outlet	Comparatively large	Comparatively small
Subpubic angle	Approx 80–90 degrees	50–60 degrees
Obturator foramen	Triangular	Oval

Ligaments of the Pelvis

The vertebropelvic ligaments (see Figs. 5.6 and 5.7):

- Iliolumbar – this V-shaped ligament extends from the transverse process of L5 to the iliac crest above, and the ventral portion of the sacroiliac ligament below (lumbosacral ligament)
- Sacrospinous ligament runs from the lower lateral aspect of the sacrum and the upper lateral aspect of the coccyx to insert into the ischial spine
- Sacrotuberous ligament is extremely strong opposing the forward tilting of the sacral promontory. It also originates from the lower lateral aspect of the sacrum and the upper lateral aspect of the coccyx inserting into the inner aspect of the ischial tuberosity.

The sacrospinous and sacrotuberous ligaments convert the greater and lesser sciatic notches into foramina (see Fig. 5.7).

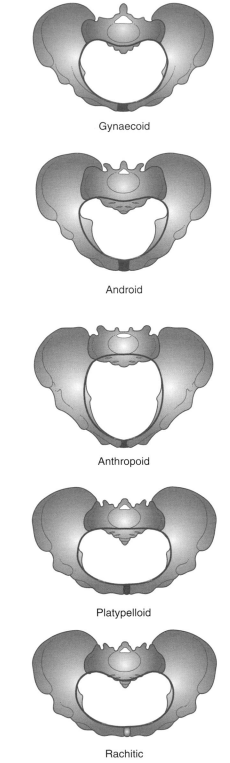

Fig. 5.8 Diagrammatic representation of different pelvic shapes.

The Fetal Skull

The skull base develops in cartilage, the vault in membrane. The fetal cranium consists of two frontal bones, two parietal bones and one occipital bone. These are separated by

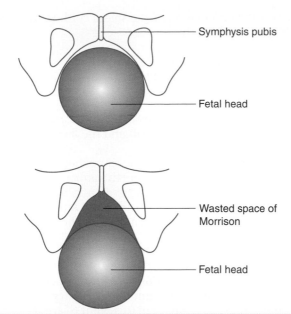

Fig. 5.9 Illustration of the effect of a narrow subpubic arch and the waste space of Morrison.

sutures and fontanelles and provide landmarks for defining the presentation of the fetal head in labour:

- Occiput describes the area behind the posterior fontanelle
- The vertex describes the parietal eminences between anterior and posterior fontanelles
- The bregma is the area around the anterior fontanelle
- The sinciput is the area in front of the anterior fontanelle which is further divided into brow and face (above and below the root of the nose).

The presenting diameter of the fetal skull varies according to its presentation:

- Occipital and face presentations have the smallest diameters (suboccipitobregmatic and submentobregmatic, respectively) both being of the order of 9.5 cm
- Vertex is most common with the occipitofrontal diameter of 11.5 cm
- Brow is the largest with the mentovertical diameter of 13 cm.

Moulding during labour slides the parietal bones under each other and the occipital and frontal bones under the parietal bones and can reduce dimensions by 1 to 1.5 cm (Fig. 5.10).

Relevant Regional Anatomy of the Thorax

SURFACE ANATOMY

Knowledge of the surface anatomy of the chest can be extremely valuable clinically:

- *The angle of Louis*, which is the ridge produced by the manubriosternal joint, lies at the level of thoracic

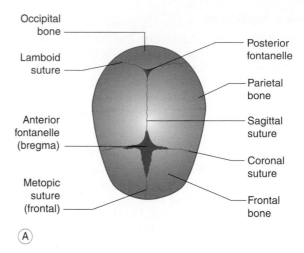

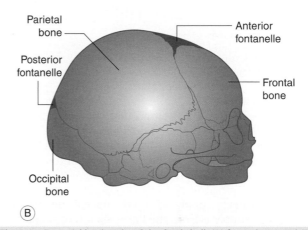

Fig. 5.10 Essential landmarks of the fetal skull: (A) from above and (B) lateral view.

vertebra T4, but more useful is the site of the second costochondral junction marking the second rib from which subsequent intercostal spaces can be defined. These features also mark the upper limit of the surface markings of the heart.
- *The 4th intercostal space* marks the dome of the diaphragm and the uppermost edge of the liver.

RIBS

Ribs generate a negative pressure for respiration (−5 to −15 mmHg)

- True ribs (ribs 1 to 7) articulate with the sternum
- False ribs (8 to 10) – their costal cartilages articulate with the rib above
- Floating ribs (11 and 12) have muscle attachments only.

The intercostal muscles which comprise three layers – external, internal and innermost – run between neighbouring ribs. The neurovascular bundles run along the lower inside border of each rib (i.e. superiorly in each intercostal space) between the internal and innermost intercostal muscles.

Clinical Application

- When aspirating or inserting a chest drain, the position of the neurovascular bundle should be remembered and access should be achieved by running the needle or drain over the rib rather than under it. The fifth intercostal space in the mid-axillary line is usually used, but in pregnancy it is best to go up one space to allow for the raised diaphragm
- The higher level of the diaphragm in pregnancy is also relevant in situations of trauma to the chest which is more likely to involve intra-abdominal organs
- The parietal pleura is innervated segmentally from the intercostal nerves and therefore when inflamed produces pain which is referred to the cutaneous distribution of that nerve. Thus anterior abdominal wall pain can arise from pleural irritation mimicking an abdominal event.

THE DIAPHRAGM

This is a musculotendinous structure which separates the thorax from the abdomen. It arises from:

- The xiphisternum
- The lower six ribs and their costal cartilages
- The medial and lateral arcuate ligaments
- The first three lumbar vertebrae on the right/first two on the left (right and left crus) and fuses into a trifoliate central tendon below the pericardium.

The motor nerve supply is from the phrenic nerve (C3-5), and sensory supply is from the lower six intercostal nerves. The blood supply comes from the lower intercostal arteries superiorly, and the phrenic arteries (branches of aorta) inferiorly.

The three main openings in the diaphragm and their vertebral levels are as follows:

1. The aortic opening at the level of T12 transmits the aorta with the thoracic duct and the azygous vein (from left to right).
2. The oesophageal opening which passes through the right crus of the diaphragm at the level of T10, and also transmits the left gastric artery and both vagi.
3. The IVC runs through the central tendon at the level of T8 together with the right phrenic nerve.

Other structures which penetrate the diaphragm include the greater and lesser splanchnic nerves and the sympathetic chain.

The Abdomen

SURFACE ANATOMY

The transpyloric plane is an important landmark because of its anatomical relationships. It lies a patient handbreadth below their xiphoid and is at the level of the first lumbar vertebra and the ninth costal cartilage and

marks the termination of the spinal cord. Structures in this plane include the:
- Pylorus of stomach
- Duodenojejunal flexure
- Fundus of the gall bladder
- Renal hila
- Neck of pancreas.

The subcostal plane joins the lowest costal margins on both sides and marks the tenth rib and the level of the third lumbar vertebra.

The plane of the iliac crests marks the bifurcation of the abdominal aorta at the level of the fourth lumbar vertebra.

The umbilicus is an inconsistent landmark, but in the slim adult lies at the lower part of the third lumbar vertebra, the third part of the duodenum and the origin of the inferior mesenteric artery.

McBurney's point lies two-thirds laterally along a line drawn from the umbilicus to the anterior superior iliac spine. It guides the positioning for an appendicectomy incision (non-pregnant) and needle entry for a paracentesis must pass lateral to this point to avoid the inferior epigastric vessels.

Langer's (cleavage or tension) lines of the skin result from the collagen fibre arrangements, and incisions placed along these heal with minimum scarring. On the anterior abdominal wall, they lie transversely.

The dermatomes of the anterior abdominal wall are relevant in situations of referred pain, and in the assessment of regional anaesthesia. They are illustrated in Fig. 5.3.

THE ABDOMINAL WALL

This is essentially muscular, maintaining tone and imposing a positive intra-abdominal pressure ($+5\,mmHg$), despite respiration.

- A muscular cylinder joins two bony rings (costal margin and pelvis) which are joined/splinted apart by the vertebral column
- The superior bony ring is closed off by the muscular diaphragm
- The inferior ring is closed off by the muscular pelvic 'diaphragm'/pelvic floor.

Clinical Application

At laparoscopy the intra-abdominal pressure should always be noted together with its fluctuation with respirations. The Veress needle and trocar should be angled inferiorly at 45 degrees from the umbilicus in the midline, thus avoiding the aorta (which has already terminated) and the iliac vessels (which have diverged).

The muscles of the abdominal wall can be thought of as straight (anterior and posterior) and flat (lateral) muscles (Fig. 5.11).

Straight Muscles

Posteriorly: Quadratus Lumborum.
ATTACHMENTS.
- Medial half of the lower border of the 12th rib
- Transverse processes of L1–5
- Iliolumbar ligament and posterior aspect of iliac crest.

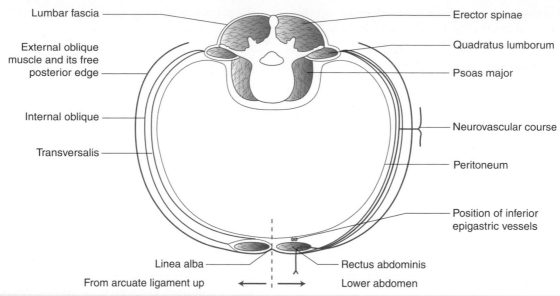

Fig. 5.11 Transverse section through the abdomen showing the muscular arrangements and fascial coverings of the rectus abdominis muscle at different levels (see text) and illustrating the neurovascular plane and course.

NERVE SUPPLY.
- Segmental from T12 to L4 ventral rami.

Anteriorly: Rectus Abdominis.
ATTACHMENTS.
- 5th to 7th costal cartilages plus xiphisternum in horizontal plane
- Pubic crest (and interdigitates across the midline)

NERVE SUPPLY.
- Segmental T7–T12.

Pyramidalis is a vestigial muscle absent in 20% of the population, which lies anterior to the lower fibres of the rectus abdominis muscle within the rectus sheath. It is supplied by the subcostal nerve.

Flat (Lateral) Muscles (All Innervated Segmentally From T7 to L1)

External Oblique. Runs downwards, forwards and medially (like the direction your hands take when in your pockets).

ATTACHMENTS.
- Angles of lower eight ribs
- Anterior half of iliac crest and anterior superior iliac spine
- Pubic tubercle and pectineal line on ipsilateral side (lacunar ligament)
- Contralateral pubic tubercle (reflected part of the inguinal ligament – this forms the floor of the inguinal canal).

THE EXTERNAL OBLIQUE MUSCLE HAS TWO FREE EDGES.
- Posteriorly
- Inferiorly (the inguinal ligament).

Internal Oblique. Runs upwards, forwards and medially (i.e. at 90 degrees to external oblique).
ATTACHMENTS.
- Anterior two-thirds of iliac crest

- Internal border of lateral two-thirds of inguinal ligament (conjoint tendon)
- Lower 3 to 4 ribs and their costal cartilages.

Transversus (Transverse Abdominis/Transversalis). Runs across laterally.
ATTACHMENTS.
- Inner aspects of costal cartilages of lower six ribs
- Anterior two-thirds of iliac crest
- Internal border of lateral third of inguinal ligament (conjoint tendon).

The conjoint tendon forms from the fibres of internal oblique and transversus abdominis which extend from their inguinal ligament attachment to arch medially and insert into the pubic crest lying behind the superficial inguinal ring.

The neurovascular plane lies between transversalis and internal oblique muscles, and the segmental lateral cutaneous nerves pierce the internal and external oblique muscles laterally to supply the external oblique muscle and skin. The nerve/vessel then continues anteriorly to enter the rectus sheath, supplying it and the anterior skin.

The Rectus Sheath

The rectus sheath is formed from the aponeuroses of external oblique, internal oblique and transversalis and ends in the linea alba in the midline which extends from the xiphisternum to pubic symphysis.

Superiorly, the internal oblique aponeurosis splits lateral to the rectus muscle (posteriorly it fuses with the aponeurosis of transversus abdominis passing behind rectus abdominis, anteriorly it fuses with the aponeurosis of external oblique and passes in front of rectus abdominis), rejoining in the midline at the linea alba. Midway between the umbilicus and symphysis this arrangement changes and all the aponeuroses pass in front of the rectus; the free edge of the lower posterior aponeurosis at this level is called the *arcuate ligament*. Inferiorly, the posterior aspect of the rectus muscle is separated in the lower third from the peritoneum only by the extraperitoneal connective tissue in which the inferior epigastric vascular bundle travels (see Fig. 5.11).

Contents of the Rectus Sheath (See Fig. 5.11)

- Rectus abdominis muscle
- Pyramidalis muscle
- Superior epigastric artery and vein (from internal thoracic)
- Inferior epigastric artery and vein (from external iliac)
- Lower six thoracic nerves and posterior intercostal vessels.

Inferior Epigastric Artery

The inferior epigastric artery is important for four reasons:

1. It is vulnerable to trauma if a finger is hooked under the rectus muscle when exposing peritoneum on entering the abdomen or when inserting the lateral laparoscopic port.
2. It is an important landmark for inguinal hernia (direct herniae are medial to this vessel, and the deep inguinal ring lies lateral to it (see Fig. 5.13).
3. In 20% of people an abnormal obturator artery arises from it.
4. Can become arteriosclerotic and fracture causing iliac fossa pain (diagnostic problem).

THE INGUINAL REGION

The free inferior edge of the external oblique aponeurosis (between its attachments to the iliac spine and the pubic tubercle) comprises the inguinal ligament. The inguinal canal extends from the deep inguinal ring (which is a defect in the transversalis fascia) to the superficial inguinal ring (which is formed by the diverging fibres of external oblique) overlying the pubic tubercle.

Surface markings of inguinal area (Fig. 5.12):

- *The mid-inguinal point* is halfway between the anterior superior iliac spine and the symphysis pubis, and is

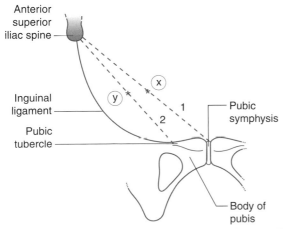

Fig. 5.12 Surface markings of the inguinal area. (1) Straight line from anterior superior iliac spine to pubic symphysis. (2) Straight line from anterior superior iliac spine to pubic tubercle. *x*, Mid-inguinal point; *y*, midpoint of the inguinal ligament.

the point at which the external iliac artery becomes the femoral artery

- *The midpoint of the inguinal ligament* is halfway between the anterior superior iliac spine and the pubic tubercle and marks the deep inguinal ring. *Note* that this is lateral to the femoral artery, but medial to the inferior epigastric artery.

The Inguinal Canal

Contents of the inguinal canal:

- Round ligament or spermatic cord
- Ilioinguinal nerve (supplies the labia)
- Genital branch of the genitofemoral nerve (supplies the labia).

The Spermatic Cord

The spermatic cord is formed when the testis passes through the inguinal canal descending into the scrotum. It has three coverings: the internal spermatic fascia derives from transversalis fascia, the cremasteric fascia derives from internal oblique and the external spermatic fascia derives from external oblique. The cord consists of:

- Vas deferens (ductus deferens)
- Three nerves
  - genital branch of genitofemoral (supplies cremaster muscle)
  - ilioinguinal (supplies scrotum and groin)
  - sympathetic
- Three arteries
  - testicular (from aorta)
  - artery to the vas (from inferior vesical)
  - cremasteric (from inferior epigastric)
- Lymphatics (which drain to para-aortic nodes)
- Pampiniform venous plexus
- Processus vaginalis (this is the obliterated peritoneal connection with the tunica vaginalis of the testis).

Fig. 5.13 illustrates the left inguinal region from behind and demonstrates the inguinal triangle (of Hesselbach) which is the position of direct inguinal herniae which are always acquired (compared with congenital indirect herniae which pass through deep inguinal ring).

THE FEMORAL REGION

In the femoral region (see Fig. 5.13), the femoral vessels pick up fascia from transversalis (anteriorly) and psoas (posteriorly) as they pass beneath the inguinal ligament to enter the leg producing the femoral sheath. The femoral nerve lies lateral to (and outside) the sheath, while medial to the femoral vein within the sheath is a space called the femoral canal, which contains the lymph node of Cloquet draining the clitoris or glans penis. The femoral ring is the superior opening to the femoral canal and the site through which herniation can occur.

The borders of the femoral ring are:

- Inguinal ligament anteriorly
- Lacunar ligament medially
- Pectineus muscle posteriorly
- Femoral vein laterally.

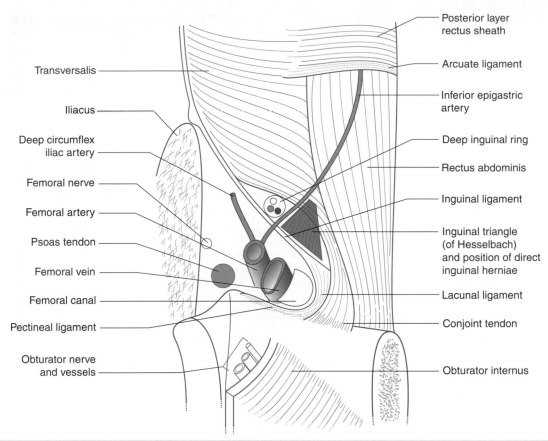

Fig. 5.13 The posterior aspect of the left anterior abdominal wall showing the relationship of the structures described in the text and illustrating the course of the inferior epigastric artery and the relative positions of the deep inguinal ring and the femoral sheath and canal.

The Femoral Triangle

The femoral triangle is bordered by the inguinal ligament, the medial edge of sartorius and the medial border of adductor longus. The adductor longus, pectineus, iliacus and psoas major form the floor of the triangle which contains the femoral vein and artery, the femoral nerve and its branches, and fat and lymph nodes. The apex of the triangle leads on under sartorius to the adductor (subsartorial or Hunter's) canal.

DEEPER POSTERIOR ABDOMINAL MUSCLES

Psoas

This triangular muscle arises from the transverse processes of the lumbar vertebrae, lies on quadratus lumborum and passes across the posterior abdominal wall diagonally inferolaterally to exit under the inguinal ligament and insert into the lesser trochanter of femur. Its nerve supply is from the ventral rami of the first three lumbar nerves.

The Relations of Psoas (Fig. 5.14)

Posteriorly.
- Lumbar arteries and external vertebral venous plexus.

Anteriorly.
- Ureter
- Sympathetic trunk
- Genitofemoral nerve
- Gonadal vessels

Within. Lumbar plexus: the nerves having three main routes of exit:

- Medially: obturator and lumbosacral trunk
- Through the centre: genitofemoral nerve
- Laterally: iliohypogastric, ilioinguinal, femoral, lateral cutaneous nerve of thigh.

PERITONEAL REFLECTIONS

The peritoneum lines the abdomen and its contents and tends to fuse with underlying viscera (serosa) while remaining loosely attached to the internal abdominal wall (parietal peritoneum). With the development of intra-abdominal structures the peritoneum is reflected or folded producing:

- Folds – on the posterior surface of the anterior abdominal wall (where obliterated umbilical vessels and urachus run)
- Mesentery – which are double layers of peritoneum which have been reflected off the dorsal surface of the abdomen by developments of the gut. They include the mesenteries to the small intestine, transverse and sigmoid colons, and the appendix, and they all contain vessels and nerves to supply the gut suspended from them
- The lesser omentum – which connects the stomach to the liver, while the greater omentum hangs down from the stomach lying over the transverse colon, and fusing with its mesentery (Fig. 5.15)
- Ligaments – these double layers of peritoneum are associated with the liver, stomach and spleen, and the uterus (broad ligament).

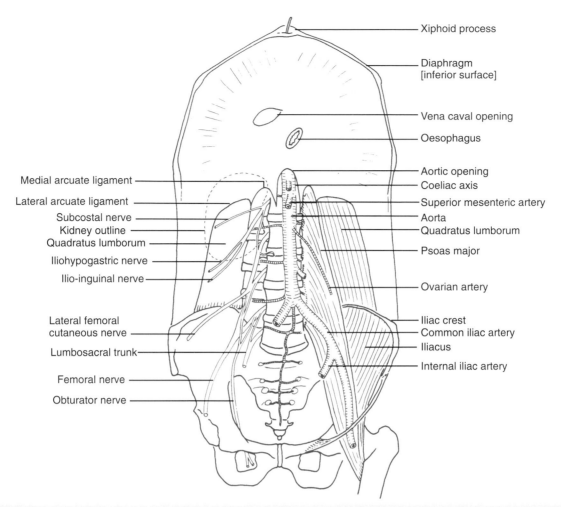

Medial arcuate ligament
Lateral arcuate ligament
Subcostal nerve
Kidney outline
Quadratus lumborum
Iliohypogastric nerve
Ilio-inguinal nerve
Lateral femoral cutaneous nerve
Lumbosacral trunk
Femoral nerve
Obturator nerve

Xiphoid process
Diaphragm [inferior surface]
Vena caval opening
Oesophagus
Aortic opening
Coeliac axis
Superior mesenteric artery
Aorta
Quadratus lumborum
Psoas major
Ovarian artery
Iliac crest
Common iliac artery
Iliacus
Internal iliac artery

Fig. 5.14 The posterior abdominal wall and pelvis showing the relative positions of the muscles, vessels and nerves.

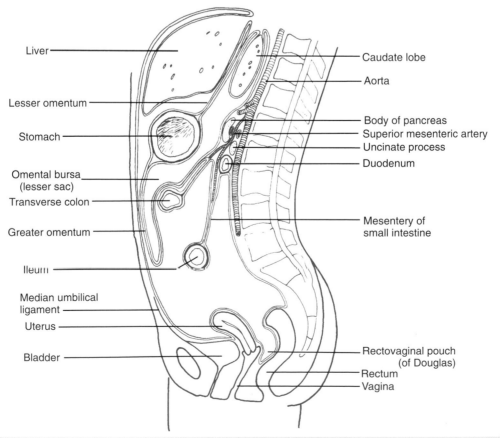

Liver
Lesser omentum
Stomach
Omental bursa (lesser sac)
Transverse colon
Greater omentum
Ileum
Median umbilical ligament
Uterus
Bladder

Caudate lobe
Aorta
Body of pancreas
Superior mesenteric artery
Uncinate process
Duodenum
Mesentery of small intestine
Rectovaginal pouch (of Douglas)
Rectum
Vagina

Fig. 5.15 Longitudinal section through the abdominal cavity illustrating the peritoneal reflections.

The final arrangement of the intra-abdominal structures distinguishes those things which are plastered down by their peritoneal covering (retroperitoneal) from those which are suspended from a mesentery (see Figs. 5.15 and 5.16).

Retroperitoneal Structures (See Fig. 5.16)

- The bare area of the liver
- Duodenum
- Ascending colon
- Descending colon
- Rectum (almost entirely)
- Kidneys and ureter
- Adrenals
- Major vessels (IVC, aorta, iliac)

Clinical Application.

- Structures suspended from a mesentery can twist but the sigmoid volvulus with its narrow base is most prone to this in the abdomen. In the pelvis, testicular torsion is a well-recognised surgical emergency, but ovaries can similarly twist (although this is most commonly associated with ovarian cysts, it can also occur with normal ovaries)
- Aortic compression is rarely needed but is a potentially life-saving manoeuvre in the management of massive post-partum haemorrhage. If the abdomen is already open, the small bowel needs to be pushed up towards the right hypochondrium together with its mesentery and pressure placed on the abdominal aorta just below the mesentery (if the abdomen has not been opened then pressure applied above the forwardly tilted fundus of the uterus at the approximate level of the umbilicus can also be effective)
- If bleeding from vessels within the broad ligament occurs, rather than producing any sort of tamponade the peritoneal layers just peel away and massive haemorrhage can occur relatively silently (concealed bleeding with minimal if any intra-abdominal pain).

THE GREATER AND LESSER SACS

The abdominal cavity comprises the general peritoneal cavity (or greater sac) and the omental bursa (or lesser sac) which lies behind the stomach and its peritoneal attachments (see Fig. 5.15).

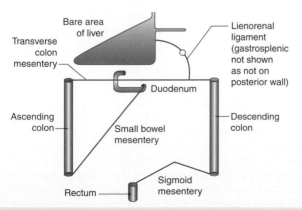

Fig. 5.16 Diagrammatic illustration of the retroperitoneal structures and the position of the roots of the mesenteries produced by the peritoneal reflections off the posterior abdominal wall.

Lesser Sac

Relations of the lesser sac:

Anteriorly.

- The stomach centrally
- Lesser omentum superiorly
- Greater omentum inferiorly
- Gastrosplenic part of greater omentum on left side
- Caudate lobe of liver on right side.

Posteriorly.

- The fused posterior greater omental layer with the transverse mesocolon
- Peritoneum over the neck and body of pancreas
- Left adrenal gland.

Laterally.

- Limited to the left by the lienorenal ligament
- Opens into the greater sac by the epiploic foramen (of Winslow) on right.

The Epiploic Foramen (Fig. 5.17)

This 2.5 cm vertical slit affords communication between the greater and lesser sac. Its borders are:

Superiorly
- The caudate process of the liver.

Inferiorly
- The first part of the duodenum.

Posteriorly
- The IVC.

Anteriorly
- The right free edge of the lesser omentum which contains:
  - the portal vein
  - the hepatic artery
  - the common bile duct
  - autonomic nerves
  - lymphatics and nodes.

The Liver

This is the largest gland in the body weighing approximately 1500 g which forms from an outgrowth of foregut. It develops in the septum transversum and protrudes into the abdomen dividing the ventral mesentery into two: anteriorly the falciform ligament is produced, posteriorly the lesser omentum.

The liver is divided into the larger right lobe and the small left lobe, and between these two on the visceral (inferior) surface lie the quadrate lobe anteriorly and the caudate lobe behind. The porta hepatis lies across this visceral junction between the lobes and comprises from – in front backwards – the common hepatic duct, the hepatic artery and the portal vein.

The Alimentary Tract

The foregut extends from the mouth to the point where the bile duct enters the duodenum. The midgut continues on

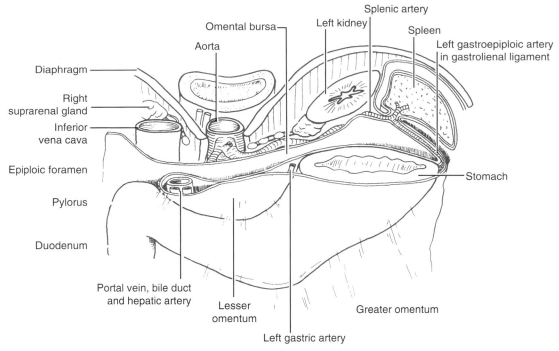

Fig. 5.17 The relations of the lesser sac and the epiploic foramen.

from this point to two-thirds of the way along the transverse colon. The hindgut continues from here to the rectum.

BLOOD SUPPLY TO THE GUT

Blood supply to the gut is directly from the ventral branches of the aorta:

1. *The coeliac axis* supplies the abdominal portion of the foregut. It is surrounded by the sympathetic coeliac plexus and branches almost immediately into the:
   - Left gastric artery which passes left then curves round lesser curve of stomach
   - Common hepatic artery which passes right and gives off the right gastric artery (which anastomoses with the left gastric) and the gastroduodenal artery which divides into the right gastroepiploic artery (which passes round the greater curve of the stomach) and the superior pancreaticoduodenal artery
   - Splenic artery which passes over the pancreas giving off short gastric arteries and then the left gastroepiploic artery which anastomoses with its right namesake.
2. *The superior mesenteric artery* supplies the midgut. It arises behind the body of the pancreas and the splenic vein anterior to the left renal vein and passes inferiorly over the third part of the duodenum towards the root of the small bowel mesentery. Its branches in order are:
   - Inferior pancreaticoduodenal artery
   - Middle colic, right colic and ileocolic
   - Jejunal and ileal branches from within the mesentery.
3. *The inferior mesenteric artery* supplies the hindgut. It arises below the duodenum and passes on the left psoas muscle

inferiorly diagonally across the left infracolic compartment giving off the left colic and sigmoid arteries. It then enters the pelvis crossing the bifurcation of the left common iliac vessels where it lies medial to but is separated from the ureter by the inferior mesenteric vein. It terminates as the superior rectal artery (which anastomoses with the middle rectal from the internal iliac and the inferior rectal from the internal pudendal artery).

Fig. 5.18 shows the relations of these vessels near their origins.

SPECIFIC FEATURES OF NOTE IN THE ALIMENTARY TRACT

Meckel's Diverticulum

A Meckel's diverticulum exists in 2% of the population. This antimesenteric ileal diverticulum occurs about 30 cm proximal to the ileocaecal valve and is usually about 5 cm long. The remains of the vitellointestinal duct may persist as a fibrous band which runs from the tip of the diverticulum to the umbilicus.

The Appendix

The peritoneal attachments have already been described, but although the ascending colon is retroperitoneal the caecum is often freely mobile being covered with peritoneum which has been reflected off the posterior abdominal wall. The vermiform appendix, which arises from the posteromedial aspect of the caecum just distal to the ileocaecal junction, can lie in this retrocaecal recess. The appendix has its own small triangular mesentery (mesoappendix) containing the appendicular vessels, nerves, lymph vessels and often a lymph node (Fig. 5.19).

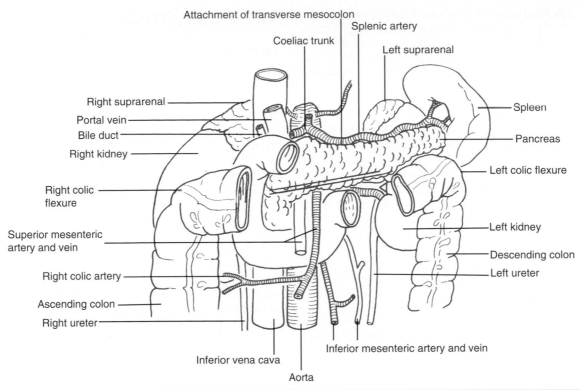

Fig. 5.18 Diagrammatic view of the upper abdominal contents and their relations with the major arteries of the alimentary canal.

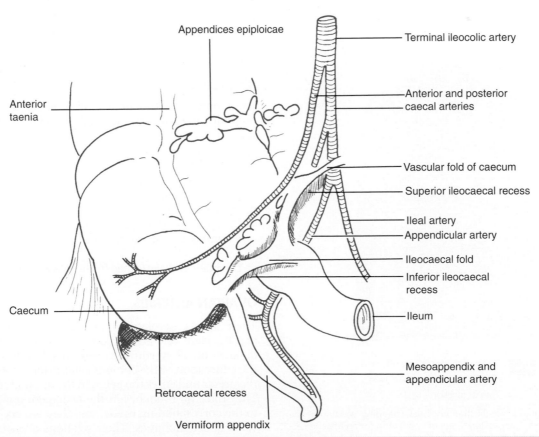

Fig. 5.19 The arrangements of the peritoneal folds and blood supply of the caecum and appendix.

Clinical Applications. Due to the different positions of the appendix, the clinical presentation of acute appendicitis can vary (e.g. retrocaecal is relatively sealed versus the freely mobile appendix which can produce frank intra-abdominal peritonitis). In pregnancy, this is further complicated because:

- Signs can be relatively subtle
- Progression of pathology can be rapid due to the failure of the omentum to 'access' the problem and seal it off.

The upward displacement of the caecum by the gravid uterus can mean that the problem is localised in mid or even upper abdomen. The surgical incision for appendicectomy in pregnancy should therefore be over the point of maximum tenderness (Fig. 5.20).

Retroperitoneal Organs

ADRENAL GLANDS

The medulla originates from neural crest cells (ectoderm) which develop into chromaffin cells that secrete catecholamines, while the larger cortex originates from mesoderm and secretes adrenocortical hormones.

The blood supply comes from branches of the phrenic and renal arteries and a small branch direct from the aorta. Venous drainage is by a single vein which passes into the IVC on the right, and the renal vein on the left. Lymphatic drainage is to the para-aortic nodes.

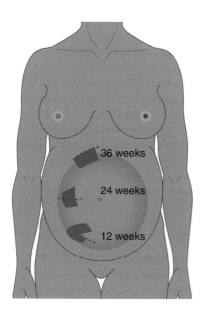

36 weeks

24 weeks

12 weeks

▬ Area of tenderness and maybe rebound tenderness

----- Site of incision

Fig. 5.20 Diagrammatic illustration of the changing position of the appendix (and the approximate site of an incision for an appendicectomy) as pregnancy advances.

The Urinary Tract

KIDNEYS

The kidneys lie on the posterior abdominal wall within fat of the retroperitoneum. They lie between T12 and L3 with the right kidney being slightly lower than the left. The suprarenal glands sit on their superomedial poles. The hilum is a deep vertical slit on the medial aspect transmitting from anterior to posterior the renal vein, renal artery and the renal pelvis, as well as lymphatics and sympathetic nerve fibres.

Papillae of renal tissue indent each of a dozen or so minor calyces where urine drains from the collecting tubules, and these in turn drain into two or three major calyces which drain into the renal pelvis and thence via the ureter to the bladder.

Each kidney receives its blood supply directly from the aorta by means of the paired right and left renal arteries. The right renal artery passes behind the IVC to reach the right kidney. Venous drainage by the accompanying renal veins passes straight into the IVC. The left renal vein is longer than the right passing in front of the aorta below the origin of the superior mesenteric artery to reach the IVC.

Lymphatic drainage passes directly to para-aortic nodes.

URETER: ITS COURSE AND RELATIONS IN THE ABDOMEN

The ureter is retroperitoneal throughout its course extending from hilum of kidney to the bladder with abdominal, pelvic and intravesical portions. In the abdomen, it passes inferiorly from the renal pelvis on the medial border of psoas (in line with the tips of the transverse processes of L2–5) to enter the pelvis anterior to the common iliac bifurcation in front of the sacroiliac joint.

Blood Supply

As it descends, the ureter takes its supply from small branches, in turn from the renal, gonadal, internal iliac and inferior vesical vessels.

Nerve Supply

- Sympathetic via T10–12 (renal, aortic, superior hypogastric plexuses)
- Parasympathetic via S2–4
- Lymphatic drainage includes internal, external and common iliac and para-aortic nodes.

The bladder is described in the pelvic section.

OVARIAN ARTERIES

These arise anterolaterally just below the renal branches and the right one passes posterior to the third part of the duodenum. They run retroperitoneally inferiorly towards the bifurcation of the common iliac artery where they cross the ureter and enter the pelvis in the infundibulopelvic fold. They have no branches in the abdomen, but supply twigs to the corresponding ureter, and they are accompanied by veins and lymphatics. Their relations are summarised in Table 5.4.

Table 5.4 The Relations of the Ovarian Arteries	
The right artery crosses the inferior vena cava and is crossed by:	The left artery is crossed by:
▪ The middle colic vessels ▪ The caecal vein ▪ Terminal ileal vein ▪ Ileocolic vein	▪ The left colic and sigmoid branches of the inferior mesenteric vessels ▪ The descending colon
The right veins drain into the inferior vena cava	The left vein ends in the left renal vein

The Common Iliac Arteries

The common iliac arteries lie retroperitoneally anterior to the common iliac veins and the sympathetic trunk on the psoas muscles. The left artery is crossed by the superior rectal vessels and both are crossed by the ureter as they divide into internal and external iliac arteries (see Fig. 5.22). The latter are crossed near their origin by the ovarian vessels and then by the genital branch of the genitofemoral nerve, the deep circumflex iliac vein and the round ligament before passing under the inguinal ligament to become the femoral artery.

The Inferior Epigastric and Deep Circumflex Iliac Arteries

The inferior epigastric and deep circumflex iliac arteries arise immediately above the inguinal ligament before the external iliac becomes the femoral artery. The inferior epigastric artery passes up and medially behind the conjoint tendon to run deep to the rectus abdominis muscle to enter the rectus sheath and anastomose with the superior epigastric artery (a terminal branch of the internal thoracic). The deep circumflex iliac artery runs laterally up to the anterior superior iliac spine and thence along the crest.

The Femoral Vessels

The femoral vessels have four cutaneous branches arising just below the inguinal ligament:

▪ *Superficial circumflex iliac* (runs upwards deep to the inguinal ligament to anastomose at the anterior superior iliac spine)
▪ *Superficial epigastric* (passes superficial to the inguinal ligament to run towards the umbilicus)
▪ *Superficial external pudendal* (passes medially anterior to the round ligament to supply the labium majus)
▪ *Deep external pudendal* (passes medially behind the round ligament to supply the labium majus).

There are accompanying veins of the same names which drain into the great (long) saphenous vein, which in turn drains into the femoral vein approximately 3 cm inferolateral to the pubic tubercle.

LUMBAR PLEXUS

Fig. 5.21 illustrates the lumbar plexus which involves the anterior primary rami from L1 to L5, and Fig. 5.14 illustrates its anatomical relations on the posterior abdominal wall.

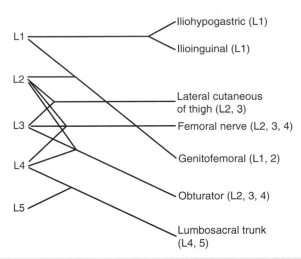

Fig. 5.21 The lumbar plexus represented diagrammatically as it forms from the anterior primary rami of the lumbar nerve roots.

This plexus forms in the substance of the psoas major muscle and all except the subcostal nerve emerge to lie on quadratus lumborum underneath the anterior lumbar fascia. All nerves emerge from the lateral border of psoas except:

▪ The genitofemoral nerve which emerges anteriorly
▪ The obturator nerve and the lumbosacral trunk which emerge medially.

The lumbar plexus supplies:

▪ The thigh muscles
▪ Sensory to the parietal peritoneum
▪ Anterior abdominal wall (via iliohypogastric and ilioinguinal).

Iliohypogastric and Ilioinguinal Nerves

The iliohypogastric and ilioinguinal nerves pass from the lateral border of psoas anterior to quadratus lumborum behind the kidney. Both perforate the transversus aponeurosis to run between that and the internal oblique, giving off lateral cutaneous branches and ending as cutaneous branches: the iliohypogastric terminating above the pubis, the ilioinguinal, running at a lower level, passing via the inguinal canal to the mons and labium majus.

Genitofemoral Nerve

The genitofemoral nerve pierces the psoas anteriorly to run retroperitoneally on its anterior surface behind the ureter. Its genital branch passes through the deep ring to enter the inguinal canal, while the femoral branch runs on the external iliac artery to pass beneath the inguinal ligament to enter the femoral sheath, which it pierces to supply the skin over the femoral triangle. Its relations are summarised in Table 5.5.

Lateral Cutaneous Nerve of the Thigh

The lateral cutaneous nerve of the thigh pierces the inguinal ligament just medial to the anterior superior spine.

Femoral Nerve

The femoral nerve (L2–L4) emerges from the psoas to run in the gutter between it and iliacus deep to the iliac fascia and supplying both muscles. It passes behind the inguinal ligament lateral to the femoral artery into the thigh to supply the quadriceps muscles and overlying skin.

Obturator Nerve

The obturator nerve emerges medial to psoas at the pelvic brim and passes under the internal iliac vessels on obturator internus to continue along the side wall of the pelvis to the obturator foramen which it passes through above the obturator vessels to supply the adductor compartment of the thigh and both the hip and the knee.

Lumbosacral Trunk

The lumbosacral trunk (L4, 5) emerges from the medial border of psoas, crosses the ala of the sacrum, the sacroiliac joint and the upper border of piriformis where it joins S1.

Clinical Applications

- The lateral cutaneous nerve of the thigh can be vulnerable to a nerve entrapment syndrome (like carpal tunnel) as it pierces the inguinal ligament due to oedema in pregnancy
- The obturator nerve, separated from the normally situated ovary only by peritoneum, can be irritated by ovarian pathology causing referred pain down the inside of the thigh (Fig. 5.22).

The Pelvis

SURFACE ANATOMY

Bilateral dimples above the buttocks

- Centre of the sacroiliac joint
- Posterior superior iliac spine

Table 5.5 Structures Which Cross the Genitofemoral Nerve

Right	Left
Ureter	Ureter
Gonadal vessels	Gonadal vessels
Ileocolic artery	Left inferior colic artery
Mesentery of the small intestine	Inferior mesenteric vein
Right infracolic compartment	Left infracolic compartment

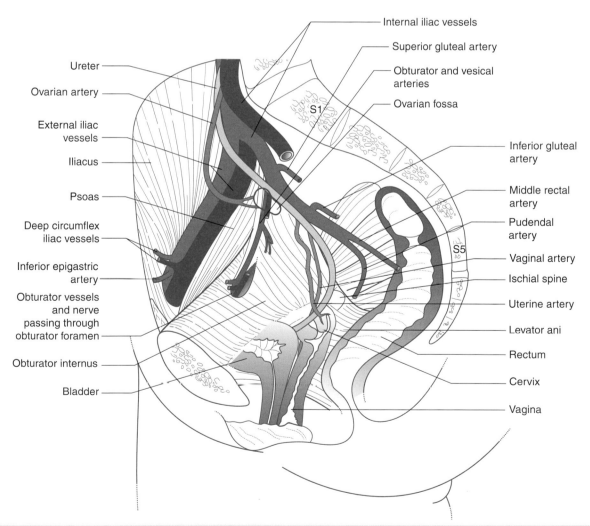

Fig. 5.22 The side wall of the female pelvis showing the course and relations of the ureter, vessels, nerves and the ovarian fossa.

- Level of S2
- Level of the end of the dural canal and of the spinal meninges.

Relations of the Sacroiliac Joint
- Psoas muscle/tendon
- Genitofemoral nerve
- Common iliac bifurcation
- Ureter
- Inferior mesenteric artery and apex of sigmoid mesocolon on the left
- Iliac branches of iliolumbar artery.

BLOOD SUPPLY TO THE PELVIS (SEE FIG. 5.22)

For descriptive purposes the arterial tree is described, but the venous drainage mirrors this pattern.

Internal Iliac Artery

The internal iliac artery passes into the pelvis between the internal iliac vein and the ureter, to divide into posterior and anterior divisions at the upper margin of the greater sciatic foramen. The posterior trunk has three branches which are all parietal: the ascending iliolumbar and the lateral sacral branch off before the largest superior gluteal artery passes with the superior gluteal nerve through the greater sciatic foramen above piriformis to supply the buttock.

Anterior Trunk

The anterior trunk continues towards the ischial spine and has nine branches:

1. Three vesical:
   - The superior vesical (supplies the lower ureter and upper bladder)
   - This continues as the obliterated umbilical artery (medial umbilical ligament) to the umbilicus
   - The inferior vesical artery (supplies the ureter and base of the bladder).
2. Three other visceral:
   - The middle rectal (supplies muscle of the lower rectum)
   - Vaginal arteries
   - The uterine artery – passes medially in the base of the broad ligament where it crosses the ureter to reach the cervix from where it passes upwards in the broad ligament to supply the uterus and tube ending by anastomosing with the tubal branch of the ovarian artery.
3. Three parietal branches:
   - The obturator artery runs with its nerve (above) and vein (below) to the obturator foramen
   - The internal pudendal artery passes out of the pelvis through the greater sciatic foramen below piriformis to curve round the ischial spine to enter the perineum through the lesser sciatic foramen and pudendal canal
   - The inferior gluteal artery passes out of the pelvis to the buttock below piriformis through the greater sciatic foramen.

Sacral Plexus

Forms on piriformis and converges and divides on route to the greater sciatic foramen.

Posterior Divisions.
- Superior gluteal (L4–5, S1) ⎫
- Inferior gluteal (L5, S1–2) ⎪ *These supply the extensor compartment of the lower limb*
- Common peroneal part of sciatic (L4–5, S1–2) ⎬
- Posterior cutaneous nerve of thigh (S1–3) ⎪
- Perforating cutaneous nerve (S2–3)   *(goes through the sacrotuberous ligament)*
- Piriformis (S2).

Anterior Divisions.
- Tibial component of sciatic (L4–5, S1–3) ⎫ *These supply the flexor compartment of the lower limb*
- Nerve to quadratus femoris (L4–5, S1) ⎬
- Nerve to obturator internus (L5, S12) ⎭
- Pudendal nerve (S2–4)
- Perineal branch of S4
- Parasympathetic visceral S2–4 pelvic splanchnics (nervi erigentes).

MUSCLES OF THE PELVIS

These comprise two groups:

1. Those of the lower limb (piriformis and obturator internus).
2. The pelvic floor (pelvic diaphragm and the superficial muscles).

Pelvic Muscles of the Lower Limb

Piriformis. Piriformis arises from the lateral mass of the middle three sections of sacrum. The sacral plexus lies on it as it passes transversely leaving the pelvis through the greater sciatic foramen to enter the buttock and then insert into the greater trochanter. It serves to help stabilise the hip and is innervated by its named nerve from the posterior division of the sacral plexus.

Obturator Internus. Obturator internus arises from the inner surface of most of the anterolateral wall of the pelvis including the thick membrane which covers most of the obturator foramen. This fan-like muscle then converges into a tendon which passes out of the pelvis into the buttock through the lesser sciatic foramen to insert into the greater trochanter. It is innervated by its named nerve from the anterior division of the sacral plexus.

Pelvic Diaphragm

The floor of the pelvis (Fig. 5.23), the pelvic diaphragm, is a muscular sling supporting the pelvic contents and exerting sphincteric actions on the rectum and vagina which pass through it. Its deep aspect relates to the pelvic viscera, while superficially its perineal aspect forms the inner wall of the ischiorectal fossa (see Fig. 5.25). It arises from the:

- Body of the pubis
- Ischial spines
- Fascia over obturator internus.

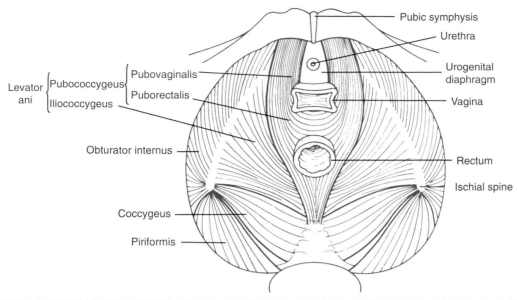

Fig. 5.23 View of the pelvic floor from above.

Levator Ani

The levator ani is comprised of two parts:

Pubococcygeus. This arises from the pubis and anterior half of the 'white line' obturator internus fascia in front of the obturator canal. It has three parts:

1. The more posterior fibres insert into the coccyx and anococcygeal raphe.
2. More anterior fibres sling around the rectum producing puborectalis (no raphe).
3. Anterior fibres insert into the perineal body producing pubovaginalis/levator prostate.

Iliococcygeus. Arises from the posterior half of the 'white line' fascia over obturator internus and some ischium and inserts into the anococcygeal body and raphe and the coccyx.

Coccygeus has the same attachments as the sacrospinatous ligament – this degenerating muscle used to wag the tail.

The Perineum (Fig. 5.24)

UROGENITAL TRIANGLE

The anterior perineum (urogenital triangle) lies superficial to the anterior pelvic diaphragm and is bordered by a line joining the ischial tuberosities (this passes just anterior to the anus) and ischiopubic rami.

The perineal membrane is a tough fascia sheet which attaches to the sides of this triangle and is penetrated by the urethra and by the vagina in the female. The space between this membrane and the levator ani comprises the deep perineal pouch, which contains the:

- External urethral sphincter
- Deep transverse perineal muscles
- The glands of Cowper (in the male)
- Areolar tissue.

The superficial perineal pouch exists superficial to the perineal membrane and contains:

- Bulbospongiosus muscle (pierced by the vagina with the Bartholin's glands in the female, and surrounding the corpus spongiosum in the male)
- Ischiocavernosus muscles
- Superficial transverse perineal muscle.

PERINEAL BODY

The perineal body is a fibromuscular pyramid-shaped mass (base inferiorly) which lies in the midline at the junction of anterior and posterior perineum separating the lower vagina from the anal canal and is the point of attachment for:

- The external anal sphincter
- Bulbospongiosus
- Transverse perineal muscles (superficial and deep)
- Pubococcygeal fibres of the levator ani.

ANAL TRIANGLE

The posterior perineum (anal triangle) lies between the ischial tuberosities and the coccyx and comprises:

- The anus and its sphincters
- The levator ani
- The ischiorectal fossae.

The Ischiorectal Fossae (Fig. 5.25)

The ischiorectal fossae occur bilaterally but communicate posteriorly behind the rectum with each other. Their borders are as follows:

- Superficially, skin
- Anteriorly, the anterior perineum
- Posteriorly, the sacrotuberous ligament and gluteus maximus

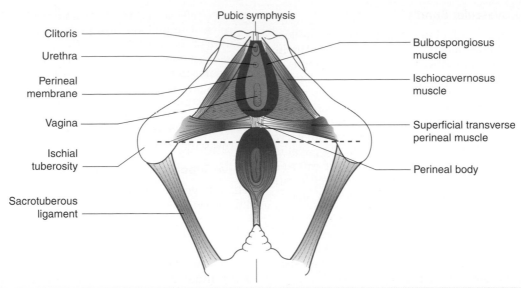

Fig. 5.24 Diagrammatic representation of the perineum showing the urogenital triangle (anterior to the ischial tuberosities) and the anal triangle (posteriorly) and the arrangements of the superficial muscles.

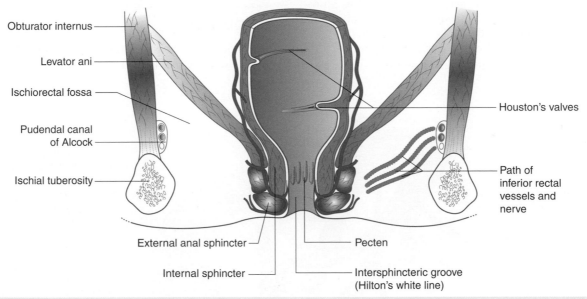

Fig. 5.25 Illustration of the relations of the ischiorectal fossae and a coronal section of the rectum and anal canal.

- Medially, the fascia over levator ani and the external anal sphincter
- Laterally, the ischial tuberosity with obturator internus and its fascia which contains the pudendal canal (of Alcock) with the pudendal vessels and nerve.

Contents:

- Ischiorectal pad of fat
- Pudendal canal (laterally)
- Transversely, the inferior rectal vessels/nerves (pudendal branches)
- Posteriorly, perineal branch S4 and perforating cutaneous nerve.

Clinical Application

- Vaginal delivery can cause trauma in this area with haemorrhage which can be concealed – beware of pain out of proportion to the apparent level of injury sustained and examine carefully for fullness and tension which can be felt through the skin between anus and ischial tuberosity, or through vaginal deviation anteriorly towards contralateral side
- Such haemorrhage can be exceedingly difficult to identify and staunch, and vaginal packing and/or embolisation may be needed
- As these spaces are essentially full of fat they are vulnerable to infection which can pass from one side to the other.

Pudendal Neurovascular Bundle

The pudendal neurovascular bundle supplies the pelvic floor and perineum. The pudendal nerve (S2–4) lies medial to the internal pudendal artery as they exit the pelvis through the greater sciatic foramen, curving round the sacrospinous ligament to re-enter the pelvis through the lesser sciatic foramen, and thence run medial to the ischial tuberosity on the fascial thickening over obturator internus (the pudendal canal) to the deep perineal pouch. The inferior rectal nerve and artery branch off at the posterior end of the canal to travel through the ischiorectal fossa to supply the external anal sphincter, anal canal and perianal skin. Thence, the neurovascular bundle continues anteriorly to pass superficially into the urogenital region giving off:

- Perineal branches (supplying skin of the posterior two-thirds of vulva [scrotum] and mucous membranes of urethra and vagina and supplying the perineal muscles of the deep and superficial perineal pouches)
- Dorsal nerve and dorsal and deep artery to the clitoris (penis).

Clinical Application

- Pudendal nerve block is carried out by guiding a protected needle through the vagina and palpating the ischial spine. The needle is then inserted just behind the spine and withdrawn to check a vessel has not been entered before injecting the local anaesthetic. A good test of efficacy is loss of the anal reflex, relaxation of the pelvic floor and loss of sensation to the vulva and lower third of the vagina (Fig. 5.26).
- Sacrospinous fixation for recurrent vault prolapse secures the vaginal vault to either one or both sacrospinous processes. The ligament is identified after reflecting the rectum away and burrowing across the ischiorectal fossa digitally. It is then grasped approximately 2 cm posteromedially from the spine to avoid damage to the neurovascular bundle.

Nerve Supply to the Pelvic Floor

This is largely the pudendal nerve (S2–4) as described above but also includes:

- Perineal branch of S4 (passes through between coccygeus and iliococcygeus to supply the skin over the ischiorectal fossa)
- Obturator nerve (L2–4) L3 fibres supply the pelvic peritoneum explaining referred pain to the thigh.

Lateral Pelvic Wall

PELVIC URETER

The pelvic ureter crosses over the common iliac bifurcation to enter the pelvis and passes round the lateral wall

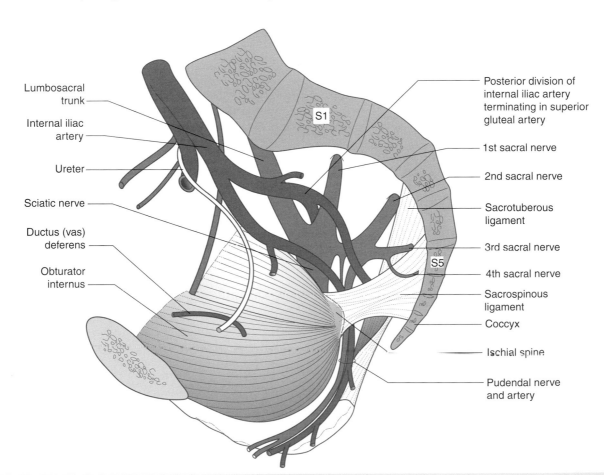

Lumbosacral trunk

Internal iliac artery

Ureter

Sciatic nerve

Ductus (vas) deferens

Obturator internus

Posterior division of internal iliac artery terminating in superior gluteal artery

1st sacral nerve

2nd sacral nerve

Sacrotuberous ligament

3rd sacral nerve

4th sacral nerve

Sacrospinous ligament

Coccyx

Ischial spine

Pudendal nerve and artery

S1

S5

Fig. 5.26 The side wall of the pelvis showing the relative positions of nerves and vessels and highlighting the course of the pudendal neurovascular bundle.

anterior to the internal iliac artery crossing the superior vesical vessels, lying in close proximity to the obturator nerve, and passing just lateral to the base of the infundibulopelvic fold (suspensory ligament of the ovary). Once it reaches the ischial spine it turns anteromedially to pass above the lateral fornix of the vagina, lateral to the cervix and below the broad ligament and the uterine vessels, to enter the bladder. In either sex, the ureter is crossed by only one structure through its course in the pelvis: the vas in the male, and the uterine artery in the female (see Figs. 5.22 and 5.26; Tables 5.6 and 5.7).

Table 5.6 Relations of the Ureters

Right Ureter	Left Ureter
Lies behind the second part of the duodenum	
In the abdomen is crossed by:	
■ Ovarian (or testicular) vessels	■ Ovarian (or testicular) vessels
■ Right colic vessels	■ Left colic vessels
■ Ileocolic vessels	■ Mesosigmoid
In the pelvis is crossed by:	
■ Vas deferens in the male	■ Vas deferens in the male
■ Uterine vessels in the female	■ Uterine vessels in the female

Table 5.7 The Relations of the Ductus Deferens and Ureter on the Pelvic Side Wall

Ductus Deferens Crosses	Ureter Crosses
External iliac artery	External iliac artery
External iliac vein	External iliac vein
Obliterated umbilical artery	Obturator nerve
Obturator nerve	Superior vesical artery
Obturator artery	Obturator artery
Obturator vein	Obturator vein

Pelvic Organs

OVARY

Each oval gland is approximately $2 \times 3 \times 4$ cm weighing approximately 8 g during adult reproductive life. The long axis lies vertically with the infundibulopelvic fold suspended off the upper pole with the ovarian ligament connecting the lower pole to the uterine cornu. The mesovarium from the posterior aspect of the broad ligament supplies the ovary anteriorly and its posterior border lies free. Laterally, the peritoneum lines the ovarian fossa on the lateral pelvic wall adjacent to (Fig. 5.27):

- The bifurcation of the common iliac artery above
- The ureter and the internal iliac artery and vein behind
- The obturator vessels and nerve laterally
- The ampulla of the uterine tube (curls round the top of the ovary so the ostium and fimbriae come to lie on its medial surface)
- Coils of ileum and, on the right side, the appendix.

Histology

This varies with age and the time in the sexual cycle, but the ovary has an inner medulla of loose connective tissue (blood vessels, lymphatics and nerves), while the outer cortex contains richly nucleated connective tissue stroma and follicles. The germinal epithelium covers the cortex and the dense collagenous tunica albuginea lies underneath.

At birth, there are about 2 million primordial follicles, each containing an oocyte, but follicular degeneration continues throughout life (approximately 300,000 follicles exist in a pre-pubertal girl) until the menopause, by which time no follicles remain. Each month throughout sexual life a follicle matures to become a Graafian or vesicular follicle reaching up to 2 cm in diameter. Following ovulation the follicle collapses, the granulosa cells enlarge and multiply taking on a yellow pigment, lutein and fatty material, to form the corpus luteum which persists in the event of

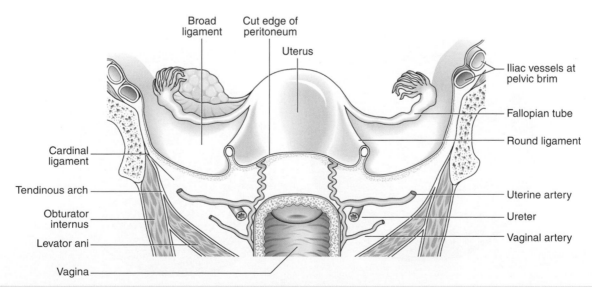

Fig. 5.27 Coronal section through the female pelvis viewed from in front illustrating the ovarian relations to the broad ligament and tube and highlighting the relations of the uterine and vaginal vessels with the ureter lateral to the upper vagina and cervix.

fertilisation for a few months. In the absence of fertilisation, the corpus luteum functions for just under 2 weeks before degenerating to form a pale corpus albicans.

FALLOPIAN TUBE (OVIDUCT)

These fibromuscular cylinders suspend the broad ligament which forms their mesentery (mesosalpinx). Medially they open into the uterus at the uterine ostia and the thin intramural portion of the tube passing through the uterine wall continues for approximately 3 cm before expanding a little into the isthmus of the tube which is a similar length. Then the tube expands into a wide and long ampulla which becomes the infundibulum opening into the peritoneal cavity at the abdominal ostia surrounded by finger-like fimbria (Fig. 5.28).

Histology

A muscular coat (inner circular and outer longitudinal smooth muscle) surrounds a folded mucous membrane. The epithelial lining cells are low columnar but they are increasingly ciliated laterally (Fig. 5.29).

UTERUS

This pear-shaped organ weighs approximately 50 g and measures approximately $8 \times 5 \times 3$ cm in adulthood (see Figs. 5.27 and 5.28). Its walls are 1 to 2 cm thick surrounding the triangular endometrial cavity whose anterior and posterior walls lie in close apposition. The whole uterus grows in pregnancy but a notable development occurs in the second half of pregnancy where the upper portion of the cervix expands upwards to accommodate the growing

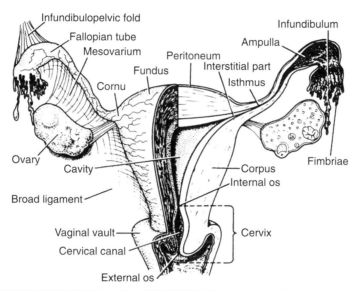

Fig. 5.28 Posterior view of the uterus and its relations.

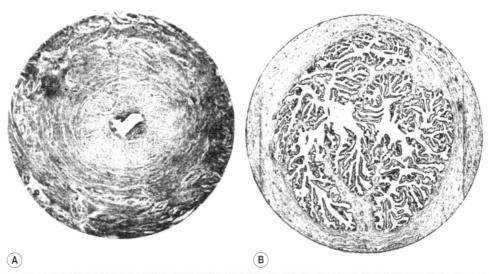

Fig. 5.29 Sections through the fallopian tube: (A) through the isthmus, (B) through the ampulla.

pregnancy and becomes the lower segment of the uterus, while the body of the uterus becomes the upper segment.

Relations of the uterus (see Fig. 5.15) are:

- Anteriorly the peritoneum is reflected from the bladder to the front of the uterus at the level of the isthmus (the junction of the cervix and uterine body) to form the uterovesical pouch. It is loosely attached to the uterus inferiorly for about 1 cm, but above this level, as with serosal peritoneum elsewhere, it is firmly adherent to the underlying organ
- Laterally the double layer of peritoneum raised by the uterine covering bilaterally produces the broad ligaments which extend to the pelvic side walls each containing a fallopian tube, round ligament and ovarian ligament. At the base of the broad ligaments the extraperitoneal adipose tissue (the pelvic cellular tissue) lying lateral to the vaginal vault and cervix forms the parametrium
- Posteriorly the peritoneum remains adherent as it passes down to cover the back of the cervix and the posterior aspect of the upper quarter of the vagina. It is then reflected onto the anterior aspect of the rectum, forming the recto-uterine pouch of Douglas.

Blood supply to the uterus comes from the uterine arteries while venous drainage is by means of a plexus of uterine veins which pass below the artery in the base of each broad ligament to communicate with the vesical and rectal venous plexuses before passing into the internal iliac veins.

Lymphatic drainage from the cervix and lower uterus passes to external and internal iliac and obturator nodes, the upper uterus drains to the para-aortic nodes, and the region of the cornua and round ligament drain to the superficial inguinal nodes (Fig. 5.30).

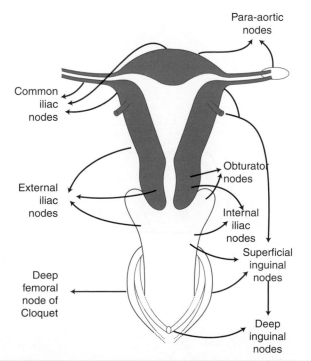

Fig. 5.30 Diagrammatic illustration of the lymphatic drainage patterns of the female genital organs.

The nerve supply to the uterus is sympathetic vasoconstrictor (T10–11) from the inferior hypogastric plexus. Pain fibres from the upper cervix and body of the uterus pass with these while pain from the cervix passes with the pelvic splanchnics.

Uterine Supports

The normal uterus is anteverted (tilted forwards on the vagina) and anteflexed (bent forwards at the isthmus) but mobile with its axis at right angles to the vagina and the cervix at the level of the ischial spines.

The Round Ligament. The round ligament arises from the body of the uterus anteroinferior to the cornua and runs laterally between the layers of the broad ligament across psoas and the external iliac vessels to pass through the deep inguinal ring and the inguinal canal to the labium majus. It is largely fibrous but has some smooth muscle fibres medially (from the uterus) and some striated fibres laterally (from the internal oblique and transversalis muscles). These latter fibres correspond to the cremaster muscle in the male.

Ligaments Formed From Pelvic Fascia. Musculofibrous bands form from condensed connective tissue over the levator ani muscles and insert into the cervix and upper vagina to form important supports to the bladder, uterus, vagina and rectum.

- The pubocervical ligament arises from fascia over the pubic bones and passes around the bladder neck
- The transverse cervical (cardinal) ligaments arise from the arcuate line on the pelvic side wall
- The uterosacral ligaments, which arise from the second sacral vertebra, are almost vertical when the woman is standing upright. As such, they pull the cervix backwards which not only supports the uterus and vagina but maintains the uterus in an anteverted position.

Clinical Applications

- The upper limit of freely mobile peritoneum on the anterior surface of the uterus is a good reliable landmark identifying the junction of lower and upper segments of the uterus at caesarean section
- Lateral to the inferior portion of the cervix, the ureter lies under the uterine vessels as it passes forwards and medially to enter the bladder. As it is within 1 to 2 cm of the lateral vaginal fornix, care must be taken to identify, reflect and avoid damage to it at hysterectomy (see Fig. 5.27)
- In the fetus, the round ligament is surrounded by a tube of peritoneum, the processus vaginalis, which is usually obliterated at birth, but may remain patent as the canal of Nuck, the rare indirect inguinal hernia in females.

Histology

The uterus may be divided into the body of the uterus and the uterine cervix. In the body of the uterus the myometrium consists of smooth muscle fibres held together by connective tissue with blood vessels and lymphatics throughout. In pregnancy there is hyperplasia and hypertrophy of the muscle fibres but as the pregnancy grows the uterus stretches and the wall actually gets thinner.

The endometrium is in constant flux:

- Permanent thin basement membrane left after menstruation
- Regeneration by proliferation due to the influence of oestrogen
- By midcycle, endometrium thickness is 2 to 3 mm (columnar epithelial cells invaginate into the endometrial stroma forming tubules or glands which reach the myometrium and remain after menstruation giving rise to a basal layer from which re-epithelialisation may occur)
- The secretory phase follows under the influence of progesterone (from the corpus luteum), which thickens the endometrium further (approx. 6 mm). The glands become increasingly elongated, tortuous and sacculated and the spiral arterioles are in abundance
- Ischaemia followed by necrosis results in the endometrium shedding
- If pregnancy occurs, menstruation does not take place and the endometrium continues to thicken (10 to 12 mm). The secretory changes continue and stroma cells are converted into large glycogen-laden decidual cells
- After the menopause the endometrium is thin and atrophic.

The cervix is largely fibrous but there is smooth muscle encircling the cervix with an outer longitudinal layer. The mucosa is of tall columnar cells which meet the stratified squamous epithelium at the external os.

THE VAGINA

This fibromuscular tube passes up and back from the vestibule to the cervix and lies at right angles to the axis of the uterus. Like the endometrial cavity, its anterior and posterior walls lie in apposition, with the posterior wall being slightly longer. As the cervix projects into the apex of the vagina, the resultant pockets produce the anterior, posterior and two lateral fornices.

Relations

The anterior vaginal wall lies adjacent to the bladder base, the termination of the ureters and, in its lower two-thirds, to the urethra. The posterior wall is covered by peritoneum in its upper portion, its middle third is separated from the rectum by the rectovaginal septum, while its lower third is separated from the anal canal by the perineal body. At the junction of the middle and lower third of the vagina the levator ani muscles blend with the lateral vaginal walls.

Blood supply to the upper two-thirds is supplied by the uterine and vaginal branches of the internal iliac arteries while the lower one-third is supplied by the perineal artery and dorsal artery of the clitoris which are both branches of the pudendal artery.

The venous drainage consists of an interconnecting venous plexus which follows the course of the arteries draining back into the internal iliac veins.

Lymphatic drainage occurs in three ways: its upper third drains with the cervix (to internal and external iliacs and obturator), its middle third drains to the internal iliac nodes, and its lower third drains with the vulva and perineum to the superficial inguinal nodes (see Fig. 5.30).

Histology

The vagina is lined by a non-keratinised stratified squamous epithelium which is surrounded by smooth muscle and then fibrous tissue containing erectile venous plexuses, nerves and lymphatics. There are no muscularis mucosae and no glands.

THE VULVA

The vulva (Fig. 5.31) is comprised of fatty folds covered by skin: the labia majora lie externally and contain hair follicles, sebaceous and apocrine (modified sweat) glands, while the smaller labia minora are similar (except they are devoid of adipose tissue and contain no hair follicles) and meet anteriorly to form a prepuce over the clitoris.

The vestibule describes the area between the clitoris anteriorly, the labia minora laterally, the fourchette posteriorly and the hymen superiorly. The urethra opens into its anterior portion with the para- and peri-urethral ducts of Skene. Posteriorly is the vaginal introitus with the ducts of the greater vestibular glands of Bartholin opening at 5 and 7 o'clock posterolaterally. These mucoid alkaline secreting glands of Bartholin are arranged as lobules and consist of alveoli lined by cuboidal or columnar epithelium.

The clitoris consists of two small erectile corpora cavernosa which terminate in the sensitive glans. They are attached to the medial aspects of the ischiopubic rami. The bulbospongiosus muscles lie deep to the labia and insert into the dorsum of the clitoris. They are surrounded by erectile tissue at the sides of the vestibule (the bulb of the vestibule).

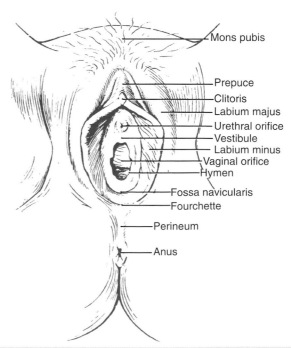

Fig. 5.31 Diagrammatic representation of the vulva.

The blood supply is via the internal and external pudendal arteries, while venous drainage is from an extensive plexus draining to surrounding areas.

The lymphatic drainage includes superficial and anterior areas draining to the superficial inguinal nodes and the lymph node of Cloquet, and posterior and deeper areas draining via the inferior rectal plexus to the internal iliacs (see Fig. 5.30). *The nerve supply* is from the iliohypogastric and ilioinguinal nerves (mons and labia majora) and branches of the pudendal nerve.

The nerve supply is from the iliohypogastric and ilioinguinal nerves (mons and labia majora) and branches of the pudendal nerve.

The Rectum

This segment of large bowel continues on from the sigmoid colon in front of the third sacral vertebrae and ends in the anal canal being approximately 15 cm long. The rectum descends following the sacral curve but has an acute angulation in its midportion produced by the muscle sling of puborectalis, which divides it into two anteroposterior curves, and it also has three lateral curves producing small folds in the canal (valves of Houston). It lies behind the middle third of the vagina from which it is separated by the rectovaginal septum. Like the large bowel, it is lined by columnar mucosa and has an outer longitudinal and an inner circular layer of smooth muscle but, unlike the rest of the large intestine, has no taeniae or appendices epiploicae.

The rectum is largely retroperitoneal: in its upper third it is covered with peritoneum anterolaterally, in its middle third it is covered anteriorly, while in its lower third it lies below the level of the peritoneum (see Fig. 5.25).

RELATIONS OF THE RECTUM

- Posteriorly lie the sacrum and coccyx with the middle sacral vessels and lower sacral nerves
- Anterosuperiorly the pouch of Douglas usually contains loops of small bowel or sigmoid colon
- Anteroinferiorly the fascia of Denonvilliers separates it from the vagina (or prostate and bladder in the male)
- Laterally it is supported by the levator ani.

Blood supply and venous drainage are via the superior (inferior mesenteric), middle (internal iliac) and inferior (internal pudendal) rectal vessels which all anastomose freely.

Lymphatic drainage is mostly upwards via the pararectal nodes and thence along the inferior mesenteric vessels to the pre-aortic nodes, but the lower rectum drains to the internal iliac nodes (via the middle and inferior rectal vessels).

Clinical Application

In obstetric injury when a fourth-degree perineal tear has occurred, the important feature to distinguish is whether the height of the anorectal mucosa tear extends above the pelvic floor. Puborectalis is the obvious sling that can normally be felt on rectal examination, which causes the acute angulation of the rectoanal junction, but this can be disrupted during parturition, or the pelvic floor can be relaxed by regional anaesthesia, making assessment more difficult. If the damage extends beyond this level, peritoneal contamination may occur and a coloproctologist should be called in for help as a defunctioning colostomy may be needed.

The Anal Canal

The anal canal (see Fig. 5.25) is the terminal part of the alimentary canal and is 4 cm long. Its internal sphincter is an expanded portion of the circular layer of smooth muscle of rectum and involuntary while the external sphincter is a continuation of the striated voluntary levator ani muscle. The puborectalis sling produced by the levator ani which produces an acute angle in the rectum is important in continence.

The conjoint longitudinal coat is a continuation of longitudinal smooth muscle which becomes fibrous and separates external from internal sphincter attaching to the intersphincteric groove (Hilton's white line).

The upper third of the anal canal is occupied by:

- Anal columns (ridges of mucous membrane covering venous channels)
- Anal valves (connect columns of anastomosing veins)
- Anal sinuses where mucous glands open.

The pectinate line is level with the anal valves, while the pecten is the smooth part of the anal canal. The mucosa below this gradually changes from columnar to squamous epithelium which becomes keratinised and pigmented at the anal orifice, where it also contains hairs, sebaceous and sweat glands.

Arterial blood supply to the anus is from the superior rectal artery above and down to the level of the intersphincteric groove, and from the inferior rectal artery (from the pudendal artery) below this. The middle rectal and the median sacral arteries supply muscle layers.

Venous drainage follows the arterial pattern but unlike the arterial supply communicates widely, together providing portosystemic communications.

Lymphatic drainage above the intersphincteric groove is to the rectum; below the groove drainage is to the superficial inguinal nodes.

Nerve supply to the external (voluntary) sphincter is via the inferior rectal branch of pudendal nerve. The internal sphincter (involuntary smooth muscle) has a sympathetic nerve supply from the inferior hypogastric plexus (contracting the internal sphincter) and has a parasympathetic supply from nervi erigentes (relaxing it).

The Bladder

This acts as a reservoir for urine (normal capacity 500 mL) and is best visualised as the bow of a boat (see Fig. 5.22). It has inferolateral surfaces, is relatively sharp anteriorly (with the urachus attached from it – medial umbilical ligament), a superior surface (closely adherent to parietal peritoneum), and a flat posterior vertical surface referred to as its base. The lowest portion of the base is the trigone which is a smooth triangular area whose three points include the two ureters superiorly and the urethral orifice inferiorly. The ureters enter at an angle after tunnelling a small way through the bladder and their orifices are approximately 2 to 3 cm apart. The bladder is retroperitoneal and as it fills and enters the abdomen it strips off the peritoneum from the anterior abdominal wall.

Blood Supply.
- Two vesical (superior and inferior)
- Two visceral (vaginal and uterine)
- Two parietal (internal pudendal and obturator).

Venous Drainage. Via vesico (prostatic) plexus to the internal iliacs.

The Lymphatic Channels. Follow the arteries draining to internal iliac nodes.

Nerve supply.
- Parasympathetic supply via the pelvic splanchnics (S234) is motor to the detrusor (*para pees*) and inhibitory to the sphincter, and these also carry pain fibres and sensory fibres relaying bladder fullness
- Sympathetic (T11–L2) is motor to the internal sphincter, inhibitory to the detrusor.

Histology

The bladder is lined by transitional epithelium surrounded by elastic areolar tissue (except at the trigone) to accommodate bladder expansion during filling. The smooth involuntary detrusor muscle becomes organised at the bladder outlet to form outer and inner longitudinal and a middle circular layer.

THE URETHRA

This musculoelastic tube which drains the bladder originates from the pelvic portion of the urogenital sinus and is endodermal in origin. It is 3 to 4 cm long in the adult female and is lined by transitional epithelium proximally and stratified squamous epithelium distally. This distal portion contains small mucous glands (Skene's glands). There is an inner longitudinal urethral smooth muscle (which shortens during micturition) and an outer voluntary striated circular muscle which has a role in urinary continence.

Blood Supply.
- Inferior vesical artery and the internal pudendal artery.

Venous Drainage.
- Vesical plexus.

Lymphatics.
- To the internal iliac nodes
- External urethral meatus drains to the superficial inguinal nodes.

Nerve Supply.
- The smooth muscle of the urethra is predominantly innervated by the parasympathetic splanchnic nerves, which cause a rise in intraurethral pressure on stimulation
- The striated voluntary urethral muscle is innervated by the somatic fibres of S2–3 via the perineal branch of the pudendal nerve.

The Breast

The breast is a modified apocrine sweat gland (exocrine compound gland).

Pre-Pubertal

Fully formed areola and small nipple. Composed of ducts embedded in fibrous tissue (no alveoli).

DEVELOPMENT OF THE BREAST AT PUBERTY

- Commences between 9 and 12 years of age (thelarche)
- General maturation is promoted by GH, parathyroid hormone, thyroid hormone, cortisol and insulin
- Duct growth is stimulated by oestrogen
- Alveolar (glandular) development is stimulated by progesterone
- Nipple grows, areola stays the same (no fat under either)
- Increased size due to fat deposition
- Few alveoli
- 15 to 20 main (lactiferous) ducts:
  - Each drains directly onto nipple surface
  - Each has dilatation or 'ampulla' under the areola
  - Each drains a lobe
  - Divided into approx. 30 lobules by fibrous septae
  - Each lobule drains 10 to 100 alveoli.

CHANGES WITH PREGNANCY

The weight of the breast and its blood supply doubles. In the first trimester alveoli bud off the duct system (progesterone stimulates glandular development/oestrogen stimulates duct growth). From the second trimester prolactin secretion increases fourfold and this with human placental lactogen stimulates colostrum formation. In the third trimester colostrum production increases and fat droplets accumulate in the alveolar cells. Postpartum, the fall in sex steroids releases the inhibition on prolactin which results in milk synthesis within a few days. This causes the breast to increase further in weight and volume as lactation establishes.

Exocrine gland milk production:

- Merocrine secretions (i.e. exocytosis – proteins)
- Apocrine secretion (i.e. membrane-bound droplets – lipids).

Position

The base of the breast lies over the second to sixth rib in the mid-clavicular line extending to the parasternal margin medially and the mid-axillary line laterally. It gains its support from the ligaments of Astley Cooper (fibrous tissue connecting deep fascia to the dermis).

Blood Supply

Arterial Supply.
- Medially: perforating branches of the internal mammary artery
- Laterally: the lateral thoracic artery (from the axillary artery)
- Inferiorly: the anterior and lateral branches of the intercostal arteries.

Other Supplies Include.
- The pectoral branch of the acromiothoracic artery
- The external mammary artery
- The superior thoracic artery.

Venous Drainage

An anastomotic circle of veins expands from the base of the nipple draining mainly to the internal mammary and axillary veins.

Lymphatic Drainage
- Lateral two-thirds to the axilla
- Medial one-third via internal thoracic to lymph trunk in root of neck and across midline draining to the mediastinum
- Superiorly drains into the infraclavicular nodes

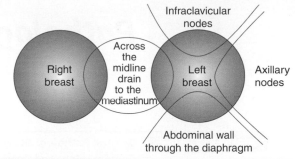

Fig. 5.32 Lymphatic drainage patterns of the breast.

- Inferiorly drains through the diaphragm to the mediastinum.
- Free communication exists between the drainage channels but essentially:
- Superficial to subareolar plexus thence largely to axillary nodes
- Deep to submammary plexus which can go to the axillary nodes but also to the internal mammary and subdiaphragmatic nodes (Fig. 5.32).

Nerve Supply
- Supraclavicular nerves (C3 and C4)
- Medial and lateral cutaneous branches of the intercostal nerves (T4–T6).

6 Pathology

NEIL J. SEBIRE

General Pathological Principles

Adequate understanding of the underlying pathophysiological disease processes associated with the range of obstetric and gynaecological presentations is essential for the rational evaluation of appropriate investigations, therapies and outcomes. Huge volumes of literature are available on almost all of the topics covered in this chapter, but the most important essential points are summarised in the sections below. A basic understanding of general pathological principles is covered in the first section of the chapter, with the pathologies of some important examples of obstetric and gynaecological entities described later.

Cellular Injury and Death

There is a limited cellular repertoire of response to injury from a variety of causes including hypoxia (lack of oxygen supply), ischaemia (lack of blood supply), metabolic insults, mechanical trauma, immunological reactions, infections and toxins. Such insults may cause either a temporary impairment of cellular function followed by complete recovery, structural cellular damage with survival but ongoing impairment or, if severe or prolonged, may result in widespread cell death. Control of cellular proliferation and death is also essential for normal tissue turnover regulation and all aspects of embryonic development. The maintenance of normal tissue architecture, whether normal or neoplastic, is dependent upon the balance between cellular proliferation and cell death. At the basic cellular level there are two major types of cell death which may occur in association with the type, severity and timing of insult, namely necrosis and apoptosis.

Necrosis essentially represents a process of severe widespread cellular damage with marked cell swelling and rupture of the membrane. It usually affects sheets of adjacent cells causing disruption of normal tissue architecture with release of mediators and associated inflammation; necrosis is always pathological. Apoptosis, in contrast, essentially represents the controlled or selective death of individual or selected cells within tissues, without significant tissue destruction or associated inflammatory response, and is an essential process in both embryonic development and normal tissue turnover. The process of necrosis is mediated within the cell by rising intracellular calcium concentration, with massive cellular swelling and uncontrolled activation of intracellular enzymes, whereas apoptosis is mediated by controlled activation of specific intracellular enzyme pathways (caspases, transglutaminases and endonucleases) which result in a controlled destruction of the cell and its subsequent phagocytosis and removal.

RESPONSE TO TISSUE INJURY

Following injury due to any mechanism, at a tissue, rather than cellular, level, there are three basic tissue responses which may be stimulated depending on the type and severity of the insult: acute inflammation, wound healing and chronic inflammation.

Acute Inflammation

Acute inflammation is the common and stereotyped tissue response to injury from a wide range of insults. Five classical clinical features are described including redness, heat, swelling, pain and loss of function. The acute inflammatory response is mediated by the activation of a range of vasoactive and chemotactic pathways which result in local vasodilatation, with increased blood flow to the affected area resulting in redness and heat; increased vascular permeability, resulting in exudation of fluid into the interstitial tissue and swelling; and release of numerous mediators which recruit further inflammatory cells to the site and cause pain and loss of function. The primary inflammatory cell mediator of acute inflammation is the neutrophil in the early stage, followed by the macrophage with resolution. Huge numbers of mediators have now been described in association with acute inflammation including histamine, prostaglandins, leukotrienes, bradykinins and complement components in addition to an ever-expanding list of cytokines produced by the inflammatory cells themselves, such as interleukin and tumour necrosis factor families. With removal or reduction of the inciting agent, the later stages of acute inflammation merge imperceptibly with the process of tissue repair and wound healing described below. Fig. 6.1 shows acute inflammation in fetal membranes in a pregnancy complicated by chorioamnionitis.

Tissue Repair and Wound Healing

The process of tissue repair or healing may involve either regeneration of the tissue to its original state by replacement of dead or damaged cells by proliferation of cells of the same type, or repair and organisation, in which new connective or scar tissue replaces the original tissue. The type of process to occur depends upon the timing, severity and extent of the insult, in addition to the underlying characteristics of the tissues involved.

An example of this process is the healing of skin wounds. In wounds with closely opposed edges, healing can occur by first intention, in which an initial blood clot forms followed by cellular proliferation and migration of the marginal epidermis across the clot to bridge the defect with proliferation of blood vessels and fibroblasts into the wound edges in the underlying connective tissue to form loose granulation-type tissue which is then remodelled over time. In skin wounds in which the edges are widely separated (healing by secondary

intention), there is similar, but more extensive, formation of granulation tissue but since the epithelial proliferation cannot rapidly bridge the defect, there is ongoing remodelling, with wound contraction secondary to the presence of myofibroblasts and replacement of the original tissue by scarring. The process of wound healing is further influenced by additional factors such as the local blood supply, the presence of infection or foreign bodies, excessive movement at the site or other systemic factors such as metabolic abnormalities. Defective wound healing may therefore result in either inadequate union and wound dehiscence or excessive production of scar tissue such as hypertrophic scars or keloid formation. It is clear that the control of the process of wound healing is complex and dependent upon large numbers of mediators such as transforming growth factor beta and epidermal growth factor, the manipulation of which may allow novel interventions in the future. It should also be noted that there are marked differences in the potential responses to injury between different tissues and at different stages in development, with fetal wound healing and remodelling, for example, occurring very rapidly.

Chronic Inflammation

Histologically, chronic inflammation is defined as an inflammatory process that is occurring simultaneously with attempted healing, rather than a simple sequential process following acute inflammation. It should therefore be noted that it may often be clinically impossible to distinguish between ongoing acute and chronic inflammation, the two potential mechanisms being persistence of a low-grade inflammatory stimulus that initially induced an acute inflammatory response, or a process involving chronic inflammation from its outset. The characteristic histopathological features of chronic inflammation are the presence of predominant mononuclear inflammatory cells, in particular lymphocytes, plasma cells and macrophages, in association with fibroblast proliferation. Many immunological diseases are associated with such chronic inflammatory responses from their outset. A specific type of chronic inflammation is termed granulomatous inflammation, which represents prominent collections of epithelioid macrophages within tissues as a consequence of either an immunological reaction or the presence of foreign organisms or material which cannot be digested and removed by macrophages (Fig. 6.2). It should be noted that granulomatous inflammation and granulation tissue are entirely different processes.

CONTROL OF CELL AND TISSUE GROWTH OR DIFFERENTIATION

In normal tissue there is very strict control of cellular growth, proliferation, death and differentiation. Several types of abnormal tissue response may occur.

- Hyperplasia represents an increase in the number of cells in a tissue or organ, which may be physiological, such as during pregnancy, or pathological, such as with oestrogen-induced endometrial hyperplasia
- Hypoplasia is a reduction in cell number within an organ or tissue, which may also be physiological or pathological
- Atrophy represents a potentially reversible reduction in mass of the tissue, with atrophic cells usually being

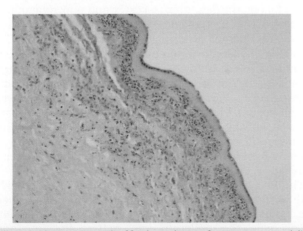

Fig. 6.1 Photomicrograph of fetal membranes from a pregnancy delivered spontaneously at 25 weeks of gestation demonstrating numerous polymorphs infiltrating the fetal membranes (chorioamnionitis); an example of acute inflammation (H&E, ×100).

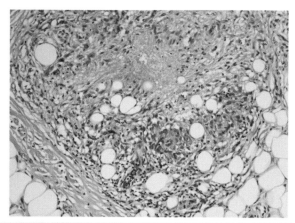

Fig. 6.2 Photomicrograph of a subcutaneous lesion demonstrating granulomatous inflammation with numerous epithelioid macrophages surrounding an area of necrosis, with numerous mononuclear inflammatory cells in the surrounding tissue (H&E, ×250).

smaller than normal. This may also be physiological, such as in postmenopausal endometrial atrophy, or pathological, such as tissue atrophy following damaged nerve or blood supply

- Hypertrophy represents a potentially reversible increase in cell size, which may be physiological, such as the uterus in pregnancy, or pathological, such as myocardial hypertrophy in hypertension
- Metaplasia represents the change in cellular phenotype from one fully differentiated state to another, and usually occurs from stem cells in epithelia, the most common example being columnar to squamous metaplasia of the transformation zone of the cervix (see later)
- Epithelial dysplasia represents the presence of cytological changes associated with malignancy but in the absence of abnormalities of underlying tissue architecture with an intact basement membrane. For many tumours, there is thought to be a clear pathway of progression from low-grade to high-grade dysplasia through to invasive carcinoma, the primary example of which being cervical intraepithelial neoplasia (CIN) as a forerunner of invasive squamous cell carcinoma of the cervix (see later)
- Neoplasia represents the process of new growth of cells
- Tumour represents a distinct mass lesion, and hence not all tumours are neoplasms
- Tumours may be simply classified as benign or malignant, and primary (arising at the site) or secondary (metastatic from another site), with specific subtyping, grading and staging on the basis of clinical and histopathological features.

Neoplasms may be benign or malignant. In general terms, benign neoplasms are usually localised, do not exhibit local destructive infiltration, do not metastasise and are often composed of relatively well differentiated cells. Malignant neoplasms demonstrate local destructive invasion of the surrounding normal tissue and the ability to metastasise (grow at sites distant from the site of origin). Despite these apparently clear-cut definitions, in a range of clinical situations, the precise distinction between a benign and malignant neoplasm may be extremely difficult, although most

of these are not of significance to the obstetrician and gynaecologist.

The terminology commonly used for many neoplasms implies their benign or malignant nature from the nomenclature. For example, benign mesenchymal neoplasms usually have the suffix 'oma', such as a leiomyoma, whereas malignant mesenchymal neoplasms usually have the suffix 'sarcoma', such as a leiomyosarcoma. Malignant epithelial neoplasms are termed carcinomas and many paediatric malignancies that mimic embryonal tissues are termed blastomas. Malignant neoplasms of haematological stem cells in the bone marrow are termed leukaemias, whereas other malignancies of lymphoid tissue are termed lymphomas. There are well described specific and detailed classification systems and staging systems (extent of spread) for all described malignancies from the World Health Organization (WHO) and, in the context of gynaecological malignancies, the International Federation of Gynecology and Obstetrics (FIGO).

Malignancies are defined histopathologically on the basis of abnormalities of tissue architecture and cytological features. There is loss of the normal well-defined microarchitecture, with destruction of the underlying basement membrane in the case of carcinomas, and invasion of the surrounding tissue by malignant cells. Cytological features of malignancy in general include abnormal nuclear shape and size, abnormal mitoses and an increased nuclear to cytoplasmic ratio. In addition, many malignant cells demonstrate reduced or abnormal differentiation. (It should be noted here that the cell of origin of a tumour is not necessarily the same as the phenotype to which it is differentiating.) Neoplasms are a consequence of abnormalities in the normal cellular proliferation and differentiation control mechanisms, the majority of which are associated with either activation of oncogenes or loss of function of tumour suppressor genes.

HISTOLOGY AND PATHOLOGY OF THE GENITAL TRACT

The female genital tract essentially almost entirely develops from the müllerian duct system embryologically, with part paired and part fused areas, resulting in development of the fallopian tubes, uterus, cervix and upper vagina, in addition to the embryologically distinct ovaries. The female genital tract is lined by a range of different types of epithelium along its length ranging from vaginal squamous epithelium, through uterine columnar epithelium and tubal ciliated epithelium. The ovary is composed of a mixture of germ cells (oocytes) among ovarian stroma and covering epithelium. The range of pathologies encountered may therefore be related to any of the above elements depending on the specific site, age and other aetiological factors, with the most common tumours being related to the underlying histological structures.

The male genital tract is also composed of paired gonads, with germ cells surrounded by epithelium and connective tissue, connected to the external by a tubal system, but in males the müllerian ducts regress, the functional ductal system being developed from the wolffian system. Therefore, although the potential spectrum of pathologies which may affect male and female gonads is similar, the specific types and distributions of neoplasms significantly differ; for example, across all ages in males, testicular germ cell tumours in younger men represent the most common neoplasms, whereas the predominant neoplasm in females is ovarian carcinoma in older women.

Pathology of Gynaecological Tumours

The basic principles of neoplasia, tumorigenesis and benign versus malignant tumours have been introduced above. A wide variety of examples of such pathologies may be encountered in the female genital tract and the characteristic pathological features of some common examples are described below. Similar to most tumours in adults, by far the commonest group of malignant lesions are epithelial derived (carcinomas), the specific subtypes of which are primarily dependent on the type of epithelium normally present at that site, although it should be noted that, since the majority of the female genital tract is derived from müllerian structures, carcinomas developing at any point may essentially recapitulate any type of müllerian derived epithelium. Mesenchymal malignancies are rare at these sites but many of the benign neoplasms commonly encountered are derived from connective tissue components such as uterine fibroids (leiomyoma) arising from the myometrium.

VULVA

The vulva is covered by squamous epithelium, and squamous cell carcinoma accounts for more than 90% of malignancies at this site and about 5% of all female genital tract cancers. This is primarily a disease of elderly women and presents with an ulcerated or thickened area on the vulva. There is local invasion and lymphatic spread, first to the inguinal lymph nodes. In an analogous manner to the cervix (see below), preinvasive epithelial changes have now been recognised, and grading described, termed vulval intraepithelial neoplasia (VIN). In this condition, there are mitoses, often abnormal, above the normal basal layers in association with other features of cytological atypia such as nuclear pleomorphism and a high nuclear to cytoplasmic ratio, but with an intact basement membrane.

VAGINA

The vagina is normally lined by non-keratinising squamous epithelium, and neoplasms of the vagina are rare. When they do occur, most are squamous cell carcinomas in elderly women, which usually present as an ulcerating or fungating mass lesion in the upper third, with local and lymphatic spread. In a similar manner to the cervix and vulva, vaginal intraepithelial neoplasia (VAIN) has also now been described, often in women with previous cervical malignancy, the process probably representing a premalignant 'field change'. Glandular structures may sometimes be present in the subepithelial stroma of the vagina, termed vaginal adenosis, occurring either sporadically or in association with females exposed prenatally to diethylstilbestrol. Such adenosis is usually asymptomatic but may predispose

to the development of clear cell adenocarcinoma of the vagina. In young girls, usually in the first 5 years of life, the vagina may also be a relatively common site of embryonal rhabdomyosarcoma, which develops in the subepithelial stroma and may present as a polypoid lesion with discharge.

CERVIX

The normal ectocervix is covered by non-keratinising squamous epithelium, whereas the endocervix and endocervical canal is lined by columnar type epithelium. During puberty, the squamocolumnar junction may become situated onto the anatomical ectocervix, and the exposed endocervical epithelium undergoes squamous metaplasia forming the transformation zone. Due to this mixture of epithelial types present, squamous cell carcinoma, adenocarcinoma and sarcoma may all occur in the cervix, although the commonest neoplasm by far is squamous cell carcinoma affecting the area of the transformation zone. It is hypothesised that during the process of metaplasia the epithelium at this site shows increased susceptibility to oncogenic agents such as smoking and human papilloma virus (HPV) infection, and it is increasingly clear that infection with certain subtypes of HPV is a significant risk factor for the subsequent development of cervical carcinoma.

Abnormal changes in the epithelium of the cervix are often apparent many years before the development of invasive carcinoma, i.e., there are cytological abnormalities, but the changes are confined to the epithelium and have not breached the basement membrane. These pre-invasive changes are termed CIN, which may be graded according to increased severity of architectural and cytological changes, from grade 1 to grade 3. Invasive carcinoma of the cervix may follow high-grade CIN and initially spreads locally, often presenting as a fungating or ulcerated lesion, and then by lymphatic spread. The peak age for development of invasive squamous cell carcinoma of the cervix is around 60 years, with CIN developing around 20 years earlier.

ENDOMETRIUM

The endometrium is composed of numerous glands set within a background stroma, the structure of which varies with age and throughout the menstrual cycle due to the sensitivity of the endometrium to the steroid hormones oestrogen and progesterone. Oestrogen, in the absence of progesterone, leads to proliferation of the endometrial epithelium, a normal finding in the first half of the menstrual cycle. Metaplasia of endometrial epithelium may occur but is extremely uncommon compared with metaplasia occurring in the cervix and is not required for the development of endometrial malignancy. As expected from the nature of its normal structure, the commonest malignancy at this site is endometrial adenocarcinoma, which again, due to its derivation from müllerian epithelium, may differentiate towards various epithelial phenotypes. The proposed precursor lesion of endometrial adenocarcinoma is endometrial hyperplasia which may occur in high oestrogen states, the risk being greatest for atypical complex hyperplasia in which there are both architectural and cytological abnormalities. Endometrial adenocarcinoma usually presents with abnormal vaginal bleeding in a peri- or postmenopausal woman and often remains confined to the uterus at presentation, although may spread locally or by lymphatics. Histologically, endometrial adenocarcinoma demonstrates abnormal, closely packed glandular structures with cytological abnormalities including nuclear enlargement, hyperchromasia and abnormal mitoses. Rarely, endometrial stromal sarcomas or malignant mixed müllerian tumours may occur with a malignant component derived from the stroma.

MYOMETRIUM

The connective tissue elements of the female genital tract only rarely give rise to neoplasms, the commonest by far being benign smooth muscle tumours of the myometrium (leiomyomata or fibroids). These occur as single or multiple intramyometrial lesions composed of interlacing bland spindle cells, which may show secondary changes such as infarction or myxoid degeneration. The other lesion that may commonly present as intramyometrial pathology, although not a true neoplasm, is adenomyosis, characterised by nests or nodules of endometrium within the myometrium (or at other extrauterine sites).

OVARY

The pathology of the ovary varies somewhat from the remainder of the female genital tract since, in addition to being covered with müllerian derived surface epithelium and containing a stromal component, the ovary also contains germ cells. The three major groups of primary tumour of the ovary may therefore be classified into those derived from epithelium, sex cord stromal tumours and germ cell tumours.

About 90% of malignant ovarian tumours are derived from the surface epithelium and are therefore carcinomas. Analogous to carcinomas from other sites in the female genital tract, ovarian carcinomas may differentiate along various pathways normally taken by müllerian epithelia, and hence may be serous, mucinous or endometrioid adenocarcinomas, although other rare types may of course also occur. Ovarian adenocarcinoma generally affects elderly women and, due to the lack of direct communication with a lumen, presentation is often with non-specific features, the disease being of advanced stage at diagnosis. Benign epithelial tumours may also occur (cystadenomas), and a group of epithelial tumours of intermediate malignancy have also been described (borderline tumours).

Sex cord stromal tumours represent neoplasms of specialised stromal cells, such as granulosa cells, Sertoli cells, theca cells and Leydig cells or specialised fibroblasts. Since these cells are often hormone-producing, such tumours may present with the consequences of abnormal hormone levels.

Germ cell tumours are relatively common in the ovary, especially in younger patients and represent a diverse group which may show minimal phenotypic differentiation, such as dysgerminomas, or extreme degrees of differentiation along all three embryonic pathways, such as mature teratomas. In addition, differentiation may be towards extraembryonic developmental elements such as trophoblast in choriocarcinoma (Fig. 6.3) or yolk sac structures in yolk sac tumour. Teratomas are the commonest ovarian neoplasms,

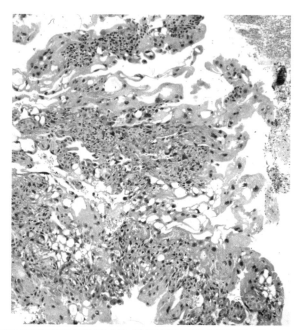

Fig. 6.3 Photomicrograph of fragments of choriocarcinoma demonstrating abnormal trophoblast with biphasic architecture and cellular features of malignancy such as nuclear pleomorphism, nuclear hyperchromasia and apoptotic debris (H&E, ×250).

most being mature teratomas in which a wide range of well-differentiated histological tissue types are present with associated generally benign behaviour. Some teratomas may contain immature elements such as neuroepithelial tubules, with an increased risk of malignant behaviour, and other teratomas may contain frankly malignant elements such as embryonal carcinoma or yolk sac tumour. Pure malignant germ cell tumours of the ovary, such as pure yolk sac tumour, may also occur, and are the commonest ovarian malignancies in young children.

Pathology of Miscarriage and Gestational Trophoblastic Disease

For the purposes of this chapter, miscarriage will be defined as the loss of the conception prior to viability. This is a relatively common event, occurring in around 15% of clinically recognised pregnancies. The underlying causes of miscarriage are varied and, although epidemiological studies have shed light on possible associated underlying categories of factors, the cause often cannot be determined with certainty in an individual case.

CHROMOSOMAL ABNORMALITIES

The commonest demonstrable underlying abnormality in first- and early second-trimester miscarriage is fetal chromosomal abnormality, including trisomies, polyploidy and other abnormalities such as monosomy. In cases in which karyotyping has been carried out, up to 50% of first-trimester miscarriages may be chromosomally abnormal, varying with underlying predisposing factors such as maternal age.

INFECTION

Obstetric and pathological literature from several decades ago suggested that infection was a common and important underlying cause of miscarriage. More recent data suggest that, although some infections may be teratogenic or cause miscarriage in early pregnancy, underlying infection is in reality an uncommon cause of first-trimester pregnancy loss. In contrast, ascending genital tract infection with either localised inflammation overlying the cervical os or frank chorioamnionitis is the commonest cause of late second-trimester spontaneous miscarriage.

MATERNAL DISEASE

Miscarriage has been reported in association with a wide range of underlying maternal diseases or exposure to external agents such as drugs or radiation. However, documented and identifiable maternal disease represents the underlying cause of only a tiny proportion of spontaneous miscarriages.

OTHER FACTORS

It will be clear from the above discussion that the underlying aetiology in many miscarriages cannot be determined with certainty, despite appropriate investigation. Pathological examination of the miscarriage specimen may be of use in identifying certain specific underlying causes, such as molar pregnancies (see below), or to suggest an underlying fetal abnormality or chromosomal defect, in a minority of cases. However, data from various sources, including pathological examination, have demonstrated that a relatively common mechanism involved in first-trimester pregnancy loss is defective trophoblastic invasion of the decidual and uterine vasculature with subsequent excessive blood flow to the developing conceptus in early pregnancy and secondary mechanical or oxidative damage. It is likely that such defective trophoblastic invasion represents a final common pathway of many conditions that may be associated with miscarriage, such as the presence of thrombophilic maternal conditions (e.g., antiphospholipid antibody syndrome) or other proposed maternal immunological factors.

The causes of second-trimester miscarriage and intrauterine death in the third trimester are similarly varied, with the major underlying aetiological categories being fetal abnormality, ascending genital tract infection and defects of uteroplacental and intervillous flow secondary to impaired trophoblastic invasion (see below).

GESTATIONAL TROPHOBLASTIC NEOPLASIA

A related group of abnormalities characterised by abnormal trophoblast proliferation are encompassed by the term gestational trophoblastic neoplasia (GTN), and include partial and complete hydatidiform mole, invasive mole, choriocarcinoma (see Fig. 6.3) and placental site trophoblastic tumour. The commonest of these entities, partial and complete hydatidiform moles, occur in 1 in 500 to 1000 pregnancies and usually present with first-trimester miscarriage, the diagnosis of mole being suspected at ultrasound examination or following routine pathological examination of the evacuated products of conception. Both partial and complete hydatidiform moles are characterised by abnormal trophoblastic proliferation in association with abnormal fetal development due to defective imprinting as a consequence of an abnormal chromosomal constitution with an excess of paternal genomic material. Complete hydatidiform moles are diploid, but with both sets of chromosomes derived from the father following fertilisation of an anucleate oocyte, whereas partial hydatidiform moles are triploid, with the extra set of chromosomes derived from the father following fertilisation of a normal oocyte by two sperm. In both cases, the relative excess of paternal chromosomal material results in overgrowth of the trophoblast of the placenta and impaired embryonic development.

In addition to presenting clinically as miscarriage, the main clinical consequence of partial and complete hydatidiform moles is the possibility of their developing into persistent GTN, occurring in around 0.5% and 15% of cases, respectively. Should it occur, such persistent disease may represent localised invasive mole; malignant, and often metastatic choriocarcinoma; or the rare placental site trophoblastic tumour. Cases of hydatidiform mole should therefore undergo surveillance by measurement of maternal serum hCG concentrations (produced by the proliferating trophoblast) in order to detect persistent disease at an early stage when it is highly responsive to chemotherapy. The malignant forms of GTN, choriocarcinoma and placental site trophoblastic tumour, although orders of magnitude more common following molar pregnancies, may also rarely complicate non-molar pregnancies, and even those resulting in live birth require specialist management.

Pathology of Common Congenital Abnormalities and Teratogenesis

A huge range of congenital abnormalities are now described with a corresponding entire subspecialty dedicated to their pathogenesis and management. An understanding of the appropriate terminology makes their classification more intuitive and improves understanding of the literature in this field.

- An anomaly is defined as any deviation from the expected normal type of structure, form or function which is interpreted as abnormal
- A malformation is a morphological defect of an organ or region of the body as a consequence of an intrinsically abnormal developmental process
- Dysplasia, in the context of congenital abnormality, is defined as an abnormal organisation of a tissue, or defective histogenesis
- A disruption represents a morphological abnormality of an organ or region of the body resulting from extrinsic interference with an originally normal developmental process
- A deformation is defined as an abnormality in shape or position of part of the body due to mechanical forces
- A sequence is a term used for a pattern of multiple abnormalities derived from a single presumed prior factor

- A syndrome represents multiple associated abnormalities thought to be pathogenically related but not representing a sequence
- An association is a non-random occurrence of multiple morphological abnormalities not identified as a sequence or syndrome
- A developmental field defect is a combination of abnormalities as a result of disturbed development of an embryonic morphogenic field.

It will be apparent from the above terms that a wide range of underlying aetiological factors may therefore result in the phenotype of congenital abnormality, the most common of which include chromosomal abnormalities, single gene defects, polygenic defects, mitochondrial defects, imprinting abnormalities, triplet repeat sequence defects and a large number of disruptions due to teratogens, metabolic diseases, immunological reactions and infections. The recurrence risk may therefore theoretically range from essentially 0% to 100% depending on the underlying aetiology. It should however be noted that the vast majority of human congenital abnormalities appear to be sporadic, with low empirical recurrence risks, presumably the cause of an interaction of genetic factors and environmental factors (so-called multifactorial defects) which do not fit neatly into the other categories listed above.

Congenital abnormalities can also be classified according to the presumed stage of human development which is primarily affected to lead to the phenotype. These include abnormalities of pregenesis, blastogenesis, embryogenesis or phenogenesis, examples of each being fetal aneuploidy such as trisomy 18, holoprosencephaly, isolated limb defects and deformations such as talipes secondary to oligohydramnios, respectively.

Normal human embryological development represents a complex sequence of events resulting in the formation and differentiation of body structures, organs, tissues and cell types. Precise details controlling such development remain uncertain but there is now extensive evidence demonstrating involvement of numerous genes leading to complex cell–cell and cell–matrix interactions. Teratology represents the study of abnormalities of normal embryonic development, and a substance or condition may be considered teratogenic when its exposure at certain stages of development results in structural or functional abnormality. The effects may be related both to timing and dose with well documented teratogens, including maternal medications, infections and other agents such as ionising radiation.

Pathology of the Placenta

In order to understand the pathology which may affect the placenta, an understanding of normal placental development, anatomy and physiology is required, which is covered in other parts of the text. In summary, however, the human placenta is a discoid, haemomonochorial, multivillous organ in which fetal blood perfuses the vascular bed within the branching chorionic villous tree, whereas maternal blood directly enters the intervillous space to surround the villi. In later pregnancy, focally only a single layer of trophoblast and basement membrane separates the maternal and fetal circulations, which in normal circumstances never come into direct contact. The anatomy and physiology of the placenta changes throughout gestation and both developmental and acquired disease processes may occur.

A potentially wide range of pathologies may affect the placenta, just as any other organ, including neoplastic (choriocarcinoma), infective (chorioamnionitis) and inflammatory (autoimmune) processes; however, the vast majority of the important conditions in which there are specific placental pathological features represent either ascending genital tract infection leading to preterm delivery or abnormalities in uteroplacental, intervillous or fetal blood flow through the organ. Such abnormalities may simply be classified as those affecting primarily the fetal circulation, such as fetal stem vessel thrombosis, and those affecting primarily the uteroplacental or intervillous flow, such as uteroplacental vascular disease (see below) or massive perivillous fibrin deposition. Although the human placenta has moderate functional reserve capacity, a significant reduction in uteroplacental or intervillous flow can result in reduced oxygen delivery and hence reduced oxygen transfer, with concomitant reduction in the delivery or transport of other substances in addition to secondary consequences on fetoplacental flow.

INTRAUTERINE GROWTH RESTRICTION AND PRE-ECLAMPSIA

It is now clear that the underlying pathophysiological basis for a wide range of pregnancy complications such as miscarriage, intrauterine growth restriction (IUGR) and pre-eclampsia is related to abnormal, defective, trophoblastic invasion of decidual and uterine vessels, with consequent significant impaired or abnormal uteroplacental blood flow and therefore perfusion of the intervillous space, as pregnancy advances (maternovascular malperfusion). In normal pregnancies, there is early trophoblastic invasion of the decidua with coordinated invasion of the decidual arterial branches which are completely or partially occluded by trophoblastic 'plugs' in early pregnancy. With advancing gestation into the second trimester and beyond, the interstitial and endovascular trophoblastic invasion progresses to involve deeper uterine vessels with conversion of the muscular uterine artery branches into the relatively flaccid and low-resistance uteroplacental vessels normally encountered in later pregnancy. Such physiological changes are thought to prevent excessive blood flow during the implantation period but allow a dramatic increase in uteroplacental blood flow with advancing gestation in association with significant reductions in the vascular reactivity of these uteroplacental vessels.

Pathological studies have clearly demonstrated that defective trophoblastic invasion and conversion of uterine arteries to uteroplacental vessels is the common underlying mechanism in cases of severe asymmetrical IUGR and pre-eclampsia, with or without superimposed acute vascular changes such as atherosis or thrombosis with infarction (Figs. 6.4 and 6.5). More recently, this defective haemodynamic process has been identified by Doppler ultrasound imaging of the uterine arteries in midgestation, manifest by the presence of a notch in the Doppler flow velocity waveform or increased resistance indices. Although the

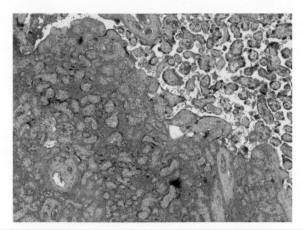

Fig. 6.4 Photomicrograph of placenta from a case of severe intrauterine growth restriction demonstrating an area of evolving villous infarction, indicating severe reduction in uteroplacental blood flow (H&E, ×40).

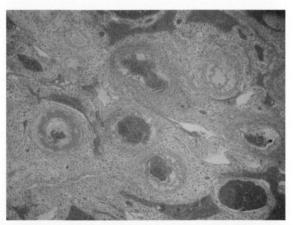

Fig. 6.5 Photomicrograph of the decidual basal plate from a patient with severe pre-eclampsia demonstrating numerous abnormal vessels, many of which exhibit foam cells within their walls (atherosis), indicating severely impaired trophoblastic invasion (H&E, ×25).

underlying defect is a marked reduction in uteroplacental blood flow, there are autoregulatory and compensatory mechanisms within the fetal part of the placenta which allow a degree of fetal compensation, but when severe may lead to characteristic pathological changes within the structure of the placenta, such as vasoconstriction of the fetal stem vessels in association with the presence of small, poorly branched and poorly vascularised chorionic villi. Such changes lead to secondary abnormalities of fetoplacental flow with high fetoplacental resistance, which can be identified antenatally by Doppler ultrasound imaging of the umbilical arteries, manifest as increased pulsatility index and absent or reversed end-diastolic frequencies. It should be noted that, although this mechanism is the presumed underlying pathophysiological mechanism for the majority of cases of asymmetrical IUGR, other mechanisms for growth restriction also exist in specific circumstances.

Although the underlying pathophysiological changes in the placenta appear to be similar in cases of classical IUGR and pre-eclampsia, the difference in maternal phenotype is probably a consequence of the maternal response to the haemodynamic changes, which appears to be related to both fetal and maternal characteristics. The underlying concept central to the development of pre-eclampsia is probable release of an as yet unidentified, vasoactive substance by the placental tissue which leads to widespread maternal vasoconstriction and abnormal vascular permeability.

In response to a severe reduction in uteroplacental flow, and hence oxygen and nutrient delivery, the fetus demonstrates several haemodynamic compensatory responses, together commonly known as 'fetal brain sparing' or 'redistribution'. This response is characterised by reduced flow resistance and increased blood flow to the brain in association with reduced blood flow to the abdominal viscera and limbs. Such fetal redistribution of blood flow is mediated by vasoactive responses to fetal hypoxia and acidosis. In association with severe and long-standing uteroplacental IUGR, secondary haemodynamic changes occur in the fetal venous system, which probably represent cardiac dysfunction and are indicators of advanced stages of the condition, preceding intrauterine fetal death. Determination of a combination of these haemodynamic fetal factors using Doppler sonography can allow optimal management and timing of delivery in fetuses with severe IUGR.

ASCENDING GENITAL TRACT INFECTION

Although bacteria are always present within the vagina, the uterine cavity is usually sterile during pregnancy. Infection may be transmitted to the placenta and fetus by several potential mechanisms, including direct inoculation (e.g., at the time of amniocentesis), haematogenous spread or infection ascending along the cervical canal. The cervix is normally plugged by mucus and is closed anatomically. Development of ascending genital tract infection probably requires a combination of factors including the type of bacteria present in the vagina, loss of the normal cervical mucous plug and cervical shortening and dilatation. Once it occurs, ascending infection causes a supracervical inflammatory reaction with local production of mediators such as prostaglandins and cytokines which can initiate the cascade of events leading to delivery. Hence, depending on the timing, ascending genital tract infection may lead to spontaneous miscarriage or extremely pre-term delivery. Furthermore, the infection may pass into the amniotic cavity with resulting fetal infection, further compromising the prematurely delivered infant. Finally, due to the inflammatory mediators associated with infection combined with the complications of pre-term delivery, chorioamnionitis has been suggested as a significant risk factor for the development of cerebral palsy.

Only a minority of cases of ascending genital tract infection will manifest with maternal systemic symptoms and signs of sepsis, the majority leading to the onset of labour without systemic upset. Histologically, ascending genital tract infection is characterised by infiltration of the fetal membranes with neutrophil polymorphs, most marked in the area overlying the cervix.

Placental Implantation Abnormalities

In addition to the rare development of placental site trophoblastic tumours as part of gestational trophoblastic disease and the impaired placentation associated with maternovascular malperfusion, other abnormalities of implantation may result in abnormal placental shape, abnormal placental position (for example placenta previa) and abnormally deep placental invasion (placenta accreta, in which there is focal absence of normal decidua with chorionic villi directly invading into myometrium). Uterine abnormality such as previous caesarean section scar significantly increase the likelihood of these types of abnormal placental implantation.

Pathology of Ectopic Pregnancy

The process of fertilisation with subsequent normal early placental implantation and trophoblastic invasion depends on a complex interaction between factors expressed by the invading trophoblast and maternal factors related to the normal uterine and decidual environment, including the presence of specific subtypes of uterine inflammatory cells. If there is damage or impaired function of the normal fallopian tubes, implantation may attempt to occur outside of the normal uterine environment resulting in an ectopic pregnancy, most commonly tubal. In such circumstances, the tissue into which the early trophoblast invades does not have a normal decidual structure or function, therefore, normal placentation cannot occur to support the ongoing pregnancy and trophoblast invasion is often destructive resulting in local complications such as haemorrhage and rupture.

7 Microbiology and Virology

JULIAN R. MARCHESI, GEOFFREY L. RIDGWAY AND PAUL TAYLOR

Bacteriology, Mycology and Parasitology

Introduction

Bacteria are the smallest organisms capable of a free-living existence. That is, with the exception of a few highly evolved examples, they are able to take up nutrients from the environment, grow and self-replicate independently of other living cells. Their basic biochemical pathways are similar to those of other organisms, and while they are morphologically less complex than the cells of higher organisms, they are orders of magnitude more metabolically diverse. The niches in which they are found are also hugely diverse, ranging from kilometres below the sea floor to extremes of both temperature and pH, and have even been to the moon and back, as unforeseen passengers in the Apollo space program. Their ubiquity stems from their fast rates of growth, high levels of exchange of genetic information and their high rates of evolution. When these traits are combined it leads to the wide range of adaptations that bacteria show to allow them to colonise these niches. The adjective 'prokaryotic' distinguishes the absence of membrane-bound organelles characteristic of bacteria from the 'eukaryotic' cell characterised by the presence of a nuclear membrane.

MORPHOLOGY AND STRUCTURE

Most bacteria are 1 µm in diameter or larger, which means that they are readily visible by light microscopy and conventional bright-field illumination. However, to visualise the internal structures of the cell, the resolving power of an electron microscope is required. Fig. 7.1 is a diagrammatic representation of the internal structures of the prokaryotic cell.

Many bacteria have a capsule or loose slime around the cell wall. This capsule is an important protective mechanism. The ability of organisms such as *Staphylococcus epidermidis* to produce slime (biofilm) on the surfaces of cannulae results in the protection of the organism from the action of antimicrobial agents, and difficulty in eradicating the organism in catheter-associated sepsis.

The cell wall of bacteria is unique in its composition and plays a structural role. This macromolecule consists of a backbone of *N*-acetyl-glucosamine and *N*-acetyl-muramic acid residues linked to polypeptides, polysaccharides and lipids, and is collectively called 'peptidoglycan'. Peptidoglycan is responsible for the rigidity of the cell wall and maintenance of the characteristic shape of an organism. Gram stain differentiates bacteria into those that take up and retain a complex of crystal violet and iodine, and those that do not. This ability is a function of the cell wall. Gram-positive organisms (stained blue/black) have a cell wall consisting largely of peptidoglycan linked to teichoic acids. In contrast, the cell wall of Gram-negative organisms (usually counterstained pink) is far more complex with an outer membrane of lipoprotein and lipopolysaccharide (LPS; also unique to bacteria), separated from the peptidoglycan layer by the periplasmic space. This arrangement has important consequences for the ability of Gram-negative bacteria to neutralise the activity of certain antimicrobial agents such as the cell wall active β-lactams (e.g. penicillins and cephalosporins) and prevents glycopeptides (vancomycin) from entering the cell and stopping peptidoglycans from being fully synthesised. Peptidoglycan is synthesised with the assistance of transpeptidases, also known as penicillin-binding proteins (PBPs), which are a target for β-lactams. This group of antibacterial agents is therefore acting against a metabolic pathway unique to bacteria, with consequent low toxicity to eukaryotic cells. The presence of β-lactamases in the periplasmic space may result in the bacteria being resistant to these agents. Mycoplasmas are unique among bacteria in not having a rigid cell wall, while the chlamydiae lack peptidoglycan. Not surprisingly, these bacteria are essentially resistant to β-lactams-based antibiotics.

The cell wall of acid-fast bacteria such as the mycobacteria and *Nocardia* spp. contains a high lipid content. They are difficult to stain by most stains, but a solution of hot phenolic carbol fuchsin, or the fluorochrome auramine, which binds to the lipid, will resist decolouration with sulphuric acid, and stain the organism.

The nucleus is a tightly coiled circular double strand of DNA, which replicates by fission. Other units of straight or circular DNA termed 'plasmids' may occur loosely in the cytoplasm. These may code for non-essential features such as antibiotic resistance or ability to ferment certain sugars such as lactose. The ability of bacteria to transfer plasmid DNA between bacteria of the same or different species may result in the spread of antimicrobial resistance (plasmid mediated). Bacteria may also transfer genetic material from the nucleus (the so-called 'jumping gene'), leading to stable, chromosomally mediated resistance.

Projecting through the cell wall may be flagellae, fimbriae or pili. Flagellae are long whip-like structures associated with motility. Fimbriae form a fringe around bacteria allowing gliding movement. Pili are longer than fimbriae, and more numerous than flagellae. They are associated with conjugation between bacteria of the same or different species, during which the exchange of genetic material, and hence transferable antibiotic resistance, can occur.

Bacteria are morphologically constrained, they are either rod-shaped (bacilli), spherical (cocci), spirillum (actually helical and not a spiral) or vibrios (curved or comma shaped), budding and filamentous (actinomycetes). Cocci may be in chains (e.g. streptococci) or in clusters (e.g. staphylococci). However, in smears, lactobacilli which are morphologically similar may appear to branch, leading to confusion in the evaluation of cervical specimens for actinomycosis. Some members of the Actinobacteria (i.e. the genus *Bifidobacteria* form 'Y'-shaped cells). Many members of the Gram-positive bacteria are also able to produce endospores, a highly resistant resting and survival phase, and can be seen in genera such as *Bacillus* and *Clostridium*.

CLASSIFICATION AND TYPING

The classification of bacteria was complicated by the lack of clear-cut morphological relationships between different members, however in the late 1970s Carl Woese and George E. Fox (Woese and Fox, 1977) proposed a new topology for the tree of life based on DNA. For the first time a rationale framework for classifying bacteria had been devised which did not require biochemical tests or morphological phenotypes. It also maintained the Linnean hierarchy of species, genus, family, order, etc. and preserved grouping of organisms with shared characteristics. However, fine characteristics were not discernible, for example, *Escherichia coli* strains are indistinguishable in phylogenetic trees which are created from the DNA sequences of the small subunit ribosomal RNA (rRNA) gene, also known as the 16S rRNA gene. This lack of resolution means that it is not possible to determine if you have isolated a pathogen (e.g. *E. coli* O157) or have a probiotic (e.g. *E. coli* Nissle (1917)). Such information has obvious clinical implications. Despite this, knowledge of an organism's classification/taxonomy is, however, important for a number of reasons. It enables communication between scientists, gives a broad picture of how the organism may behave in vitro and in vivo, and may give some indication of the likely efficacy of proposed antimicrobial chemotherapy.

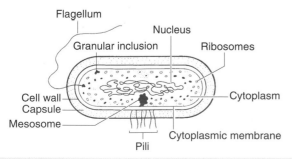

Fig. 7.1 Prototype bacterial cell.

With the cost of DNA sequencing plummeting and currently heading towards 0.1 pence or cent per base, whole genome sequencing (WGS) has become the main tool to characterise and classify bacteria. With a WGS project costing around £30 to 40 for the raw sequence (2021), it is possible to obtain a draft genome which shows the main properties and functions of the organism of interest. The use of WGS is also making its way into public health systems for tracking pathogen outbreaks, including viral pathogens and for fast classification of pathogen virulence factors and antibiotic resistance profiles.

The naming of newly discovered bacterial isolates follows the conventional Latin binomial system, which is overseen by an international body that applies strict rules. The genus is always written with a capitalised first letter and followed by the specific epithet commencing with a lower-case letter. Both components are written in italics – thus, *Staphylococcus* spp. and *Staphylococcus aureus*. The generic name may be abbreviated after first use, thus *S. aureus*, or if confusion is likely to arise, *Staph. aureus*. All other references to the specific bacterial taxonomic lineage (e.g. family names such as 'Staphylococcaceae' and order 'Bacillales') should also be italicised, however, this practice is not enforced by many journals. Trivial names such as 'coliform', or adjectives such as 'staphylococcal' or 'staphylococci' are not written in italics and are not proper nouns. Table 7.1 is a simple classification of medically important bacteria based on these characteristics.

In addition to a need to classify bacteria, it is often necessary to distinguish between infecting organisms of the same species, for example when trying to trace the source of a staphylococcal outbreak or confirming the chain of infection in a case of alleged sexual abuse. A variety of methods are available, some more applicable to some species than others. With the advent of WGS and DNA-based approaches the majority of strain typing is based on molecular approaches. Where an organism can be isolated to purity, WGS offers a cheap and relatively quick approach for source tracking in nosocomial outbreaks (Quainoo et al., 2017). For organisms which are harder to grow nucleic-acid based approaches are the most feasible assay, and the Center for Disease Control recommends the use of DNA-based approaches to identify and type *Chlamydia*.

PATHOGENESIS

The distinction between commensal and pathogenic organisms is far from clear-cut. Indeed, many of the organisms associated with common infections are part of the normal or transient microbiota of the body. Mere isolation of the organism from a specimen does not necessarily equate with disease. Rather isolation of an organism from a site normally considered sterile is more indicative of infection and disease. For example, the presence of *E. coli* in the small intestine reflects its normal habitat, but its presence in bladder urine indicates a urinary tract infection. *Haemophilus influenzae*, *Streptococcus pneumoniae* and *Moraxella catarrhalis* are all normal inhabitants of the upper respiratory tract, but each are capable of causing lower respiratory tract infection.

All bacterial species complexes have a Dr Jekyll and Mr Hyde persona, with examples of non-pathogenic strains and highly virulent strains. Examples include the plague bacillus, *Brucella* spp. and *Treponema* spp., however in general

Table 7.1 A Simple Classification of Medically Important Bacteria

FREE LIVING ORGANISMS

Gram-positive cocci
  Aerobic
    Staphylococcus spp.
    Streptococcus spp., *Enterococcus* spp.
  Anaerobic
    Peptostreptococcus
Gram-positive bacilli
  Aerobic
    Spore forming
      Bacillus spp.
    Non-spore forming
      Lactobacillus spp.
      Corynebacterium spp., *Listeria* spp.
  Anaerobic
    Clostridium spp.
Gram-negative cocci
  Aerobic
    Neisseria spp., *Moraxella* spp.
  Anaerobic
    Veillonella spp.
Gram-negative bacilli
  Aerobic or facultative anaerobic
    Small rod-shaped
      Legionella spp., *Haemophilus* spp.
      Bordetella spp., *Brucella* spp.
      Pasteurella spp., *Bartonella* spp.
    Comma-shaped
      Vibrio spp.
    Helically curved
      Campylobacter spp., *Helicobacter* spp.
    Large rod-shaped
    Fermentative
      Escherichia spp., *Klebsiella* spp.
      Enterobacter spp.
      Salmonella spp., *Shigella* spp., *Yersinia* spp.
    Non-fermentative
      Pseudomonas spp., *Stenotrophomonas* spp.
  Anaerobic
    Bacteroides spp.
    Prevotella spp.
Gram-variable coccobacilli
  Mobiluncus spp., *Gardnerella* spp.
Stain with acid-fast stains (e.g. Ziehl–Neelsen)
  Mycobacterium spp., *Nocardia* spp.
OBLIGATE INTRACELLULAR ORGANISMS
  Chlamydia spp., *Rickettsia* spp., *Coxiella* spp.

these genera are considered to be predominantly pathogenic. At the other extreme are organisms that are usually referred to as 'Generally regarded as safe' or 'GRAS' and are considered quite innocuous unless the host's defences are markedly impaired. These include 'opportunistic' organisms, such as *Pseudomonas aeruginosa*, which are often associated with sepsis in the immunosuppressed. There are also case reports of probiotic species causing pathologies when an opportunity arises (Boumis et al., 2018). Since it is not possible to continuously maintain a biological surface as sterile in an open system, the surface (e.g. an initially sterile burn) will soon become colonised with whatever organisms are in close proximity. In addition, if the biological surface has become selective because of antibiotic administration, the colonising organism is likely to be resistant to that antibiotic. The concept of creating the selective medium is important; it is, after all, what the laboratory does to select a single organism from a mixture – merely an in-vitro version of what the clinician may unwittingly be doing in vivo.

While a breakdown in the host immune system may lead to commensal organisms causing disease, bacteria have evolved a number of mechanisms to enhance their disease-causing potential and allow them to evade the immune system. Resistance to lysis by serum is a feature of the *Enterobacteriaceae*, associated with the presence of LPS at the cell surface. Initial contact with the host may be facilitated by a variety of adhesions. Once attached, the presence of a capsule, with or without antigenic similarity to the host, or the production of a protective biofilm may protect the organism against the host's immune system. More sophisticated evasive mechanisms include the production of proteases that cleave IgA, a feature of pathogens invading via mucosal surfaces such as *Neisseria* spp., or coating with host proteins, such as fibronectin as found in *T. pallidum*. *Chlamydia trachomatis* is able to prevent the fusion of lysosomes to the intracellular phagosome containing the infectious elementary body (EB); thus the host protects the invading organism from destruction. To initiate an infection of a clean wound with *Staph. aureus*, some 10^5 organisms are required. However, the presence of a foreign body, be it traumatic or a medically inserted cannula, reduces the required inoculum by 99% to 10^3. Such numbers are small by microbiological standards.

Iron is an important growth factor for many bacteria, which enables them to fix iron-binding proteins either through specific receptors for lactoferrin or transferrin (e.g. *Staph. aureus*), or by producing extracellular chelators such as siderophore (e.g. enterobactin from *E. coli*). Other extracellular products such as hyaluronidase and the ureases of *Proteus* spp. and *Helicobacter pylori* may also contribute to pathogenesis.

Toxin production is important for the ability of many pathogens to cause disease (virulence). These toxins may be found extracellularly as exotoxins or released upon cell death as endotoxins. Exotoxins are a feature of Gram-positive and Gram-negative organisms. Examples of the action of exotoxins include the neuromuscular effects of *Clostridium botulinum* and *Cl. tetani* toxins, gastrointestinal symptoms of cholera, *E. coli*, *Shigella* spp. and *Staph. aureus*, and skin necrosis from *Staph. aureus*. Some toxins require the infection of the bacteria with a phage for expression, such as diphtheria toxin, which affects the heart and lungs, and the erythrogenic toxin of *Str. pyogenes* (Group A streptococcus). Staphylococcal toxic shock syndrome toxin is a potent pyrogen. Some exotoxins can be formalin fixed to produce toxoids, which are used as vaccines (e.g. tetanus toxoid).

Endotoxin, otherwise known as LPS, is a feature of the Gram-negative cell wall. An important component of LPS is lipid A, which links it to the outer membrane. Lipid A seems to be responsible for the inflammatory responses associated with the endotoxic shock found in severe Gram-negative septicaemia. While the LPS of the *Enterobacteriaceae* are among some of the most potent triggers of inflammatory responses there are many other endotoxins that are often overlooked including flagellin, peptidoglycan and lipoteichoic acid (Gram-positive cell wall component). Some of these antigens are also triggers of the innate immune system and need to also be considered as they can influence a host's response to some of the more canonical antigens such as LPS from *E. coli*.

Laboratory Identification

SPECIMEN COLLECTION

The quality of the specimen is particularly important in microbiology. A poor specimen transported to a laboratory under less-than-ideal conditions could lead to a result that is at best, unhelpful, and, at worst, highly misleading. In general, specimens from sites thought to be infected will be collected for microscopy, culture and antigen or genome sequencing. In addition, serum samples may be sent for antibody determination. While the pressures on a clinician are appreciated, it is important that full clinical details including any current or intended antimicrobial therapy are also provided. Such information informs how clinical microbiology laboratories will undertake tests and interpret results.

Specimens should almost always be taken before treatment is commenced. Sensitive bacteria will not survive in the presence of antibiotics (unless the agent is bacteriostatic rather than bactericidal), and even if clinically resistant may not be recoverable on artificial media. The correct transport medium should always be used for swabs, to maintain the balance of organisms as similar to that observed at the site and time of sampling, and to ensure survival of pathogens. Because organisms will continue to divide at ambient temperature, specimens should be kept at $+4°C$ and transported to the laboratory as soon as possible. Some organisms are highly sensitive to storage conditions. For example, while conventional deep freeze at $-20°C$ is satisfactory for preserving many species, it is lethal to chlamydiae and many viruses, which survive better when stored below $-70°C$. Some fastidious organisms such as the gonococcus, which do not survive well out of their in vivo niche, should be either direct plated at the bedside or rapidly transported to the laboratory. To increase the likelihood of a positive result, liquid pus should always be preferred to a swab dipped in the pus. Different antigen or genome tests require different collection media, even where the same organism is being detected. It is therefore necessary to check with the laboratory before sending these specimens. If the possibility of sexual abuse arises, it is vital to set up a formal chain of evidence with the laboratory, or the evidence may not be admissible in court.

CULTURE

The majority of bacteria are still identified by culture on solid agar media in public health and clinical microbiology laboratories, however, there is a slow adoption of culture-independent assays which expedite identification. Using culture means that a minimum of 18 hours will elapse before even presumptive results are available. Microscopy will assist in some cases, but where there is a high abundance of normal microbiota, such as in the respiratory tract, identification of potential pathogens will be challenging and will thus facilitate some form of DNA or biomarker approach. It is never possible to speciate organisms by microscopy. Thus, intracellular Gram-negative cocci are not necessarily synonymous with *Neisseria gonorrhoeae* and should never be reported as such until confirmatory results are available. Culture of organisms is necessary in most circumstances to define a full picture of the organisms colonising or infecting a particular site. Sites that are considered to contain very low levels of microbial biomass, such as blood and cerebrospinal fluid, should present little problem to the laboratory as any organism cultured ought to be significant. However, the possibility of contamination of the specimen during collection, even under optimal conditions, may make interpretation of the results difficult. The problem is much greater with specimens from a site with a normal microbiota, because, as previously stated, many potentially pathogenic organisms may also be part of the normal microbiota. Further, it is not yet routinely possible to predict sensitivity to antibiotics without exposing actively divided organisms to them. However, developments in shotgun metagenomics offer a promising approach to meet the challenge of providing clinicians with timely and germane information, without the need to culture. Extraction of bacterial DNA for sequencing on third-generation sequencing platforms such as the Nanopore MinION and bioinformatic analyses may facilitate identification of the predominate strain present and its predicted antibiotic susceptibilities, within 5 hours of the sample being delivered to the laboratory.

ANTIGEN DETECTION

While no microbiological test is 100% sensitive, the specificity of culture approaches 100%. The same may not be true of antigen-detection systems, although even here the tendency is to concentrate on good specificity over sensitivity. This aim is because a false-positive diagnosis is more likely to mislead than a false-negative one. In the latter situation clinical impression will override the negative report from the laboratory. Non-culture detection tests provide two useful functions. First, they may be used in situations where rapid diagnosis has important therapeutic and public health consequences (e.g. meningitis). Second, the tests are useful to diagnose pathogens that are difficult or slow to isolate in the laboratory. A good example of this is in the diagnosis of chlamydial infection. Because of the need for cell culture to isolate the organism, the development of non-culture detection tests has served to highlight the prevalence and importance of the organism, and also to make diagnostic facilities more widely available. The disadvantage is that the tests are of variable sensitivity, and in some hands, specificity is less than optimal. Direct immunofluorescence tests are of good sensitivity but are subjective; in contrast enzyme-immunoassay systems are of high specificity, but generally of lower sensitivity. The importance of this discussion is that, in low prevalence populations, a low sensitivity (around 90%) may lead to a positive predictive value of under 50%. That is, one in two positive results may be a false positive.

NUCLEIC ACID DETECTION

Molecular technology has revolutionised diagnostic microbiology. Tests based on the amplification of DNA such as the polymerase chain reaction (PCR) and the closely related ligase chain reaction (LCR) are now established in the routine diagnosis of certain pathogens (e.g. *Neisseria meningitidis* and *C. trachomatis*). However, because of their extreme sensitivity, these techniques are subject to contamination problems. Only validated tests should ever be used for routine diagnostic purposes. Biological inhibitors may reduce the sensitivity of these tests in practice. The use of WGS is becoming much more routine as a tool to classify and characterise both viral and bacterial pathogens. In part this adoption has been accelerated by the ever-decreasing cost of DNA sequencing and the ease of access to second-generation sequencing platforms such as the Illumina HiSeq, Nextseq500 and MiSeq. In the future it will be much more commonplace for public health microbiology laboratories to rely on WGS and bioinformatic tools to classify a bacterial sample rather than culture-based approaches.

ANTIBODY DETECTION

Antibody detection tests have the theoretical advantage that all that is required is a sample of clotted blood. Unfortunately, in practice, it is unusual for a definitive diagnosis to be made on a single sample of serum. The antibody rise takes a minimum of 10 to 14 days, and in some infections (e.g. chlamydial infections) more than 3 weeks may elapse. The safest criterion for the diagnosis of infection using serology is a greater than fourfold rise in specific antibody titre in at least a pair of sera. The exceptions are diseases where antibodies to the organism in question are rare in the normal population, or the organism cannot be cultured. An example of the former is plague, and of the latter syphilis. In the case of syphilis, several different tests are carried out on a single specimen in an attempt to confirm the treponemal infection, and also to define the stage of the disease.

Bacteria and Disease

NORMAL MICROBIOTA

The relationship between humans and their microbes is complex, and it represents a shared co-evolutionary history. Products synthesised by one organism may assist the growth of another organism, which may in turn produce factors which will protect the host from invasion by extraneous organisms. Constant stimulation of the host immune system by resident bacteria will lead to early recognition and elimination of related, but potentially pathogenic, organisms, as well as contributing to the control of potentially neoplastic host cells by virtue of antigens similar to aberrant host ones. Intestinal microorganisms are capable of synthesising vitamins. The interactions of the various species of organism found on the skin are important for maintaining a healthy integument by production of fatty acids and other substances that inhibit the growth of potential pathogens. Disruption of this delicate balance will result in symptoms; for example, antibiotics that affect the normal gut microbiota will result in a change in the proportion of different bacterial species, with overgrowth of some at the expense of others. This imbalance is manifest by diarrhoea. A more sinister consequence may be the proliferation of *Clostridioides difficile*, an anaerobic spore-former present in 2% to 3% of the population, leading to toxin-mediated pseudomembranous colitis.

However, it was recently discovered that the opportunity for *C. difficile* to propagate and to cause infection is most probably due to the use of antibiotics that remove the ability of other bacteria in the community to create colonisation resistance. If the functions of these bacteria are re-introduced, for example, through the use of faecal microbiota transplantation, *C. difficile* can no longer thrive.

The interaction of aerobic organisms with anaerobic organisms is particularly intriguing. The aerobes serve to consume oxygen, thus lowering the oxygen tension (eH) to very low levels and allowing the proliferation of strictly anaerobic organisms. The anaerobes outnumber the aerobes by 10:1 to 100:1 on the skin, rising to over 1000-fold excess in the large intestine. One gram of faeces contains some 10^8 aerobic organisms and 10^{11} anaerobic organisms. Maintenance of the anaerobic gut microbiota is essential for health, and the use of anaerobe-sparing antibiotics (e.g. ciprofloxacin) where indicated is less likely to lead to diarrhoea as a side-effect.

The predominantly Gram-positive resident microbiota of the skin is supplemented by transient organisms, usually from the environment, and often Gram-negative. They are unable to establish themselves but may survive for several hours. This period is long enough for transfer to occur to susceptible individuals via the examining fingers.

NORMAL GENITAL TRACT MICROBIOTA OF WOMEN

Lactobacillus species have long been recognised as being predominant members of the genital tract microbiota. More recently, metataxonomic approaches have indicated that there exists 5 major vaginal bacterial profile types or community state types (CST), 4 of which were dominated by species from the genus *Lactobacillus* and a fourth CST which is dominated by strictly anaerobic and low levels of lactic acid bacteria. Specifically, CST I, II, II and V are dominated by *L. crispatus*, *L. gasseri*, *L. iners* and *L. jensenii* respectively, and are considered to be low diversity communities. CST IV is a relatively high diversity community colonised by species from the *Prevotella*, *Megasphaera*, *Atopobium* and *Sneathia* genera, for example. Several groups have now independently replicated these findings in different patient cohorts and identified interesting correlations between these CSTs and pre-term birth and cervical cancer, thus identifying the potential for interventions that modulate the vaginal microbiota and abrogate these issues.

The normal microbiota of the vagina changes under the influence of circulating oestrogens. The presence of oestrogen leads to an environment rich in glycogen, and the release of glucose via vaginal α-amylase activity favours the growth of lactobacilli and other acid-tolerant organisms. The metabolism of glycogen breakdown products to lactic acid, results in a pH less than 4.5. Other bacteria commonly present include anaerobic cocci, diphtheroids, coagulase-negative staphylococci and α-haemolytic streptococci. In addition, a number of organisms that are also potential pathogens may colonise. These include β-haemolytic streptococci including *Str. agalactiae* and *Actinomyces* spp. The balance between health and disease in the vagina is delicate. Factors leading to alteration of this balance will lead to overgrowth of organisms at the expense of the lactobacilli leading to bacterial vaginosis. Specific disease can be caused by yeast-like fungi (e.g. *Candida* spp.) or infection with the protozoon *Trichomonas vaginalis*. Gonococcal and chlamydial infections affect the cervix, causing genital discharge. Bacterial vaginosis, gonococcal and chlamydial infections all predispose to ascending infection resulting in endometritis and salpingitis, with the attendant sequelae of ectopic pregnancy or infertility. Bacterial vaginosis also appears to be a factor in the pathogenesis of pre-term labour.

GRAM-POSITIVE AND GRAM-NEGATIVE BACTERIA

Table 7.2 lists some of the more medically important bacteria. *Staph. aureus* is distinguished from other staphylococci by production of coagulase. Increasingly, these organisms are proving to be resistant to the anti-staphylococcal β-lactam antibiotics (penicillins and cephalosporins). Such strains are designated methicillin-resistant *Staph. aureus* (MRSA) after the now obsolete antibiotic used as a laboratory test to detect them. Strains are frequently also multi-resistant, and some are able to spread easily through clinical areas (epidemic MRSA – EMRSA). MRSA are usually no more virulent than other coagulase-positive staphylococci, and frequently colonise wounds and carrier sites. However, when they do cause infection the antibiotic choice is considerably limited compared with methicillin-sensitive strains.

Streptococci are divided into three broad groups based on their haemolysis of horse blood agar. Strains producing partial haemolysis (resulting in a greenish pigmentation of the agar) are termed α-haemolytic. This group comprises a number of commensal strains found particularly on the skin and in the mouth ('viridans' streptococci), but they are also important pathogens in deep-seated abscesses and endocarditis. The pneumococci and enterococci (*Enterococcus (Streptococcus) faecalis* and *Ent. faecium*) are also important members of this group. Pneumococci are showing increasing resistance to penicillin. The enterococci are frequent super-infecting organisms, particularly associated with cephalosporin therapy. Glycopeptides (vancomycin and teicoplanin) are often required to treat enterococcal infection; consequently the emergence of vancomycin- and teicoplanin-resistant strains (VRE) is a major worry. Complete haemolysis is termed β-haemolysis. Organisms in this group are further subdivided into the Lancefield Groups A to O. Some α-haemolytic strains also have Lancefield antigens (e.g. the enterococcus is Lancefield Group D). The major human pathogens are in Groups A, B, C and G. However, members of these four groups may also occur as normal human microbiota. The Group A streptococcus is the most important pathogen (*Str. pyogenes*) and remains fully sensitive to penicillin. The third broad group is the non-haemolytic streptococci, which are commensal organisms, although anaerobic streptococci may cause wound infections.

The corynebacteria are Gram-positive rods widely distributed over the skin and upper respiratory tract. It is important to differentiate rapidly the pathogenic *C. diphtheriae* strains from the commensals, and to determine whether the former are toxin-producing strains. *C. jeikeium* strains have achieved some notoriety by their ability to colonise intravenous cannulae, particularly in the immunosuppressed. Strains are frequently multiply resistant, and may require glycopeptide therapy, or removal of the cannula.

Table 7.2 Bacterial Species of Medical Importance

Group or Genus	Important Species	Diseases Caused, Comments
GRAM-POSITIVE COCCI		
Staphylococci	*Staphylococcus aureus*	Wound infections, abscess, bacteraemia/septicaemia, osteomyelitis, tampon-associated toxic shock syndrome, food poisoning
	S. epidermidis	Vascular cannula-associated infection
	Staph. saprophyticus	Urinary tract infections
Streptococci (α-haemolytic)	*Streptococcus milleri*	Normal mouth microbiota, deep-seated abscesses, endocarditis
	S. pneumoniae	Lobar pneumonia
	Enterococcus (Streptococcus) faecalis	Normal bowel microbiota, urinary tract infection, opportunistic wound infection
Streptococci (β-haemolytic)	*S. pyogenes* (Group A)	Bacterial upper respiratory tract infection, wound infection, abscesses, bacteraemia/septicaemia, puerperal sepsis, necrotising fasciitis, scarlet fever, septic arthritis
	S. agalactiae (Group B)	Normal vaginal microbiota, neonatal bacteraemia/septicaemia and meningitis
Peptostreptococcus	*P. anaerobius*	Anaerobic abscesses
GRAM-POSITIVE BACILLI		
Bacillus spp.	*B. anthracis*	Anthrax
	B. cereus	Normal microbiota of air, food poisoning with diarrhoea and vomiting
Lactobacilli	*Lactobacillus casei*	Normal vaginal microbiota
Corynebacteria	*Corynebacterium diphtheriae*	Diphtheria
	C. jeikeium	Skin microbiota, line- (cannula/vascular) associated bacteraemia/septicaemia
Listeria	*L. monocytogenes*	Maternal and neonatal listeriosis
Clostridium spp.	*C. perfringens*	Gas gangrene
	C. tetani	Tetanus
Actinomycetes	*Actinomyces israelii*	Pelvic actinomycosis
Nocardia	*N. asteroides*	Chronic infection in transplant patients
GRAM-NEGATIVE COCCI		
Neisseriae	*Neisseria gonorrhoeae*	Gonorrhoea, pelvic inflammatory disease, arthritis, bacteraemia/septicaemia, infertility, neonatal ocular infection
	N. meningitidis	Meningitis
Moraxellae	*Moraxella (Branhamella) catarrhalis*	Respiratory microbiota, exacerbations of chronic bronchitis
Veillonella	*Veillonella* spp.	Normal oropharyngeal microbiota
GRAM-NEGATIVE BACILLI		
Haemophilus spp.	*H. influenzae*	Respiratory microbiota, exacerbations of chronic bronchitis
Legionella spp.	*L. pneumophila*	Atypical pneumonia
Pasteurella spp.	*P. multocida*	Animal bites
Yersinia	*Y. pestis*	Plague
	Y. enterocolitica	Mesenteric adenitis
Comma-shaped	*Vibrio cholerae*	Cholera
Helically curved	*Campylobacter fetus*	Normal microbiota of chickens, food poisoning with diarrhoea
	Helicobacter spp.	Gastritis and peptic ulcers
Bartonellae	*Bartonella henselae*	Cat-scratch disease, bacillary peliosis, bacillary angiomatosis
Enterobacteriaceae	*Escherichia coli, Klebsiella pneumoniae, Enterobacter cloacae*	Urinary tract infection, abdominal sepsis, wound infection, bacteraemia/septicaemia, nosocomial respiratory infection
	Proteus mirabilis	Enteric fever
	Salmonella typhi, Salmonella enteritidis	Food poisoning with diarrhoea
	Shigella dysenteriae	Dysentery
Pseudomonads	*Pseudomonas aeruginosa*	Nosocomial urinary tract infection and respiratory infection, opportunistic wound infection, bacteraemia/septicaemia
	Stenotrophomonas maltophilia	
Anaerobic Gram-negative bacteria	*Bacteroides fragilis*	Normal gut microbiota, abdominal sepsis, pelvic inflammatory disease
	Prevotella melaninogenica	Respiratory tract infection
	P. bivia	Normal vaginal microbiota, abdominal sepsis, pelvic inflammatory disease
	Fusobacterium nucleatum	Severe oral sepsis

Continued

Table 7.2 Bacterial Species of Medical Importance – Cont'd

Group or Genus	Important Species	Diseases Caused, Comments
OTHERS		
Gram-variable coccobacilli	*Mobiluncus curtisii*	Normal vaginal microbiota, but predominant in bacterial vaginosis
	Gardnerella vaginalis	Associated with clue cells
Mycobacteria	*Mycobacterium tuberculosis*	Tuberculosis
	M. avium-intracellulare	Chronic respiratory infection and bacteraemia in severely immuno-suppressed patients
Spirochaetes	*Treponema pallidum*	Syphilis
	T. pertenue	Yaws
	Leptospira interrogans	Leptospirosis
	Borrelia recurrentis	Relapsing fever
Mycoplasmas	*Mycoplasma pneumoniae*	Atypical pneumonia
	M. hominis	Normal vaginal microbiota, pyelonephritis, pelvic inflammatory disease
	Ureaplasma urealyticum	Normal vaginal microbiota, non-gonococcal non-chlamydial urethritis, neonatal respiratory infection
Chlamydiae	*Chlamydia trachomatis*	Non-gonococcal urethritis, cervicitis, endometritis, pelvic inflammatory disease, infertility, neonatal ocular and respiratory infection
	C. pneumoniae	Atypical pneumonia, possible association with coronary heart disease
	C. psittaci	Animal pathogen, atypical pneumonia in humans
Rickettsiae and *Coxiella* spp.	*Rickettsia prowazekii*	Typhus
	Coxiella burnetii	Q fever

Listeria monocytogenes is of particular importance in obstetrics. It is a motile Gram-positive rod widely distributed in nature. The organism is capable of active division at low temperatures (e.g. in display and domestic refrigerators). Depending on regional, occupational and animal exposure, between 5% and 70% of the population carry the organism in the bowel, and strains can be isolated from soil, vegetables, salads and dairy products, and uncooked or partly cooked chicken. Of the 13 serovars, only two are of importance in human disease. Infection in adults is an important cause of meningitis. Maternal infection usually occurs late in pregnancy, and symptoms range from mild 'flu-like' to chills, fever and back pain and bacteraemia. Neonates infected during pregnancy are ill at or soon after birth. Symptoms are non-specific, but respiratory distress is common, with bradycardia, jaundice and hepatosplenomegaly; neurological symptoms and skin rashes are also found. The characteristic lesions found in the placenta and at postmortem examination of infected neonates are miliary granulomata with focal necrosis. Routine macroscopic inspection of the placenta to exclude these macroscopic lesions should be encouraged. Intrapartum neonatal infection will lead to predominantly meningitic symptoms with an incubation period of 5 to 7 days.

The only bacteria to show branching are the actinomycetes. These organisms colonise the mouth, gut and female genital tract and may also colonise intrauterine devices. Pelvic actinomycosis is a rare chronic granulomatous disease. The diagnosis can be made by observing the yellow mycelial masses (sulphur granules) in tissue. Symptoms may mimic pelvic neoplasia, and the distinction is important because actinomycosis may be treated with extended courses of appropriate antibiotics such as amoxicillin or co-trimoxazole. Cytologists frequently report *Actinomyces*-like organisms seen on cervical smears. This statement is not synonymous with actinomycosis. The organisms seen are usually commensal lactobacilli, which are also long Gram-positive rods and may appear to show branching in smears.

Clostridium perfringens is a component of normal bowel microbiota. Resistant spores are produced under certain conditions, which may survive inadequate disinfection or sterilisation. The organism will proliferate in necrotic or poorly perfused tissue, giving rise to gas gangrene. The source is almost always the patient's own microbiota. *C. difficile* is also found in the adult normal bowel in small numbers, and in neonates in large numbers (Jangi and Lamont, 2010). Antibiotics lead to an overgrowth of this organism, and production of exotoxins which gives rise to pseudomembranous colitis and toxic megacolon. Practically all antimicrobials may lead to this condition, but it is particularly associated with clindamycin, cephalosporins and more recently ciprofloxacin. Neonatal tetanus may be encountered in areas of poor hygiene, acquired via the umbilical stump wound. *Cl. botulinum* produces a powerful neurotoxin. The disease in adults results from ingestion of the pre-formed toxin, but neonatal botulism may develop from bacteria growing in the gut.

The Gram-negative cocci of medical importance are contained within the genus *Neisseria*. Both *N. gonorrhoeae* and *N. meningitidis* are fastidious organisms, and care is necessary with specimen collection to ensure that the organisms remain viable. The organisms are usually found within inflammatory exudate cells. *N. meningitidis* is a common nasopharyngeal commensal, and the commonest bacterial cause of meningitis. Both organisms are capable of causing genital infection. *N. gonorrhoeae* infects columnar cells; it is therefore a parasite of the cervix, not the vagina. *M. catarrhalis* strains are usually resistant to penicillins, which may compromise treatment of exacerbations of chronic bronchitis.

The enteric Gram-negative rods comprise a large group of morphologically identical organisms located in the gut. The simplest classification divides them into those that ferment lactose, and those that do not. The lactose fermenters include *E. coli*, *Enterobacter* spp. and *Klebsiella pneumoniae*. The non-lactose fermenters include the enteric pathogens such as *Shigella* spp. and the salmonellae. There are over 2000 types of salmonella, including enteric fever-causing typhoid and paratyphoid, and the common species associated with food poisoning such as *Salmonella typhimurium* and *Salmonella enteritidis*. Other important Gram-negative aerobic bacilli include *Pseudomonas* spp. and *Acinetobacter* spp. These are predominantly environmental organisms that will colonise and infect wounds opportunistically – that is, wounds in patients who are debilitated, immuno-suppressed or on long-term inappropriate broad-spectrum antibiotics.

The anaerobic Gram-negative bacilli are non-sporing. Although their growth requirements are very precise, they are widely distributed in the body, colonising small-intestine and to a lesser extent the large intestine, oropharynx and vagina. They may contribute to the formation of abscesses in association either with other anaerobes, or with aerobic organisms.

The precise cause of bacterial vaginosis is unknown. However, the effect is a change in the balance of the bacterial species making up the normal microbiota. The normally predominant Gram-positive lactobacilli are replaced by Gram-variable coccobacilli. These organisms characteristically adhere to the squamous cells and are called 'clue cells' when seen in vaginal smears. The organisms include the anaerobic *Mobiluncus* spp. and the microaerophilic *Gardnerella vaginalis*. The term 'vaginosis' implies that there is no inflammation of the vaginal wall, but a fishy smelling, watery vaginal discharge is produced with a pH greater than 5.0.

SPIROCHAETES, MYCOPLASMAS, CHLAMYDIAE AND OTHER BACTERIA

Treponema pallidum, the spirochaete that causes syphilis, cannot be easily cultivated in the laboratory and needs to be grown with tissue culture cells. It is also serologically indistinguishable from the spirochaetes that cause yaws and pinta. In consequence, the laboratory can only provide evidence of current or past treponemal infection. It cannot diagnose syphilis. This unsatisfactory state means that if there is any doubt as to the cause of serum treponemal antibodies, the patient must be assumed to have active syphilis and be treated accordingly. Syphilis in pregnancy will affect the fetus, resulting in a number of characteristic clinical features such as rashes, snuffles, teeth abnormalities, hepatosplenomegaly, proceeding over months and years to osteochondritis and gummata. Specific treatment at any time in pregnancy will result in a healthy neonate.

Mycoplasmas are widely distributed throughout plants and animals. There are more than a dozen species colonising humans, in the oropharynx, bowel and genital tract. The majority of these strains are commensal, and their role in disease is controversial. *Mycoplasma pneumoniae* is an important cause of atypical pneumonia. *Mycoplasma hominis* is found in some 20% of sexually active women and may be associated with bacterial vaginosis and pelvic inflammatory disease (PID); it causes some cases of pyelonephritis. *Ureaplasma urealyticum* is present in up to 80% of sexually active women. Its role in disease is less clear. Both *U. urealyticum* and *M. hominis* have been isolated from

chorioamnionitis. Mycoplasma should be considered as a cause of postpartum pyrexia and treatment with tetracyclines considered if the fever does not settle. *M. hominis* differs from other mycoplasmas infecting humans by being resistant to macrolides (e.g. erythromycin), but sensitive to clindamycin. *Mycoplasma genitalium* is difficult to isolate in the laboratory for routine purposes, but there is evidence from molecular studies that it plays a role in pelvic inflammatory disease.

The chlamydiae have a complex life cycle, as they are obligate intracellular parasites with a unique life cycle involving an extracellular transport phase – the EB – and an intracellular phase – the reticulate body (RB). The life cycle is about 48 hours, during which the EB is taken up into a phagosome within the host cell, and transforms into a RB. Division of the RB leads to an inclusion full of daughter RBs, which condense to form the much smaller EBs. Release of the EBs by rupture of the host cell allows infection of further cells. The organisms cannot be cultured on artificial media, requiring living cells. This makes their laboratory isolation inconvenient. Culture has for routine purposes been superseded by antigen detection (e.g. direct immunofluorescence or enzyme immunoassay) or by molecular technology using PCR. Serology is of limited use in the diagnosis of acute chlamydial genital infection owing to cross-reaction of *C. trachomatis* with the commoner respiratory species *C. pneumoniae*. As with *N. gonorrhoeae*, *C. trachomatis* also infects columnar epithelium, and so is found in cervical cells.

Killing Bacteria

ACTION OF ANTIBIOTICS

The unique structure of the bacterial cell wall has led to the development of chemotherapeutic agents with specific antibacterial activity and low host toxicity (see also Chapter 12). The β-lactam antibiotics comprise two main groups – the penicillins and cephalosporins – each of which contains a large number of members giving an antibacterial spectrum, at least in theory, spanning the bacterial genera of medical importance. Other members of the class include the monobactams and carbapenems (e.g. imipenem). All act selectively on the PBPs unique to the region of the bacterial cell wall. Glycopeptides such as vancomycin and teicoplanin are also important inhibitors of the cell wall construction, preventing incorporation of new units.

The cell membrane structure of all living organisms is very similar, so polymyxins, which are active at the bacterial cell membrane, are toxic to humans and rarely used systemically. The antifungal agents nystatin and amphotericin B act on the unique sterol-containing membrane of fungi but are in themselves also toxic to animals. The azole antifungals block sterol synthesis and are less toxic.

Similarities of the basic metabolic and nucleic acid synthesising pathways of plants, animals, fungi and bacteria also causes problems of selective toxicity. Consequently, it is necessary to exploit differing enzyme affinities or alternative pathways to kill infecting organisms selectively with minimal adverse effects on the host. The 70S ribosomes of bacteria are different to the 80S ribosomes of mammals, so that antibiotics affecting bacterial protein synthesis are likely to be ineffective against the host's mechanism.

Examples include the macrolides (e.g. erythromycin) and lincosamides (e.g. clindamycin), tetracyclines, aminoglycosides (e.g. gentamicin), fusidic acid and chloramphenicol.

Antibiotics can also affect nucleic acid synthesis. Differing enzyme affinities ensure that toxicity to humans is minimised. The quinolones inhibit the α-subunit of bacterial DNA gyrase, preventing supercoiling of the DNA. The ansamycins (e.g. rifampicin) inhibit bacterial DNA-dependent RNA polymerase. Bacteria need to synthesise folic acid in the same way as other organisms. Sulphonamides and trimethoprim act at different points along the folic acid pathway. Bacteria must synthesise folic acid, while mammalian cells require pre-formed folate, and hence are not affected by sulphonamides, which inhibit folic acid formation. Further along the pathway, the reduction of dihydrofolate to tetrahydrofolate requires the action of dihydrofolate reductase. Trimethoprim, the anti-protozoal pyrimethamine and the anti-cancer drug methotrexate all act at this site. Selective toxicity reflects selective affinity for the relevant enzyme.

The actual site of action of nitroimidazole drugs such as metronidazole is unknown. However, the active compound is known to be a reduced form of the drug which is produced only at the very low oxygen tension (eH) produced in the cells of anaerobic bacteria. The action of this active form is thought to be against the nucleus.

Bacterial resistance may be mediated by one of four mechanisms:

1. The antibiotic may not get into cells (e.g. vancomycin and Gram-negative organisms).
2. It may be rapidly eliminated by efflux mechanisms (e.g. tetracycline resistance).
3. Enzymes may destroy the antibiotic, such as β-lactamases and aminoglycoside-modifying enzymes.
4. The target site may be increased, altered or blocked, such as by rifampicin or quinolone resistance.

What is apparent is that the ingenuity of the bacterial cell knows no bounds when it comes to the battle for survival. The antibiotic that has no resistance to it has not yet been discovered. Multi-resistant bacteria are becoming more common, and more difficult or even impossible to treat with currently available drugs.

PHYSICAL METHODS

The technological advances in medicine have resulted in a vast array of different materials being used to manufacture devices for insertion into the body for therapeutic purposes. Ever since antisepsis was first demonstrated to reduce postoperative sepsis by Joseph Lister in 1867, it has been axiomatic that devices should be pathogen free. Antisepsis was replaced by asepsis at the turn of the century, but the comment that is ascribed to the surgeon Berkeley Moyhnihan (1865 to 1936) that 'every operation in surgery is an experiment in bacteriology' remains as true today as in the 1920s.

Sterilisation/Disinfection

Sterilisation is the removal of all microorganisms including spores and is defined internationally as a viable organism count of less than 10^{-6}. That is, a single viable organism in one of a batch of 1 million surgical packs would mean that sterile conditions had not been achieved. Disinfection is the removal of all actively dividing organisms and may not necessarily include spores of fungi or bacteria, nor viruses or prions (such as the spongiform encephalopathy agents). It equates to a reduction in bacterial load in excess of 10^5. The difference between the two concepts is crucial. Sterilisation is not easy to obtain reliably, and disinfection may be adequate in some circumstances if done properly. Sterilisation is always preceded by disinfection, in order to reduce the bioburden. The three components of disinfection are: (1) cleaning, (2) heat and (3) chemicals.

Heat

Heat results in coagulation of proteins and loss of viability. Heat can be in the form of dry heat, which penetrates surfaces poorly, or moist heat in the form of pure steam. The process of sterilisation by heat requires a heating-up period, a sterilising time at the correct sterilising temperature, a further safety period at this temperature, to give a total holding time at the sterilising temperature, and a cooling period. The entire process time is the cycle time and will depend on the method of sterilisation and the type of load (e.g. an open tray of instruments or a wrapped operative pack containing metal and other materials).

Dry heat is of limited use in surgical practice because it requires a holding time of 1 hour at 160°C, giving a cycle time of over 2 hours. At this temperature, materials other than metal may char. The use of pure steam is considerably more efficient, requiring lower temperatures for shorter holding times. The basic time/temperature used in the UK is 134°C to 137°C held for 3 minutes. This equates to a cycle time of some 10 minutes and should not be confused with the American standard of 137°C with a holding time of 10 minutes. Two basic forms of steam steriliser are in use. The downward displacement autoclave relies on the incoming steam to displace air from the load. Any combination of air and steam will result in sterilising conditions not being achieved. Therefore, a downward displacement autoclave using the UK cycle cannot be used to sterilise wrapped loads or loads with narrow lumens, such as liposuction cannulae. To achieve reliable air removal and steam penetration, a vacuum autoclave is required, which draws a high pre-vacuum before steam is introduced to the autoclave chamber. It is important that the instruments placed in a downward displacement autoclave are packed loosely, not placed within impervious containers. In contrast a high vacuum autoclave is packed tightly to physically remove the bulk of air in the chamber. Recently, benchtop vacuum autoclaves have been developed. These allow small-wrapped loads or a few items with lumens to be processed away from sterile service departments. These machines must not be overloaded. The quality of water used to generate the steam is also important. Water for irrigation should be used in benchtop autoclaves and changed at least daily; this prevents the build-up of pyrogens such as endotoxin, which may remain despite the organisms being killed. It is important that autoclaves are properly maintained, with daily, weekly, quarterly and annual checks being performed relevant to the machine and type of cycle and an audit loop of recording these checks.

Disinfection by heat usually involves the use of machines called washer disinfectors. These are in use for disinfection of crockery, as bedpan washers and for processing instruments before sterilisation. The key is obtaining a temperature of at least 80°C for 1 minute. The load is usually heat-dried to avoid the use of drying cloths.

Chemicals

The inappropriate use of chemicals is a potential source of infection. Chemicals are incapable of reliable sterilisation, except under very carefully controlled circumstances, seldom reached in clinical practice. The term 'high-grade disinfection' describes attempts to achieve chemical sterilisation of articles that cannot be sterilised by conventional means. Chemicals are markedly affected by a number of factors, including:

- Spectrum of activity
- Temperature of use
- Presence of organic debris
- Contact time and penetrability
- Dilution
- Stability at in-use dilution
- Inactivators (such as plastics and hard water).

Many disinfectants are odourless and have the 'disinfectant' smell added. 'Pine fluid' has practically no disinfectant action. Cetrimide is widely used in the laboratory as a selective medium for growing *P. aeruginosa*. It is vital that the correct disinfection process is used for the proposed task. Prior cleaning must always occur. For the processing of endoscopes, this should involve a mechanical washer because cleaning is likely to be more efficient than manually, reducing the chances of biofilm build up in the lumens. All disinfectants are toxic to humans and require care in use. Many disinfectants are corrosive, and it is prudent to ensure that the manufacturer has confirmed that the intended process will not damage the instrument and will be effective in decontamination. The machines used to clean scopes must also be fully maintained to avoid their becoming colonised and recontaminating the scopes at the end of the process.

Other Methods and Approaches to Sterilise and Disinfect

Ethylene oxide gas may be used to sterilise heat-sensitive devices. The process is difficult to control and requires a prolonged aeration phase after sterilisation. More recently, gas plasma has become practical. Thoroughly cleaned and dried instruments are placed in a chamber with hydrogen peroxide. Low-frequency radio waves are used to generate a plasma, which converts the hydrogen peroxide to lethal superoxide and super hydroxyl ions. The process is suitable for heat-sensitive items. Radiation is used to sterilise single-use items such as syringes after manufacture. It has little practical role in medical practice.

Mycology

Fungi are generally larger than bacteria and are commonly multicellular. Fungal cell walls do not contain peptidoglycan but owe their rigidity to fibrils of chitin embedded in a matrix of protein and the polysaccharides mannan or glucan.

Most fungi that infect humans grow at a wide range of temperatures, although the optimal temperature for the majority is between 25°C and 30°C. The dermatophytes responsible for skin infections, such as ringworm, grow best between 28°C and 30°C, while organisms such as *Candida albicans* or *Aspergillus fumigatus*, which are responsible for systemic infections, grow best at 37°C. Fungi are predominantly aerobic, but many yeasts can produce alcohol by fermentation as an end-product of anaerobic metabolism. Virtually all fungi have the potential to reproduce by production of asexual spores. These may be conidia, produced in large numbers by moulds, such as aspergillus or the dermatophytes, or the chlamydospores produced in small numbers for survival in extreme conditions by fungi such as *C. albicans*.

The majority of fungi pathogenic to humans were thought to lack a sexual phase in their life cycle and were therefore classified as 'fungi imperfecti'. A sexual phase has now been demonstrated in the laboratory for many of these pathogenic fungi, allowing them to be more accurately classified; however, it is convenient in the medical context to leave them under a single grouping of 'fungi imperfecti'.

PATHOGENIC FUNGI

There are four main groups of pathogenic fungi:

1. Moulds (filamentous fungi)
2. True yeasts
3. Yeast-like fungi
4. Dimorphic fungi.

Most pathogenic fungi are easily cultured in the laboratory, using Sabouraud dextrose agar, with and without supplements. *Candida* spp. and many other pathogenic fungi will also grow on blood agar.

Moulds

These grow as long, branching filaments called 'hyphae', which intertwine to form a 'mycelium'. Reproduction is by spores, including sexual spores, which are characteristic and are important in identification. The fungi often appear as powdery colonies on culture owing to the presence of abundant spores. Included in this group are the dermatophytes, responsible for common superficial skin, nail and hair infections, and belonging to the genera *Trichophyton*, *Microsporum* and *Epidermophyton*, and also the moulds causing systemic infections in the immunocompromised, for example *A. fumigatus* or *Mucor* spp.

True Yeasts

These are unicellular, round or oval fungi. Reproduction is by budding from the parent cell. Characteristically, cultures show creamy colonies. The major pathogen in this group is *Cryptococcus neoformans*, which has a large polysaccharide capsule. Encapsulated yeasts seen in biological fluids are diagnostic of cryptococcal infection.

Yeast-Like Fungi

Like yeasts, these appear as round or oval cells and reproduce by budding. They also form long branching filaments known as 'pseudohyphae'. *Candida* is the characteristic genus in this group with *C. albicans* being the major pathogen. Formation of germ tubes in serum broth distinguishes *C. albicans* from other members of the genus for practical purposes. *C. albicans* may be normal microbiota of the gastrointestinal tract, vagina or skin. Vaginal carriage is increased in pregnancy. Vaginal candidosis (thrush) is a common cause of vaginal discharge. Systemic candidal infection is a feature of the immunosuppressed, or severely ill patient on broad-spectrum antibacterial therapy.

Dimorphic Fungi

These grow as yeast forms in the body and at 37°C on culture media, and in a mycelial form in the environment or on culture media at 22°C. *Histoplasma capsulatum* is a well-known member of this group. Infection is usually asymptomatic but may produce calcified lung lesions. Chronic infection may lead to lung cavities, but a rare acute progressive disease involving widespread infection of the reticuloendothelial cells is usually fatal.

Pneumocystis carinii was originally considered to be an uncommon parasite until, as a result of DNA analysis, it was re-classified in 1988 as an unusual fungus which is very difficult to culture. The human form of *Pneumocystis* was named *P. jirovecii* in 2002, although the acronym PCP for the respiratory disease caused has been retained.

Parasites

PROTOZOA

These are unicellular eucaryotic organisms. They are able to reproduce by simple asexual binary fission, or by a more complex sexual cycle with the formation of cystic forms. Among the parasitic protozoa, both forms may occur in a single host.

The protozoa of medical importance are usefully classified into three groups: the sporozoa (containing the non-flagellate blood and tissue parasites), the amoebae and the flagellates (containing the trypanosomes that cause sleeping sickness, *Giardia lamblia* and *T. vaginalis*). A list of some medically important species is given in Table 7.3. The two protozoa of importance in obstetrics and gynaecology are *T. vaginalis* and *Toxoplasma gondii*.

T. vaginalis infects the vagina. The organism is sexually transmitted, and although men may become colonised they generally clear the organism from the urethra within a few days. The organism is similar in size to a white blood cell (10 to 20 μm), and readily identified by flagella movement in wet preparations under a ×40 microscope objective. The organism has three free flagella, and a fourth is embedded in an undulating membrane along the anterior two-thirds of the cell. The organism may cause an irritant, purulent vaginal discharge, with a pH greater than 5.0. The vaginal wall may be erythematous. In the USA, some 5% to 10% of men with a non-gonococcal urethritis (NGU) are infected with *T. vaginalis*. Treatment is with metronidazole.

T. gondii is an intracellular protozoon with a worldwide distribution, causing infection in humans and a wide range of animals. The asexual phase of the organism (bradyzoite) is able to develop in the tissues of a wide variety of vertebrate hosts, including humans. The definitive host is the cat, both domestic and wild cats, in which the sexual cycle occurs in the intestine. Human infection rates may be as high as 90% in some populations. Infection is most often acquired by ingesting bradyzoites in undercooked meat. It may also follow ingestion of oocysts containing tachyzoites resulting from the sexual cycle in the intestine of a cat, which are excreted in its faeces. Cat litter trays and garden soil contaminated with cat faeces are a likely source to be avoided in pregnancy. After ingestion, the tachyzoites are distributed to many organs and tissues via the bloodstream and invade nucleated cells in all parts of the body and fetus. They multiply within the host cells, disrupting them by producing tissue cysts containing large numbers of slowly metabolising bradyzoites. Focal areas of necrosis occur in many organs, particularly the muscles, brain and eye. Human infection is usually subclinical but may produce a glandular fever-like syndrome or choroidoretinitis. Transplacental infection may occur during an acute infection in the mother, which may not be diagnosed but may result in serious disease in the fetus. Infection early in pregnancy may result in a stillbirth, or the birth of a live baby with disseminated infection. Features include: choroidoretinitis, microcephaly or hydrocephalus, intracranial calcification, hepatosplenomegaly and thrombocytopenia. Maternal infection during the third trimester can also be transmitted to the fetus, but at this stage of development it usually causes no damage. Controversy surrounds the benefits of antenatal screening. Maternal infection may go undetected unless serological screening is carried out, but a single estimation of antibody may give rise to unnecessary anxiety because of infection before pregnancy began, which carries no risk to the fetus. A rise in the mother's toxoplasma antibody titre during pregnancy or the finding that she has IgM antibodies, indicating recent infection, raises the question of whether to treat the infection, given that treatment does not guarantee the infant will be unaffected, or to terminate the pregnancy even though it is not certain that the fetus has been damaged. Spiramycin (a macrolide) is the drug of choice for treatment of the mother and her fetus.

HELMINTHS (WORMS)

The helminth parasites of humans belong to three zoologically distinct groups: trematodes (flukes), cestodes (tapeworms) and nematodes (roundworms (e.g. hookworm) *Ascaris lumbricoides*). None of the infections has particular significance during pregnancy other than as a cause of chronic anaemia with intestinal infection.

Table 7.3 Some Protozoal Parasites of Humans

Protozoa	Site of Infection
Entamoeba spp., *Giardia lamblia*, *Cryptosporidium parvum*	Intestine
Trichomonas vaginalis	Vagina
Plasmodium spp.	Blood
Trypanosoma spp.	Blood and tissue
Toxoplasma gondii	Tissues

Virology

Introduction

The layperson (and some doctors) thinks of viruses as being 'small germs'. Although most viruses are indeed very small, size is not a distinguishing feature since some of the larger viruses (e.g. pox viruses) are larger than small bacteria. An idea of the size of viruses may be obtained by comparing the size of an animal cell to a lecture theatre seating about 200 people; in such circumstances, a polio virus would be about the size of a squash ball, rubella virus the size of a tennis ball, and measles virus the size of a football.

Viruses are distinguished from other microorganisms by their nucleic acid content and method of replication. Microorganisms other than viruses are really cells; they contain both forms of nucleic acid, but DNA is their repository of genetic information. They have their own machinery for producing energy and can synthesise their own macro-molecular constituents (i.e. nucleic acid, proteins, carbohydrates and lipids). They all multiply by binary fission. Viruses generally contain no ribosomes, mitochondria or other organelles; they are dependent on the host cell machinery for protein synthesis and energy metabolism. Consequently, they are totally dissimilar from other microorganisms; they can reproduce themselves from a single nucleic acid molecule and are predatory parasites.

Viral Nucleic Acid

Viruses contain either DNA or RNA as their genetic material, usually as single molecules, but never both. In contrast, all other microorganisms contain both forms of nucleic acid. Viral nucleic acid may be either single-stranded (ss) or double-stranded (ds) and the nucleic acid may be in the form of a single piece or it may be segmented, as in influenza and rotaviruses. The nucleic acid content of viruses is very small when compared with that of the cell (e.g. influenza viruses have about one-hundredth of the nucleic acid of the cells they infect). RNA viruses (riboviruses) represent the only form of 'life' utilising RNA as genetic material.

REPLICATION

Viruses can only replicate in living cells, which may be of plant, bacterial (infecting viruses being termed bacteriophage or 'phage') or animal origin. The result of infection of a cell is twofold: first, and most usually, the formation of new virus particles and, second, some change in the cell (often but not always resulting in its destruction). Thus, viruses may establish latent infection in the cells they infect (e.g. the herpes group of viruses, papovaviruses and some adenoviruses). Alternatively, some viruses (e.g. papillomaviruses and the Epstein–Barr virus) may induce malignant transformation in the cells they infect. The bi-phasic lifestyle is also reflected in the viruses of bacteria. Bacteriophage can be either lytic or lysogenic. Lytic bacteriophage infect a specific strain of bacteria, replicate and lyse the cell when they complete their life cycle. Lysogenic bacteriophage infect the host and integrate their genomes into the host's genome, sometimes bringing new phenotypes to the host or remaining dormant until an environmental trigger causes them to excise and complete the lytic cycle.

The host cell provides the source of all the machinery required for viral reproduction; the invading virus introduces specific information relating to its own structure and constitution, as well as that required to divert cellular mechanisms to viral ends and for the construction of enzymes needed to manufacture viral products. This information is contained, in coded form, in the sequence of bases in the viral nucleic acid. Thus, infection with the virus results in the introduction into the living cell of an infective and foreign nucleic acid with specific biological properties. Once the virus particle has been taken into the cell, the virus merges its identity with it and the whole entity becomes a new and different cell which may be considered as 'a virus–cell complex'.

Details of the method by which different viruses replicate can be found in standard textbooks. In simple terms for DNA viruses, viral messenger RNA is transcribed from the parental virus DNA within the host cell, and codes for the formation of virus-specific proteins. For RNA viruses, the viral genome acts as a template for the synthesis of new viral RNA. SS RNA viruses are classified as positive or negative strand according to the way in which coding information is stored in the viral genome. With positive-strand RNA viruses, the viral genome is of the same polarity as messenger RNA, and may itself act as messenger RNA, being translated into code for virus-specific proteins. With negative-strand viruses, a complementary RNA copy of the viral genome, or part of it, acts as messenger RNA. One further group of RNA viruses known as reversi viruses replicates by reverse transcription of viral genomic RNA to form a DNA intermediate, from which both messenger RNA and progeny viral genomes are transcribed. This group includes retroviruses, such as the human immunodeficiency virus (HIV), and hepadnaviruses, such as hepatitis B virus (HBV).

STRUCTURE OF VIRUSES

Even before negative staining techniques by electron microscopy were available to determine the fine structure of viruses, x-ray diffraction studies indicated that viruses displayed distinct symmetry properties. Because of the limited genetic information available and for reasons of economy, Crick and Watson postulated that the nucleic acid of viruses would code for a virus coat (capsid) consisting of identical subunits arranged in a single repetitive form; negative staining techniques have confirmed these findings. There are two main types of symmetry: cubic and helical. Helical symmetry is generally associated with rod-shaped viruses and cubic symmetry with the more spherical ones.

In its simplest form, a virus consists of nucleic acid and a protein coat, and it is this protein coat which contains the regular assembly of protein molecules. Some viruses (e.g. viruses of the herpes group and myxoviruses, influenza) are surrounded by an envelope, which is derived from the host cell membrane during release of the virus particles. The capsid consists of numerous identical smaller units, designated capsomeres, which are constant in number and identical in shape. Fig. 7.2 illustrates cubic symmetry and Fig. 7.3 helical symmetry. The nucleic acid and capsid (nucleocapsid) of viruses exhibiting helical symmetry bear

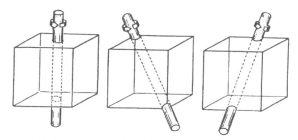

Fig. 7.2 Axes of symmetry of a cube: fourfold, threefold, twofold.

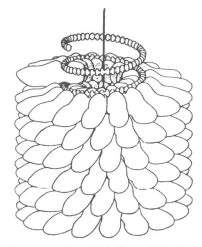

Fig. 7.3 Capsomeres arranged helically around central nucleic acid. Model of tobacco mosaic virus. (Reproduced from Advances in Virus Research 1960;7:274.)

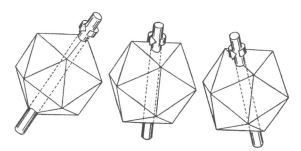

Fig. 7.4 Axes of symmetry of an icosahedron: fivefold, threefold, twofold.

a resemblance to a spiral staircase. Each step bears a constant relationship to its neighbours around a central axis which could be represented by the well of the staircase. Cubic symmetry is more complex and describes a group of regular units which have symmetry properties in common with a cube. Specifically, for viruses, it includes the tetrahedron, octahedron and icosahedron. Most viruses exhibiting cubic symmetry that infect humans have icosahedral symmetry (Fig. 7.4). The particle is three-dimensional with 20 identical faces with 12 vertices; each face is in the form of an equilateral triangle. Fig. 7.5 illustrates the fine structure of some of the viruses discussed in this chapter. No satisfactory electron micrographs of the hepatitis C virus have been published to date and, although an electron micrograph of Japanese B virus is not included, it is somewhat similar in its fine structure to the rubella virus.

DIAGNOSIS OF VIRAL INFECTIONS

An understanding of the nature, including the structure, of viruses is of importance in the diagnosis of viral infections. Viruses may be identified by demonstrating the effect they induce in living cells (cell culture), which can be visualised by low-power light microscopy. Different viruses induce different changes (cytopathic effects) in different cell lines and the virus may be identified by neutralising the virus infectivity in cell culture by specific antisera.

Whole virus may also be visualised by electron microscopy, but high virus concentrations are necessary and electron microscopy cannot distinguish viruses which are morphologically identical within a single group (e.g. different members of the herpesvirus group). Nevertheless, electron microscopy may rapidly identify a herpesvirus from a vesicular lesion, which may be all that is necessary for clinical purposes. Another virus belonging to the herpes group (cytomegalovirus (CMV)) may be visualised in the urine of congenitally infected infants.

Using specific antibodies, most usefully monoclonal antibodies, the presence of viral antigens may be identified directly from clinical samples. Alternatively, non-structural proteins may also be identified in clinical samples. Such techniques are used for the identification of respiratory syncytial virus in children with respiratory infections, and CMV in the blood and urine of patients with suspected CMV infection. More recently, techniques of considerable sensitivity and specificity have been employed to identify viral nucleic acid. Thus, nucleic acid hybridisation and gene amplification techniques (particularly the PCR) are now frequently used in diagnosis to identify a number of viral infections, including infections by the herpes group of viruses, enteroviruses, hepatitis C, hepatitis B and HIV viruses. These methods can also be used to quantify the amount of virus in specimens. This quantification is useful for monitoring virus infections in patients who are immunosuppressed or receiving antiviral therapy.

Serological techniques can be used to determine evidence of immunity to viruses, usually by detecting the presence of virus-specific IgG responses. Diagnostically, a significant rise in antibody titre (greater than fourfold) between acute and convalescent sera is significant for determination of recent infection. However, more frequently, evidence of current, recent or persistent infection may be detected by a virus-specific IgM response directed towards viral capsid proteins. Such responses are useful in the diagnosis of intrauterine and some perinatal infections (e.g. rubella), CMV and parvovirus B19 infections.

Viruses of Importance in Obstetrics and Gynaecology

Rather than provide basic information on different groups of viruses, attention will be focused on the importance of viruses which may induce severe infections in pregnancy, as well as intrauterine, perinatal and gynaecological infections. The classification and properties of these viruses is shown in Table 7.4. Some of these viruses, such as the influenza virus, cause classical acute infections, characterised by a rapid onset of symptoms and a brief period of viral replication, followed by clearance of the virus and

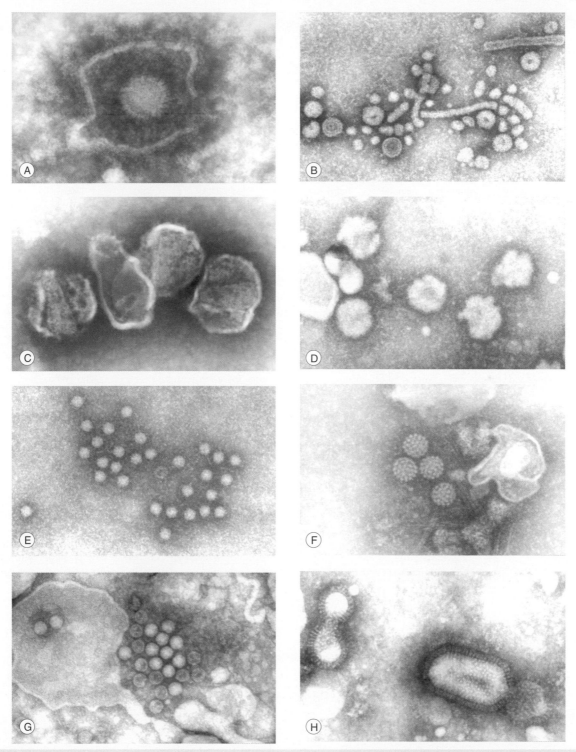

Fig. 7.5 Electron micrographs of common viral types. (A) Herpes simplex virus from a vesicular lesion from a patient with herpes simplex. (B) Hepatitis B virus showing 42 nm virions – the 'Dane' particles – and 22 nm HBsAg spheres and filaments. The serum sample was from an HIV-positive male, hence the large proportion of intact virions. (C) Human immunodeficiency virus. (D) Rubella virus. (E) Human parvovirus. The serum sample was from an HIV-positive male. (F) Human papillomavirus. (G) Enterovirus. (H) Influenza virus. *HBsAg*, HBV surface antigen.

resolution of symptoms. Naturally acquired infection with a particular strain of influenza A or B results in long-term immunity to that strain, but not those influenza strains which have exhibited major antigenic changes (antigenic shift) or even minor degrees of variation (antigenic drift). Others cause persistent infections, in which the patient often remains infected for life. Persistent infections may be characterised by an acute phase of infection, which may or may not be symptomatic, followed by life-long latency, where the virus persists in a non-replicative form with restricted viral gene expression. Subsequent reactivations of infection may occur, although in the immunocompetent person reactivated infection is usually more limited than primary infection and may be asymptomatic. This

Table 7.4 Classification and Characteristics of Viruses of Significance in Pregnancy

Virus	Maternal, Intrauterine or Perinatal Infection	Classification	Properties of Virus			
			Genome	Symmetry	Diameter (nm)	Envelope
Herpes simplex virus types 1 and 2	Perinatal	Herpesvirus[a]	dsDNA	Cubic	120–300	Yes
Varicella-zoster virus	Maternal, intrauterine	Herpesvirus[a]	dsDNA	Cubic	180–200	Yes
Cytomegalovirus	Intrauterine	Herpesvirus[b]	dsDNA	Cubic	150–200	Yes
Hepatitis B virus	Perinatal	Hepadnavirus	dsDNA	Cubic	40–42	Yes
Hepatitis C virus	Perinatal	Hepacivirus	(+) ssRNA	Cubic	Not known	Yes
Hepatitis E virus	Maternal	Uncertain	(+) ssRNA	Cubic	27–34	No
Human immunodeficiency virus types 1 and 2	Intrauterine, perinatal	Retrovirus	(+) ssRNA	Cubic	110	Yes
Human T cell lymphotropic virus type 1	Perinatal (breastfeeding)	Retrovirus	(+) ssRNA	Cubic	110	Yes
Rubella virus	Intrauterine	Rubivirus	(+) ssRNA	Cubic	58	Yes
Human parvovirus B19	Intrauterine	Parvovirus	(+) or (−) ssDNA	Cubic	18–26	No
Human papillomavirus	Perinatal	Papovavirus	dsDNA	Cubic	55	No
Enteroviruses	Intrauterine, perinatal	Picornavirus	(+) ssRNA	Cubic	24–30	No
Influenza virus A and B	Maternal	Orthomyxovirus	(−) ssRNA	Helical	120	Yes
Japanese B virus	Maternal	Flavivirus	(+) ssRNA	Cubic	40–60	Yes
Lassa fever virus	Maternal	Arenavirus	Ambisense ssRNA	Cubic	90–110	Yes

[a]Herpes simplex viruses and varicella-zoster viruses are subclassified as alphaherpesviruses. These herpesviruses have a variable host range, grow rapidly in cell culture, destroy infected cells efficiently and establish latency in vivo in primarily sensory ganglia.
[b]Cytomegalovirus is subclassified as a betaherpesvirus. These herpesviruses usually have a restricted host range and grow slowly in cell culture; infected cells often show cytomegalic inclusions both in vivo and in vitro. They establish latency in a variety of tissues including secretory glands, the kidney and lymphoreticular cells.

Table 7.5 Virus Infections That May Be Severe or Fatal in pregnancy

Virus Infection	Comments	Prevention
Influenza A (B)	Increased mortality in 1918 and 1957 associated with chronic heart disease	Influenza vaccine (inactivated)
Varicella	Mortality associated with pneumonia among adults. Possibly more severe in pregnancy	Varicella-zoster immune globulin preferably within 72 h of contact (treat established infections if severe with aciclovir systemically). Varicella vaccine for specific at-risk groups
Poliomyelitis	Spinal paralysis increases with gestational age	Polio vaccine (attenuated or inactivated) for travellers to any remaining endemic areas
Measles	Increased mortality and complications in pregnancy	In the absence of previous vaccination or history of measles give normal human immunoglobulin
Hepatitis E	12%–18% mortality rate with fetal death in last trimester. Endemic in many developing countries	Trials in progress with recombinant-derived vaccines
Lassa fever	70%–90% mortality rate with fetal death in last trimester. Endemic in West Africa	Prophylactic ribavirin to pregnant household contacts (treat patient with ribavirin systemically)
Japanese B encephalitis	20%–40% mortality rate; higher in pregnancy with fetal death. Widely distributed in South-East Asia and the Far East	Vaccine available on named-patient basis for travellers to endemic areas

pattern of persistence is typical of herpesviruses such as herpes simplex virus (HSV) and varicella-zoster virus (VZV). Other persistent viral infections such as HIV and hepatitis B and C viruses (HBV and HCV) are characterised by ongoing virus replication and chronic, evolving disease.

VIRUSES WHICH MAY INDUCE SEVERE INFECTION IN PREGNANCY

The features of these viral infections, together with preventive measures where applicable, are listed in Table 7.5. Some infections may be prevented by immunisation (e.g. influenza

A and B) and poliomyelitis, and recombinant-derived vaccines are under trial for the hepatitis E virus, which carries a high mortality rate among pregnant patients in developing countries. Although there is some doubt as to whether varicella is more severe in pregnancy, infection is often severe and occasionally fatal among adults generally, particularly those who smoke. Thus, pregnant women who give no history of varicella, or in whom screening tests for VZV antibodies indicate susceptibility, should be protected by the administration of varicella-zoster immune globulin (VZIG) within 72 hours of an exposure. Aciclovir treatment should also be used for pregnant women with established infection as they are at increased risk of varicella pneumonia, and this has a high mortality rate. Japanese B encephalitis is one of the more widely distributed arbovirus infections, being present in Asia. Although subclinical infection is common, those exhibiting clinical features may experience a mortality rate of up to 20% in outbreaks. Fetal death is common. An inactivated vaccine is available on a 'named-patient basis', but since it may be reactogenic is not recommended in pregnancy. Lassa fever may be particularly severe in the latter stages of pregnancy, and the fetal death rate is high. Recently the zoonotic Zika virus, transmitted by mosquitos (*Aedes aegypti* and *A. albopictus*), has become a serious issue for pregnant women. This RNA virus, which is a member of the virus family Flaviviridae, along with Japanese B encephalitis, can cross the placental barrier and infect the developing fetus, causing microcephaly, severe brain malformations and other birth defects.

SEVERE ACUTE RESPIRATORY SYNDROME AND OTHER CORONAVIRUSES

Severe acute respiratory syndrome (SARS) is caused by a coronavirus that first emerged in the southern Chinese province of Guangdong in November 2002. Pregnant women with SARS appear to have a worse prognosis and a higher mortality rate. Therefore, early delivery or termination of pregnancy should be considered in those who are seriously ill. The following criteria for early delivery have been proposed:

- Maternal rapid deterioration
- Failure to maintain adequate blood oxygenation
- Difficulty with mechanical ventilation due to the gravid uterus
- Multi-organ failure
- Fetal compromise
- Other obstetric indications.

There seems to be no reason for elective pre-term delivery in those women who are relatively well with SARS infection. Pregnant women should be treated empirically since a laboratory diagnosis may be prolonged. It has been suggested that the treatment of pregnant women with SARS should be without the use of ribavirin. Infections due to other coronaviruses are relatively mild and have not been reported as causing problems during pregnancy.

In 2019, severe acute respiratory syndrome coronavirus (SARS-CoV-2) that causes the respiratory illness coronavirus disease 2019 (COVID-19) emerged out of Wuhan, China. In March 2020, the World Health Organisation declared the outbreak a pandemic. The impact of COVID-19 on pregnancy outcomes continues to be investigated. However, at the time of publishing, research indicated that COVID-19 infection was not associated with stillbirth, small for gestational age infants or early neonatal death, but was associated with increased risk of premature birth.

INTRAUTERINE INFECTIONS

Viruses which may damage the fetus are shown in Table 7.6. The rubella virus, and two viruses belonging to the herpesvirus group – CMV and VZV – as well as human

Table 7.6 Viruses Which May Infect or Damage the Fetus

Virus Infection	Birth Defects	Persistent Infection	Fetal Death
Rubella	Yes	Yes	Yes
CMV	Yes	Yes	Yes
Varicella	Yes	Possible	Yes
Parvovirus B19	No	Yes	Yes
HIV-1 and -2	No	Yes	Yes
Hepatitis C	No	Yes	Unknown
Hepatitis E	No	? Yes	Yes
Poliomyelitis	No	No	Yes
Coxsackie B virus	No	No	Yes
Japanese B encephalitis	Unknown	Unknown	Yes
Lassa fever	No	No	Yes

CMV, Cytomegalovirus; *HIV*, human immunodeficiency virus.

parvovirus B19 may induce persistent infections in the fetus.

Rubella

As a result of immunisation programmes against rubella now being directed against pre-school children of both sexes and rubella-susceptible adult women, only about 2% of women of childbearing age born and brought up in Britain are susceptible to infection. However, susceptibility rates equivalent to or higher than those observed in developed countries during the pre-vaccination era are present in many developing countries. Congenitally acquired rubella is now rare in Britain and most industrialised countries, although rubella-induced defects have been reported with varying frequencies in other parts of the world.

Rubella virus produces an anti-mitotic protein and consequently, if infection occurs during the critical phase of organogenesis (i.e. during the first 8 weeks of pregnancy), severe and multiple defects are likely to occur. If infection occurs during the first trimester, fetal infection is almost invariable, and 75% to 80% of conceptuses are damaged. After the first trimester, the incidence and spectrum of defects is much less. Although congenital heart disease, eye defects (particularly cataracts) and deafness are the commonest manifestations of congenitally acquired infection if maternal infection is acquired in early pregnancy, rubella induces a generalised and persistent infection with multi-organ involvement, and a wide spectrum of defects may be present at birth or evolve in infancy.

Cytomegalovirus

About 40% to 50% of women of childbearing age in Britain have no serological evidence of previous CMV infection. In contrast with rubella, primary maternal CMV infection is often asymptomatic, but may result in fetal infection and damage throughout pregnancy. The viral transmission rate to the fetus is of the order of 30% to 40%, but fetal damage occurs in only about 10% of infected conceptuses. Nevertheless, the burden induced by congenitally acquired CMV infection is considerable; it has been estimated that somewhere in the order of 300 to 400 CMV-damaged babies are born in the UK each year. CMV is the commonest microbial cause of psychomotor retardation, although deafness may be the sole manifestation of congenitally acquired disease. Recurrent CMV infection or reactivation is rarely associated with fetal damage.

Varicella

Although very few Indigenous adult women born in the UK are susceptible to varicella, the proportion may be considerably higher – up to 35% – among those born and brought up in rural areas of developing countries. The overall risk of congenitally acquired disease following maternal varicella is restricted to the first 20 weeks of gestation, but, in contrast to rubella and CMV, the risks are low (about 1% overall); the incidence is greater between 13 and 20 weeks of gestation (2%) than between 1 and 12 weeks (0.4%). Defects involve the CNS and musculoskeletal system; limb hypoplasia and cicatricial scarring may be present.

If acquired towards term, the infant may develop varicella after delivery. If maternal varicella occurs 8 days or more before delivery, neonatal varicella is usually mild. In contrast, maternal varicella infection that occurs less than 1 week before delivery may be severe and, without treatment, occasionally fatal. VZIG should therefore be given to infants whose mothers develop varicella 8 days or less before delivery; aciclovir may be given if neonatal infection is severe, despite administration of VZIG. Varicella-susceptible pregnant women exposed to infection during the last 3 weeks of pregnancy should be given prophylactic VZIG.

Parvovirus B19

About 40% of women of childbearing age in Britain are susceptible to parvovirus B19 infection. Human parvovirus may induce a rubella-like rash, sometimes accompanied by arthralgia, although infection may also be asymptomatic. The fetus is infected in about 33% of cases and in about 10% of these, spontaneous abortion may occur, usually in the second trimester. Parvovirus B19 binds to a globoside (P antigen) expressed on the membrane of erythrocytes and fetal heart, and this results in a reduction of fetal erythroid progenitor cells, which may result in a severe fetal anaemia, leading to heart failure and development of hydrops fetalis. Heart failure may also result from viral myocarditis. However, developmental defects have not been recorded. Parvovirus infection is therefore not a reason for therapeutic abortion. Fetal anaemia and hydrops may be 'rescued' by fetal blood transfusion.

Human Immunodeficiency Virus (HIV-1 and -2)

WHO estimates that, globally, 38.0 million adults and 2.3 million children were living with HIV at the end of 2005. In developing countries, infection is usually contracted heterosexually. In Britain, HIV infection tends to be concentrated in London. In its inner-city areas, up to 0.5% of pregnant women are now HIV-1 positive. In the absence of treatment with a combination of antiretroviral drugs, HIV-1 is transmitted to the fetus of infected mothers in about 12% to 15% of cases. Combination antiretroviral therapy has reduced the HIV transmission rate, and studies suggest that chemotherapy together with delivery by caesarean section further reduces the risk of transmission to 1% to 2%. Infection may be transmitted *in utero* but occurs more frequently during delivery, or when breastfeeding. In contrast to HIV-1, HIV-2

is transmitted in only about 1% of cases, and this is almost certainly a manifestation of the much lower maternal viral load present. If HIV infection occurs *in utero*, it is usually possible to establish a diagnosis during the first few weeks of life. If infection occurs during delivery or via breastfeeding, or in infants born to mothers on antiretroviral treatment, it may take considerably longer to establish a diagnosis of HIV infection in infancy. Diagnosis of HIV infection in infancy is usually made by detecting the virus by molecular techniques; serological techniques are of limited value since maternal antibody may persist for up to 18 months.

Enteroviruses (Polioviruses, Coxsackie A and B Viruses, Echoviruses)

Most developed countries are now free of poliomyelitis, and the WHO Expanded Programme of Immunisation has resulted in a marked decline in poliomyelitis cases in developing countries. Very occasionally, maternal poliomyelitis results in the delivery of infants with limb paralysis. Maternal infection by other enteroviruses may result in the delivery of infants with severe generalised infections in which myocarditis and central nervous system (CNS) disease are prominent features. Scandinavian studies suggest that enterovirus infection, if acquired *in utero*, may be associated with the subsequent development of insulin-dependent diabetes mellitus (type 1 diabetes) in childhood. Infection may also be acquired during delivery, transmission occurring via contamination with enterically shed maternal virus. Infected babies may also transmit infection nosocomially.

PERINATAL INFECTIONS

Viruses which may cause severe infection if acquired perinatally or during the neonatal period are listed in Table 7.7. A range of diagnostic methods may need to be employed to confirm viral infection in such cases including qualitative and quantitative molecular techniques.

Herpes Simplex Virus

About 75% of genital infections are caused by HSV-2 and about 25% by HSV-1. Infants may be infected by maternal genital lesions, fetal scalp monitoring, maternal non-genital lesions or contact with HSV-infected nursery staff or visitors. Primary maternal lesions carry a much higher risk of infection than recurrent lesions since primary infections are associated with high concentrations of virus over a long period.

The incidence of neonatal herpes in Britain is estimated to be of the order of 1.6 per 100,000 deliveries, whereas in Sweden and USA it is considerably higher (5 and 7 per

Table 7.7   Perinatal Infections
Herpes simplex virus (HSV)
Varicella-zoster virus (VZV)
Cytomegalovirus (CMV)
Hepatitis B
HIV
Enteroviruses
Papillomaviruses
Human T cell leukaemia virus (HTLV-1)

100,000, respectively). The presence of maternal lesions at or within 6 weeks of birth is an indication for caesarean section provided membranes are intact or ruptured less than 6 hours before delivery. Infants delivered via an infected birth canal should be given prophylactic aciclovir intravenously. Although it is recommended that women with evidence of a recurrent lesion at delivery should deliver by caesarean section, transmission is rare; studies from the Netherlands have shown that the risks of acquiring neonatal HSV following caesarean section and vaginal delivery are not significantly different. Testing mothers with a history of recurrent herpes, or whose partners give a history, is no longer recommended, since virus shedding in late pregnancy does not correlate with transmission to the neonate. There is some evidence to suggest that treatment of mothers with oral aciclovir who have a history of recurrent genital herpes during the last month of pregnancy may reduce the incidence of lesions at delivery and consequently the necessity for caesarean section.

Clinical manifestations may be delayed until 10 to 14 days after birth. Infants may present with lesions of the skin and mucous membranes (60% will disseminate), CNS involvement or generalised infection.

Hepatitis B

There are 350 to 400 million HBV carriers worldwide, the highest rates being in South-East Asia (~15%) and sub-Saharan Africa (~10%). In some inner-city areas in Britain, the HBV carrier rate among pregnant women is about 1%. Pregnant women with acute HBV infection are likely to transmit infection to newborn infants perinatally. Infants delivered of mothers who are HBV surface antigen (HBsAg) and 'e' antigen (HBeAg) positive should be protected by the administration of hepatitis B immune globulin (HBIG) and HBV vaccine (active/passive immunisation) at birth. Provided a full course of vaccine is given (three doses and a booster), this procedure will effectively reduce the risk of persistent HBV infection in the infant by about 95%, thereby reducing the risk of long-term chronic liver damage and primary hepatocellular carcinoma. Infants delivered of mothers who have antibody to HBeAg (anti-HBe) should be given HBV vaccine without HBIG. Infants whose mothers are HBsAg positive without 'e' markers, or where the 'e' marker status has not been determined, or whose mothers had acute hepatitis B during pregnancy, should be given active/passive immunisation. There is currently a debate on whether using molecular methods to detect HBV DNA in mothers with anti-HBe may detect those with high levels of viraemia, whose children should be given active/passive vaccination.

Hepatitis C

It is estimated that there are about 170 million HCV carriers worldwide, with relatively high carrier rates (2.5% to 5%) occurring in some developing countries, particularly in sub-Saharan Africa, Asia and Latin America. In Britain, infection is common among multi-transfused persons, injecting drug users and those from countries with a high prevalence. The prevalence among pregnant women in some inner-city areas in London is about 0.25%. Infection

may be transmitted *in utero* if acute maternal infection occurs in the last trimester of pregnancy, but mothers who are carriers may also occasionally transmit *in utero* since HCV RNA has been detected in neonates at birth, and caesarean section may not prevent transmission. Neonatal infection occurs in about 6% of infants delivered of mothers who are HCV carriers and who are HCV RNA positive, but in mothers co-infected with HIV the transmission rate is 30% to 35%. Mothers who are HCV antibody positive but HCV RNA negative are very unlikely to transmit infection. HCV-infected infants are likely to develop persistent HCV infection which may in due course result in chronic liver damage.

Human Papillomavirus

About 100 different genotypes have been identified, of which at least 30 are found in the genital tract. Human papillomavirus (HPV) types 6 and 11 cause genital warts and are known as 'low risk' types as they are rarely found in cancers. HPV types 16, 18, 31 and a few other types are designated as 'high risk' as they are associated with pre-malignant and malignant cervical disease; viral DNA can be detected in ~95% of cancers, often integrated into host cell chromosomes, and virus-encoded oncoproteins, which bind to and inactivate the p53 and pRB tumour suppresser proteins, are expressed.

HPV 6 and 11 may be transmitted from mother to infant at delivery and may cause juvenile laryngeal or genital warts, but this is rare. High-risk types may also be transmitted at birth and may persist in infancy, but they are not associated with obvious disease and the consequence of these infections is unknown. Girls aged 12 to 13 years are now vaccinated with HPV vaccine to protect against cervical cancer.

Human T Cell Lymphotropic Virus Type 1

This virus is endemic in South-West Japan, the South Pacific, parts of West Africa, the Caribbean basin, southern USA and parts of South America. Persons who have emigrated from these areas may also be carriers. The prevalence of antibodies among antenatal patients in London and Birmingham is 0.14% to 0.26%. Studies in Japan and the Caribbean have shown that this virus is transmitted via breast milk. Of the carriers of this retrovirus, 2.5% to 4.0% who have not acquired infection through blood transfusion may develop adult T cell leukaemia or tropical spastic paraparesis 10 to 30 years after infection.

References

Boumis, E., Capone, A., Galati, V., et al., 2018. Probiotics and infective endocarditis in patients with hereditary hemorrhagic telangiectasia: a clinical case and a review of the literature. BMC Infectious Diseases 18, 65.

Jangi, S., Lamont, J.T., 2010. Asymptomatic colonization by Clostridium difficile in infants: implications for disease in later life. Journal of Pediatric Gastroenterology and Nutrition 51(1), 2–7.

Quainoo, S., Coolen, J.P.M., van Hijum, S.A.F.T., et al., 2017. Whole-genome sequencing of bacterial pathogens: the future of nosocomial outbreak analysis. Clinical Microbiology Reviews 30(4), 1015–1063.

Woese, C.R., Fox, G.E., 1977. Phylogenetic structure of the prokaryotic domain: the primary kingdoms. Proceedings of the National Academy of Sciences of the United States of America 74(11), 5088–5090.

8 Immunology

ANDREW J. T. GEORGE AND UDAY KISHORE

Introduction

The immune system exists to protect the organism from the consequences of infectious disease and, to a lesser extent, neoplasia. It does this by having a complex system of organs, cells and molecules that are distributed throughout the body. Most of the cells involved are highly motile, adding to the complexity of the system. The importance of the immune system in health and disease is highlighted by rare congenital abnormalities of components of the system, which in many cases result in early death due to uncontrollable infections.

The immune system plays an important role in a number of conditions of pregnancy including spontaneous abortion, pre-eclampsia and hypersensitivity reactions that damage the fetus. Pregnancy can also result in changes in the severity of autoimmune diseases. In addition, one of the most interesting questions in immunology is why a fetus is not recognised by the mother's immune system and destroyed; if an equivalent organ were transplanted into a woman without massive immunosuppression, it would be rapidly rejected. This might seem an academic question, of little practical importance. However, new strategies for preventing graft rejection are being developed based on our knowledge of how the fetus/placenta blocks rejection.

The Immune System

Frequently, the immune system is characterised as differentiating between 'self' (anything originating from the organism) and 'foreign' (anything that is not self), and destroying anything it recognises as foreign. However, this is a gross simplification. When the immune system is first introduced to a foreign molecule or organism, it needs to decide whether to respond or not. Frequently it does not – we normally fail to produce immune responses to the large amounts of foreign antigen that we ingest as food or are present as commensal organisms in our gut. Having decided to mount an immune response, there is a secondary decision – what sort of response should be initiated? Different pathogens need to be dealt with in different ways, and an inappropriate immune response will not only be ineffective but may also damage the organism.

The decision-making is vital because there are important consequences to mistakes. The failure to mount an immune response when needed may cause uncontrolled infection or malignancy. However, mounting an immune response to foreign material when it is not needed can result in pathology, for example allergies. Immune responses against self can result in autoimmunity. Choice of inappropriate types of immune response will result in tissue damage. Even appropriate immune responses frequently damage the organism; the necessary immune responses against *Mycobacterium tuberculosis*, the bacteria that cause the deadly disease tuberculosis, result in scarring. In the context of pregnancy, the immune response against an infection may result in miscarriage of the fetus, although the consequences of failing to respond would be more serious.

There are two main parts to the immune system: the innate and the adaptive immune systems. The innate immune system contains both cells and soluble molecules and is often thought of as the first line of defence against pathogens. Unlike the adaptive immune system (see below), it does not recognise specific antigens on the pathogens, but rather responds to general common features of pathogens (for example sugar molecules expressed on the surface of bacteria but not mammalian cells). Every pathogen has a particular surface structure due to patterns of carbohydrates, lipids and charge distribution, collectively termed as pathogen-associated molecular patterns (PAMPs). A number of innate immune cells such as macrophages and dendritic cells have PAMP-recognising receptors (PRRs). PAMP–PRR engagement can thus lead to uptake of pathogens (phagocytosis), and/or generate an inflammatory reaction that would involve mobilisation of immune cells and proteins at the site of infection.

The innate immune system is always present and ready to recognise and destroy pathogens (though it can become more active during inflammation). The adaptive immune system, in comparison, recognises specific antigens using receptors (antibody and T-cell receptors (TCRs)). When first faced with a pathogen, the adaptive immune response must first select and then amplify cells bearing the appropriate receptors (clonal selection; see below). Only then can it produce a specific immune response, resulting in a delay of several days before it is effective.

The adaptive immune response is characterised by its memory; once it has responded to an antigen it will mount a rapid and vigorous secondary immune response if it is re-exposed to the antigen (Fig. 8.1). This is the basis of both immunisation and protection by prior infection.

However, the divide between the adaptive and innate immune system masks the considerable interactions that occur. This is both at the level of regulation of the immune response (the innate immune system is essential in instructing the adaptive response), and at the level of effectors where components of the adaptive immune response amplify and focus the effector mechanisms of the innate system onto their targets.

Here, we will look first at the cells and molecules of the adaptive and innate immune systems. We will then go on to consider some examples of how they interact to control immune responses. Finally, we will turn to look at areas of particular interest to reproductive immunology.

Adaptive Immune Systems

The main cells of the adaptive immune system are the bone marrow-derived lymphocytes. There are two main categories of lymphocyte: the B lymphocyte (or B cell) and the T lymphocyte (T cell). B cells are responsible for producing the soluble antigen-specific effector molecule of the immune system, the antibody. T cells have two roles; one is to regulate the immune system (T helper cells and T regulatory cells) and the other is to kill virally infected or neoplastically transformed cells (cytotoxic T cells).

ANTIBODY MOLECULES

The main role of the B cell is to produce antibody molecules, or immunoglobulins (Fig. 8.2). Immunoglobulins have a basic structure consisting of four polypeptide chains: two identical heavy chains and two identical light chains. When different antibody molecules are compared, most of the antibody is similar. However, the N-terminal regions of the heavy and light chains are variable in sequence. These come together to form, for each antibody, a unique three-dimensional shape. It is this part of the antibody that binds to the antigen. Because each antibody has a different antigen binding site, it binds to a different antigen.

The antibody molecule has three main functions (Fig. 8.3). One of these is to act as the B cell receptor for antigen. The second is to bind directly to toxins, viruses and other molecules and block their ability to bind to a target cell (neutralising antibodies). This is how anti-toxin (diphtheria/tetanus) antibodies work. The third function of antibodies is to recruit effector mechanisms to the target cell. It does this with the part of the molecule that does not vary (the constant region – in particular the upright 'stalk' of the molecule, called the Fc region). The Fc region binds to

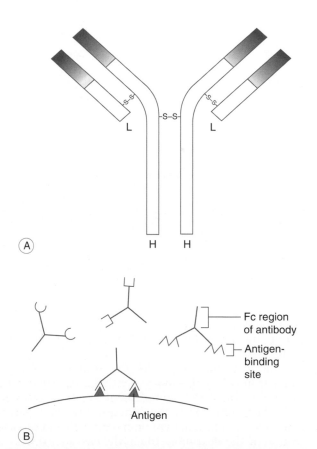

Fc region of antibody

Antigen-binding site

Antigen

Fig. 8.2 The antibody molecule. (A) The antibody molecule is made up of four polypeptide chains: two identical heavy chains *(H)* and two identical light chains *(L)*, held together with disulphide bonds. Within any one antibody class or subclass the sequence of most of the antibody is the same. However, the N-terminal parts of the molecule *(shaded)* vary between antibodies. The result is that every antibody molecule has a unique antigen binding site, as shown in cartoon form in (B), where the antibodies are depicted as a simple Y-shaped molecule with each antibody having a different antigen binding site. Where the antibody has a complementary structure to the antigen (e.g. of the surface of a pathogen), it can bind to the molecule.

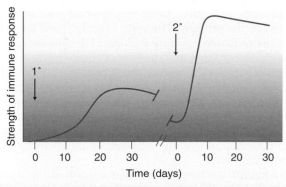

Fig. 8.1 Immunological memory. A cardinal feature of the adaptive immune system is its memory. When the immune system is first exposed to antigen (primary 1° exposure, indicated by *arrow*) it takes a number of days for the immune response to get going. However, a secondary exposure (2°) to the same antigen results in a more rapid and stronger immune response. This is the basis of protection found following immunisation or a primary infection.

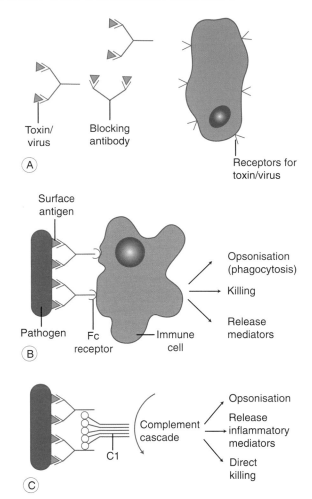

Fig. 8.3 Antibody function. Antibodies can serve to block the binding of toxins and viruses to receptors on the surface of cells (A). They can also direct immune cells bearing Fc receptors to antibody-coated cells, the result of which depends on which cells are targeted but can include opsonisation of the pathogen (preparing it for phagocytosis), killing, or the release of soluble mediators (B). In addition, the first component of the complement cascade *(C1)* can bind to the Fc regions, activating the complement cascade. This results in opsonisation of the coated target, release of inflammatory mediators and direct killing of the target cell (C).

receptors (Fc receptors) on cells of the innate system, such as macrophages, neutrophils and eosinophils, and focuses them onto the target that carries the antigen recognised by the antibody.

In addition to targeting cells, the antibodies can also recruit a group of soluble molecules that are present in the circulation, termed the 'complement system.' This consists of a large number of components that are organised in a cascade such that activation of one molecule leads to activation of the next molecule in the cascade (similar in many respects to the blood clotting system). Activation of the complement cascade results in the production of inflammatory proteins that cause increased vascular permeability, vasodilatation and recruitment of inflammatory cells. In addition, components of the complement cascade are coated onto the target cell. There they can act as recognition elements for cells of the immune system (phagocytes such as macrophages) and can also directly kill some pathogens. Complement can be activated in several

manners, including innate recognition of pathogens. However, antibodies will also activate the complement system by binding of the first component of the cascade, C1q, to the Fc region of antibodies. This route of complement activation, called the classical pathway, is ably supported by two other complement pathways, termed the alternative and lectin pathways. In the alternative pathways, spontaneous recognition of charge surfaces by complement component C3 can complete the cascade, while in the lectin pathway, the recognition subcomponent is the carbohydrate pattern recognising Mannan-binding lectin (MBL). The recognition process in all three pathways is followed by generation of opsonins (that decorate the target cell surface and enhance phagocytosis), anaphylatoxins (which recruit more immune cells) and membrane attack complex (a cluster of terminal complement components which can punch holes in the pathogen in a similar manner to the secretory products of CD8$^+$ cytotoxic T cells).

There are five different classes of antibody: IgM, IgG, IgD, IgA, IgE (in addition, there are subclasses of IgG and IgA). The different antibody classes have different functions. Thus, the different Fc regions recruit different effector responses – IgE, for example, binds strongly to mast cells and basophils and is important in allergic responses seen in asthma. IgA is found in mucosal secretions and provides protection for mucosal surfaces. IgM, which consists of five basic antibody units joined together, is important early in the immune response where the ability to bind to 10 antigen molecules simultaneously increases the strength of binding.

B CELLS

The adaptive immune response controls the production of antibody by a mechanism termed clonal selection (Fig. 8.4). During development, a large number (10^8 in the mouse, 10 to 100 times more in the human) of B cells are generated, each of which makes a unique antibody molecule. These early (termed naive or virgin) B cells do not secrete their antibody molecules but express them on the surface of the cell as a receptor for antigen. These B cells are resident in the lymph nodes and spleen. When an antigen is introduced into the system (following infection or immunisation), it is 'shown' to the different B cells there. Most B cells will not recognise the antigen, but given the vast number of different antibody molecules, there will by chance be some that do bind to the antigen. The cells bearing these antibodies will start to divide, forming a clone of B cells recognising the antigen, resulting in a swelling of the lymph node. After a period of clonal expansion, the B cells start to differentiate, no longer expressing the antibody on their surface but secreting it. In addition, some of the B cells become memory cells, so that the next time the system encounters the antigen there is an increased pool of cells capable of recognising the antigen, providing the basis for the memory of the immune response.

In addition, the B cell will, under control of the T helper cell (see below), change the class of antibody that it makes. Initially all the antibodies are IgM, but if, for example, the antibody is needed on a mucosal surface, then the class will switch to IgA.

During the course of a response, the immune system will also mutate the sequence of the antigen binding site of the

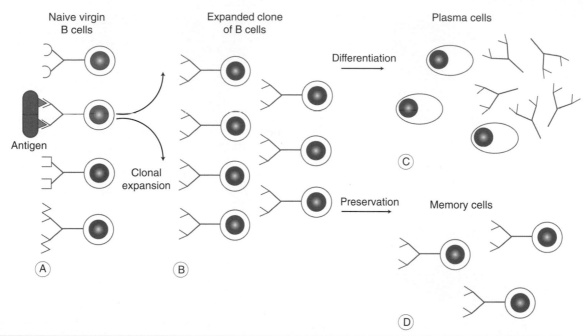

Fig. 8.4 Clonal selection theory. The clonal selection theory states that there are a large number of virgin, naive B cells, each of which expresses a different antibody on its surface – four are shown in (A). If antigen is introduced into the system, any B cell that has an antibody receptor that binds the antigen is activated and undergoes clonal expansion, resulting in a large number of B cells, all with the same antibody molecule (B). Some of these cells then differentiate into plasma cells, which secrete soluble antibody that can act as an effector molecule (C), while others persist to act as memory cells and form the basis of a rapid response upon re-exposure to antigen (D). Clonal selection also operates on T cells.

antibody, selecting molecules that bind better to the antigen. This process is known as affinity maturation and improves the ability of the antibody to recognise the antigen.

T CELLS

Antigen Recognition

The T cells are so called because they mature in the thymus. They recognise antigen through the TCR. In the thymus, T cells are educated to ignore or not react to self-antigens prior to being exported to the circulation. Like the antibody molecule, the TCR has a variable region that binds to antigen. In a similar manner to the B cell, the T cell with an appropriate TCR specificity undergoes clonal selection during an immune response. However, unlike the antibody, the TCR is only a cell surface receptor and is never secreted by a cell.

The way in which the TCR recognises antigen is more complex. The TCR does not bind directly to pathogen-derived antigens, but rather recognises the antigen in association with molecules of the major histocompatibility complex (MHC, also known as HLA in human). There are two types of MHC molecule involved in TCR recognition: class I molecules that are expressed on all nucleated cells and class II molecules that, under normal conditions, are expressed only on B cells and specialised antigen presenting cells (such as macrophages and dendritic cells, see below). Both MHC class I and class II molecules have a structure which allows them to bind to short peptides derived from the antigens (Fig. 8.5), and the TCR recognises a combination of the foreign peptide and the MHC molecule, and is unable to recognise either individually.

The two MHC molecules present their peptides to different types of T cell, and also vary in how the peptide gets into the binding groove of the MHC molecule. Thus MHC class I molecules present peptide to cytotoxic T cells (Fig. 8.6A). The peptide is derived from within the cell and may result from a viral infection or be an antigen associated with neoplastic transformation of the cells (e.g. a mutated oncogene). These proteins are made in the cytoplasm, where they are chopped into small peptides by a molecular complex termed the proteosome. The peptides are then pumped into the endoplasmic reticulum by the T cell-activating protein (TAP) molecule, where they are loaded into the MHC class I peptide binding groove. The complex is then exported to the surface of the cell.

The T cells capable of recognising antigen in the context of MHC class II are the helper and the regulatory T cells (Treg) (see below) (see Fig. 8.6B). In this case, the antigens are acquired from outside the cell, and are taken up by the antigen presenting cell. They are then degraded into peptides that are loaded onto MHC class II molecules before being exported to the cell surface.

Function of T Cells

T cells can be differentiated in terms of both their function and markers expressed on their surface. Cytotoxic T cells express the molecule CD8 on their surface. Helper and Treg express CD4.

The role of CD8+ cytotoxic T cells is to kill the target cells expressing the appropriate peptide in the context of MHC class I. In most cases this peptide will be derived from a virus or be a mutated oncogene.

CD4+ T cells recognise peptide in the presence of MHC class II, which is only expressed on the surface of antigen

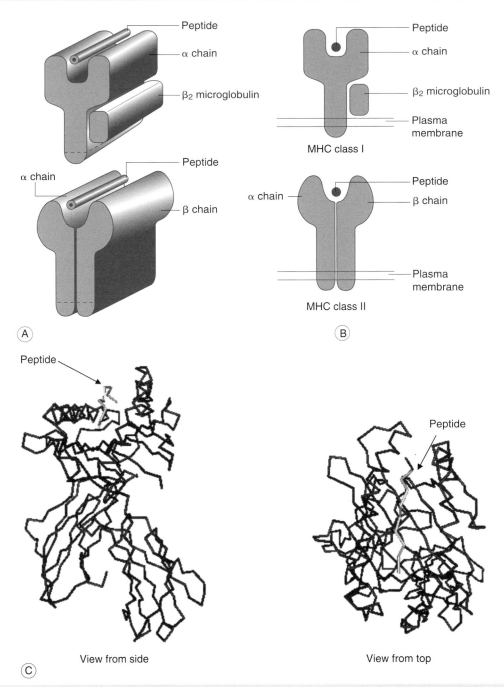

Fig. 8.5 Major histocompatibility complex *(MHC)* molecules. (A and B) MHC molecules are transmembrane molecules that bind peptide. The MHC class I molecule consists of one transmembrane chain (α chain) complexed to β_2 microglobulin. The MHC class II molecule contains two transmembrane chains, α and β. In both class I and class II molecules there is a similar binding site, or groove, which holds short linear peptides. The T cell receptor (TCR) 'recognises' the combination of MHC and peptide. (C) The MHC molecules act to hold short linear antigenic peptides in a peptide binding groove of the molecule. The figure shows the structure of an MHC class I molecule binding a virus-derived peptide. The peptide is shown in light colour and the backbone of the MHC molecule in black. The left-hand figure shows a side view, with the peptide binding groove at the top. The right-hand figure shows a view from the top of the molecule, as would be 'seen' by a TCR docking – the TCR would 'recognise' both the MHC and the peptide together. The structure of the MHC class II peptide binding groove is similar.

presenting cells. There are two main roles of CD4$^+$ cells. The majority of CD4$^+$ cells are helper cells that serve to amplify the responses of other cells, both of the adaptive and innate immune systems. Indeed, in general the action of cytotoxic T cells and B cells are dependent upon such help. The T helper cells operate both by cell surface contact and, more generally, by secreting molecules termed cytokines that act on nearby cells. Thus, secretion of cytokines such as tumour

necrosis factor (TNF) by helper T cells can activate macrophages, neutrophils and other cells to generate inflammatory responses.

The action of T helper cells is more subtle than just turning on immune responses. Different types of helper cell can be induced under different conditions, which by secreting different cytokines can determine the nature of the immune response. The two main types of helper cell characterised

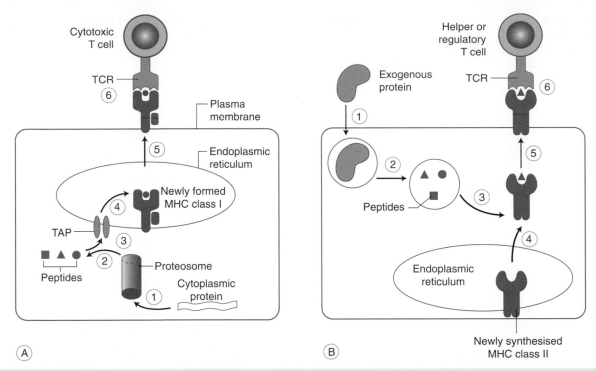

Fig. 8.6 Loading of peptides onto major histocompatibility complex *(MHC)* molecules. (A) The MHC class I molecule binds peptides derived from cytoplasmic proteins. These are degraded by the proteosome (1) to form peptides (2), which are then transported by the T cell-activating protein into the endoplasmic reticulum (3) and loaded onto newly formed MHC class I molecules (4), which are then transported to the cell surface (5) for recognition by cytotoxic T cells (6). (B) The MHC class II molecule binds peptides derived from extracellular (exogenous) proteins. The proteins are taken up and internalised by the antigen presenting cell (1), before being chopped up into peptides (2) and then associating (3) with MHC class II molecules that have been newly synthesised in the endoplasmic reticulum (4). The complex of peptide and MHC class II is then exported to the plasma cell membrane (5) where it can be recognised by T helper or regulatory cells (6). *TCR*, T-cell receptor.

are Th1 and Th2 cells. The Th1 cells secrete interleukin (IL) 2, interferon gamma (INF-γ), TNF-α and, in general, help inflammatory responses. Th2 cells secrete IL-4, IL-5, IL-10 and IL-13, which help antibody-mediated responses. The cytokines secreted by helper cells can also modify the nature of the antibody response, for example IL-4 instructs B cells to switch antibody class to IgE production.

While Th1 and Th2 are the main types of T helper cell, there are more subsets that are being defined, such as Th9, Th17 and Th22. These have particular functions, so for example Th17 cell subset is characterised by production of IL-17 and is important in the pathogenesis of some autoimmune diseases.

The other type of CD4+ cell is a regulatory T cell. These cells damp down immune responses, and have been shown to be responsible, in part, for blocking the action of T cells that recognise self-antigen, thus preventing autoimmunity. As with the helper cells, T regulatory cells operate by secreting cytokines (such as IL-10 and TGF-β) and by self-surface contact. As we shall discuss later, T regulatory cells have a role in preserving the fetus from immunological rejection.

Cells of the Innate Immune System

There are many cell types in the innate immune system, and we shall discuss only the most central. Indeed, many cells in the body that are not normally thought of as being immune cells can participate in immune responses by secreting cytokines and altering the expression of cell surface molecules. Thus, endothelial cells are involved in the recruitment of inflammatory cells, and many parenchymal cells can secrete cytokines that modify the immune cells in their locality.

NATURAL KILLER CELLS

The natural killer (NK) cell is a lymphocyte; however, unlike T and B cells, it does not have receptors for specific antigens. Its main role is to kill target cells, in a manner similar to cytotoxic T cells. The NK cell recognises its targets either by virtue of their being coated by an antibody (NK cells carry Fc receptors that allow them to recognise the antibody), or by receptors that recognise alterations in the cell surface molecules of the target cell. The most notable of these are receptors that recognise MHC class I molecules, expressed on all nucleated cells. If a cell downregulates its MHC class I expression then the absence of the class I molecules is detected by the NK cell, which kills it. This is an important mechanism because an obvious way for a virally infected or malignant T cell to escape from being killed by a cytotoxic T cell would be to downregulate expression of MHC class I molecules – preventing recognition of the antigenic peptide. However, NK cells circumvent this strategy as they wipe out class I-negative cells.

MACROPHAGES

Macrophages are mononuclear phagocytic cells that take up and ingest foreign material and damaged cells. They recognise their targets either by general receptors on the surface (e.g. against carbohydrates expressed on bacteria), or because they are coated with antibody or complement components. Macrophages also express MHC class II, and so are capable of presenting antigen derived from the phagocytosed material to T helper cells, which in turn can secrete cytokines that activate the macrophages – an example of the intimate cooperation between adaptive and innate immune systems.

Macrophages are members of the monocyte family. Other closely related members of the family include the Kupffer cells that line the sinusoids of the liver and phagocytose circulating antibody-coated antigens.

GRANULOCYTES

The granulocytes, so called because they have granules in their cytoplasm, include the neutrophil, eosinophil and basophil. These are capable of recognising foreign material directly, but also can be focused by antibody and complement components. All granulocytes are capable of killing target cells by secreting toxic molecules present in granules and the production of reactive oxygen species, and also of inducing and amplifying inflammation by secreting soluble cytokines and other molecules. The most common is the neutrophil, which is important in controlling bacterial infections and is recruited in large numbers in inflammatory sites. The other cells have more specialised roles; for example, the eosinophil kills parasites.

THE DENDRITIC CELL

The dendritic cells are responsible for initiating adaptive immune response because they are the only cells that stimulate naive T cells. Dendritic cells, in the form of Langerhans cells, are present in most tissues, such as the skin. In their resting state, they continually take antigens up from their surroundings and process and present them on MHC class II molecules. In this state, the dendritic cell is known as an immature dendritic cell. However, if the dendritic cell is activated (by a pathogen or danger signal, see below) then it stops taking up antigen and moves rapidly to the lymph nodes where it can stimulate the response of an antigen-specific T cell.

Regulation of the Immune System

THE DANGER THEORY

As indicated above, the immune system has considerable control mechanisms. However, one control system, popularised as the 'danger theory', is fundamental to our understanding of immune responses. This suggests that the most important decision the immune system has to make is when to respond, and that questions about specificity (i.e. about what antibodies and TCRs recognise) are secondary. The immune system is activated to respond only where there is evidence that there is a damaging event happening, as indicated by the presence of 'danger signals'. These signals are caused by the presence of tissue damage and dead cells, as well as by the presence of some components derived from pathogens. If these signals are not present, then the immune system does not respond, even in the presence of foreign antigen.

The central interaction that mediates the danger signal is that involving the dendritic cell and the T cell (Fig. 8.7). The immature dendritic cell, which as described above expresses low levels of MHC class II, is resident in the tissues and trafficks only slowly to the draining lymph nodes. When it reaches the lymph nodes, it is incapable of stimulating T cell proliferation (indeed it 'turns off' or anergises T cells, see below), because it does not express a series of molecules called co-stimulatory molecules. However, if there are danger signals, for example tissue damage caused by a pathogen infection, a surgeon's scalpel or stepping on a rusty nail, then receptors on the dendritic cell are engaged by the resulting danger signals. The dendritic cell is then activated into a mature dendritic cell and upregulates expression of both MHC class II and co-stimulatory molecules, and rapidly moves to the lymph node where it can activate T cells specific for any foreign antigen that it has picked up.

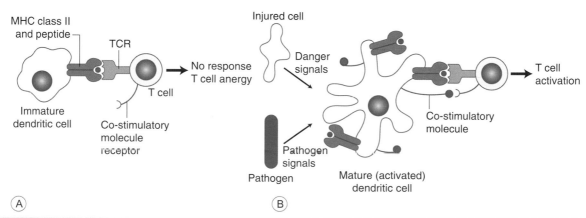

Fig. 8.7 Dendritic cell–T cell interactions and the danger signal. (A) Immature dendritic cells express low levels of major histocompatibility complex *(MHC)* class II and co-stimulatory molecules. If T cells interact with these antigen presenting cells they are not activated, but rather are rendered anergic (refractory to further stimulation). This is because a T cell needs signals both from the T-cell receptor *(TCR)* engagement of MHC and peptide, and from engagement of co-stimulatory molecules. (B) However, if the dendritic cell is activated either by danger signals from injured cells or by pathogen-derived signals then it undergoes a shape change, upregulates expression of MHC class II and co-stimulatory molecules, and rapidly migrates to the lymph node. Now if an antigen-specific T cell encounters the dendritic cell it is activated, as it receives signals both through the TCR and by binding co-stimulatory molecules.

The importance of the danger theory is that it allows us to understand when the immune system responds. It also explains why in some circumstances damage to tissues by infection or trauma can initiate immune responses in settings where normally there would be no such response.

TOLERANCE

While the danger theory can explain when the immune system responds, it is not enough to prevent autoimmunity, when there is an immune response against self. If the danger theory was the only control process, then every time we cut ourselves with a kitchen knife, causing danger signals, we would initiate an autoimmune response against skin antigens. There are many mechanisms that prevent autoimmunity, the most fundamental of which is deletion of autoreactive cells.

The main time in which autoreactive lymphocytes are deleted is soon after they are formed. There is a window after the generation of a new B cell in the bone marrow when, if it recognises self antigen, it is killed. T cells develop in the thymus, where the same process of deletion occurs.

However, some autoreactive cells escape from the bone marrow or thymus, either by chance or because the antigen that they recognise is not found there (e.g. tissue-specific molecules). These cells are controlled by several additional mechanisms. One is the presence of Treg which turn off cell responses. These regulatory cells can be generated in the thymus, but also can be made in lymph nodes and other tissues.

Autoreactive T cells can also be turned off when they encounter antigen presented in particular ways. The most important example is when autoreactive T cells encounter an immature dendritic cell presenting a self-antigen (e.g. a tissue-specific antigen) and they become anergic (unresponsive to future stimulation). This means that an encounter with antigen in the absence of a danger signal will turn off an immune response.

The Fetus as an Allograft

One major focus of immunological research is in transplantation. It is important to understand some of the issues of transplantation when considering reproductive immunology because, from an immunological point of view, the fetus is a form of transplanted tissue.

If an organ is transplanted from one individual to another without any drug treatment, it is rapidly recognised by the mother's immune system and destroyed. This alloresponse (between different members of the same species) is very strong because MHC molecules are highly polymorphic, showing considerable variability between individuals. These differences are recognised by a high frequency of T cells, termed alloreactive T cells.

Clinically, the rejection of allografts is minimised by attempting to match the MHC types of the donor and recipient (HLA matching). While it is realistically impossible (except in the case of twins) to obtain a perfect match, the better the match, the weaker the rejection response. The second approach is to immunosuppress the recipient, using drugs, antibody or (not commonly in the clinical setting)

irradiation. In the experimental laboratory setting, it is also possible to 're-educate' the immune system not to recognise the donor tissue, and to be tolerant of the transplanted organ. These strategies are being moved into the experimental clinical setting.

The fetus is a semi-allogeneic graft; half of its MHC molecules come from the mother and half from the father. It therefore presents a major target for the mother's immune system. It is thus interesting to understand why the fetus is not normally rejected. It is now recognised that there are active processes by which fetal tissues (in particular at the placental interface between the mother and fetus) prevent cells of the maternal immune system from rejecting the fetal tissue.

SYSTEMIC CONTROL MECHANISMS

These processes have both a systemic and local action. At the systemic level, there is an increase in Treg during pregnancy, as well as a shift in the responses from a Th1 to a non-inflammatory Th2 type. The absence of Treg in animals leads to failure of gestation in mothers carrying allogeneic but not syngeneic (MHC identical) fetuses, indicating their role in preventing rejection. The presence of a Th1 type response in the placenta is associated with miscarriages and can be caused by infection or stress. The factors responsible for Th2 bias in the immune responses include hormones and cytokines secreted by the placenta, including progesterone. Thus, a successful pregnancy is compatible with Th2 polarisation. The increase in the number of Treg and the alteration in the Th1/Th2 balance are likely to be important reasons why several Th1-dependent autoimmune diseases (such as multiple sclerosis and rheumatoid arthritis) are mitigated during pregnancy, with the symptoms getting worse after delivery. However, women with autoantibody-driven autoimmune diseases, such as myasthenia gravis and systemic lupus erythematosus, can undergo mild to moderate 'flares' during pregnancy or immediately after, possibly because Th2 responses (autoantibodies) are important in the pathogenesis of these diseases.

When the fetus is rejected by the immune system, it need not involve direct killing mechanisms. Thus, Th1 cytokines can act on trophoblastic cells to induce a pro-coagulant phenotype in the placental circulation, clotting off the maternal circulation.

LOCAL IMMUNOMODULATION

More local immunomodulation may be the result of expression of molecules by cells at the interface between the mother and fetus. A key cell is the syncytiotrophoblast, which forms the fetal-derived boundary between the mother and fetal cells. These cells have no or little expression of MHC molecules. As such, they might be a target for attack by maternal NK cells. However, they express an alternative MHC molecule (HLA-G in the human) that binds to NK cells, giving them a negative signal that prevents activation (Fig. 8.8). The cells also express an enzyme, indoleamine 2,3-dioxygenase (IDO), that catabolises tryptophan. This is an essential amino acid, and T cell responses are inhibited by both low concentrations of tryptophan and by the

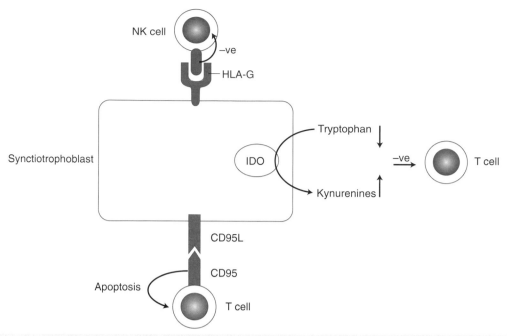

Fig. 8.8 Local immunomodulation by syncytiotrophoblasts. Syncytiotrophoblasts are capable of modulating immune responses in a variety of ways. The expression of HLA-G inhibits natural killer (NK) cell activity. Expression of the enzyme indoleamine 2,3-dioxygenase *(IDO)* catabolises tryptophan, and both deprivation of tryptophan and the production of metabolites (kynurenines) inhibit T cell activation. Finally, expression of CD95L (FasL) results in apoptosis of inflammatory cells that express CD95 (Fas).

metabolites (kynurenines) generated by IDO breakdown of tryptophan (see Fig. 8.8). Syncytiotrophoblasts also express CD95-ligand (CD95L, also known as FasL). This is the receptor for CD95 (Fas) which is expressed by activated leukocytes. Engagement of CD95 on the leukocytes by CD95L induces apoptosis in any fetus-recognising alloreactive T cells (see Fig. 8.8).

Antibodies and Pregnancy

Antibodies are important in pregnancy. In some cases, this is because of the damage that they cause, for example in rhesus incompatibility and anti-phospholipid syndrome. Importantly, antibodies are actively transported from the maternal circulation into the fetal circulation, where they are responsible for much of the immunity of the infant post-partum.

Maternal anti-fetal antibodies can be induced during pregnancy or may be pre-existing (such as the ABO blood group antibodies). In order to prevent damage to placental cells that bind these antibodies, there are high levels of complement regulatory molecules expressed on trophoblastic cells, which prevent activation of complement by antibody coating these cells.

Anti-phospholipid syndrome, in which there are circulating antibodies against molecules such as cardiolipin or phosphatidylserine, is associated with early and late fetal loss, as well as intrauterine growth retardation and other fetal morbidities. While there is still debate about how the antibodies cause disease, the anti-phospholipid antibodies may have a direct effect on trophoblast development, with a failure to establish a good feto-placental circulation being responsible for early pregnancy losses. In later pregnancy, the pro-inflammatory and pro-thrombotic effects of the

antibody on the endothelial cells (probably in combination with complement) may be responsible for the pathologies associated with this syndrome.

At birth, the neonate has almost no endogenous antibodies. One of the roles of the placenta is to transport maternal immunoglobulin into the fetus. Following birth, this maternal antibody provides temporary immunity while the infant's own immune system matures. In many other mammals, the maternal antibody is predominantly provided through milk rather than via the placenta (in the human IgA antibodies in the maternal milk are important in protecting the infant's gut). The maternal antibody is transported through the syncytiotrophoblast layer, probably via the neonatal Fc receptor (FcRn), which binds to the Fc region of the antibody, internalises it in an endosome and deposits it on the other side of the cell. Immune complexes between antibodies and antigens, and antibodies reactive with paternal HLA molecules are absorbed in the stroma, and the antibody then crosses the fetal endothelial cells.

Maternal antibodies can damage the fetus and/or newborn infant. This is seen when the mother has an antibody-mediated autoimmune disease, such as Graves disease or myasthenia gravis, where transfer of autoantibody results in disease in the infant (which remits as the maternal antibody is cleared). These pathogenic antibodies can be removed by plasmapheresis and the newborn is exempted from the disease aetiology and symptoms.

The classic case of maternally derived antibodies damaging the infant is haemolytic disease of the newborn, resulting in general from incompatibilities in the rhesus blood group antigen. RhD-negative women carrying an RhD-positive fetus have no problems with their first pregnancy. However, at birth the passage of fetal blood to the mother can immunise her, resulting in an anti-RhD antibody response. In subsequent pregnancies, the anti-RhD antibodies can cross into the fetal circulation prior to birth, leading to lysis of red blood cells. This can be treated by intrauterine blood transfusions or prevented by administration to RhD-negative women of anti-RhD antisera at the time of each birth (or invasive procedure). These antibodies mop up the fetal blood, preventing maternal immunisation.

OTHER IMMUNOLOGICAL INTERACTIONS WITH THE FETUS

In addition to killing pathogens, the immune system is important in tissue repair and remodelling. Many of the immune system's pathophysiological roles in pregnancy do not involve killing of the fetal allograft, and that active involvement of the immune system is important for successful gestation. There are a number of immune cells that play an important role during pregnancy and their dysregulation can lead to a range of pregnancy-associated complications, such as recurrent pregnancy loss, preterm delivery and pre-eclampsia.

One such example is the interaction between maternal NK cells and fetal trophoblasts that penetrate the maternal decidua and are necessary for the remodelling of the spiral arteries. This remodelling is required to increase blood flow to the placenta and the fetus. The NK cells in this process do not have a cytotoxic role, but their recognition, in particular of MHC antigens (HLA-C, -E, and -G in the human) on the trophoblasts, results in the secretion of cytokines and growth factors that are necessary for the action of the cytotrophoblasts. Failure of this recognition can result in poor remodelling of the spiral arteries and inadequate placentation – leading ultimately to pre-eclampsia or intrauterine growth retardation. The importance of this pathway is supported by genetic findings demonstrating that pre-eclampsia is more common when the receptors on the maternal NK cells are poor at being stimulated by the fetal MHC molecules. The immunological component may also explain why pre-eclampsia is more common in first pregnancies. Altered decidual NK cell number is linked with weak vascular growth and angiogenesis and reduced trophoblast invasion. NK cell-deficient mice show reduced placental blood flow compared to normal mice.

Uterine NK cells can be recruited from the blood to the uterus followed by their further differentiation, in addition to the presence of uterine precursor NK cells. Thus, the uterine NK cells may have multiple origins, but contribute equally to a successful pregnancy. Decidual NK cells express on their surface receptors for HLA-C, HLA-E and HLA-G. Killer Immunoglobulin Receptors (KIR) are highly expressed on decidual NK cells which are skewed towards recognising HLA-C during pregnancy. Additional inhibitory receptors interact with HLA-E present on maternal cells and trophoblasts, thus preventing their cytolysis.

A diverse range of immune cell interactions take place during fetal-maternal interaction. Decidual NK cells can modulate other maternal immune cells locally. Their production of IFN-γ can upregulate IDO which in turn can suppress T cell activation and instead expand Treg. The same NK cell derived IFN-γ can inhibit pro-inflammatory Th17 differentiation at the fetal-maternal interface. Low numbers of IFN-γ producing decidual NK cells have been associated with recurrent pregnancy loss and implantation failures, highlighting the importance of decidual NK cells in the maintenance of maternal tolerance via IFN-γ mediated suppression of Th17 cells and inflammatory response.

Decidual macrophages play an important role in vascular remodelling, trophoblast invasion and parturition. In the initial phase of pregnancy, they are of classic M1 phenotype (phagocytic and pro-inflammatory), as opposed to immunosuppressive M2 macrophages, which transition into a mixed M1/M2 phenotype during the first and early part of second trimester. After full blown placental development, the decidual macrophages acquire M2 phenotype. Another set of M2 macrophage-like Hofbauer cells, present with chronic villi, have been considered important in placental remodelling and angiogenesis.

As described earlier, Treg contribute heavily towards maternal immune tolerance by suppressing effector T cells via a range of direct and indirect mechanisms. Treg cells are found to be in low numbers in cases of recurrent miscarriage, spontaneous abortion and pre-eclampsia. Removal of Treg cells in mice leads to gestation failure in mice.

Conclusion

The immune system is a complex network of cells and molecules that are tightly controlled. In pregnancy, this control ensures that the fetus is not destroyed or damaged. While the main role of the immune system may be to protect the organism against pathogens, it is also involved in tissue remodelling and repair, and these functions may be crucial in pregnancy. It is clear that immune cells, as expected, play a very crucial role in the acceptance of the allograft (i.e. the fetus) and subsequent maintenance of the tolerance during pregnancy. Decidual NK cells are located nearby decidua and its receptor interaction with trophoblast HLA-E prevents cytolysis of the fetal tissue, while NK cell alternative receptor interaction with trophoblast HLA-G can release inflammatory and angiogenic factors required for tissue remodelling. Secretion of IFN-γ by decidual NK cells, encouraged by IL-15 producing decidual antigen presenting cells, can selectively expand immunosuppressive Treg cells. Macrophages, during the early part of the pregnancy, have phagocytic and pro-inflammatory M1 phenotype to facilitate clearance of pathogens and apoptotic cells. However, slowly, there is a shift towards immunosuppressive M2 phenotype after early part of the second trimester. Although early pregnancy decidual macrophages have M1 phenotype, they express low levels of co-stimulator molecules suggesting their poor capacity to activate effector T cells. Thus, an interplay between various immune cells is crucial for a successful pregnancy.

9 — Biochemistry

FIONA LYALL, NIAMH SAYERS AND NICK DIBB

Structure and Function of the Normal Cell

All cells possess certain basic structural features, regardless of their location, type and function (Fig. 9.1). The major division is into nucleus and cytoplasm.

NUCLEUS

The nucleus contains the chromosomes (see Chapter 1) and is surrounded by a nuclear envelope consisting of an inner and outer membrane, both of which are formed from a lipid bilayer. The nuclear envelope has pores which are used for the transport of RNA from the nucleus into the cytoplasm and for the import of nuclear proteins (which are made in the cytoplasm). Within the nucleus, one or more nucleoli are present. These sites mark the site of transcription of ribosomal RNA, which is a key component of ribosomes and is required in large amounts. In addition, ribosomal proteins are imported into nucleoli where they are assembled with ribosomal RNA to form ribosomes, which are then exported to the cytoplasm. The splicing machinery, or spliceosomes, are also located within the nucleus (see below). The messenger RNA (mRNA) is transported from the nucleus to the cytoplasm for translation. Nuclear RNA is a precursor of cytoplasmic ribosomal RNA (see Chapter 1).

CYTOPLASM

The remainder of the cell is comprised by the cytoplasm. It is enclosed within a single cell or plasma membrane that is also a lipid bilayer and when stained has a distinctive trilaminar structure. The cell membrane has a very complex biochemical structure, including many proteins and lipids; it is not rigid, but can alter its shape in response to various stimuli. The major function of the cell membrane is control and maintenance of the appropriate intracellular electrolyte and biochemical environment by energy-requiring active transport mechanisms (e.g. sodium removal by the sodium pump). It also provides adhesion between adjacent cells and displays the individual cell's major histocompatibility (transplant or human leukocyte antigen (HLA)) antigens. In some cells (e.g. polymorphs), it determines motility and phagocytosis.

The cytoplasm contains many organelles:

1. *Mitochondria* are elongated, enzyme-rich bodies; each has a continuous external limiting membrane and an inner membrane folded into septa (cristae), which create partial subdivisions of the matrix. Oxidative phosphorylation occurs within mitochondria, which are able to oxidise proteins, carbohydrates and fats into energy, store it as adenosine triphosphate (ATP) and subsequently release it when required by the cell.

Animal Cell

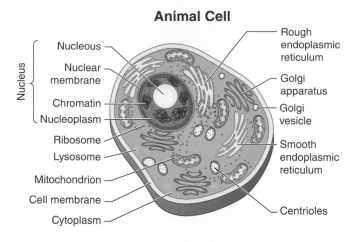

Nucleous

Nuclear membrane

Chromatin

Nucleoplasm

Nucleus

Ribosome

Lysosome

Mitochondrion

Cell membrane

Cytoplasm

Rough endoplasmic reticulum

Golgi apparatus

Golgi vesicle

Smooth endoplasmic reticulum

Centrioles

Organelle	Function
Nucleus	Contains chromosomal material and apparatus for cell division
Nucleolus	RNA and ribsosome production
Lysosomes	Degradation of macromolecules
Golgi apparatus	Modification of proteins and their secretion and re-cycling
Endoplasmic reticulum	Membrane system for protein synthesis
Ribosomes	Catalyse peptide bond formation in protein synthesis
Mitochondria	Contain many enzymes involved in metabolism and energy production

Fig. 9.1 Structure of a cell.

2. *Ribosomes* are small ribonucleic acid protein particles (RNPs) that contain ribosomal RNA and ribosomal proteins. The ribosomal RNA and proteins are encoded by a large family of different genes within the nucleus. Ribosomes catalyse the synthesis of all proteins including those for intracellular metabolism. Aggregates of ribosomes are designated polysomes or polyribosomes.

3. *Spliceosomes* are also RNPs that contain small nuclear RNAs and many proteins. They act upon pre-messenger RNA (pre-mRNA) to generate mRNA which is transported to the cytoplasm. Pre-mRNA is larger than mRNA and 90% of gene transcripts contain introns, which are removed by spliceosomes. Spliceosomes can also generate alternative mRNA transcripts from pre-mRNA which allows a single gene to encode multiple protein isomers.

4. *The endoplasmic reticulum* (ER) is a complex network of intercommunicating narrow tubules and vesicles (cisternae) and is mainly responsible for N-linked glycosylation and the transport of certain proteins to the Golgi apparatus. Two continuous types of ER exist: rough ER, where ribosomes are attached to the outer surface, and smooth ER where ribosomes are absent. The rough ER is continuous with the outer membrane

of the nucleus. The smooth ER is involved in the synthesis of lipids, including cholesterol and phospholipids. In certain cell types, the smooth ER plays an important role in the synthesis of steroid hormones from cholesterol.

5. *The signal recognition particle* (SRP) is another ribonucleic acid particle and is responsible for identifying those proteins that need to be secreted into the lumen of the ER for subsequent transport to the Golgi apparatus and to different parts of the cell. Proteins that enter the ER lumen usually contain a signal recognition peptide at their N-terminal that is recognised by the SRP, which directs the protein/ribosome complex to the ER for translocation (Fig. 9.2).

6. *The Golgi complex* is a stack of flattened membranous sacs and is the major sorting centre of the cell. Proteins are transported from the Golgi complex to lysosomes, secretory granules or the cell membrane according to signals within their amino acid sequences and how they associate with other proteins and lipids. The Golgi apparatus also adds O-linked sugars to proteins and may modify the N-linked sugars that arrive from the ER.

7. *The centrosome* is a relatively clear area, usually near the cell centre, containing two centrioles. *Centrioles* are hollow cylindrical bodies, 0.3 to 0.7 μm in length, which replicate before mitosis and orientate the mitotic spindle.

8. *Lysosomes* are round or oval membrane-bound bodies containing proteolytic enzymes (acid hydrolases) for digesting unwanted endogenous and phagocytosed exogenous material.

9. *Phagosomes* are membrane-bound bodies containing material ingested by phagocytosis. To effect digestion, phagosomes combine with lysosomes to produce phagolysosomes. When indigestible material remains, residual or dense bodies are formed.

10. *Filaments*. Cells have microfilaments (made of actin and 7 nm in diameter), intermediate filaments (made of one or more of the family of over 50 intermediate proteins, 8 to 10 nM in diameter) and microtubules (made of tubulin, 25 nM in diameter). Filaments are of indefinite length and have a variety of functions. For example, tonofibrils are a type of intermediate filament that converge on intercellular junctions (desmosomes) to promote cell adhesion; actin microfilaments interact with myosin to generate force in muscles cells or interact with myosin motors in other cell types to effect cell movement or vesicle transport; microtubules radiate from centrioles and are important for mitosis and vesicle transport.

11. *Clathrin coated pits*. Cells use a variety of mechanisms to endocytose cell surface proteins and lipids and the use of clathrin coated pits is one of the best characterised processes. Some cell surface proteins, such as transferrin, are selectively endocytosed in a network of clathrin, known as a clathrin pit. The endocytosis of transferrin allows the entry of iron into a cell. Low-density lipoproteins are also endocytosed via clathrin pits.

12. *Vesicles* are small spheres containing specialised cytoplasm that is enclosed by a lipid bilayer. They are used for transport and communication between different

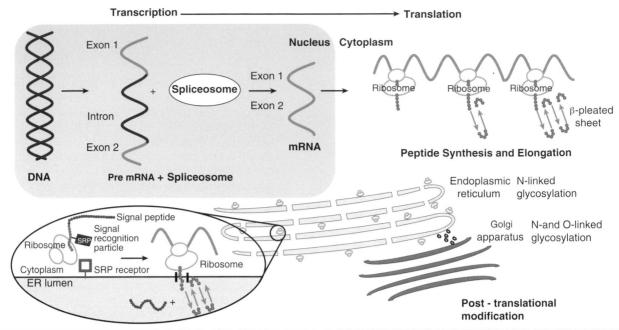

Fig. 9.2 Sequence of events in protein synthesis.

parts of the cells. For example secretory vesicles (exosomes) are used to transport proteins from the ER to the Golgi and to secrete proteins. Vesicles known as endosomes are essential for endocytosis and transport proteins from outside the cell to the cytoplasm or to lysosomes.

13. *Proteasomes* are large protease complexes within the cytoplasm that degrade proteins into amino acids, which are recycled. Protein degradation is regulated by the attachment of a small highly conserved protein called ubiquitin which directs the tagged protein to the proteasome.

Specific structures are unique to, and characteristic of, specialised cells (e.g. myofilaments in muscle cells and melanosomes in melanocytes). Several other structures may also be seen, including glycogen granules, lipofuscin granules, myelinoid bodies, siderosomes and lipid droplets.

CELL TYPES

The human body contains over 200 mature cell types that are sometimes classified into four tissue types: epithelial, connective, muscle or nervous. Alternative classifications place more emphasis upon the origin of a mature cell type from the three layers of the early embryo, namely ectoderm, endoderm or mesoderm. Tissue membranes are composed of either epithelial or connective cells.

Epithelial cells cover or line body surfaces and internal cavities; in addition, most glands are epithelial, being derived embryologically from body surfaces. Epithelial cells therefore act as selective and protective barriers and synthesise most secretions.

Connective tissue cells are derived largely from the embryonic mesoderm. Connective tissue exists in many types, and its composition varies in different parts of the body, depending on local requirements. Its main function is to provide structural support, generally as fibrous tissue and specifically as bone, cartilage, muscle and tendon. It is probably also responsible for body defences since leucocytes and mononuclear phagocyte (reticuloendothelial) system cells are usually considered connective tissue in origin.

INTERCELLULAR MATRIX

The intercellular matrix refers to the non-living material filling the space between cells. This varies considerably in amount; very little is seen between epithelial cells, whereas connective tissue cells are often quite widely separated by matrix, the exact nature of which may provide the unique connective tissue structure (e.g. bone and cartilage). Interstitial extracellular fluid is located in the intercellular matrix.

The epithelial intercellular matrix is a narrow, mucopolysaccharide-rich layer traversed by intercellular junctions. Formerly a designated cement substance, it is now thought, in some instances, to be an integral component of the cell membrane's external surface.

Connective tissue intercellular matrix contains ground substance and fibres. The ground substance is a gel of variable consistency and viscosity, containing mucoproteins, glycoproteins and mucopolysaccharides; it is probably mainly secreted by fibroblasts. Collagen is one of the most important fibres and provides structural rigidity. It has a trihelical structure derived from a soluble precursor (procollagen), secreted by fibroblasts and osteoblasts via an insoluble intermediate (tropocollagen). Four collagen types, encoded by different structural genes, are known: collagen type I is the form found in bone, collagen type II is found in cartilage and collagen type IV is found in the basement membranes of epithelia. Collagen type III is found in the tissues of the fetus but this is replaced by type I following birth. Adults have little type III, although it does reappear during the wound response. Collagen type I is a major component of bones, skin and a number of other tissues and this single protein comprises more than 50% of the total protein in the body.

Proteins, Peptides and Amino Acids

Each of the many cell types in the body makes a unique set of proteins. There is considerable variation in the types of protein made by each cell type and a particular cell synthesises is only a part of the total human protein repertoire. For example, despite the large amount of albumin present in blood plasma, it is only synthesised in adults by hepatocytes in the liver. This is despite the fact that every cell contains within its nucleus a copy of the gene for albumin along with a copy of every other human gene. During development and differentiation, the DNA within each cell type comes under a regulatory mechanism such that some genes are expressed and others are repressed. This mechanism underlies the concept of 'totipotency', which refers to the ability of totipotent stem cells to generate all of the many different mature cell types during differentiation. In the case of some proteins, expression does not occur all the time but does so in response to a specific signal such as a hormone. The control of protein expression is aberrant in many tumours and inappropriate proteins are produced.

The proteins synthesised by a cell play a number of different roles. Some proteins have a structural role. For example, there are proteins that provide the structural basis for the membrane around the cell and the membranes around the nucleus, mitochondria and the other discrete subcellular organelles (see Fig. 9.1).

Other proteins such as enzymes have non-structural roles. The human genome encodes many thousands of proteins which act as enzymes for specific reactions; these include synthesis reactions, degradative reactions, energy-producing reactions and energy-storing reactions. Very few biochemical reactions occur in the absence of enzymes and thus this catalysis is essential for life.

Other non-structural proteins include hormones, neurotransmitters and transport proteins, all of which are found in plasma. One of the functions of albumin is to transport free fatty acids, and the plasma protein transferrin carries iron from the gut to tissues. In blood, there are different classes of lipoprotein that carry lipids in circulation; chylomicrons carry triglycerides from the gut to adipose tissue and the liver. Low-density lipoproteins carry much of the cholesterol that is required by tissues; some of the cholesterol comes from dietary sources but most has been synthesised in the liver.

Some proteins in plasma play a hormone-binding role. Other major constituents of plasma are the immunoglobulins (antibodies) and complement proteins that are part of the immune system.

AMINO ACIDS

There are 21 amino acids used in the synthesis of proteins. The generalised structure of an amino acid is shown in Fig. 9.3; each amino acid has a characteristic R group or side chain. Fig. 9.4 shows the chemical structure of each amino

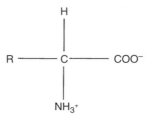

Fig. 9.3 General structure of an amino acid. R is a side chain that defines the amino acid. (See also Fig. 9.4.)

acid used by humans, along with its three-letter and one-letter designation. Every amino acid has a mirror image form but only L amino acids (not the D amino acids) are constituents of proteins. Similarly, monosaccharides such as glucose have mirror image forms but conversely the six carbon sugars used in nature are D-isomers not L-isomers.

Selenocysteine is a recently discovered and unusual 21st amino acid. It has the same structure as cysteine except that it has selenium instead of a sulphur atom (Fig 9.3). Unlike the other 20 amino acids, there is not a dedicated codon (or codons) that encodes selenocysteine. However, for the small number of human proteins that contain selenocysteine, this amino acid is encoded by a UGA stop codon (see Chapter 1) but only when a selenocysteine insertion sequence is also present in the mRNA. Not all amino acids can be synthesised *in vivo*. Those that can be synthesised are referred to as the 'non-essential amino acids' and comprise the following:

- Alanine
- Aspartic acid
- Asparagine
- Glutamine
- Cysteine
- Glutamic acid
- Glycine
- Proline
- Serine
- Tyrosine.

The essential amino acids are:

- Arginine
- Histidine
- Isoleucine
- Leucine
- Lysine
- Valine
- Methionine
- Phenylalanine
- Selenocysteine
- Threonine
- Tryptophan.

The situation is slightly more complex than this since cysteine can be synthesised if there is sufficient methionine present; similarly, tyrosine can be synthesised if there is sufficient phenylalanine present. Histidine and arginine are not strictly essential but are required for normal growth. The essential amino acids are required in the diet. A simple estimate of total protein will not indicate sufficiency. For example, if the diet contained insufficient

AMINO ACID	STRUCTURE	SYMBOL
Basic amino acids		
Arginine	H—N—CH$_2$—CH$_2$—CH$_2$—CH—COO$^-$ ‖ C=NH$_2^+$ NH$_3^+$ ‖ NH$_2$	Arg (R)
Lysine	CH$_2$—CH$_2$—CH$_2$—CH$_2$—CH—COO$^-$ ‖ NH$_3^+$ NH$_3^+$	Lys (K)
Histidine	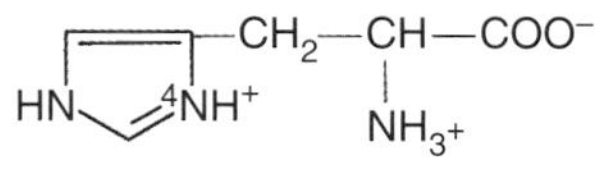 ┌─────┐—CH$_2$—CH—COO$^-$ HN─┘ ^{4}NH$^+$ NH$_3^+$	His (H)
Acidic amino acids		
Aspartic acid	$^-$OOC—CH$_2$—CH—COO$^-$ ‖ NH$_3^+$	Asp (D)
Glutamic acid	$^-$OOC—CH$_2$—CH$_2$—CH—COO$^-$ ‖ NH$_3^+$	Glu (E)
Asparagine	H$_2$N—C—CH$_2$—CH—COO$^-$ ‖ ‖ O NH$_3^+$	Asn (N)
Glutamine	H$_2$N—C—CH$_2$—CH$_2$—CH—COO$^-$ ‖ ‖ O NH$_3^+$	Glu (Q)
Aromatic amino acids		
Phenylalanine	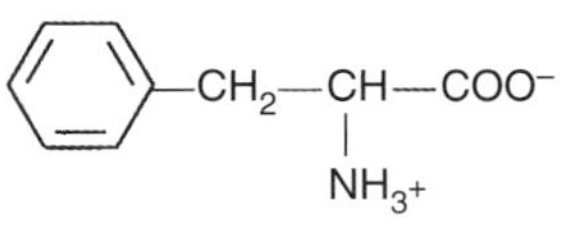 ⬡—CH$_2$—CH—COO$^-$ ‖ NH$_3^+$	Phe (F)

Fig. 9.4 Structures of the amino acids.

valine, then the total protein content would be immaterial since protein synthesis cannot continue in the absence of valine. This leads to the concept of qualitative and quantitative dietary sufficiency. A diet is only satisfactory if it contains adequate concentrations of all the essential amino acids. A protein is a sequence of amino acids that are chemically coupled by the enzyme activity of ribosomes.

The sequence of events that occurs in the synthesis of a protein is depicted in Fig. 9.2. The sequence of amino acids for a protein is encoded in the gene for that protein. This genetic information is stored in the form of DNA. The structure of DNA is that of a double helix of two long nucleotide chains. Each chain has a deoxyribose phosphodiester backbone carrying a covalently linked sequence

AMINO ACID	STRUCTURE	SYMBOL
Aromatic amino acids		
Tyrosine	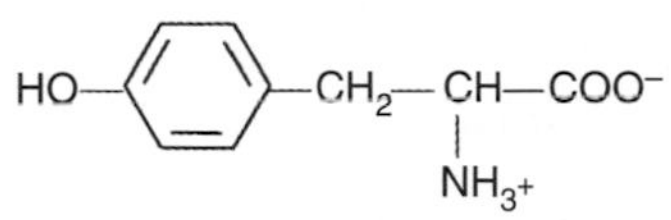 HO—⟨ring⟩—CH$_2$—CH—COO$^-$ with NH$_3{}^+$	Tyr (Y)
Tryptophan	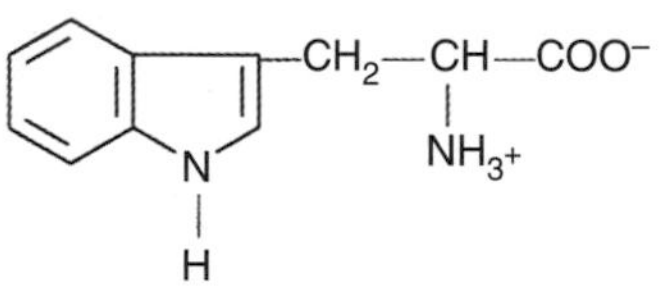 ⟨indole ring with N—H⟩—CH$_2$—CH—COO$^-$ with NH$_3{}^+$	Try (W)
Amino acids with aliphatic chains		
Glycine	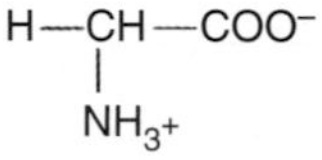 H—CH—COO$^-$ with NH$_3{}^+$	Gly (G)
Alanine	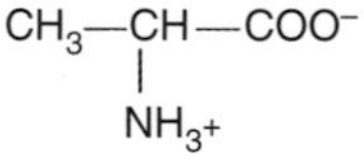 CH$_3$—CH—COO$^-$ with NH$_3{}^+$	Ala (A)
Valine	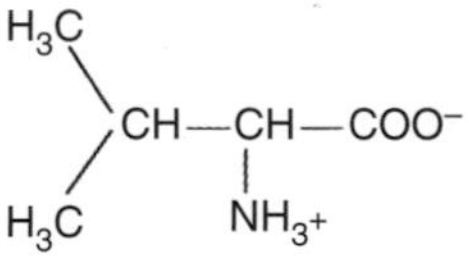 H$_3$C, H$_3$C >CH—CH—COO$^-$ with NH$_3{}^+$	Val (V)
Leucine	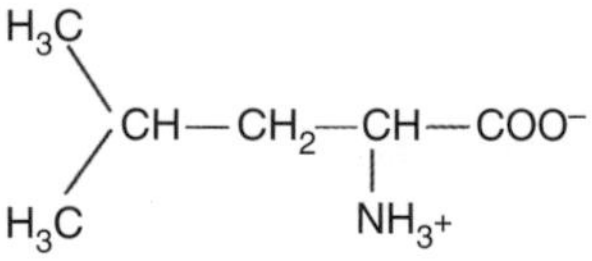 H$_3$C, H$_3$C >CH—CH$_2$—CH—COO$^-$ with NH$_3{}^+$	Leu (L)
Isoleucine	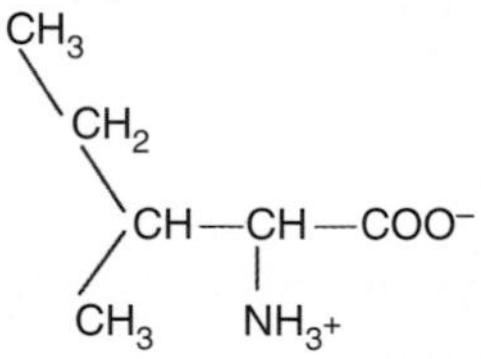 CH$_3$—CH$_2$ >CH—CH—COO$^-$ with CH$_3$ and NH$_3{}^+$	Iso (I)

Fig. 9.4 Cont'd

of the nucleotides or bases that make up the genetic code. There are four bases, namely, adenine, cytosine, guanine and thymine. The strands of DNA are held together tightly by hydrogen bonding between bases on each strand. The base adenine bonds to thymine and cytosine bonds to guanine. This complementarity provides accurate and strong pairing and is the basis of the famous discovery by Watson and Crick of the structure of DNA.

There are many hundreds of genes on each chromosome and they are found on both DNA strands. A gene has a specific sequence and number location within each chromosome. The first stage in the production of a protein is transcription; this is the term used to denote the process by which a complementary copy of the gene is made. The initial transcription product is called pre-mRNA, which is rapidly processed to mRNA by splicing. mRNA is a single-stranded

AMINO ACID	STRUCTURE	SYMBOL
Amino acids with hydroxyl groups		
Serine	CH_2—CH—COO^- $\mid$ $\mid$ OH NH_3^+	Ser (S)

Threonine	CH_3—CH—CH—COO^-
	      $\mid$ $\mid$
	     OH NH_3^+
		Thr (T)

Amino acids with sulphydryl groups		
Cysteine	CH_2—CH—COO^- $\mid$ $\mid$ SH NH_3^+	Cys (C)
Methionine	CH_2—CH_2—CH—COO^- $\mid$ $\mid$ S—CH_3 NH_3^+	Met (M)
Imino acids		
Proline	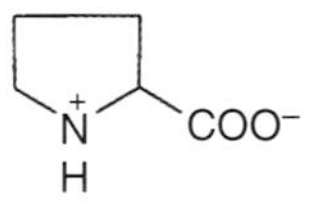 $\overset{+}{N}$H COO^-	Pro (P)

Fig. 9.4 Cont'd

nucleic acid that has ribose rather than deoxyribose in the phosphodiester backbone. Like DNA it contains the bases cytosine, guanine and adenine but, in contrast to DNA, contains uracil rather than thymine. The terminology of the bases is complex. The terms 'adenine', 'cytosine', 'guanine', 'thymine' and 'uracil' are used to describe the bases. When these are linked to the sugar ribose they are called 'adenosine', 'cytidine', 'guanosine', 'uridine' and 'thymidine'. If they are linked to deoxyribose, the prefix 'deoxy' is used.

When mRNA is transported out of the nucleus, it becomes attached to ribosomes. Each functional ribosome is composed of two subunits (known as large and small or 50 S and 30 S), each of which contains a number of different proteins and RNA species. Together this complex is responsible for the recognition of all the substrates and factors that are required for protein synthesis. Ultimately, the function of the ribosome is to couple together successive pairs of amino acids through the formation of peptide bonds (Fig. 9.5) in accordance with the genetic code. Ribosomal RNA is expressed by all animal and plant species and is highly conserved. The comparison of ribosomal RNA sequence between species is the basis of many taxonomy and phylogenetic studies.

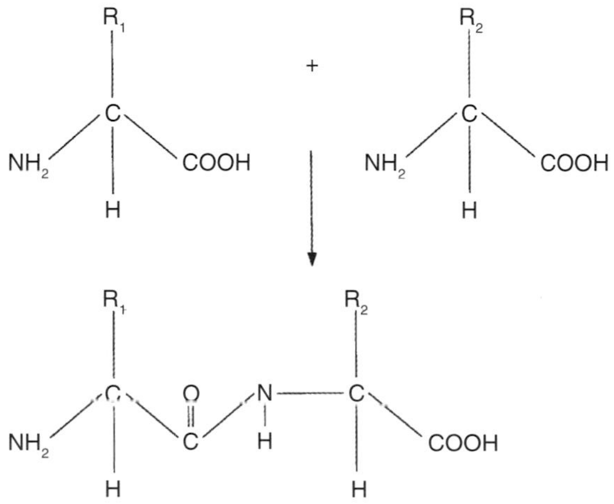

Fig. 9.5 Formation of a peptide bond.

STRUCTURE OF PROTEINS

Proteins vary greatly in size. Small proteins are referred to as 'peptides' and some of these have fewer than 10 amino acids in their sequence and have molecular weights of about 1000 Da. Examples of peptides include the hormones oxytocin and vasopressin. At the other end of the spectrum, some proteins are close to 1 million Da in molecular weight and have hundreds of amino acids in their sequence. Examples of larger proteins would be α_2-macroglobulin, an important anti-protease found in plasma, and the IgM class of immunoglobulins, which play a role in the early defence reaction against infecting organisms.

Proteins have primary, secondary, tertiary and often quaternary structures. The primary structure is the simplest description of the protein and refers to the linear sequence of amino acids, which is encoded by the gene for that protein. The primary sequence begins with an amino acid with a free amino terminal (*N*-terminus) and concludes with the last amino acid, which will have a free carboxyl group (*C*-terminus). All the intervening amino acids lose their free amino and carboxyl groups during the formation of the peptide bonds (see Fig. 9.5). Some proteins are modified at the *N*-terminus. For example, some of the proteins involved in the blood-clotting cascade have the *N*-terminal glutamic acid modified to become a γ-carboxyglutamic acid residue. The blocking of the *N*-terminus in this case involves an enzyme cascade that requires vitamin K. Warfarin acts by inhibiting this pathway. Proteins that enter the lumen of the ER often have signal peptides of about 20 amino acids that are recognised by the SRP and are then subsequently removed by signal peptidase (see Fig. 9.2).

The tertiary structure of a protein is the three-dimensional arrangement of a single protein and this structure is determined by the linear or primary amino acid sequence. There has been considerable progress in the prediction of the three-dimensional protein structure from the linear gene sequence but experimental verification through techniques such as x-ray crystallography are still essential. Nuclear magnetic resonance can also be used to determine the structure of smaller proteins. The tertiary structure of a single protein can be subdivided into elements of secondary structures, namely alpha helices, beta sheets, turns and loops. Alpha helices and beta sheets are stabilised by regular hydrogen bonding between the repeating CO and NH groups of the peptide backbone. This leaves the amino acid side chains sticking out which allows them to interact with each other (by hydrogen bonding or ionic attraction) or to catalyse chemical reactions. The side chains of the amino acid cysteine can form covalent disulphide bonds; these are commonly found on proteins on the outside of a cell. The overall tertiary structure of a protein is determined by the interaction of its secondary structures and in addition the tertiary structure of a soluble protein is also stabilised by its hydrophobic core, which is formed by the interaction of amino acids with hydrophobic side chains. Loop regions are less structured and are nearly always found at the cell surface, these regions often contain amino acids that have key catalytic functions. Turns are so named because they stabilise a change in direction of a peptide chain.

Many proteins, such as haemoglobin, are composed of subunits. These can be identical or dissimilar. The subunits are held together by non-covalent forces which are most commonly charge–charge interactions. The three-dimensional structure of all the subunits comprising a protein is referred to as its quaternary structure. A new technique called cryo-electron microscopy can be used to determine the structure of higher-order protein complexes.

PURIFICATION AND ANALYSIS OF PROTEINS

There are several techniques available for the separation of proteins. Most can be used for the preparative purification of a single protein to homogeneity as well as analytically in order to determine the degree of purity of a protein.

Some methods separate proteins on the basis of size. Thus, gel permeation chromatography involves the use of beds of resin beads that contain pores of a predetermined size. Some proteins will diffuse into these pores while other proteins are too large and are excluded. Large proteins are eluted from the bed before the smaller ones. A second method involving size is gel electrophoresis. A support of agarose or polyacrylamide is used and the protein solution is exposed to an electric field. In the absence of detergent, the proteins will move according to their mass/charge ratio. If a detergent such as sodium dodecyl sulphate is added to the system, the proteins move at a rate proportional to their size alone.

Ion-exchange chromatography involves the use of resins that contain at their surface positively or negatively charged groups. Proteins contain negatively charged carboxyl groups and positively charged amino groups. The proteins will bind to the resin and can then be eluted by changing either the pH or the salt strength of the buffers used. Individual proteins have unique patterns of charge and can be separated from one another if gradients of buffer strengths are used.

Another technique called affinity chromatography can often be used to achieve complete purity of a protein in a single step. Here a chemical moiety is coupled to a bed of support beads. The agent that is coupled binds with high specificity to the protein that is to be purified. When a mixture of proteins in solution is passed through the bed, only the target protein binds to the beads and, after washing off all non-specifically bound material, a high salt concentration or change of pH is used to elute the protein. The types of ligand that can be coupled to the beads are antibodies or substrate for an enzyme.

MODIFICATION OF PROTEIN STRUCTURE

Very few proteins are composed purely of amino acid chains and most have carbohydrate chains covalently attached. This is referred to as post-translational modification because, after the protein has been synthesised on the ribosomes, the peptide passes to the ER and then the Golgi apparatus, where enzymes assemble chains of sugars onto the protein.

The carbohydrate is always linked to specific amino acids in the protein chains, namely serine, threonine or asparagine. In the case of serine or threonine, the carbohydrate is linked via the oxygen of the hydroxyl groups and is hence referred to as *O*-linked carbohydrate. In the case of asparagine, it is linked to the nitrogen of the amino group and is referred to as *N*-linked carbohydrate. N-linked glycosylation occurs in both the ER and Golgi, whereas O-linked glycosylation occurs in the Golgi.

There is considerable diversity in terms of the size and nature of the carbohydrate that is attached to protein and it appears to serve different functions. Proteins that are part of membranes are heavily glycosylated (the term used to denote the attachment of sugar residues) and the oligosaccharide chains play a role in maintaining the proteins in the correct orientation within the membrane. Proteins in the cytosol are also often glycosylated.

Proteins found in plasma are also often highly glycosylated and in this case the sugar plays a regulatory role in controlling turnover. While sugar chains remain intact, the protein continues to circulate in plasma. When the sugar chains become cleaved or modified, then the proteins are removed from circulation and degraded. The liver has a most efficient mechanism for detecting altered circulating proteins. There are in the newly formed proteins no terminal galactose residues; there is a sialic acid residue after the galactose. If the galactosyl groups are revealed following damage to the protein, it is immediately removed from circulation by hepatocytes which contain at their surface a receptor for the terminal galactose.

Metabolism

OVERALL ENERGY METABOLISM

Every cell has to maintain an adequate supply of energy. Dietary lipids, carbohydrates and proteins are all sources of energy because each has an intrinsic energy that is released when the molecule is broken into smaller parts. Nature has evolved a mechanism by which this energy can be harnessed to produce ATP, which is used to drive most biological reactions. Which particular energy source is used depends upon a number of parameters such as dietary status, circadian rhythm, etc. In this section, the individual metabolic pathways will be described as will the controls that operate and the interrelationships between the pathways.

The metabolism of carbohydrates (sugars), fats (fatty acids and glycerol) and protein begins with pathways that are specific for each energy source. The products from these pathways then feed into common pathways. The overall interaction of the pathways is shown in Fig. 9.6.

Sugars, fatty acids and amino acids are all metabolised to produce acetate in the form of acetyl coenzyme A (acetyl-CoA). The acetyl group has to be covalently linked to CoA for stabilisation.

The acetyl-CoA then enters the tricarboxylic acid (TCA) cycle, which is also known as the 'citric acid cycle' or the 'Krebs cycle', after the biochemist who was involved in its discovery. The TCA cycle results in the complete degradation of acetyl groups. The products are carbon dioxide, which is breathed out by the lungs, and water. During this process hydrogen becomes available in the form of nicotinamide adenine dinucleotide (NADH) and flavin adenine dinucleotide (FADH$_2$). NADH and FADH$_2$ are fed into the respiratory chain (also known as the electron transport chain) inside the mitochondrion in order to produce ATP from adenosine diphosphate (ADP). This reaction within the respiratory chain requires molecular oxygen, hence the name 'respiratory chain'.

The overall oxidation of glucose is:

$$\longrightarrow C_6H_{12}O_6 + 6O_2 \rightarrow 6CO_2 + 6H_2O$$

That is, the complete oxidation of a molecule of glucose to carbon dioxide and water. Nature has evolved an efficient sequence of reactions and much of the energy within the glucose molecule is utilised in the production of ATP from ADP. A single molecule of glucose can result in the net formation of 2 ATP molecules by glycolysis and a further 28 molecules of ATP are generated by oxidative phosphorylation within the mitochondria. The chemical combustion of glucose in the presence of excess oxygen yields 686,000 cal/mol.

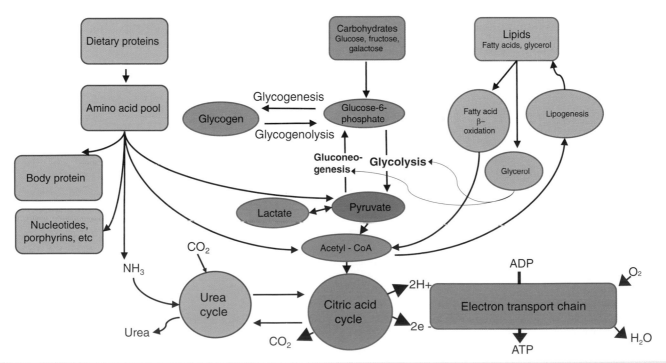

Fig. 9.6 Processing of dietary constituents. *ADP*, Adenosine diphosphate; *ATP*, adenosine triphosphate.

Each time an ADP molecule is converted to one of ATP, 7300 cal are captured. Because there is a net profit of about 30 molecules of ATP, this indicates that the process is approximately 32% efficient. The remaining energy is released as heat.

GLYCOLYSIS

The enzymes of the glycolytic pathway are found in the cytoplasm of the cell. The glycolytic pathway converts a molecule of glucose that contains six carbon atoms to two molecules of pyruvic acid, each containing three carbon atoms. The pathway for glycolysis is shown in Fig. 9.7 and it can be seen that in the first few steps the glucose becomes doubly phosphorylated; this consumes ATP and is thus energy dependent. Glucose is converted to glucose 6-phosphate, which is in turn isomerised to fructose 6-phosphate. Here, isomerisation refers to the rotation of two bonds around a carbon atom. The fructose 6-phosphate is then phosphorylated to fructose 1,6-diphosphate and this is then hydrolysed to produce one molecule of 3-phosphoglyceraldehyde and one of dihydroxyacetone phosphate.

The next step is the conversion of the dihydroxyacetone phosphate into 3-phosphoglyceraldehyde. Thus, two molecules of 3-phosphoglyceraldehyde have been generated from one molecule of glucose. These two molecules are then converted to pyruvic acid via the intermediate stages 1,3-diphosphoglyceric acid, 3-phosphoglyceraldehyde and

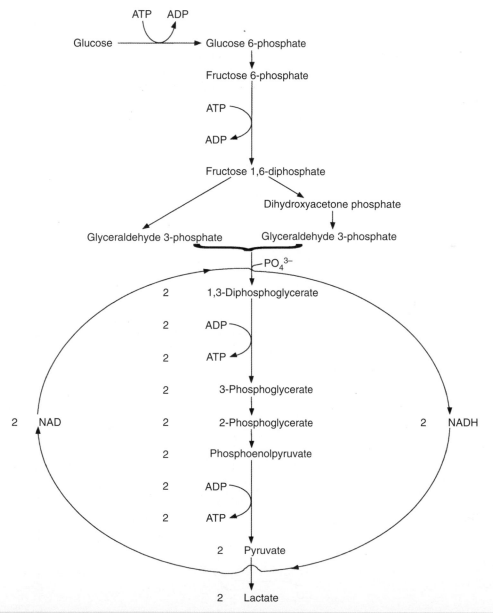

Fig. 9.7 Glycolysis, a metabolic rearrangement in which hexose sugars are converted to pyruvate or lactate. The major attack is the cleavage of fructose 1,6-diphosphate to two trioses. *Note* that two molecules of ATP are used up in the phosphorylation reactions in the first half of glycolysis, while two pairs of ATP molecules are produced in the second half, for an overall gain of two ATP molecules. Two NAD$^+$ molecules are converted to NADH in the oxidative phosphorylation of glyceraldehyde 3-phosphate. Under anaerobic conditions the NADH is used to reduce pyruvate to lactate, which regenerates NAD$^+$. In aerobic glycolysis the NADH molecules enter the TCA cycle. *ADP*, Adenosine diphosphate; *ATP*, adenosine triphosphate; *NAD*, nicotinamide adenine dinucleotide; *TCA*, tricarboxylic acid.

phosphoenolpyruvic acid. The two steps involving the metabolism of 1,3-diphosphoglyceric acid and phosphoenolpyruvic acid are worthy of note. In both cases, the phosphate group that is transferred is of a 'high-energy' type (this means that the phosphate bonding has high internal energy). These groups are transferred to ADP to generate ATP.

Although more ATP is formed during glycolysis than ATP expended, there is a net production of only two molecules of ATP. Unlike the respiratory chain which is where the bulk of cellular ATP is produced, the glycolytic pathway does not require oxygen. Thus, for short periods of time the cell can survive without consuming oxygen by generating ATP via glycolysis. In the absence of oxygen, pyruvate is converted to lactate in order to regenerate NAD^+. The lactate generated by anaerobic glycolysis is often secreted by cells and can be used by the liver to make glucose by gluconeogenesis (Cori cycle). Alternatively lactate is used as a fuel for the TCA cycle by cells undergoing aerobic glycolysis.

CITRIC ACID CYCLE

The enzymes that carry out the citric acid cycle are located inside the mitochondria. Pyruvate is transported into the mitochondrion and is oxidatively decarboxylated by the pyruvate dehydrogenase complex to form Acetyl CoA; this process also generates CO_2 and NADH

$$Pyruvate + CoA + NAD^+ \rightarrow acetylCoA + CO_2 + NADH + H^+$$

NADH can be viewed as a molecule containing high intrinsic energy. The NADH feeds into the respiratory chain and in the presence of oxygen will provide the energy for production of most of the ATP that is produced by any cell. Fig. 9.8 shows how the TCA cycle operates and which steps release CO_2 and hydrogen atoms. The hydrogen is used to reduce NAD or FAD to produce NADH or $FADH_2$; these enter the electron chain in the mitochondria to produce ATP.

The pyruvate is supplied into the cycle as a two-carbon molecule in the form of acetyl-CoA (one of pyruvate's three carbons is lost as CO_2), which is combined with oxaloacetate (four-carbon structure) to yield the six-carbon citric acid. After a rearrangement to isocitric acid, α-ketoglutaric acid is produced with the formation of carbon dioxide and NADH. The next step also generates a molecule of carbon dioxide and of NADH when succinic acid is formed. There is then a series of rearrangements to fumaric and then to malic acid. In the final part of the citric acid cycle, a further

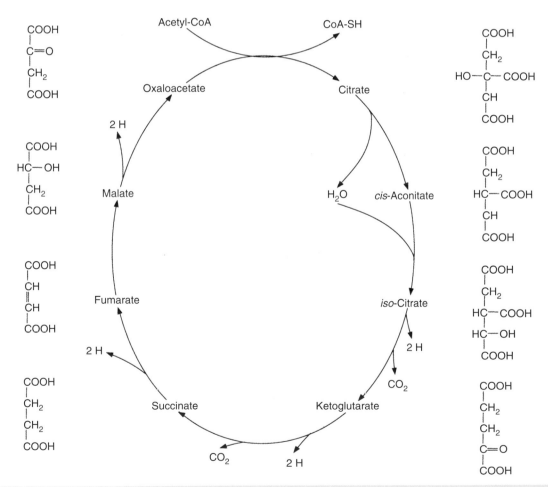

Fig. 9.8 Tricarboxylic acid cycle. For each turn of the cycle, at four points, two hydrogen atoms become available, these are used to reduce NAD^+ or FAD, which then enter the electron transport chain in order to generate ATP. At two points, carbon dioxide is released; this accounts for the complete combustion of the acetyl group of acetyl-CoA, while oxaloacetate is again ready to accept another molecule of acetyl-CoA. A single molecule of GTP (which is readily converted to ATP) is also generated directly by the TCA cycle. *acetyl-CoA*, acetyl coenzyme A; *ATP*, adenosine triphosphate; *FAD*, flavin adenine dinucleotide; *TCA*, tricarboxylic acid.

molecule of NADH is produced as malic acid is converted to oxaloacetate. Thus, the starting substrate has been regenerated and another molecule of acetyl-CoA (derived from pyruvate) can now react to initiate another round of the cycle. The net reaction of the citric acid cycle is:

$$AcetylCoA + 3NAD^+ + FAD + ADP + P_i + 2H_2O$$

$$\longrightarrow$$

$$2CO_2 + 3NADH + FADH_2 + ATP + 2H^+ + CoA$$

RESPIRATORY CHAIN

The respiratory chain, otherwise known as the electron transport chain, also resides in the mitochondria. The chain consists of a series of electron carriers which generate a proton gradient during the oxidation of NADH or $FADH_2$ to produce water plus NAD^+ and FAD (Fig. 9.9). The proton gradient drives the generation of ATP from ADP through the flow of protons through ATPases. NADH is also generated during glycolysis (see Fig. 9.7) and also by the decarboxylation of pyruvate (see above) and each citric acid cycle generates three molecules of NADH and one molecule of FADH (see Fig. 9.8). All of these can enter the electron transport chain to generate ATP (see Fig. 9.9). In addition, a molecule of ATP is generated during the conversion of ketoglutarate to succinate (see Fig. 9.8). The amount of ATP generated by NADH and $FADH_2$ via the proton gradient has been revised and is now concluded to be 2.5 ATPs for each NADH and 1.5 ATPs for each $FADH_2$. The ATP generated by the two molecules of NADH that are made by glycolysis in the cytoplasm is less (1.5 ATPs for each) because of the energy expenditure required for the NADH to enter the mitochondria.

FATTY ACID OXIDATION

Many tissues produce most of their energy by the oxidation of fatty acids. Tissues such as the heart and other muscles only derive limited energy from glucose and rely on circulating free fatty acids. Parts of the kidney are completely unable to utilise glucose or other carbohydrates as energy sources and therefore depend upon a source of fatty acids.

Triacylglycerols (triglycerides) are stored in adipose tissue and, in response to one of a variety of signals, a lipase enzyme becomes activated that cleaves the three fatty acids from the glycerol molecule. The free fatty acids then travel to other tissues bound to albumin; fatty acids are insoluble in water and therefore have to be transported by albumin. The glycerol that is formed as a result of triglyceride hydrolysis is converted to pyruvate or glucose in the liver.

Once a free fatty acid has reached the cell in which it is going to be used, it is subjected to a pathway called β-oxidation. Fig. 9.10 shows the sequence of reactions involved. The fatty acid is activated by combination with CoA. There are then four enzymic steps in which the fatty acyl-CoA is reduced, hydrolysed, reduced again and finally hydrolysed to yield a molecule of acetyl-CoA and a molecule of acyl-CoA where the acyl group is now two carbon atoms shorter than the original. The acetyl-CoA feeds into the citric acid cycle and the acyl-CoA goes through the process repeatedly until it is completely degraded. Thus, a

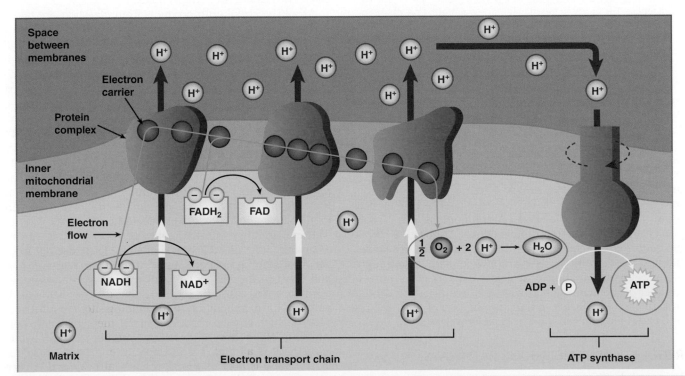

Fig. 9.9 Oxidative phosphorylation. NADH or FADH2 are oxidised to generate NAD+ or FAD and water. This process also causes the translocation of protons into the mitochondrial intermembrane space. The subsequent return of protons through ATP synthase drives the generation of ATP, so explaining how phosphorylation is coupled to oxidation, as first envisaged by Peter Mitchell. Electrons from NADH or FADH2 are transported by proteins that constitute the electron transport chain and this electron flow allows the same proteins to pump protons into the intermembrane space. *ADP*, Adenosine diphosphate; *ATP*, adenosine triphosphate; *FAD*, flavin adenine dinucleotide; *NAD*, nicotinamide adenine dinucleotide; *TCA*, tricarboxylic acid.

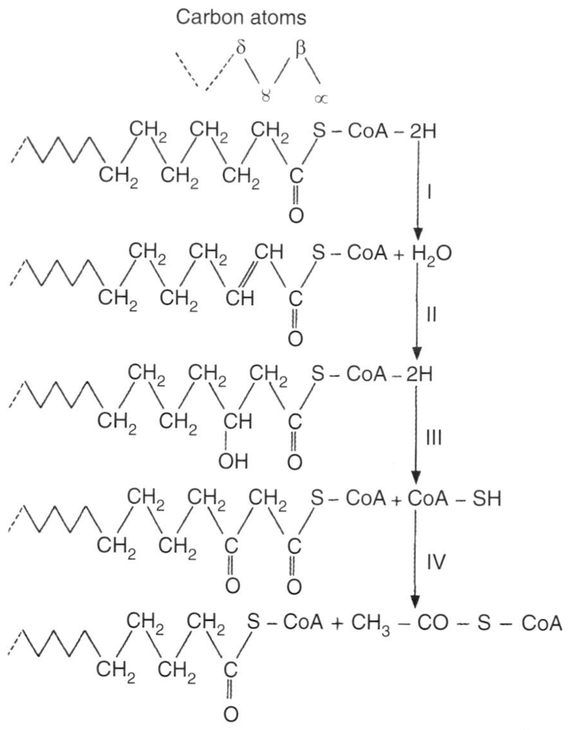

Carbon atoms

Fig. 9.10 β-Oxidation of even-numbered long-chain fatty acids. Reaction I, the initial attack on the α- and β-carbon atoms, with removal of a hydrogen atom from each and the formation of a double bond between them, is catalysed by fatty acetyl coenzyme A (acyl-CoA) dehydrogenases with an electron-transferring flavoprotein as co-factor. Next (reaction II) comes hydration of this double bond, followed by reaction III, oxidation of the secondary alcoholic group to a keto group on the β-carbon atom, catalysed by a β-hydroxy fatty acyl-CoA dehydrogenase. The final step (reaction IV) is cleavage with CoA, catalysed by β-thiolase, to give acetyl-CoA. The resulting fatty acyl-CoA is in the same form as the starting material, and can undergo reaction I again, but is two carbon atoms shorter. Ultimately, the fatty acid is completely disassembled to two carbon acetyl-CoA units.

molecule of palmitic acid which has 18 carbon atoms will be degraded to nine molecules of acetyl-CoA, which will be further metabolised to produce ATP.

The metabolism described earlier refers to saturated fatty acids only, that is, those with no unsaturated double bonds. There are three polyunsaturated fatty acids which are essential for health. Linoleic acid has 18 carbon atoms and two double bonds, while linolenic acid has 18 carbon atoms and three double bonds. Arachidonic acid is 20 carbon atoms long with four double bonds. Although all three are required by cells, since humans can synthesise linolenic and arachidonic acids from linoleic acid, an adequate dietary supply of linoleic acid is sufficient. There are a number of biochemical pathways that require the essential unsaturated fatty acids, and the production of leukotrienes and prostaglandins has been especially well studied.

REGULATION OF METABOLIC PATHWAYS

In an adult, there is turnover within tissues and so the diet has to provide the nutrients for replacement as well as energy utilisation. The nutritional requirement includes amino acids, vitamins, salts and trace elements. There are considerable differences in the rates at which tissues turn

over. A tissue such as bone has a very slow rate of turnover and the macromolecules in the matrix will be degraded and renewed with half-times measured in weeks if not months. In contrast, the surface of the gut has a high rate of turnover and renewal. Like most epithelia, there is a constant movement and desquamation of cells. This must be balanced by replacement within the germinal layers.

An individual exists in different metabolic states throughout the day, and while at one point in time energy may be derived from carbohydrate, at another ATP might be produced exclusively from oxidation of fatty acids. Following a meal, the body is in an absorptive state and there will be high levels of free glucose, triglycerides and amino acids in the bloodstream. The tissues will use some of these components, but most will be stored. The liver becomes active and will take up glucose and convert some to the storage polymer glycogen (see Fig. 9.6). The arrows in Fig. 9.6 show that excess amino acids or glucose can feed into the indicated pathways in order to make glycogen (in the liver and muscle) or fatty acids (in the liver). By contrast, fatty acids cannot be converted to glycogen, although glycerol can and as shown can be used for either gluconeogenesis or glycolysis.

Triglyceride travels in the circulation in the form of chylomicrons, which are aggregates of lipid and a small amount of protein. Some of the triglyceride in chylomicrons is taken up directly into adipose tissue, while some is taken up in the liver, where the triglycerides are used to make other types of lipoprotein. Very low-density lipoprotein and low-density lipoprotein contain different proportions of triglyceride, phospholipid, cholesterol and protein. Both forms of lipoprotein are secreted from the liver and then circulate to all the tissues where they supply lipids.

As all the circulating products from digestion are taken up into cells, the body turns to a postabsorptive state. Most tissues cannot store adequate amounts of carbohydrate and lipid for their energetic needs and so during the postabsorptive state, the liver and adipose tissue release glucose and triglyceride for use by other tissues. It is often not appreciated that the glycogen in the liver is only able to provide glucose for a matter of 1 to 2 hours and (apart from the brain and red blood cells) most tissues use fat in the form of free fatty acids as their energy source for most of the day. The liver can also produce ketone bodies such as β-hydroxybutyrate and acetoacetic acid from fatty acids. Ketone bodies can be used as an energy source by a number of tissues, and even the central nervous system, after an adaptation period, can metabolise ketone bodies to provide ATP.

There are very effective control processes that ensure adequate levels of ATP and that the ATP is derived from the most suitable energy source. Most of the regulation of and between the metabolic pathways occurs via a mechanism known as allosteric control. Some key enzymes in each pathway have, in addition to the binding sites for substrate, sites at which other components of the metabolic pathways can bind. When these other components bind to the enzyme, its activity is altered. For example, the enzyme phosphofructokinase is part of the glycolytic pathway and is very sensitive to cellular concentrations of ATP, ADP and AMP (adenosine monophosphate). When concentrations of ATP are high, then the activity of the enzyme is downregulated since glycolysis should be slowed down in order to conserve carbohydrate stores. Phosphofructokinase is also regulated by the concentration of citrate and this provides a mechanism for regulation between different metabolic pathways. If there are high concentrations of acetyl-CoA which have been derived from fatty acid oxidation, then this will result in high levels of citrate formation. High concentrations of citrate downregulate phosphofructokinase, and thus the use of fat for energy production will have a conserving effect on carbohydrate stores.

It is now known that many metabolic enzymes can be regulated. In addition to allosteric control, the concentrations of co-factors will also regulate enzyme activity. The status of the respiratory chain will influence NAD/NADH ratios. Since the sum of NAD and NADH concentrations is held fairly constant, if there are high levels of NADH then there will be insufficient substrate for several enzymes in the citric acid cycle and it will consequently be downregulated.

An example of a control that operates in a metabolic cycle, which is important in the neonate, follows. The enzyme ATP-citrate lyase hydrolyses citrate and reverses the first step of the citric acid cycle. Although energy is consumed in this reaction, the step is important for the neonate since it ensures levels of acetyl-CoA are maintained. During growth, cellular proliferation requires adequate lipid for membrane biosynthesis. ATP-citrate lyase ensures that, at a time in development when dietary lipid can be low, fatty acids are not used too extensively as an energy source. This maintains adequate supplies for growth.

Catabolism

HAEMOGLOBIN

All the red cells, white cells and platelets in circulation originate in the bone marrow. The stem cells within the marrow divide and differentiate to form the different mature blood cells. The process is regulated by a series of peptide growth factors. Erythropoietin, for example, is the peptide that promotes the formation of erythrocytes; it is synthesised and secreted by the juxtaglomerular apparatus of the kidney and it circulates to the bone marrow where it promotes proliferation.

Erythrocytes have a half-life of about 125 days before they are removed from circulation by the spleen. In order for constant replacement of these lost cells to occur, the bone marrow is very active in erythropoiesis. As well as cellular proliferation, there has to be synthesis of haemoglobin. This oxygen-binding molecule is composed of two pairs of globin chains and a haem ring. The haem ring is synthesised in the mitochondria and cytoplasm of liver and bone marrow cells and needs a sufficient supply of iron, which can frequently become the rate-limiting step. The uptake of iron across the gut is not an efficient process and, even in the presence of sufficient dietary iron, the plasma concentration can become limiting.

Unless there is sufficient iron available, the production of the globin peptide chains is redundant. For this reason, there is a sophisticated control mechanism that operates. Only in the presence of sufficient haem does the synthesis of globin chains proceed. Protein synthesis involves a number of elongation factors whose activity is controlled by phosphorylation and dephosphorylation, and the enzymes responsible are regulated by haem levels.

When erythrocytes are degraded in the spleen (or indeed at the site of a wound response following tissue trauma), the haemoglobin is catabolised. The globin chains are degraded to amino acids, which are re-utilised. Haem cannot be re-used and is catabolised in a number of enzyme steps, which finally produce bilirubin. This all occurs at the site of erythrocyte breakdown. The bilirubin is then transferred to the liver; because it is highly insoluble, it travels to the liver bound to albumin. After diffusion into the hepatocytes, bilirubin is solubilised and detoxified by the coupling of two glucuronic acid residues. The conjugated bilirubin is then excreted into the bile.

UREA CYCLE

In the developed world, most individuals have a diet that is far in excess of requirement. Thus, an individual consumes an amount of protein, which when hydrolysed to amino acids is considerably more than will be required for normal cellular turnover. The carbon and hydrogen components of amino acids can be converted to glycogen or fatty acids and stored. The amino groups are used for the synthesis of nitrogenous compounds, but excess free amino groups will become toxic if allowed to accumulate. There is an efficient detoxification mechanism which results in more than 95% of the nitrogen being excreted via urine in the form of urea. Fig. 9.11

Fig. 9.12 shows a sequence of metabolic reactions which constitute the urea cycle. The detoxification of amino acids begins before the urea cycle, when a transaminase enzyme results in the transfer of the amino group from the acid onto α-ketoglutaric acid. The product, glutamic acid, is itself one of the amino acids, but it is through this intermediate that all amino groups are metabolised. The glutamate is oxidatively deaminated to produce ammonia, which immediately becomes an ammonium ion.

In a reaction requiring ATP, carbon dioxide and ammonium ions form carbamoyl phosphate and it is this that feeds into the urea cycle. The first step is the formation of citrulline from ornithine and carbamoyl-phosphate. Then, in another ATP-dependent reaction, a molecule of aspartic acid combines with citrulline to generate arginosuccinate. This is next hydrolysed to yield fumarate and arginine and, in the final reaction, arginase releases urea from arginine, leaving ornithine. Thus the cycle is completed.

Most amino acid detoxification in humans occurs in the liver, although small levels of the urea cycle enzymes are found in other tissues. The first few reactions occur in the mitochondria, while the latter part of the cycle takes place in the cytoplasm. The urea diffuses out of the liver into the systemic circulation. Like all small molecules, urea is filtered through the glomerulus of the kidney but, while nutrients such as glucose and amino acids are reabsorbed by the kidney tubules, urea is not and passes quantitatively into the urine. This excretory process is vital and in the case of chronic kidney failure, accumulation of urea can become a life-threatening process.

Enzymes

Enzymes are proteins that act as catalysts. They bring about the enormous range of sophisticated chemical reactions

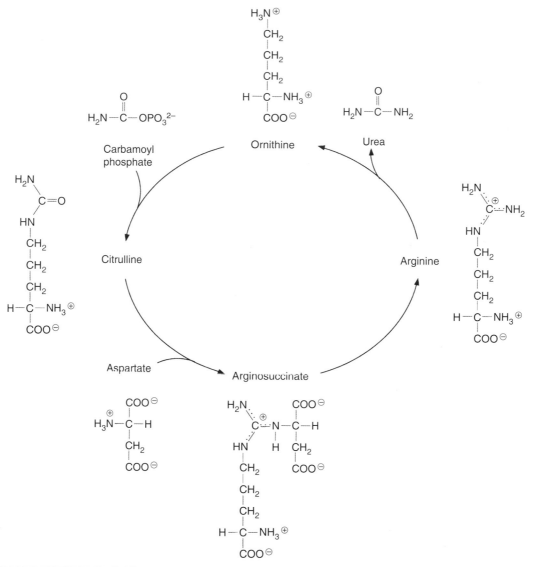

Fig. 9.11 The urea cycle.

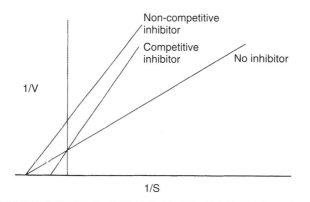

Fig. 9.12 Lineweaver–Burk plots for enzyme inhibitors. V is the reaction rate and S is the substrate concentration.

that are necessary for life. In strict thermodynamic terms, it is incorrect to state that enzymes make reactions occur. Rather, an enzyme shifts the equilibrium of a reaction so that it is more favourable for it to proceed. This is accomplished by reducing the activation energy that is needed to promote the reaction. The catalysis occurs on a part of the enzyme called the active site.

The three-dimensional conformation of an enzyme is crucial to activity and the ability to act as a catalyst can be lost if the three-dimensional shape is altered. A change of shape and resulting loss of activity is referred to as 'denaturation' and can be brought about in a number of ways. Heating an enzyme usually results in complete loss of activity. The three-dimensional structure of the protein is maintained in part by hydrogen bonds. These are fairly weak in nature and can be readily disrupted by heat. Most enzymes are destroyed at 50°C to 60°C.

Organic solvents will usually destroy enzymic activity. The solvent disrupts the internal bonding of the protein, in particular the interactions of the hydrophobic amino acids in the core of the enzyme. Even after removal of the solvent, it is rare that the protein can re-fold in such a way as to regenerate enzyme activity.

Changes in pH will also affect enzyme activity. Because amino acids are zwitterions and partially charged, the local pH will influence the degree to which they are charged. Changes in pH can thus affect the charge of amino acid residues, which in turn affects the interactions between the amino acids and can result in denaturation. Some proteins are extremely sensitive and lose activity with small pH changes; others are less sensitive.

ENZYME KINETICS

Enzymes are usually present at low concentrations inside the cell. The substrate binds to the enzyme and, by reducing the activation energy for the reaction, the enzyme brings about a shift in equilibrium and this allows formation of product. If the reaction involves only a single substrate then this can be described by:

$$\textbf{Enzyme} + \textbf{Substrate}$$
$$\rightarrow \textbf{Enzyme} - \textbf{Substratecomplex}$$
$$\rightarrow \textbf{Enzyme} + \textbf{Product}$$

The rate of reaction is dependent upon the concentrations of enzyme and substrate, but at high concentrations of substrate the enzyme will become saturated. At this point the rate of the reaction is maximal (and is depicted as V_{max}). In order to describe the activity of an enzyme, the Michaelis constant (K_m) is used and this is the concentration of substrate at which the velocity of the reaction is half-maximal. K_m is a measure of how tightly a substrate binds to the enzyme. The lower the value of K_m, the more tightly the substrate can bind. Values for the Michaelis constant are commonly in the micromolar range.

Values for K_m and V_{max} can be calculated by measuring enzyme rates of reaction at a number of different substrate concentrations. These values can either be plotted as reaction rate versus substrate concentration or alternatively they can be plotted as reciprocals. This is called a Lineweaver–Burk plot and normally produces a straight line (see Fig. 9.12), where the intercept with the vertical axis is $1/V_{max}$, the slope equals K_m/V_{max} and the intercept on the horizontal axis is $-1/K_m$.

Enzyme inhibitors can act in a competitive or non-competitive manner. In the case of competitive inhibitors, there is direct competition between the substrate and inhibitor for binding to the active site of the enzyme: K_m is increased but V_{max} is unaltered. In the case of a non-competitive inhibitor, K_m remains the same, while V_{max} is reduced because the inhibitor binds at a location away from the active site but brings about a reduction in activity of the enzyme without affecting substrate binding (see Fig. 9.12).

VITAMINS

Many enzymes require a co-factor in order to operate. The co-factors are small in comparison to the enzyme but play an essential role in the binding and activation of the substrate. Most of the co-factors cannot be synthesised by humans and the factor or its precursor have to be supplied in the diet. These dietary components are known as vitamins. To give an example, pyridoxine (also known as vitamin B_6) is a vital dietary requirement. Once it has been absorbed across the gut and transported to a tissue, it is converted enzymatically inside the cell by enzymes to pyridoxal phosphate, which is then in turn used as a co-factor for transaminase enzymes.

Vitamins are classified as water or fat soluble. The water-soluble vitamins are the B series and vitamin C, which are all used in a large number of enzymatic reactions that concern intermediary metabolism. The four fat-soluble vitamins – A, D, E and K – take part in diverse unrelated reactions ranging from formation of blood-clotting proteins (vitamin K) to formation of visual pigments (vitamin A).

The bacteria in the colon produce some of the vitamins required by humans and this can act as a limited source. Some vitamins turn over fairly rapidly and so a deficiency state can arise soon after withdrawal. In the case of other vitamins, such as vitamin B_{12}, the body maintains significant reserves of material and humans can survive for months without this particular vitamin in the diet.

ROLE OF ENZYMES IN DIGESTION

The diet contains proteins, fats and complex carbohydrates. None of these can be absorbed by the gastrointestinal tract and enzyme digestion has to occur in order to generate products that can be absorbed into the bloodstream or lymphatic circulation.

Protein

Digestion of protein begins in the stomach. The 'chief' cells secrete pepsinogen. The parietal (oxyntic) cells secrete hydrochloric acid and the resulting low pH causes the hydrolysis of pepsinogen into pepsin, which is a proteolytic enzyme. Pepsin shows specificity and causes peptide bond hydrolysis only next to three particular amino acids, namely tryptophan, phenylalanine and tyrosine; these are all amino acids with aromatic side chains. Pepsin therefore generates peptide fragments from large proteins.

The pancreas synthesises three protease enzymes in inactive precursor form. These are trypsinogen, procarboxypeptidase and chymotrypsinogen. These are secreted in inactive forms and released into the gut via the pancreatic duct. The mucosa of the proximal part of the small intestine secretes an enzyme called enterokinase, which cleaves trypsinogen, converting it to trypsin. Trypsin in turn cleaves and activates procarboxypeptidase and chymotrypsinogen. In all these cases the release of a small peptide fragment generates active enzyme.

Chymotrypsinogen is like pepsin and cleaves next to amino acids with aromatic side chains. Trypsin cleaves next to the basic amino acids, lysine and arginine, while carboxypeptidase cleaves sequential amino acids starting at the carboxyl terminus. The action of these enzymes is to convert proteins to either amino acids or very small peptides with two or three amino acids.

In the small intestine, the single amino acids are transported by the enterocytes into the systemic circulation. The microvilli of the intestinal mucosa contain peptidases that cleave the di- and tripeptides into single amino acids, which are then also transported into the bloodstream. The small intestine is highly efficient and most of the amino acids are absorbed across the wall of the duodenum and jejunum.

Carbohydrate

Most of the carbohydrate in the diet is starch, which is a large polymer of glucose. The diet will also contain some sucrose and lactose, which are both disaccharides. Sucrose is composed of glucose and fructose while lactose is composed of glucose and galactose.

The salivary glands and the pancreas both secrete amylases, which break down starch into the disaccharides, maltose and isomaltose. These two carbohydrates, along with lactose and sucrose, are then taken up by a similar mechanism. The mucosal villi contain the four enzymes maltase, isomaltase, lactase and sucrase and these break down the relevant disaccharide into monosaccharides, which are transported into the bloodstream. The transport of glucose and galactose is an active process and ATP is required; the transport of fructose is passive.

Glucose is the most utilised carbohydrate energy source. Most cells take up glucose from the circulation, and the insulin released from the beta cells of the pancreas following a meal stimulates this process. The glucose can be used immediately for energy production or it can be stored in the liver or muscle as glycogen, which is a branched polymer of glucose. When the cell requires the use of glucose stored as glycogen, then the lower glucose levels in the blood stimulates the release of the hormone glucagon from the alpha cells of the pancreas. This hormone binds to its receptors on liver cells leading to the export into the blood of glucose from glycogen and the inhibition of glycogen synthesis (Fig. 9.13). Glucose is released from glycogen as glucose-1-phosphate. Glucose-1-phosphate cannot be transported out of cells but is converted via Glucose-6-phosphate into glucose, which can be exported. Glucose is not exported by muscle cells as they lack Glucose-6-phosphatase.

Fat

The predominant dietary fat is triglyceride, that is, three fatty acids esterified to a single molecule of glycerol. It is not until the small intestine that digestion of fat begins. The first stage is the emulsification of the fats with the bile salts. The liver synthesises bile salts and acids, but they are stored in the gall bladder. In response to the hormone cholecystokinin, bile is ejected into the small intestine and causes dispersal of dietary fat into small droplets. This has the effect of increasing the surface area, thereby increasing the rate of action of the lipase enzymes secreted by the pancreas. The products are fatty acids and monoacylglycerol, and these diffuse into the epithelial cells lining the gastrointestinal tract. Inside the cell, the monoacylglycerols are broken down to fatty acid and glycerol. The epithelial cells then resynthesise triglycerides and then, along with a small amount of phospholipid, cholesterol and specific protein are assembled into chylomicron particles, which diffuse into the lacteals of the lymphatic system. The process of fat digestion in the healthy individual is also very efficient and is completed in the duodenum and jejunum.

The chylomicrons diffuse into the lymphatic lacteals and then travel along the lymphatic vessels. Ultimately, they enter the bloodstream when the lymph in the thoracic duct flows into the left subclavian vein. The triglycerides in the chylomicrons are taken up and stored by adipose tissue. When there is demand, this fat can be used by a number of organs and tissues. Free fatty acids are transported to the site of utilisation. Lipases within the adipose tissue will hydrolyse the triglycerides and the resulting fatty acids diffuse out of the adipocytes and become bound to albumin in the bloodstream.

Cell Signalling and Second Messaging

GENERAL OVERVIEW

Communication between cells is essential to regulate their development, to organise them into tissues and organs, and to allow normal physiological processes to take place. There are many methods that cells use to communicate. This part of the chapter reviews some of the most common methods used in mammals and the basic mechanisms involved. In particular, the major signalling mechanisms and second messengers (Ca^{II}, cAMP, IP_3, diacylglycerol) activated within a cell when it receives an external signal (often released from another cell) are highlighted.

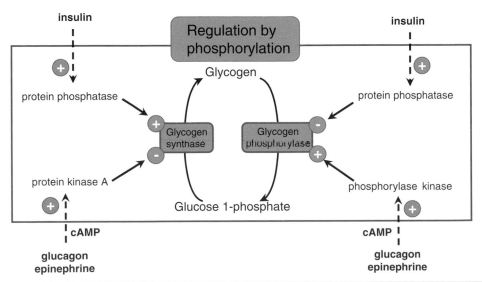

Fig. 9.13 Regulation of glycogen synthesis and breakdown. *cAMP*, Cyclic AMP.

Cells signal to each other in different ways, mainly dependent on the distance between them. If the cells are touching, signalling may simply be through pores or gap junctions in the adjoining membranes or through the interaction of a membrane-bound ligand (from the Latin *ligare*, to bind) with a receptor on the membrane of an adjacent cell. If the cells are further apart they may communicate via the release of signalling molecules that are then detected by receptors on target cells or in the case of nerve cells by the transmission of an electrical signal.

Signalling molecules include hormones, cytokines, growth factors, neurotransmitters, pheromones, photons and recently a group of molecules that include nitric oxide (NO), hydrogen peroxide (H_2O_2) and carbon monoxide (CO) have also been found to have a role in the control of cellular functions. Signalling molecules bind to specific receptors within or upon the surface of cells and have very high biological activities, some are active at only 10^{-11} to 10^{-13} molar concentrations. Signalling molecules are rarely released singly and an individual signalling molecule often stimulates the production of many other different types of signalling molecules.

Cytokines and growth factors are a group of low molecular weight proteins that are secreted by many different cell types and usually act upon either neighbouring cell in a paracrine fashion. More rarely cytokines and growth factors act upon the same cell (autocrine). Cytokines and growth factors bind to specific receptors upon the surface of target cells. Hormones are made by endocrine cells and are secreted into the blood where they are carried to distant target cells. All polypeptide hormones such as gonadotrophin bind to cell surface receptors. Some non-polypeptide hormones, such as acetylcholine or adrenalin (epinephrine) bind to cell surface receptors whereas other non-polypeptides, such as steroid hormones, can bind to intracellular receptors.

Nerve cells form specialised junctions known as synapses and secrete short-range, short-lived neurotransmitters. Information is clearly conveyed much faster by nerve cells than hormonal methods since, while nerves use electrical impulses to carry information, hormones rely on diffusion or blood flow. Hormones usually act at very low concentrations ($<10^{-8}$ M) since they become diluted in blood. Neurotransmitters are less diluted and work at much higher concentrations, for example acetylcholine in synaptic clefts acts at 5×10^{-4} M. In most other respects hormones and neurotransmitters have similar cell signalling mechanisms.

Most animal cells have characteristic and specific high-affinity receptors, allowing a range of responses. Signalling molecules can have different effects depending on the cell type they encounter. For example, acetylcholine contracts skeletal muscle but decreases heart rate force and contraction. Cells can also modulate their response by altering the number of receptors on the cell surface for a particular ligand. Some signalling mechanisms are rapid and transient, such as insulin secretion in response to raised blood sugar levels; some are even faster, such as neurotransmission. Some are slow in onset and long-lasting such as oestradiol production by the ovaries at the onset of puberty. Cells require many signalling molecules just to survive and additional signalling molecules to proliferate. When deprived of survival signalling molecules, cells may undergo programmed cell death (apoptosis).

EICOSANOID SYNTHESIS

Eicosanoids are signalling molecules which are continuously made in the plasma membrane of all mammalian tissues. They are synthesised from 20-carbon fatty acid chains (mainly arachidonic acid), which in turn are cleaved from membrane phospholipids by phospholipases. There are four major groups of eicosanoids: prostaglandins, prostacyclins, thromboxanes and leukotrienes. Prostaglandins are important stimulators of myometrium. They are formed from arachidonic acid released from membrane phospholipids (Fig. 9.14). The key enzymes in this step are phospholipase A_2 and phospholipase C; the latter releases diacylglycerol (see later), which eventually leads to arachidonic acid release. The free arachidonate is the substrate for prostaglandin H_2 (PGH_2) synthase or cyclo-oxygenase (COX), an enzyme with two activities. PGH_2 synthase has both COX activity, which converts arachidonic acid to prostaglandin G_2 (PGG_2), and a peroxidase activity which converts PG G_2 to PGH_2. PGH_2 is then converted to a range of prostaglandins including $PGF_{2\alpha}$ and PGE_2.

Until recently, there were two recognised forms of PGH_2 synthase or COX, now known as COX-1 and COX-2. These two enzymes function similarly but are the products of two distinct and different genes. The gene which encodes COX-1 is large, with large introns, and a promoter that contains transcription factor binding domains which suggest that it is generally a constitutively expressed gene. The gene for COX-2 is far smaller, with only small introns, and its promoter contains transcription factor binding domains which suggest that it is a gene which is inducible. In general, COX-1 is found in tissues which produce prostaglandins constantly, such as the stomach mucosa, whereas COX-2 is only expressed at sites of inflammation. Older non-steroidal anti-inflammatory drugs (NSAIDs) such as indomethacin inhibit both COX-1 and COX-2. More recent NSAIDs are selective for COX-2. In general, the more COX-2 selective an NSAID is, the better its side-effect profile. More recently, a COX-3 form was identified and is formed by alternative splicing of the COX-1 gene.

Aspirin inhibits both COX-1 and COX-2 (it is actually much more active against COX-1 than COX-2, hence its poor side-effect profile). Unlike most NSAIDs, which are competitive antagonists, aspirin functions by permanently acetylating the active site of the COX enzyme. It can be used at a low dose to inhibit platelet thromboxane synthesis with little effect upon vascular endothelial prostacyclin synthesis. This may be of value in thromboprophylaxis, and in the management of pre-eclampsia. A low dose of aspirin permanently disables platelet COX as the platelets pass through the hepatic portal system. Since the platelet has no nucleus it cannot synthesise new COX and so platelet thromboxane synthesis is permanently inhibited. Most of the aspirin is then inactivated within the liver. The small amount of aspirin which then passes into the general circulation may acetylate vascular endothelial COX but, since these cells have a nucleus, they can synthesise the new COX enzyme and maintain prostacyclin synthesis. High concentrations of prostanoids have been reported during normal menstruation and in particular with menorrhagia, dysmenorrhoea and endometriosis – all correlate with painful menstruation. COX-2-selective inhibitors are just as effective as NSAIDs but have fewer gastrointestinal side effects. During labour, the

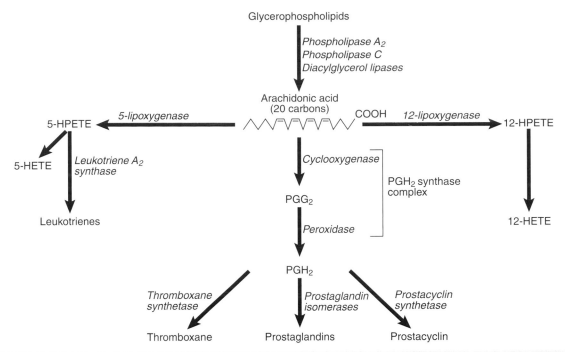

Fig. 9.14 The synthesis of eicosanoids. There are four major classes of eicosanoid: prostaglandins, prostacyclins, thromboxanes and leukotrienes, and most are made from arachidonic acid. *12-HFTE*, 12-hydroxyeicosatetraenoic acid; *5-HPETE*, 5-hydroperoxyeicosatetraenoic acid; *PGG2*, prostaglandin G2; *PGH2*, prostaglandin H2.

fetal membranes are the main source of prostaglandins. The increase in prostaglandins is thought to be due to induction of COX-2 in the fetal membranes. Bacterial products and pro-inflammatory cytokines can increase expression of COX-2 and hence prostaglandin synthesis. It is known that women with intra-amniotic infection have raised pro-inflammatory cytokines in the amniotic fluid and fetal membranes, although cytokines are also elevated in spontaneous term labour in the amniotic fluid and membranes.

In addition to the prostaglandin synthetic pathway, a 5-lipoxygenase pathway converts arachidonate to 5-hydroperoxyeicosatetraenoic acid (5-HPETE), which leads to formation of leukotrienes. A 12-lipoxygenase pathway leads to formation of 12-HPETE and a 15-lipoxygenase pathway to 15-HPETE. These lipoxygenase compounds have a direct stimulatory effect on the myometrium. Prostacyclin and thromboxanes are also formed through a cyclo-oxygenase pathway which utilises prostacyclin synthetase and thromboxane synthetase, respectively. The synthetic pathways of eicosanoids can be targeted by therapeutic drugs. For example, corticosteroid drugs such as cortisone inhibit phospholipase and are used to treat inflammatory conditions such as arthritis. NSAIDs including aspirin and ibuprofen block the first oxidation step of the fatty acid, which is catalysed by cyclooxygenase.

GAP JUNCTIONS

Gap junctions are specialised cell–cell junctions which form from a mirror image of protein units (connexons) between plasma membranes of cells. The cytoplasms of the cells are connected by narrow water-filled channels. These channels allow passage of small signalling molecules such as calcium and cyclic AMP, but not of large molecules such as proteins.

In the myometrium, gap junctions provide low-resistance pathways between the smooth muscle cells, thereby increasing their electrical coupling to allow increased coordination of myometrial contractility. During pregnancy, gap junctions are present at very low numbers in the myometrium; however labour is associated with increased numbers and size of gap junctions. This has led to the idea that gap junctions are essential, but not sufficient, for effective labour and delivery.

NITRIC OXIDE IS AN IMPORTANT SIGNALLING MOLECULE

Although most signalling molecules are hydrophilic molecules, some are small enough to pass straight into the cell where they can directly exert their effects. One such example is the gas NO. NO is produced from L-arginine by the enzyme NO synthase in the presence of co-factors and oxygen. The by-product is L-citrulline. There are three main forms of this enzyme, each the product of separate genes and sharing about 50% to 60% sequence homology. One of these enzyme isoforms was first described in endothelial cells and thus is commonly known as eNOS. It is constitutively expressed and is calcium–calmodulin dependent (see later). NO has a very short half-life (5 to 10 seconds) and is converted to nitrates and nitrites in the blood. However, when released from endothelial cells on blood vessels in response to increased shear stress or agents such as acetylcholine, NO diffuses to the underlying smooth muscle, where it reacts with iron in the active site of the enzyme guanylate cyclase to produce the intracellular mediator cGMP (cyclic guanosine monophosphate) (see later). The effects of this enzyme are rapid and result in muscle relaxation. Continual release of NO from blood vessels is therefore one of the main mechanisms for keeping blood pressure at its normal level. In pregnancy, blood pressure falls and it is thought that the vasodilatation is partly mediated by increased NO release. In contrast, evidence for reduced NO release as a cause of increased vascular resistance and hence hypertension in pregnancy or pre-eclampsia is controversial. NO is also important in regulating blood flow within the placenta and eNOS expressed on the entire syncytiotrophoblast surface is thought, just like that on blood vessels, to inhibit aggregation of neutrophils and platelets present in maternal blood in the intervillous space. In contrast the expression of another NO synthase enzyme is induced in response to inflammatory signals such as bacterial cell wall products which include lipopolysaccharides and cytokines such as γ-interferon or tumour necrosis factor-α. This enzyme is commonly known as iNOS. The activity of iNOS is calmodulin independent and is induced in activated macrophages and neutrophils. NO released from these cells helps them to kill invading microorganisms. This third NO synthase was first described in the brain and is known as bNOS. Like eNOS it is constitutively expressed and is also dependent on calcium–calmodulin for activity. NO is released by many types of nerve cell to signal neighbouring cells, for example NO released by autonomic nerves in the penis causes the local blood vessel dilatation that is responsible for penile erection. It is emerging that the distribution of NO synthase enzymes is not simple with many cells expressing more than one form. In reproductive biology, NO has also been implicated in the control of myometrial quiescence, in the onset of labour and in cervical ripening, although the evidence for some of these is certainly not conclusive. The effects of NO on blood vessels also explain the mechanism of action of nitroglycerine, which has been used for nearly 100 years to treat angina. Nitroglycerine is converted to NO, which relaxes blood vessels in the heart. Other chemicals such as gyceryl trinitrate (GTN), which breaks down to NO, have also been used in an attempt to prevent pre-term labour by relaxing myometrial smooth muscle and in ripening the cervix. These studies have met with mixed success rates. CO is another gas which also stimulates guanylate cyclase. CO is produced by the action of the enzymes haem oxygenase (HO) 1 and HO-2. HO-1 is inducible while HO-2 is constitutively expressed. The functions of CO are only now being unravelled.

CALCIUM AS AN INTRACELLULAR MESSENGER

Cells maintain low concentrations of free calcium (10^{-7} M) despite much higher extracellular concentrations in the extracellular fluid (10^{-3} M) and ER. Increases in intracellular calcium concentrations are one way in which extracellular signals are transmitted across the plasma membrane. When calcium channels are transiently opened in the plasma membrane or ER membranes, intracellular calcium concentrations rise to about 5×10^{-6} M and activate calcium-responsive proteins in the cell. Resting calcium concentrations are kept very low by several means. Calcium-ATPases in the plasma membrane pump calcium out of the cell while cells such as nerve and muscle, which use calcium much more for signalling, have an additional calcium pump (sodium calcium antiporter) in the plasma membrane which couples Na^+ influx to calcium efflux. In the ER there is also a pump (Ca^{2+}-ATPase) that also takes up calcium from the cytosol. Mitochondria can also pump calcium inside; a low-affinity high-capacity calcium pump in the inner mitochondrial membrane uses the electrochemical gradient generated across the membrane during electron transport in oxidative phosphorylation. This pump only operates when calcium levels are extremely high, usually as a consequence of cell damage. These transport mechanisms are represented in Fig. 9.15.

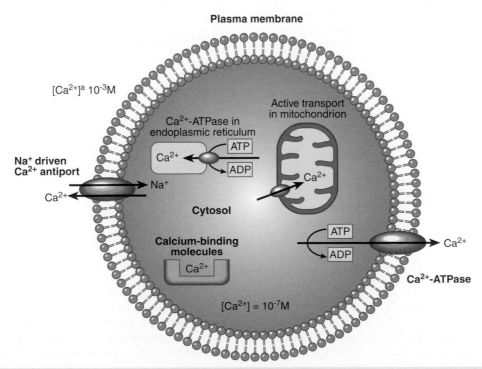

Fig. 9.15 Schematic representation of the main methods used by cells to maintain low levels of cytosolic calcium concentrations in the face of much higher concentrations of calcium outside. *ADP*, Adenosine diphosphate; *ATP*, adenosine triphosphate.

Calmodulin is a calcium-binding protein found in all eukaryotic cells. It mediates many calcium-regulated processes and undergoes a conformational change when bound to calcium. When this happens the calcium–calmodulin complex can bind to various target proteins and alter their activity. Among the calcium–calmodulin targets are various enzymes (such as eNOS and bNOS) and membrane transport proteins. Most effects of calcium–calmodulin are, however, indirect and are mediated by calcium–calmodulin-dependent protein kinases; an example of this is myosin light chain kinase, which activates smooth muscle contraction. Two pathways of calcium signalling have been well defined. One is used mainly by excitable cells; when nerve cell membranes are depolarised by an action potential, voltage-gated calcium channels open and calcium enters the cell leading to secretion of the neurotransmitter. In the other pathway, binding of extracellular signalling molecules to cell surface receptors ultimately leads to the opening of channels in the ER and a rise in intracellular calcium. The opening of these channels is brought about by an intermediate molecule known as inositol trisphosphate (see later).

SIGNALS ACTING ON INTRACELLULAR RECEPTORS

While all neurotransmitters and most hormones are water soluble, steroid hormones such as cortisol, oestrogen and progesterone, retinoids, vitamin D and thyroid hormones are not; they are small hydrophobic molecules. The latter are made water soluble for transport within the body by being transported in the blood by specific carrier proteins. Steroid hormones are released from their carrier proteins and pass through the plasma membrane where they exert their effects. Because water-soluble proteins are hydrophilic, they cannot pass directly through the lipid layer of the plasma membrane and instead bind to specific receptors on the cell surface. In addition, water-soluble molecules are usually broken down within minutes of entering the blood. Neurotransmitters are broken down even faster, within seconds or milliseconds. In contrast, steroid hormones persist in the blood for hours, thyroid hormone for days.

On reaching their target cell, steroid hormones, thyroid hormones, retinoids and vitamin D diffuse across the plasma membrane and bind to intracellular receptor proteins (Fig. 9.16). The receptors can be regarded as ligand dependent transcription factors. Some intracellular receptor proteins are held in an inactive state by being complexed with heat shock proteins, also known as chaperone proteins. When the ligand binds to the receptor, it causes a structural change that causes the heat shock proteins to dissociate, receptor dimerisation and translocation to the nucleus where the activated receptor is able to bind to specific DNA-binding sites. The end result is activation, or sometimes suppression, of gene transcription. Transcription is dependent upon the recruitment of co-activator proteins and similarly gene repression is dependent upon co-repressor proteins (see Fig. 9.16).

The activation of transcription by steroid hormones often occurs in two steps. First, there is the direct induction of transcription of a small number of specific genes within 30 minutes, and this is known as the primary response.

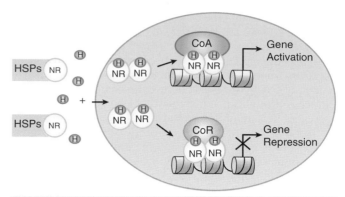

Fig. 9.16 Model of intracellular receptor activation by steroid hormones. Binding of the ligand to the receptor results in dissociation of heat shock proteins, receptor dimerisation, translocation to the nucleus, where the activated receptor is able to bind to specific DNA-binding sites. The steroid hormone–receptor complex can either activate or repress transcription according to whether it associates with co-activators or co-repressors.

Some of the primary response proteins can then turn on secondary response genes, while other primary response proteins can turn off primary response genes. Even when different cell types have the same intracellular receptor, the response in each cell may be different. This is because a combination of gene regulatory proteins must bind to the DNA and some of these are cell specific.

As stated earlier, all water-soluble signalling molecules bind to specific receptors on the surface of their target cell. Cell surface receptors act as signal transducers, that is, binding to the receptor by the ligand leads to intracellular signals which modulate the response of the cell. There are three main classes of cell surface receptor: (1) those which are ion channel linked, (2) those which are G-protein linked and (3) those which are enzyme linked.

ION CHANNELS

Ion channels are not open all the time but have 'gates' that open in response to specific stimuli. The main types of stimuli which open ion channels are changes in voltage across the plasma membrane (voltage-gated channels), mechanical stress (mechanical-gated channels) or the binding of a ligand (ligand-gated channels). The activity of many channels is additionally regulated by protein phosphorylation and dephosphorylation.

G-PROTEIN-LINKED RECEPTORS WHICH INCREASE CYCLIC AMP

The interaction between a receptor and a target protein (enzyme or ion channel) is mediated by a trimeric GTP-binding regulatory protein (G-protein). Receptors linked to G-proteins are the largest (>800) family of cell surface receptors. Many hormones, neurotransmitters and local mediators signal through G-protein-linked receptors. All G-protein-linked receptors have a similar structure consisting of a polypeptide chain that threads back and forth through the plasma membrane seven times (this feature is not shown in Fig. 9.17, which uses a simplified representation). The associated G-proteins consist of α, β and γ subunits

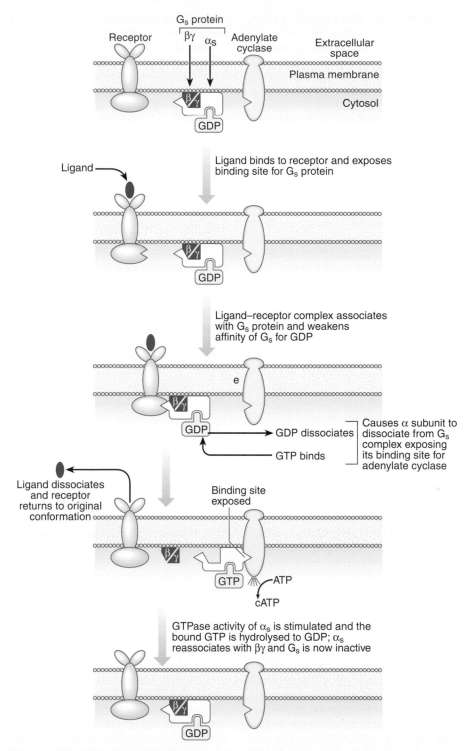

Fig. 9.17 Schematic representation of how G_s couples receptor activation to adenylate cyclase activation. As long as the ligand is bound to the receptor, the receptor can continually activate the G-protein. *ATP*, adenosine triphosphate; *cATP*, cyclic adenosine triphosphate; *GTP*, guanosine triphosphate.

and these activate intracellular signalling in response to the binding of signalling molecules to the G-protein receptor (see Fig. 9.17).

Cyclic AMP (cAMP) is synthesised from ATP by a plasma membrane-bound enzyme, adenylate (adenylyl) cyclase. cAMP is rapidly and continually destroyed by cyclic AMP phosphodiesterases. Adenylate cyclase is an example of

an enzyme, the activity of which is regulated by a trimeric G-protein. Since in this case the enzyme is activated by the G-protein, the G-protein is called a stimulatory G-protein (G_s). Some of the best studied receptors linked to adenylate cyclase are the β-adrenergic receptors.

Trimeric G-proteins are so called because they are made up of an α and a βγ subunit. In its inactive state G_s exists as a trimer with guanosine diphosphate (GDP) bound to the α subunit. When a ligand binds to the receptor, the conformation of the receptor is altered, exposing a binding site for the G_s protein complex. Association of the ligand-receptor–G_s complex is brought about by diffusion of the subunits within the membrane and results in the α-subunit changing its affinity for GDP to GTP. This causes the α-subunit to dissociate from the β- and γ-subunits and, in doing so, exposes the α-subunit's binding site for adenylate cyclase. The α-subunit then binds to and activates adenylate cyclase, which then produces cAMP. When the ligand dissociates, the receptor returns to its original conformation. The GTP is then hydrolysed to GDP by the α-subunit's GTPase activity, brought about by its binding to adenylate cyclase. This is shown schematically in Fig. 9.17. This causes it to dissociate from the adenylate cyclase and the system returns to the original inactivated state. Cholera toxin is an enzyme which alters the α-subunit so that it can no longer hydrolyse its bound GTP. The prolonged production of cAMP in intestinal epithelial cells causes a large efflux of Na^+ and water leading to severe diarrhoea characteristic of cholera.

INHIBITORY G-PROTEINS

The same signalling molecule can increase or decrease cAMP depending on the receptor it binds to. For example, when adrenaline binds to α-adrenergic receptors, it activates adenylate cyclase, whereas when it binds to $β_2$-adrenergic receptors it inhibits the enzyme. The reason for this is that these receptors are coupled by different G-proteins. An inhibitory G-protein (G_i) has a different subunit ($α_i$ rather than $α_s$). When activated, these receptors bind to G_i, causing $α_i$ to bind to GTP and dissociate from the α-complex. Both the released α-complex and the $α_i$ contribute to the inhibition of adenylate cyclase. G_i also has a role in opening K^+ channels in the plasma membrane. Pertussis toxin, made by the bacterium which causes whooping cough, alters $α_i$ to prevent it from interacting with receptors, so that it cannot inhibit adenylate cyclase or open K^+ channels.

CYCLIC AMP DEPENDENT PROTEIN KINASE (PROTEIN KINASE A)

cAMP mediates its effects mainly by activating the enzyme known as cAMP-dependent protein kinase (protein kinase A). Protein kinase A catalyses the transfer of the terminal phosphate group from ATP to a specific serine or threonine of a protein. This in turn regulates the activity of the target protein. Fig. 9.13 illustrates that enzymes such as glycogen synthase are inhibited by phosphorylation, whereas enzymes such as glycogen phosphorylase are activated by phosphorylation. Because phosphate groups can be readily added by kinases or removed by phosphatases, this provides a rapid and reversible mechanism of enzyme regulation that is widely used in cells.

In some cells, cAMP can also regulate gene transcription. Some genes contain a sequence known as the 'cyclic AMP response element' (CRE), which is recognised by a gene regulatory protein known as CRE-binding protein. When this protein is phosphorylated on a single serine residue by PKA, it is activated to turn on gene transcription. Enzymes known as serine/threonine phosphoprotein phosphatases can remove phosphate groups added by PKA and so provide a means of regulating cAMP action.

Phosphorylation is important because it is the most common way of modifying the structure of an enzyme and is often used to regulate enzyme activity. For example, glucagon acts to release glucose from glycogen and it does this by activating its glucagon receptors (GPCR) which stimulates the production of cAMP. One of the effects of cAMP is to cause the phosphorylation of glycogen synthase which inactivates it and so prevents glycogen synthesis. At the same time cAMP results in the phosphorylation of glucose phosphorylase, which activates the first step in the breakdown of glycogen to glucose (see Fig. 9.13).

INOSITOL PHOSPHATE AND DIACYLGLYCEROL SECOND MESSENGERS

Inositol phosphate (IP_3) is produced as a result of the hydrolysis of inositol phospholipids (phosphoinositides) located mainly in the inner half of the plasma membrane. It is the breakdown of one class of these inositol phospholipids known as phosphatidyl bisphosphate (PIP_2) which is most important, even though this type accounts for less than 10% of the total inositol lipids and less than 1% of all the phospholipids in the cell membrane. The breakdown of PIP_2 starts with a signalling molecule binding to its receptor in the plasma membrane. The activated receptor stimulates a G-protein, known as G_q, which in turn activates an inositide-specific phospholipase C, known as phospholipase C-β. The enzyme cleaves PIP_2 to produce two products: IP_3 and diacylglycerol (Fig. 9.18). Each of these molecules has a separate role, as will be discussed.

IP_3 is small and water soluble. It diffuses into the cytosol where it binds to IP_3-gated calcium release channels in the ER. These channels are similar to those in the sarcoplasmic reticulum of muscle cells (ryanodine receptors) which trigger muscle contraction on calcium release. In many cell types, both forms of calcium receptor are present. To end the calcium response, calcium is pumped back out of the cytosol and IP_3 is broken down by phosphatases within the cell. Some of the IP_3 is also phosphorylated to form IP_4, which may promote the refilling of the intracellular calcium stores and/or mediate slower or longer-lived responses within the cell.

Diacylglycerol has two potential fates. It can be cleaved to give arachidonic acid, which can act as a messenger or can be used in the synthesis of eicosanoids. However, its more important role is to activate a serine/threonine protein kinase (a protein kinase phosphorylates serine/threonine residues in target proteins within the cell and changes their properties). This protein is named 'protein kinase C', so called because it is calcium dependent. It is the initial rise in calcium brought about by IP_3 which causes the protein kinase C to move from the cytosol to the plasma membrane, where it is activated. At least four of the eight types of protein kinase C in animals are activated by diacylglycerol. Because diacylglycerol is rapidly metabolised, sustained protein kinase C activation for longer-term responses depends on a second wave of diacylglycerol production released this time by phospholipases which cleave phosphatidyl choline, the major phospholipid in the cell.

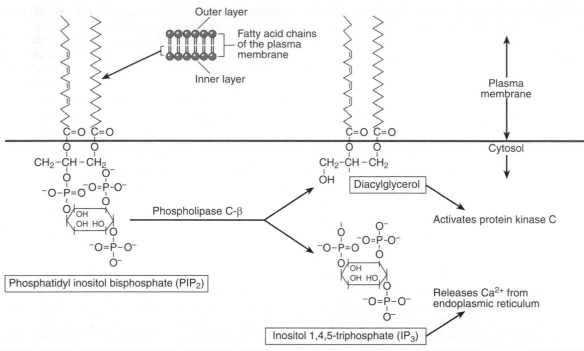

Fig. 9.18 Schematic representation of the inositol phosphate pathway. The activated receptor binds to a specific trimeric G-protein (G_q) causing the α-subunit to dissociate and activate phospholipase C-β (PLC-β). PLC-β hydrolyses PIP_2 to release IP_3 and diacylglycerol. IP_3 diffuses through the cytoplasm and releases Ca^{2+} from the endoplasmic reticulum while diacylglycerol remains within the membrane and activates protein kinase C. PLC-β is one of three classes of phospholipase (PLC-β, γ and δ). This class is activated by G-protein-linked receptors and also by tyrosine kinase and cytokine receptors.

Protein kinase C can also alter the transcription of specific genes. In one pathway, it leads to the phosphorylation of a protein kinase called mitogen activated protein (MAP) kinase, which in turn phosphorylates and activates the gene regulatory protein Elk-1; this is then bound along with another protein (serum response factor) to a short DNA sequence (called the serum response element). This leads to transcription of the gene. In another pathway, activation of protein kinase results in the release of a gene regulatory protein nuclear factor kappa-light-chain-enhancer of activated B cells (NF-κB), which then moves into the nucleus and activates the transcription of specific genes.

ENZYME-LINKED RECEPTORS

Unlike G-protein-linked receptors, enzyme-linked receptors are single-pass transmembrane proteins with (like G-proteins) the ligand-binding site outside the cell and the catalytic unit inside the cell. Instead of the cytosolic domain interacting with a G-protein, the cytosolic domain has its own enzyme activity or associates directly with an enzyme. These receptors can activate most of the cell signalling pathways that are activated by G-protein receptors, with the exception of cAMP signalling. There are five known classes of enzyme-linked linked receptor:

1. *Receptor guanylate (sometimes called guanylyl) cyclases* catalyse the production of cyclic GMP. An example of this group is the atrial natriuretic peptide (ANP) receptor. ANP is secreted by the atrium of the heart when blood pressure rises and stimulates the kidney to secrete Na^+ and water, and also induces the smooth muscle of vessel walls to relax. The binding of ANP activates the intracellular catalytic domain (guanylate cyclase) to produce cyclic GMP, which in turn binds to and activates a G-kinase; this phosphorylates serine and threonine residues on specific proteins. There are few members in this family.

2. Many receptors are *tyrosine kinases*, which auto-phosphorylate specific tyrosine residues within or outside their kinase domain upon ligand binding. The phosphorylated tyrosines on the receptor recruit intracellular signalling proteins, which leads to the activation of cell signalling pathways. Members of this family include receptors for the epidermal growth factor, fibroblast growth factor, platelet-derived growth factor, vascular endothelial growth factor (VEGF), nerve growth factor and insulin-like growth factor-1.

3. *Tyrosine kinase-associated receptors* are also known as cytokine receptors and these receptors when activated by signalling molecules associate with and activate intracellular tyrosine kinases, such as janus activated kinase (JAK) and members of the Src family.

4. *Receptor tyrosine phosphatases* remove phosphate groups from signalling molecules.

5. *Receptor serine/threonine kinases* phosphorylate specific serine or threonine residues on particular proteins. Receptors for the transforming growth factor-β superfamily receptors, which are important in development, are a member of this group.

VASCULAR ENDOTHELIAL GROWTH FACTORS

VEGFs are important regulators of vascular development during embryogenesis (vasculogenesis) as well as during blood vessel formation (angiogenesis) in the adult. VEGFs have been studied intensively in reproduction. VEGFs are thought to play important roles in many aspects of reproductive biology. They are active during menstruation, and during both implantation and placental development. The concentration of circulating VEGF falls during pregnancy and falls even more in pre-eclampsia. This is due to the free circulating VEGF being 'mopped up' by being bound to a circulating VEGF receptor. In mammals, five VEGF ligands (differently spliced variants and processed forms) have been identified to date. The VEGF ligands bind in an overlapping fashion to three receptor tyrosine kinases (RTKs), known as VEGF receptor-1, -2 and -3 (VEGFR-1–3), as well as to co-receptors that lack established VEGF-induced catalytic function, such as heparan sulphate proteoglycans (HSPGs) and neuropilins. VEGFs share some regulatory mechanisms with other well-characterised RTKs, such as the platelet-derived growth factor receptors (PDGFRs) and the epidermal growth factor receptors (EGFRs). These mechanisms include receptor dimerisation and activation of the tyrosine kinase, as well as creation of docking sites for signal transducers. VEGFRs induce cellular events that are common to many growth factor receptors, such as cell migration, survival and proliferation. Tumour growth depends on new angiogenesis and, recently, tumour therapies that are based on neutralising anti-VEGF antibodies and small-molecular-weight tyrosine kinase inhibitors that target the VEGFRs have been developed. These new treatments for cancer show the importance of understanding signal transduction pathways and their clinical relevance. It is important, when treating cancer and other diseases that are associated with pathological angiogenesis, to select therapy that preserves pathways that are important for the survival of blood vessels in healthy tissues.

Biochemistry Exam Notes

Dietary sugars: sucrose (glucose fructose dimer), lactose (galactose glucose dimer) maltose (glucose glucose dimer)

Most dietary sugars are aldoses (and hexoses) except fructose which is a ketose (and a pentose)

Sucrose is a non-reducing sugar (due to its glucose fructose bridge), rest are reducing.

Glycogen, starch, dextran and cellulose are all made of glucose chains (cross links are different). 40% starch is the lowest level found in crops (oats).

Salivary amylase breaks down starch into maltose (glucose glucose) and larger polymers. Sucrase, lactase and maltase are in the small intestine (duodenum) and break dimers into monomers.

Small intestine: duodenum responsible for digestion; jejunum responsible for majority of absorption; ileum absorbs vitamins D, A, K, E (fat soluble), B_{12} and bile salts.

Glycogenolysis – Mobilisation of glycogen into glucose and glucose-1-phosphate (readily converted to glucose-6-phosphate).

Glycogenesis – Formation of glycogen from glucose

Glycolysis – Breakdown of glucose into two molecules of pyruvate (older and perhaps more logical name is glucolysis)

Gluconeogenesis – Conversion of pyruvate (or lactate, glycerol, amino acids) into glucose

Pentose phosphate pathway (PPP) – Generation of NADPH (needed to make fatty acids) and ribose 5 phosphate (used to make DNA and RNA). PPP also called the phosphogluconate pathway and the hexose monophosphate shunt

Where do biochemical pathways occur? Cytosol: glycolysis; PPP; fatty acid synthesis. Mitochondria: Citric acid cycle (also known as Krebs and TCA cycle); oxidative phosphorylation; oxidation of fatty acids; production of ketones. Interplay of cytosol and mitochondria: gluconeogenesis and urea synthesis.

Rate limiting enzymes in metabolism:

Glycogenolysis: glycogen phosphorylase and phosphorylase kinase. The kinase activates the phosphorylase. And the kinase is in turn activated by adrenalin (epinephrine) in muscle and by glucagon in the liver. Glycogenesis; glycogen synthase. This enzyme is inhibited by adrenalin and glucagon. Glycolysis: phosphofructosekinase-1; Gluconeogenesis: fructose 1,6 bisphosphatase (this enzyme counteracts phosphofructokinase -1). TCA cycle: isocitrate dehydrogenase; PPP: glucose-6-phosphate dehydrogenase; Urea cycle: carbamoyl phosphate synthetase 1; fatty acid synthesis: acetyl CoA carboxylase; fatty acid oxidation: carnitine acyltransferase I; ketogenesis: HMG-CoA synthase; cholesterol synthesis: HMG-CoA

Anaerobic glycolysis uses two ATPs but generates four. Also uses up NAD^+, which is restored by the conversion of pyruvate to lactate.

One molecule of glucose generates two ATPs by glycolysis and 28 ATPs by oxidation to CO_2 and H_2O via the TCA cycle and electron transport chain. The TCA cycle and electron transport chain are the final common pathways for the oxidation of glucose, fatty acids and amino acids. Amino acids are also made from intermediates of the citric acid cycle (and also from intermediates of glycolysis and the PPP). Thiamine (vitB1) is a prosthetic group for the TCA enzymes pyruvate dehydrogenase *alpha-ketoglutarate dehydrogenase* and transketolase

Insulin – increases glucose uptake and glycogen synthesis in all tissues, particularly skeletal muscle. Liver is stimulated by insulin to produce glycogen from glucose. Brain and liver take up glucose independently of insulin and of Glut 4 (glucose transporter activated by insulin). Once the liver is full of glycogen it uses glucose to generate acetyl coA, which is used to make fatty acids, which are transported to adipocytes. Insulin also stimulates adipocytes to make glycerol (product of glycolysis), which together with fatty acids is used to make triglycerides. Insulin stimulates the uptake of branched chain amino acids by muscle, which favours building up muscle protein. Inhibits the intracellular degradation of proteins. Insulin activates potassium influx into many cell types.

GPCR mainly expressed in liver and kidney. Stimulate glycogen breakdown into glucose which is released into the bloodstream. Inhibits fatty acid synthesis. Stimulates gluconeogenesis.

Diabetes – far too much glucose in the blood that cannot be taken up well because of the lack of effective insulin. Body responds by breaking down a lot of fat to acetyl coA. However, can't be used well in the TCA cycle because of a lack of oxaloacetate (which requires glycolysis for production), therefore used to make ketone bodies. This causes acidosis and lowered blood pH level and dehydration.

Warburg effect. Warburg reported that cancer cells have less oxidative phosphorylation activity and more glycolytic activity than normal cells, even in the presence of sufficient oxygen.

Rcd blood cells have no mitochondria, therefore cannot metabolise fatty acids and amino acids. No nucleus, do have mRNA.

Brain can use glucose or ketone bodies (but only during starvation) to generate ATP

Skeletal muscle uses glucose, fatty acids and ketone bodies as energy, does not export glucose (lacks glucose 6 phosphatase).

Heart muscle has no glycogen stores and generates ATP aerobically via abundant mitochondria from fatty acid supplies.

Adipose tissue – makes triacylglycerols from fatty acids (from the liver) and glycerol (from glycolysis)

Liver and cardiac muscle and other tissues use fatty acids as primary fuel, so does skeletal muscle under resting or mild exercise. Liver provides fuel to other tissues. Makes glycogen from glucose, lactate, glycerol (from fat cells) and amino acids. Usually sends fatty acids to adipose tissues. Starvation converts fatty acids into ketone bodies. Synthesises fatty acids from acetylcoA.

Amino acid degradation: amino group removed as urea by the liver. Carbon skeleton converted to glucose or to ketone bodies, according to the amino acid.

Fatty acids are long hydrocarbons ending in a carboxyl group. Three fatty acids attached to glycerol are called triacylglycerols, neutral fats or triglycerides. Triacylglycerols in adipose tissue mobilised by lipases under hormonal control. Ketone bodies are made of acetoacetate and derivatives 3 hydroxybutyrate and acetone.

Animals cannot convert fatty acids into glucose, can convert glycerol into glucose.

Chylomicrons come from the intestine and carry dietary triacylglycerol. Very low density lipoproteins contain triacylglycerols plus cholesterol (which is made by the liver), LDL –main carrier of cholesterol.

Chylomicrons carry diet-derived lipids to body cells

VLDLs (very low density lipoproteins) carry lipids synthesised by the liver to body cells

LDLs (low density lipoproteins) carry cholesterol around the body

HDLs (high density lipoproteins) carry cholesterol from the body back to the liver for breakdown and excretion

BPG (2,3-bisphosphoglyceric acid) lowers the oxygen affinity of haemoglobin for oxygen 26-fold. 2,3-BPG is present in human red blood cells (RBC; erythrocyte) at approximately 5 mmol/L. It binds with greater affinity to deoxygenated haemoglobin (e.g. when the red cell is near respiring tissue) than it does to oxygenated haemoglobin (e.g. in the lungs) due to spatial changes: 2,3-BPG (with an estimated size of about 9 angstroms) fits in the deoxygenated haemoglobin configuration (11 angstroms), but not as well in the oxygenated (5 angstroms). It interacts with deoxygenated haemoglobin β subunits by decreasing their affinity for oxygen, so it allosterically promotes the release of the remaining oxygen molecules bound to the haemoglobin, thus enhancing the ability of RBCs to release oxygen near tissues that need it most. 2,3-BPG is thus an allosteric effector.

R or relaxed state has higher oxygen affinity. T or taut state has lower oxygen affinity; this is promoted by high 2,3-BPG or high CO_2 and High H+. High CO_2 and high H+ directly interact with haemoglobin and change its structure to taut.

CO_2 transported in red blood cells as bicarbonate produced from CO_2 and H_2O by carbonic anhydrase. H+ from this reaction taken up by haemoglobin (Bohr effect where acid conditions cause O_2 release) Remainder of CO_2 is carried by amino acid side chains of haemoglobin as carbamate.

Bilirubin is a breakdown product of haem. Old red blood cells broken down in spleen. The haem group is changed to bilirubin bound to serum albumin and sent to liver where it is conjugated to glucuronate (derivative of glucose) to make bile which is soluble for secretion and storage in the gallbladder and then the small intestine, where it helps to digest fats. Acute biliary obstruction prevents bile release and causes gallstones.

Water soluble – Vit C & B (eight of these)

Fat soluble A, D, E and K

Folic acid is a vitamin that is required to make DNA and RNA and certain amino acids. Deficiency causes macrocytic anaemia (red blood cell deficiency) and elevated homocysteine (precursor of cysteine). It protects against neural tube defects. Methotrexate competitively inhibits dihydrofolate reductase (DHFR), an enzyme that participates in tetrahydrofolate synthesis.

Non-essential amino acids: A to G and Pro, Ser, Tyr.

Urea and uric acid are different. Urea made in liver, uric acid is a breakdown product of purines and made not just by liver (also muscle and intestines). Both filtered and secreted by kidneys.

Liver removes two thirds of glucose, all of the remaining monosaccharides and most amino acids from the blood supply from the intestine. Remainder goes to other cells. Liver then regulates the provision of fuel (glucose, fatty acids and ketones) to other tissues. Makes glycogen from glucose, lactate, glycerol (from fat cells), alanine and other amino acids. Synthesises fatty acids from acetylcoA which are exported as fuel or for storage in adipose tissues. Starvation, converts fatty acids into ketone bodies.

Amino acids are first used for protein synthesis in all cell types. Excess amino acids are degraded and the amino group is removed as urea by the liver. The remaining part of the amino acid is broken down into carbon skeletons such as acetyl CoA acetoacetyl coA, pyruvate or one of the intermediates of the TCA cycle. These can be used to generate ketone bodies or glucose. Urea generated in the liver is transported to the kidneys for secretion in urine.

10 *Physiology*

BETHAN GOULDEN AND DAVID WILLIAMS

Biophysical Definitions

MOLECULAR WEIGHT

One mole of an element or compound is the atomic weight or molecular weight, respectively, in grams. For example, 1 mol of sodium is 23 g (atomic weight Na = 23) and 1 mol of sodium chloride is 58.5 g (atomic weight Cl = 35.5; 35.5 + 23 = 58.5). A 'normal' (molar) solution contains 1 mol/L of solution. Therefore a 'normal' solution of sodium chloride contains 58.5 g and is a 5.85% solution. This is very different from a physiological 'normal' solution of sodium chloride, where the concentration of sodium chloride (0.9%) is adjusted so that the sodium has a similar concentration as the total number of cations in plasma (154 mmol/L). The concentrations of biological substances are usually much weaker than molar. However, commonly used intravenous solutions that combine sodium chloride with glucose often contain sodium chloride 0.18% (sodium 30 mmol/L and chloride 30 mmol/L) and glucose 4%. Injudicious use of excessive volumes of this combination with 30 mmol NaCl will quickly lead to hyponatraemia.

The conventional nomenclature for decreasing molar concentrations is given below. The same prefixes may be used for different units of measurement:

$$1\,\text{millimole}\,(\text{mmol}) = 1 \times 10^{-3}\,\text{mol}$$

$$1\,\text{micromole}\,(\mu\text{mol}) = 1 \times 10^{-6}\,\text{mol}$$

$$1\,\text{micromole}\,(\mu\text{mol}) = 1 \times 10^{-6}\,\text{mol}$$

$$1\,\text{picomole}\,(\text{pmol}) = 1 \times 10^{-12}\,\text{mol}$$

$$1\,\textbf{femtomole(fmol)} = 1 \times 10^{-15}\,\textbf{mol}$$

$$1\,\textbf{attomole(amol)} = 1 \times 10^{-18}\,\textbf{mol}$$

1 equivalent (Eq) = 1 mol divided by the valency, (valency is the capacity of the atom to combine with a hydrogen atom). Thus 1 Eq of sodium (valency 1) = 23 g, and 1 mol of sodium = 1 Eq, that is, 1 mmol = 1 mEq.

However, 1 Eq of calcium (valency 2, mol wt 40) = 20 g. 1 mol of calcium = 2 Eq, and 1 mmol Ca^{2+} = 2 mEq Ca^{2+}.

Measurements in medicine are wherever possible being made in Systeme Internationale (SI) units. Under this system, the concentration of biological materials is expressed in the appropriate molar units (often mmol) per litre (L).

The units used in the measurement of osmotic pressure are considered below.

Distribution of Water and Electrolytes

A normal 70 kg man is composed of 60% water, 18% protein, 15% fat and 7% minerals. Obese individuals have relatively more fat and less water. Of the 60% (42 L) of water, 28 L (40% of body weight) are intracellular; the remaining 14 L of extracellular water are made up of 10.5 L of interstitial fluid (extracellular and extravascular) and 3.5 L of blood plasma. The total blood volume (red cells and plasma) is 8% of total body weight, or about 5.6 L.

The reference method of measuring total body water (TBW) is to give a subject deuterium oxide (D_2O), 'heavy water', and measuring how much it is diluted. Extracellular fluid volume can be measured with inulin by the same principle. Intracellular fluid volume = TBW (D_2O space) less extracellular fluid volume (inulin space). Intravascular fluid volume can be measured with Evans blue dye. Total blood volume can be calculated knowing intravascular fluid volume and the haematocrit. Interstitial fluid volume = extracellular fluid volume (inulin space) less intravascular fluid volume. TBW and distribution can now be measured noninvasively with bioelectric impedance analysis (BIA).

The distribution of electrolytes and protein in intracellular fluid, interstitial fluid and plasma is given in Fig. 10.1. Note that, for reasons of comparability, concentrations are expressed in milliequivalents per litre (mEq/L) of water, not millimoles per litre (mmol/L) of plasma.

The major difference between plasma and interstitial fluid is that interstitial fluid has relatively little protein. As a consequence, the concentration of sodium in the interstitial fluid is less and therefore, so is the overall osmotic pressure (see below). There are further major differences between intracellular fluid and extracellular fluid. Sodium is the major extracellular cation, whereas potassium and, to a lesser extent, magnesium are the predominant intracellular cations. Chloride and bicarbonate are the major extracellular anions; protein and phosphate are the predominant intracellular anions.

ANION GAP

In considering the composition of plasma for clinical purposes, account is often taken of the 'anion gap'. This is calculated by subtracting the concentrations of the two principal anions, chloride (100 mmol/L) and bicarbonate (24 mmol/L), from the principal cation, sodium (136 mmol/L). This leaves a positive balance of 12 mmol/L: normal range 8 to 16 mmol/L. The gap is considered to exist because of the occurrence of unmeasured anions, such as protein and lactate, which balance the number of cations. An increase in the anion gap suggests that there are more unmeasured anions present than usual. This occurs in such situations as lactic acidosis, or diabetic ketoacidosis, where the lactate and acetoacetate are balancing the excess sodium ions. A more complete explanation of the anion

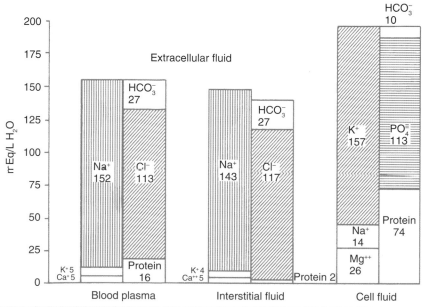

Fig. 10.1 Electrolyte composition of human body fluids.

Table 10.1 Anion Gap (mEq/L)

Cation		Anion	
Na$^+$	136	Cl$^-$	100
—		HCO$_3^-$	24
		—	
	136		124
		Gap	12
—		—	
	136		136
The gap consists of unmeasured cations and anions:			
K$^+$	4.5	Protein	15
Ca^{2+}	5	PO$_4^{3-}$	2
Mg^{2+}	1.5	SO$_4^{2-}$	1
		Organic acids	5
—		—	
	11		23
—		—	
	147		147

gap would be to consider both the unmeasured cations as well as the unmeasured anions, as in Table 10.1. Situations where the anion gap is increased include ketoacidosis, lactic acidosis and hyperosmolar acidosis, and poisoning with salicylate, methanol, ethylene glycol and paraldehyde, and hypoalbuminaemia. A decreased anion gap occurs in bromide poisoning and myeloma, which is characterised by excess immunoglobulin.

Cellular Transport Mechanisms

These mechanisms account for the movement of substances within cells and across cell membranes. The transport mechanisms to be considered include diffusion, solvent drag, filtration, osmosis, non-ionic diffusion, carrier-mediated transport and phagocytosis. Not all of these mechanisms will be considered in detail.

Diffusion is the process whereby a gas or substance in solution expands to fill the volume available to it. Relevant examples of gaseous diffusion are the equilibration of gases within the alveoli of the lung, and of liquid diffusion, the equilibration of substances within the fluid of the renal tubule. An element of diffusion may be involved in transport across all cell membranes because there is a layer of unstirred water up to 400 μm thick adjacent to biological membranes.

If there is a charged ion that cannot diffuse across a membrane which other charged ions can cross, the diffusible ions distribute themselves as in the following example:

In	*Out*
K$_i^+$	K$_0^+$
Cl$_i^-$	Cl$_0^-$
Protein$^-$	

$$\frac{\left[K_i^+\right]}{\left[K_0^+\right]} = \frac{\left[Cl_0^-\right]}{\left[Cl_i^-\right]} \text{ Gibbs – Donnan equilibrium}$$

The cell is permeable to K$^+$ and Cl$^-$ but not to protein. Since intracellular potassium (K$_i$) is about 157 mmol/L and extracellular potassium (K$_0$) is 4 mmol/L, the Gibbs–Donnan equilibrium would predict that the ratio of chloride concentration outside the cell to that inside should be 157/4 (i.e. about 40). In fact, there is almost no intracellular chloride so that the ratio *in vivo* is even greater than 40. This is because factors other than simple diffusion affect both potassium and chloride concentrations.

Solvent drag is the process whereby bulk movement of solvent drags some molecules of solute with it. It is of little physiological importance.

Filtration is the process whereby substances are forced through a membrane by hydrostatic pressure. The degree to which substances pass through the membrane depends on the size of the holes in the membrane. Small molecules pass through the holes, larger molecules do not. The renal glomerular basement membrane (GBM) has holes too small for blood cells and the majority of plasma proteins to traverse, but large enough to allow filtration of most other blood constituents. The GBM also acts as a charge-selective filtration barrier, favouring the passage of positively charged molecules.

Osmosis describes the movement of solvent from a region of low solute concentration, across a semipermeable membrane to one of high solute concentration. The process can be opposed by hydrostatic pressure; the pressure that will stop osmosis occurring is the osmotic pressure of the solution. This is given by the formula:

$$P = nRT/V$$

where P = osmotic pressure, n = number of osmotically active particles, R = gas constant, T = absolute temperature, V = volume. For an ideal solution of a non-ionised substance, n/V equals the concentration of the solute. In an ideal solution, 1 osmol of a substance is then defined such that:

1 osmol = mol wt in grams/number of osmotically active particles in solution

So for an ideal solution of glucose:

1 osmol = mol wt/1 = mol wt = 180 g

However, sodium chloride dissociates into two ions in solution. Therefore, for sodium chloride:

1 osmol = mol wt/2 = 58.5/2 = 29.2 g

Calcium chloride dissociates into three ions in solution. Therefore, for calcium chloride,

1 osmol = mol wt/3 = 111/3 = 37 g

However, the molecules or ions of all solutions aggregate to a certain degree so that interaction occurs between the ions or molecules, and they each do not behave as osmotically independent particles and do not form ideal solutions.

Freezing point depression by a solution is also caused by the number of osmotically active particles. The greater the concentration of osmotically active particles, the greater the freezing point depression. In an ideal solution, with no interaction, 1 mol of osmotically active particles per litre depresses the freezing point by 1.86°C. Therefore, an aqueous solution which depresses the freezing point by 1.86°C is defined as containing 1 osmol/L. One which depresses the freezing point by 1.86°C/1000 (i.e. 0.00186°C) contains 1 mosmol/L. Plasma (osmotic pressure 300 mosmol/L) has a freezing point of (0 to 0.00186 × 300) °C = −0.56°C.

Osmolarity defines osmotic pressure in terms of osmoles per litre of solution. Since volume changes at different temperatures, osmolality which defines osmotic pressure in terms of osmoles per kilogram of solution is preferred, though not always employed. The major osmotic components of plasma are the cations sodium and potassium, and their accompanying anions, together with glucose and urea.

The concentration of sodium is about 140 mmol/L. This, and the accompanying anions, will therefore contribute 280 mosmol/L. The concentration of potassium is about 4 mmol/L, which, with its accompanying anions, will give 8 mosmol/L. Glucose and urea contribute 5 mosmol/L each to a total of 300 mosmol/L in normal plasma. During pregnancy, due to an expansion of plasma volume this falls to below 290 mosmol/L. The mechanism of plasma volume expansion appears to relate to a resetting of the hypothalamic thirst centre, so that in early pregnancy women still feel thirsty at a lower plasma osmolality than when not pregnant.

We are now in a position to consider some of the forces acting on water in the capillaries (Fig. 10.2). The capillary membrane behaves as if it is only permeable to water and small solutes. It is impermeable to colloids such as plasma protein. There is a difference of 25 mmHg in osmotic pressure between the interstitial water and the intravascular water due to the intravascular plasma proteins (see above). This force (oncotic pressure) will tend to drive water into the capillary. At the arteriolar end of the capillary, the hydrostatic pressure is approximately 37 mmHg; the interstitial pressure is 1 mmHg. The net force driving water *out* is therefore 37 − 1 − 25 = 11 mmHg, and water tends to pass out of the arteriolar end of the capillary. At the venous end of the capillary, the pressure is approximately 20 mmHg lower, at around 17 mmHg. The net force driving water *in* the capillary is therefore 25 + 1 − 17 = 9 mmHg. Fluid therefore enters the capillary at the venous end. Factors which would decrease fluid reabsorption and cause clinical oedema are a reduction in plasma proteins, so that the osmotic gradient between the intravascular and interstitial fluids might be only 20 mmHg, not 25 mmHg, or a rise in venous pressure, for example, due to increased pressure on the inferior vena cava in the third trimester of pregnancy, so that the pressure at the venous end of the capillary might be 25 mmHg, rather than 17 mmHg.

Non-ionised diffusion is the process whereby there is preferential transport in a non-ionised form. Cell membranes consist of a lipid bilayer with specific transporter proteins embedded in it. Lipid-soluble drugs (e.g. propranolol) can cross the lipids of the blood–brain barrier or the placenta by

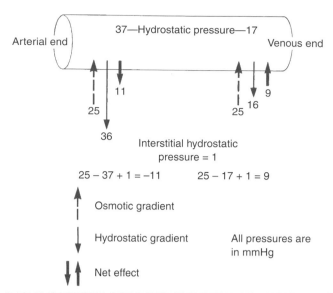

Fig. 10.2 At the arterial end of the capillary the hydrostatic forces acting outwards are greater than the osmotic forces acting inwards. There is a net movement out of the capillary. At the venous end of the capillary, the hydrostatic forces acting outwards are less than the osmotic forces acting inwards. There is a net movement into the capillary.

non-ionised diffusion. But small hydrophilic molecules such as O_2 can also diffuse across the lipid bilayer, which is also permeable to water.

Carrier-mediated transport implies transport across a cell membrane using a specific carrier. If the transport is down a concentration gradient from an area of high concentration to one of low concentration, this is known as facilitated transport (e.g. the uptake of glucose by the muscle cell) facilitated by the participation of insulin in the transport process. If the carrier-mediated transport is up a concentration gradient from an area of low concentration to one of high concentration, this is known as active transport (e.g. the removal of sodium from muscle cells by the ATPase-dependent sodium pump). The channel may be ligand gated where binding of external (e.g. insulin as earlier) ligands or an internal ligand opens the channel. Alternatively the channel may be voltage gated, where patency depends on the transmembrane electrical potential; voltage gating is a major feature of the conduction of nervous impulses.

Phagocytosis and pinocytosis involve the incorporation of discrete bodies of solid and liquid substances, respectively, by cell wall growing out and around the particles so that the cell appears to swallow them. If the cell eliminates substances, the process is known as exocytosis; if substances are transported into the cell, the process is endocytosis. In endocytosis, the Golgi apparatus is involved in intracellular transport and processing to varying extents depending on whether exocytosis is via the non-constitutive pathway (extensive processing) or the constitutive pathway (little processing). Similarly, endocytosis may involve specific receptors for substances such as low-density lipoproteins (receptor-mediated endocytosis) or there may be no specific receptors (constitutive endocytosis).

Acid–Base Balance

NORMAL ACID–BASE BALANCE

A simple knowledge of chemistry allows some substances to be easily categorised as acids or bases. For example, hydrochloric acid is clearly an acid and sodium hydroxide is a base. But when describing acid–base balance in physiology, these terms are used rather more obscurely. For example, the chloride ion may be described as a base. A more applicable definition is to define an acid as an ion or molecule which can liberate hydrogen ions. Since hydrogen ions are protons (H^+), acids may also be defined as proton donors. A base is then a substance which can accept hydrogen ions, or a proton acceptor. If we consider the examples below, hydrochloric acid dissociates into hydrogen ions and chloride ions, and is therefore a proton donor (acid). If the chloride ion associates with hydrogen ions to form hydrochloric acid, the chloride ion is a proton acceptor (base). Ammonia is another proton acceptor when it forms the ammonium ion. Carbonic acid is an acid (hydrogen ion donor); bicarbonate is a base (hydrogen ion acceptor). The $H_2PO_4^-$ ion can be both an acid when it dissociates further to HPO_4^{2-} and a base when it associates to form H_3PO_4:

$$HCl \rightleftharpoons H^+ + Cl^-$$

$$NH_3 + H^- \rightleftharpoons NH_4^+$$

$$H_2CO_3 \rightleftharpoons H^+ + HCO_3^-$$

$$H_3PO_4 \rightleftharpoons H_2PO_4^- + H^+$$

$$H_2PO_4^- \rightleftharpoons H_3PO_4^{2-} + H^+$$

pH

The pH is defined as the negative $\log_{10}$ of the hydrogen ion concentration expressed in mol/L. A negative logarithmic scale is used because the numbers are all less than 1 and vary over a wide range. Since the pH is the negative logarithm of the hydrogen ion concentration, a low pH number (e.g. pH 6.2) indicates a relatively high hydrogen ion concentration (i.e. an acidic solution). High pH numbers (e.g. pH 7.8) represent a lower hydrogen ion concentration (i.e. alkaline solutions). Because the pH scale is logarithmic to the base 10, a 1-unit change in pH represents a 10-fold change in hydrogen ion concentration.

The normal pH range in human tissues is 7.36 to 7.44. Although a neutral pH (hydrogen ion concentration equals hydroxyl ion concentration) at 20°C has the value 7.4, water dissociates more at physiological temperatures, and a neutral pH at 37°C has the value 6.8. Therefore, body fluids are mildly alkaline (the higher the pH number, the lower the hydrogen ion concentration).

A pH value of 7.4 represents a hydrogen ion concentration of 0.00004 mmol/L as seen in the following example:

$$pH = 7.4$$

$$\left[H^+\right] = 10^{-7.4} \text{ mol/L}$$

$$= 10^{-8} \times 10^{0.6} \text{ mol/L}$$

$$= 0.00000001 \times 4 \text{ mol/L}$$

$$= 0.00000004 \text{ mol/L}$$

$$= 0.00004 \text{ mmol/L}$$

$$(1 \text{ mol/L} = 1000 \text{ mmol/L} \quad)$$

Partial Pressure of Carbon Dioxide

In arterial blood, the normal P_{CO_2} value is 4.8 to 5.9 kPa (36 to 44 mmHg). It is a coincidence that the figures expressing P_{CO_2} in mmHg are similar to those expressing the normal range for pH (7.36 to 7.44).

Henderson–Hasselbalch Equation

This equation describes the relationship of hydrogen ion, bicarbonate and carbonic acid concentrations (see Equation (3) below). It can be rewritten in terms of pH, bicarbonate and carbonic acid concentrations, as in Equation (4), but carbonic acid concentrations are not usually measured. However, because of the presence of carbonic anhydrase in red cells, carbonic acid concentration is proportional to P_{CO_2} (Equation (1)). Equation (4) can therefore be rewritten in terms of pH, bicarbonate and P_{CO_2} (Equation (5)). All these data are usually available from blood gas analyses. If we know any two of these variables, the third can be calculated.

Carbonic anhydrase:

$$CO_2 + H_2O \rightleftharpoons H_2CO_3$$

$$[H_2CO_3] \rightleftharpoons H^+ + HCO_3^- \tag{1}$$

By the Law of Mass Action:

$$[H_2CO_3] = K[H^+][HCO_3^-] \tag{2}$$

$$\therefore [H^+] = \frac{1}{K}\left(\frac{[H_2CO_3^-]}{[HCO_3^-]}\right) \tag{3}$$

By taking logarithms of the reciprocal:

$$pH = K' + \log\left(\frac{[HCO_3^-]}{[H_2CO_3]}\right)$$

K' is a constant equal to 6.1:

$$pH = 6.1 + \log\left(\frac{[HCO_3^-]}{[H_2CO_3]}\right) \tag{4}$$

$$pH = 6.1 + \log\left(\frac{[HCO_3^-]}{P_aCO_2 \times 0.04}\right) \qquad (5)^*$$

Control of pH

The Henderson–Hasselbalch equation, expressed in Equation (5), indicates that the variables controlling pH are P_{CO_2} and bicarbonate concentration. Ultimately, P_{CO_2} is controlled by respiration. Short-term changes of pH may therefore be compensated for by changing the depth of respiration. Bicarbonate concentration can be altered by the kidneys, and this is the mechanism involved in the long-term control of pH. Further details of these mechanisms are given on pp. 25 and 201.

BUFFERS

A buffer solution is one to which hydrogen or hydroxyl ions can be added with little change in the pH.

Consider a solution of sodium bicarbonate to which is added hydrochloric acid (Fig. 10.3). The hydrogen ions of the hydrochloric acid react with bicarbonate ions of the sodium bicarbonate to form carbonic acid. Carbonic acid does not dissociate so readily as hydrochloric acid. Therefore the hydrogen ions are buffered. Reading from right to left in Fig. 10.3, we have a solution that starts as 100% bicarbonate ions and becomes 100% carbonic acid as hydrochloric acid is added. Initially, in the pH range 9 to 7, a very small change in bicarbonate concentration, requiring the addition of only a few hydrogen ions, is associated with a large change in pH. However, in the steep part of the curve, between pH 5 and 7, a considerable quantity of

hydrogen ions can be added, as indicated by a marked fall in the proportion of bicarbonate remaining, with relatively little change in pH. It is in that pH range that the buffering ability of bicarbonate is greatest.

The pH at which 50% of the buffer is changed from its acidic to its basic form (or vice versa) is known as the pK. For bicarbonate the pK is 6.1, making bicarbonate rather poor as a buffer for body fluids, since the pK is considerably towards the acidic side of the physiological pH range (7.36 to 7.44). The buffer value of a buffer (mmol of hydrogen ion per gram per pH unit) is the quantity of hydrogen ions which can be added to a buffer solution to change its pH by 1.0 pH unit from p$K + 0.5$ to p$K - 0.5$.

In blood, the most important buffers are proteins. These are able to absorb hydrogen ions onto free carboxyl radicals, as illustrated in Fig. 10.4. Of the proteins available, haemoglobin is more important than plasma protein, partly because its buffer value is greater than that of plasma protein (0.18 mmol of hydrogen per gram of haemoglobin per pH unit, vs 0.11 mmol of hydrogen per gram of plasma protein per pH unit), but also because there is more haemoglobin than plasma protein (15 g haemoglobin per 100 mL vs 3.8 g of plasma protein per 100 mL). These two factors mean that haemoglobin has six times the buffering capacity of plasma protein. In addition, deoxygenated haemoglobin is a weaker acid and a more efficient buffer than oxygenated haemoglobin. This increases the buffering capacity of haemoglobin where it is needed more, after oxygen has been liberated in the peripheral tissues.

Buffer Base and Base Excess

The buffer base is the total number of buffer anions (usually 45 to 50 mEq/L of blood) and consists of bicarbonate, phosphate and protein anions (haemoglobin and plasma protein).

Base excess is the difference between the actual buffer base and the normal value for a given haemoglobin and

---

*For Equation (5), because of the action of carbonic anhydrase, $[H_2CO_3]$ is proportional to P_aco_2. For the given constants of Equation (5), P_{CO_2} is expressed in mmHg.

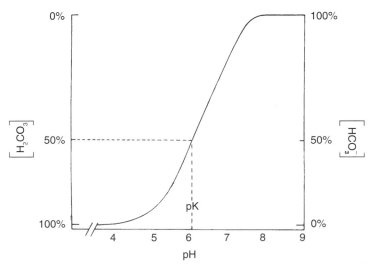

Fig. 10.3 Effect of adding H⁺ (as HCl) to an HCO_3^- solution (as $NaHCO_3$). The pH changes from 9.0 when the solution is 100% HCO_3^- and 0% H_2CO_3 to <4 when the solution is 0% HCO_3^- and 100% H_2CO_3. At the pK value when the HCO_3^- is 50% changed to H_2CO_3 the curve is steepest, indicating that there is relatively little change in the pH for a relatively large change in HCO_3^- concentration. The pK is 6.1.

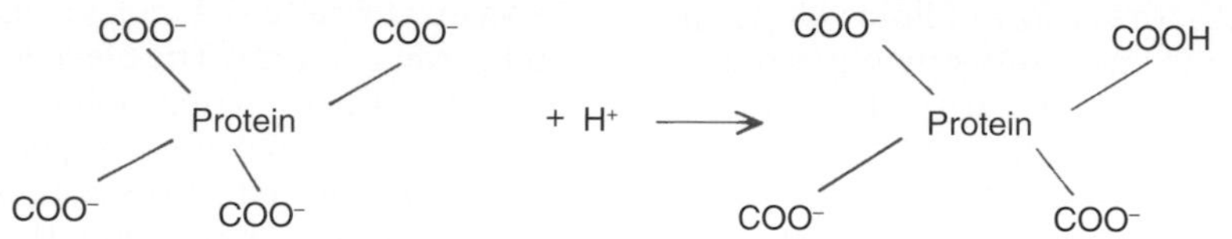

Fig. 10.4 The absorption of hydrogen ions onto free carboxyl radicals.

Table 10.2 Values of pH and Partial Pressure of Carbon Dioxide Characterising Acidosis and Alkalosis

	pH	P_{CO_2} (kPa)	P_{CO_2} (mmHg)
Normal	7.36–7.44	4.8–5.9	36–44
Respiratory acidosis	<7.36	>5.9	>44
Respiratory alkalosis	>7.44	<4.8	<36
Metabolic acidosis	<7.36	<5.9	<44
Metabolic alkalosis	>7.44	>4.8	>36

body temperature. It is negative in acidosis and is then sometimes expressed as a positive base deficit, and positive in alkalosis. It gives an index of the severity of the abnormality of acid–base balance.

Standard bicarbonate

This is the carbon dioxide content of blood equilibrated at a P_{CO_2} of 40 mmHg and a temperature of 37°C when the haemoglobin is fully saturated with oxygen. In general it represents the non-respiratory part of acid–base derangement and is low in metabolic acidosis and raised in metabolic alkalosis. The normal value for the standard bicarbonate is 27 mmol/L.

ABNORMALITIES OF ACID–BASE BALANCE

These are usually divided into acidosis (pH <7.36) and alkalosis (pH >7.44). In addition, we consider respiratory acidosis and alkalosis where the primary abnormality is in respiration (carbon dioxide control) and metabolic acidosis and alkalosis, which are best defined as abnormalities that are not respiratory in origin. Only initial, single abnormalities will be considered. For these single uncomplicated abnormalities, respiratory and metabolic acidosis and alkalosis can be defined according to Table 10.2, which gives the values of pH and P_{CO_2} characterising each abnormality.

Respiratory Acidosis

There is a low pH and a high P_{CO_2}. Here the basic abnormality is a failure of carbon dioxide excretion from the lungs. Carbon dioxide dissolves in the blood, and in the presence of carbonic anhydrase, carbonic acid is formed which dissociates into hydrogen ions and bicarbonate (Equations (1) and (2), p. 5). Respiratory acidosis may arise from abnormalities of respiration, which may range from impaired respiratory control due to excessive sedation, to chronic pulmonary disease. In the long term, respiratory acidosis is compensated by bicarbonate retention in the kidneys, which increases pH towards normal values.

Respiratory Alkalosis

There is a high pH and a low P_{CO_2}. This is induced by hyperventilation, whatever the cause. Perhaps the commonest clinical presentation is anxiety, where the acute fall in hydrogen ion concentration due to blowing off carbon dioxide may cause paraesthesiae, or even tetany. Tetany occurs because more plasma protein is ionised when the pH is high. This protein binds more calcium, lowering the ionised (metabolically effective) calcium level. However, respiratory alkalosis is also seen in the early stages of exercise, at altitude and in patients who have had a pulmonary embolus. In pregnancy, there is hyperventilation but the kidney excretes sufficient bicarbonate to compensate fully for the fall in carbon dioxide, and there is therefore no change in pH.

Metabolic Acidosis

There is a low pH and the P_{CO_2} is not elevated. This may occur because of excessive acid production, impaired acid excretion or excessive alkali loss. Examples of excess acid production are diabetic ketoacidosis and methanol poisoning, in which methanol is metabolised to formaldehyde, which subsequently forms formic acid.

Failure of acid excretion occurs in chronic renal failure, and more specifically in renal tubular acidosis, where the patients are not initially uraemic but acid excretion by the kidney is impaired. Acetazolamide is a diuretic drug which inhibits ammonia formation within the kidney, and this too causes metabolic acidosis. Excess alkali loss is seen in patients who have a pancreatic fistula or prolonged diarrhoea, since both the bodily fluids lost are alkaline.

Women with diabetes are prone to ketosis and ketoacidosis in pregnancy but even non-diabetic women may become ketotic or ketoacidotic in pregnancy during periods of starvation, particularly in the third trimester. During the second half of normal pregnancy, a relatively insulin resistant state develops secondary to increased levels of placentally derived counter-regulatory hormones such as glucagon, human placental lactogen and cortisol. In the absence of glucose and sufficient glycogen stores during fasting, adipose tissue is utilised as an energy source with fatty acid oxidation to acetyl CoA. Acetyl CoA can then be utilised by the citric acid cycle to produce ATP. If, however, the capacity of the citric acid cycle is overwhelmed, acetyl CoA will instead be converted to ketones including acetone, acetoacetate and β-hydroxybutyrate. Whilst a healthy adult would only become ketoacidotic after prolonged periods of fasting (i.e. >14 days), in the third trimester, pregnant woman can develop ketoacidosis in as little as 24 hours. When assessing ketoacidosis as a cause of metabolic acidosis, a finger prick test of capillary ketones, measuring β-hydroxybutyrate, are preferred to urinary ketones, which measure acetoacetate. β-Hydroxybutyrate is present in higher concentrations than acetoacetate and capillary testing can more accurately track response to treatment.

Metabolic Alkalosis

The pH is high and the P_{CO_2} is not reduced. This may occur due to prolonged vomiting. The mechanism is less to do with the loss of acidic fluid and more to a loss of fluid volume and a compensatory activation of the renin–angiotensin–aldosterone system. Sodium is reabsorbed at the renal tubules at the expense of potassium and hydrogen ions. Metabolic alkalosis also occurs in excessive alkali ingestion, seen in patients who take antacids for peptic ulceration. Metabolic alkalosis frequently accompanies hypokalaemia.

Cardiovascular System

Cardiac disease is now the leading cause of maternal mortality in the United Kingdom as described in successive Mothers and Babies: Reducing Risk through Audits and Confidential Enquiries across the UK (MBRRACE) reports. This section will detail the physiology of both cardiac output and the conduction system in a normal pregnancy as well as examining normal pregnant haemodynamics and the potential changes that can occur in cardiac disease.

CONDUCTION SYSTEM OF THE HEART

The heart has its own unique electrical conduction tissue (Fig. 10.5) which allows orderly coordinated activity between atria and ventricles to ensure maximum efficiency and cardiac output. The electrical impulse is generated by the sino-atrial (SA) node which is located high in the right atrium at the entry of the superior vena cava. The impulse is then transmitted across both atria by crossing adjoining cardiomyocytes of the smooth muscle via gap junctions resulting in atrial contraction. There is an electrical seal allowing no conduction between the atria and ventricles which in the normal heart is broken only by the atrioventricular (AV) node. The electrical impulse once arrived at the AV node is stored for a few milliseconds to allow maximum ventricular filling from the atria. The AV node, which sits in the AV ring, conducts the impulse through specialised conduction tissue called the His–Purkinje system. The His bundle divides into a right and left branch which innervate the right and left ventricles respectively. The right bundle is a relatively narrow group of fibres. The left bundle is a much wider sheet of fibres and divides further into fascicles. Thus right bundle branch block due to damage to the right bundle occurs relatively easily and is not necessarily of pathological significance. Left bundle branch block implies considerable additional damage to the underlying myocardium to interrupt such a wide sheet of fibres and is always pathological. Interruption or damage to the normal conduction system can lead to varying

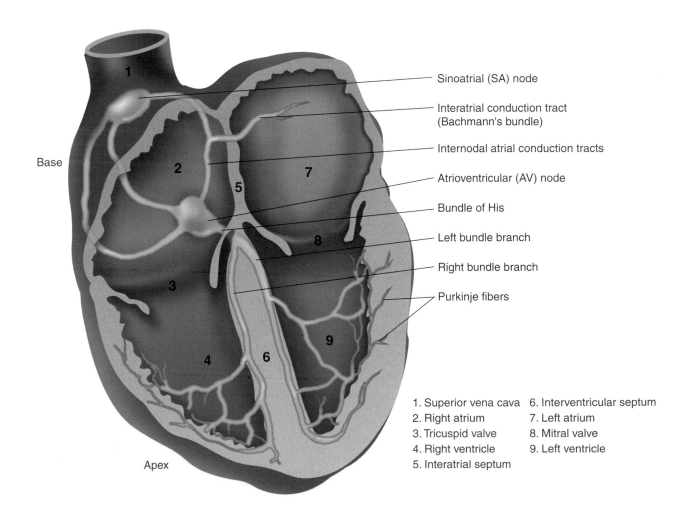

Base

Apex

Sinoatrial (SA) node

Interatrial conduction tract (Bachmann's bundle)

Internodal atrial conduction tracts

Atrioventricular (AV) node

Bundle of His

Left bundle branch

Right bundle branch

Purkinje fibers

1. Superior vena cava
2. Right atrium
3. Tricuspid valve
4. Right ventricle
5. Interatrial septum
6. Interventricular septum
7. Left atrium
8. Mitral valve
9. Left ventricle

Fig. 10.5 The conducting system of the heart. Internodal pathways in the atria are not specialised conducting tissue in normal individuals. Aberrant pathways have been found in subjects susceptible to dysrhythmias. (*Source:* From Kacmarek R., Stoller J., Heuer A., 2021. *Egan's Fundamentals of Respiratory Care*, 12th edn. Elsevier Inc, St. Louis).

degrees of heart block. In the event of failure of the SA or AV node, the ventricular tissue has the ability to contract under its own intrinsic rate, although this is usually at a much slower rate than normal.

Some patients have additional electrical pathways which cross the AV seal and can conduct impulses antegradely (from atria to ventricles) and retrogradely (from ventricles to atria). By having an additional pathway to the AV node, impulses can pass from atria to ventricles and back again to create a circuit which causes tachyarrhythmias. The most common example of this is Wolff–Parkinson–White (WPW) syndrome that predisposes to supra-ventricular tachycardia.

FACTORS AFFECTING HEART RATE

The activity of the SA node is controlled neurogenically by the sympathetic and parasympathetic nervous systems, directed by the vasomotor and cardio-inhibitory centres, respectively (see later). At rest, the dominant tone is parasympathetic, mediated via the vagus nerve (a muscarinic effect; Table 10.3).

In addition, the discharge rate from the SA node and therefore heart rate is increased by the direct actions of thyroxine, high temperature, β-adrenergic activity, and block of the dominant parasympathetic tone by atropine. Conversely, it is decreased by hypothyroidism, hypothermia, and β-adrenergic blockade. SA node activity is also decreased in ischaemia, and under these circumstances other intrinsic pacemakers (AV node, ventricles) take over pacemaker activity, albeit at a slower rate.

Cardiac Chambers

Table 10.4 shows the normal dimensions for the cardiac chambers outside of pregnancy. In pregnancy, the chambers increase to accommodate the increased circulating volume with the largest changes being seen in the left and right atrium (an increase of 5 and 7 mm, respectively) (Campos, 1996).

Table 10.3 Autonomic Receptors Affecting the Heart and Blood Vessels

Location	Receptor	Comments
Heart muscle and conducting tissue	Cholinergic	↓ Heart rate
		↓ Conduction velocity
		↓ Contractility
	α-Adrenergic	Nil
	β₂-Adrenergic	↑ Heart rate
		↑ Conduction velocity
		↑ Contractility
Blood vessels	Cholinergic (vasodilator)	Muscle
		Coronary artery
		Salivary glands
	α-Adrenergic (vasoconstrictor)	All tissues
	β₁-Adrenergic (vasodilator)	Brain
		Skeletal muscle
		Intra-abdominal

ELECTROCARDIOGRAM

Fig. 10.6 shows a normal electrocardiogram (ECG). The P wave is atrial depolarisation which leads to atrial contraction while the QRS complex is ventricular depolarisation which leads to ventricular contraction. The T wave is secondary to ventricular repolarisation. Atrial repolarisation is not seen on the surface ECG as it occurs at the same time as ventricular depolarisation, and it is too small an electrical signal to be seen within the QRS. The normal ECG is recorded at a speed of 25 mm/s, so each small square represents 0.04 seconds and each large square represents 0.2 seconds. In the vertical axis, the ECG is calibrated so that 1 cm equals 1 mV. In order to calculate the heart rate, divide 300 by N, where N is the number of large squares between successive R waves. In the event of atrial fibrillation (AF), where it is variable, an average is taken.

The normal PR interval is between 0.12 and 0.20 ms. If there is a delay, then there is a delay in conduction between the atria and ventricles and this is known as first-degree heart block. If the PR interval is short, then the electrical impulse is being transmitted between the atria and ventricles through a much faster pathway than normal, which implies aberrant conduction. This is typically seen in WPW syndrome and leads to a rapid inflection on the upstroke of the R wave known as a delta wave.

The normal QRS width should be no greater than 0.12 seconds (three small squares) and any longer is due to a delay in the impulse travelling along the His–Purkinje system. This is known as bundle branch block and, depending upon

Table 10.4 Cardiac Chamber Dimensions

	Control	Weeks 8–12	Weeks 20–24	Weeks 30–34	Weeks 36–40	Change cf Control
LVEDd	40.1	41.1	42.7	43.0	43.6	3.5
LA	27.9	29.6	31.5	33.1	32.8	4.9
RVEDd	28.5	30.1	31.9	35.5	35.5	4.4
RA	43.7	42.8	47.4	50.8	50.9	7.2

LA, Left atrium; LVEDd, left ventricular end-diastolic dimension; RA, right atrium; RVEDd, right ventricular end-diastolic dimension.
Source: Campos (1996).

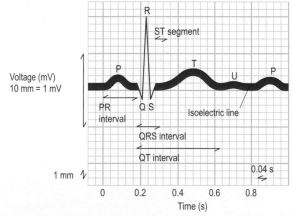

Fig. 10.6 The normal electrocardiogram. (*Source:* From Kumar P., Clark M., 2011. *Kumar & Clark's Medical Management and Therapeutics*, Elsevier Ltd., Edinburgh).

which bundle is involved, leads to a different morphology of the QRS seen best in lead V1. The QT interval is between 0.30 and 0.45 seconds and is dependent upon heart rate. It is increased in hypocalcaemia, hypokalaemia, rheumatic carditis and with a large number of drugs. It is decreased in hypercalcaemia, hyperkalaemia and digoxin.

PRESSURE AND SATURATION IN THE CARDIAC CHAMBERS

Blood enters the right side of the heart via the inferior and superior vena cava (Fig. 10.7). That which comes from the head is more desaturated than that from the rest of the body due to increased consumption by the brain, and normal mixed venous oxygen saturation in the right atrium (RA) is usually around 60%. If there is oxygenated blood abnormally entering the atrium due to a shunt or atrial septal defect, then this will lead to a step up in the saturations if sampled from high to low RA and will lead to an increased mixed venous saturation. True mixed venous blood, however, is best taken from the pulmonary artery (PA) as blood from the coronary sinus enters the right atrium and with streaming, which occurs in the right atrium and ventricle, blood is not fully mixed until it reaches the PA. Blood in the left side of the heart is 96% saturated with oxygen, giving a P_{O_2} of 90 to 100 mmHg (100 mmHg = 13.3 kPa). There is no difference in saturation in blood in the left atrium (LA) and left ventricle (LV).

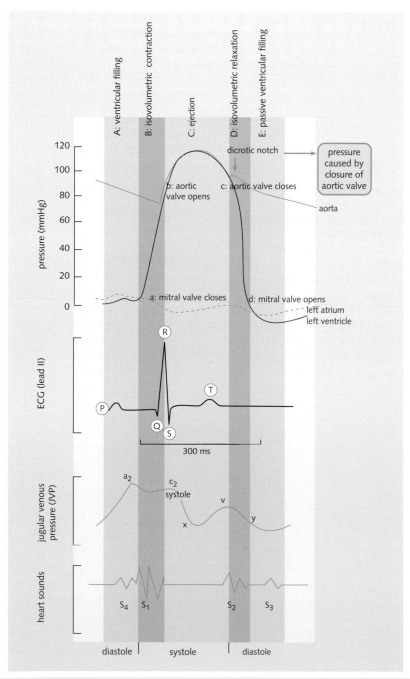

Fig. 10.7 Haemodynamic and electrocardiographic correlates of events in the cardiac cycle. (*Source*: From Evans J., Newby D.E., Horton-Szar D., 2012. *Crash Course: Cardiovascular System*, 4th edn. Elsevier Ltd., Oxford).

Table 10.5 Normal Values for Cardiac Pressure and Saturations

	Normal Pressure (mmHg)	Normal Saturation (%)
Right atrial pressure	2–6	
Right ventricle	15–25	Mixed venous saturations
Systolic	0–8	
End-diastolic		
Pulmonary artery	15–25/8–15	70–75
Systolic/diastolic	10–20	
Mean		
Pulmonary capillary wedge	6–12	
Left ventricle end-diastolic pressure (EDP)	<12	95–100
Cardiac output (L/min)	4.0–8.0	
Cardiac index (L/min per m²)	2.8–4.2	

All pressures in the circulation should be measured relative to a fixed reference point, ideally the level of the right atrium. The normal ranges are shown in Table 10.5. Using this reference point, the mean right atrial pressure is usually between 2 and 6 mmHg (average 4 mmHg). This is determined indirectly by assessing the jugular venous pressure, and more directly by measurement of central venous pressure. The pressure in the LA is approximately 10 to 15 mmHg, and this can be measured using a Swan–Ganz catheter. The catheter is placed in the PA either under direct radiological vision or the balloon tip inflated and the device floated through the right heart via a central vein. Once in the PA, the inflated balloon can be wedged into a branch of the distal PA. Providing there are no significant reasons for pressure across the lung capillaries to be raised then the pressure reflects that of the LA. The same Swan–Ganz catheter can also be used for measuring cardiac output by the thermodilution method which involves injecting a bolus of cold saline into the PA and recording the area under the curve of the temperature change over time. Essentially, the higher the cardiac output, the quicker the cold saline is replaced with warm blood and hence the area under the curve will be reduced.

HAEMODYNAMIC EVENTS IN THE CARDIAC CYCLE AND THEIR CLINICAL CORRELATES

This section describes events in the left side of the heart, although the events occurring on the right side of the heart are similar. However, left atrial systole occurs after right atrial systole and LV systole precedes right ventricular systole.

At the very beginning of ventricular systole, the mitral valve is open; the pressure in the LA is somewhat greater than that in the LV. As ventricular systole continues, the pressure in the LV exceeds that in the LA, thus closing the mitral valve. Shortly afterwards, the pressure in the LV exceeds that in the aorta, and this opens the aortic valve; ejection of blood then occurs from the LV. As the ventricle starts to relax, the pressure in the LV falls below that in the aorta; initially, the aortic valve stays open because of the forward kinetic energy of the ejected blood. With a further

fall in pressure in the LV, the aortic valve then closes. As the pressure in the LV continues to fall below and becomes lower than that in the LA, the mitral valve opens, and blood passes from the atrium to the ventricle.

In the period of rapid passive filling (early in diastole) blood falls from the atria to the ventricles. However, the remaining one-third of ventricular filling is caused by atrial systole (active filling), which, in turn, causes the *a* wave in the jugular venous pressure trace. The *c* wave coincides with the onset of ventricular systole, making the tricuspid valve bulge into the atrium and raising the pressure there. The *v* wave is due to the filling of the atrium while the tricuspid valve is shut, and the upward movement of the tricuspid valve at the end of ventricular systole. Active filling constitutes approximately 5% of cardiac output in a normal heart and is lost in AF. This may not be noticed by women with normal LV function. However, in patients with a fixed cardiac output (e.g. mitral stenosis) it may reduce cardiac output significantly.

During the early part of ventricular systole, both the mitral and aortic valves are closed. The volume of blood within the ventricle must then remain the same. This is therefore known as the period of isovolumetric contraction. As the ventricle relaxes, there is a similar period when both aortic and mitral valves are closed: the period of isovolumetric relaxation.

In those with normal hearts, valve closure is associated with heart sounds, but valve opening is not. The first sound is caused by mitral valve closure, and the second sound by aortic valve closure. Patients with abnormal valves may have an ejection click (aortic stenosis) at aortic valve opening, or an opening snap (mitral stenosis) at mitral valve opening. The third heart sound occurs at the period of rapid ventricular filling; the fourth heart sound is related to atrial systole. The fourth heart sound is therefore absent in patients with AF. Heart sounds, other than the first and second, are usually considered pathological, although the third heart sound in particular is very commonly heard in pregnancy and in young people.

The electrical events of the electrocardiograph precede mechanical ones. Thus, the P wave representing atrial depolarisation occurs before the fourth heart sound, and the QRS complex representing ventricular depolarisation occurs at the onset of ventricular systole. The T wave (ventricular repolarisation) is already occurring at the height of ventricular systole.

Alterations in heart rate are associated with changes in the length of diastole rather than the length of systole. This can be a problem in patients where filling of the ventricles is impaired, as in mitral stenosis; such patients are very intolerant of rapid heart rates.

Since right ventricular systole occurs a little later than left, the second sound is split, the second component being due to the closure of the pulmonary valve. During inspiration, the delay of ejection of blood from the right side of the heart is even greater, so that splitting of the second sound widens.

CONTROL OF CARDIAC OUTPUT

Cardiac output (CO) is the product of stroke volume (SV) and heart rate (HR), where stroke volume is the volume of blood ejected by the heart per beat and is normally 70 mL.

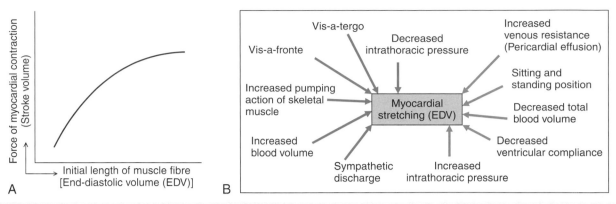

Fig. 10.8 Relation between ventricular end-diastolic volume *(EDV)* and ventricular performance (Frank–Starling curve), with a summary of the major factors affecting EDV. (*Source*: From Khurana I., Khurana A., 2015. *Textbook of Medical Physiology*, 2nd edn. Elsevier India, New Delhi).

$$\mathbf{CO\,(L/min\,) = SV\,(mL) \times HR\,(rate/min\,)}$$

Normal resting cardiac output is 4.5 L/min in females and 5.5 L/min in males. While this can be a useful measurement, it does not take into account the differences between individuals and thus an 80-year-old small woman does not have the same cardiac output as a 90-kg large man. The cardiac index is therefore a measurement which is corrected for surface area and is thus more accurate than cardiac output. It is calculated as the CO divided by the body surface area in square metres, and normal is 3.2 L/min/m².

Cardiac output can be affected by either changes in heart rate or contractility. Starling's law states that the force of contraction is proportional to the initial muscle fibre length. This initial fibre length is in turn dependent upon the degree of stretch of the ventricular muscle, or the amount that the ventricle is dilated in diastole (i.e. the venous return). As end-diastolic volume increases, the force of contraction increases until a maximum is reached after which the heart will start to fail (Fig. 10.8).

Factors affecting end-diastolic volume (also called preload) are those factors that control effective blood volume (i.e. the total blood volume), body position (pooling of blood in the lower limbs in the upright posture) and pumping action of muscles in the leg which encourages the venous return. Venous tone also affects the effective blood volume. The veins are the capacitance vessels of the circulation. If venous tone is increased, venous return is also increased. Intrathoracic pressure is also important. If intrathoracic pressure is high, as in patients who are being artificially ventilated, blood does not return so effectively to the heart. When patients have a pericardial effusion, intrapericardial pressure may be high, the heart cannot dilate and ventricular filling is impaired, so cardiac output falls. Atrial systole, as described above, contributes to one-third of ventricular filling.

Fig. 10.8 shows one curve relating ventricular performance to end-diastolic volume. However, one can also draw a series of such curves (Fig. 10.9) showing how ventricular performance may be increased without change in end-diastolic volume. Such an increase from a lower to higher curve represents an increase in contractility. This is seen in treatment with digoxin and other 'inotropic' agents such as β-adrenergic catecholamines (e.g. adrenaline (epinephrine) and isoprenaline). A decrease in contractility is seen with drugs such as β-adrenergic blocking agents (e.g. propranolol)

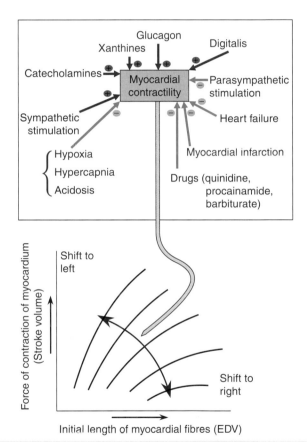

Fig. 10.9 Effect of changes in myocardial contractility on the Frank–Starling curve. The major factors influencing contractility are summarised on the right. (*Source*: From Khurana I., Khurana A., 2015. *Textbook of Medical Physiology*, 2nd edn. Elsevier India, New Delhi).

which pharmacologically depress myocardial activity and in pathological states such as hypoxia, hypercapnia, acidosis and in patients who have lost myocardial tissue after a myocardial infarction or with systolic hypertension. Systemic arterial pressure is a major component of afterload, the resistance against which the heart must work to pump out blood.

CHANGES IN BLOOD VOLUME AND CARDIAC OUTPUT DURING PREGNANCY

During pregnancy, plasma volume increases from the non-pregnant level of 2600 mL to about 3800 mL (Fig. 10.10).

This increase starts in early pregnancy and reaches a maximum around 32 weeks' gestation. The red cell mass also increases steadily until term from a non-pregnant level of 1400 mL to 1650 to 1800 mL. However, since plasma volume increases proportionately more than red cell mass, the haematocrit and haemoglobin concentration fall during pregnancy. A haemoglobin level of 105 g/L is typical during healthy pregnancy.

Cardiac output also rises by about 40% from about 4.5 to 6 L/min. This rise starts in early pregnancy and reaches a maximal plateau between 24 and 30 weeks of gestation. The rise is maintained through labour, and declines to prepregnancy levels over the next 2 to 6 weeks after childbirth. If the patient is studied lying supine, the gravid uterus constricts the inferior vena cava, and decreases the venous return, thus falsely decreasing cardiac output. This is also the mechanism of supine hypotension seen when some pregnant women lie flat on their backs at the end of pregnancy and can contribute to fetal distress.

The gestational increase in cardiac output is through a combination of increased heart rate by about 20%, and an increase in stroke volume. The increase in cardiac output is more than is necessary to distribute the extra 30 to 50 mL of oxygen consumed per minute in pregnancy. Therefore, the arteriovenous oxygen gradient decreases in pregnancy.

Fig. 10.11 indicates the distribution of the increase in cardiac output seen in pregnancy. At term, about 400 mL/min goes to the uterus and about 300 mL/min extra goes to the kidneys. The increase in skin blood flow could be as much as 500 mL/min. The remaining 300 mL would be distributed among the gastrointestinal tract, breasts and the other extra metabolic needs of pregnancy, such as respiratory muscle and cardiac muscle. Cardiac output, renal blood flow and blood flow to most other maternal organs occurs before an increase in uterine blood flow. It is the mother preparing her body for the demands of an enlarging placenta and fetus in the second half of pregnancy.

BLOOD PRESSURE CONTROL

Blood pressure is proportional to cardiac output and peripheral resistance. Peripheral resistance is controlled neurogenically by the autonomic nervous system, and directly by substances that act on blood vessels: (e.g. angiotensin II, serotonin, kinins, nitric oxide, endothelial-derived hyperpolarising factor, catecholamines, adenosine, potassium, H^+, PCO_2, PO_2 and prostaglandins).

From the Poiseuille formula the flow (f) in a tube of radius (r) and length (L) is governed by the relation:

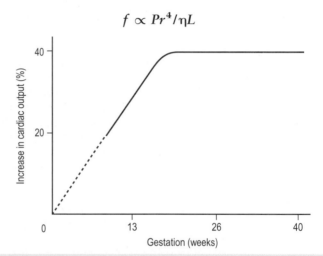

$$f \propto Pr^4/\eta L$$

Fig. 10.10 Changes in cardiac output through pregnancy. Note that cardiac output is considerably increased by the end of the first trimester, and the increase is maintained until term. (*Source*: From Rankin J., 2017. *Physiology in Childbearing: With Anatomy and Related Biosciences*, 4th edn. Elsevier Ltd, Oxford).

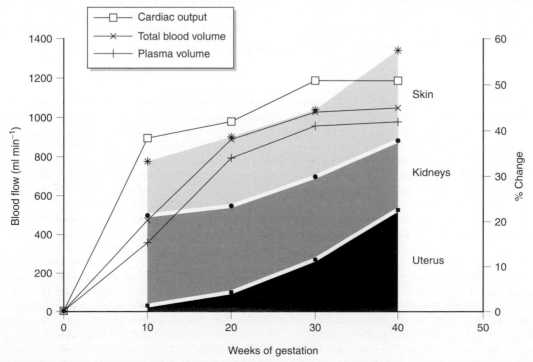

Fig. 10.11 Distribution of increased cardiac output during pregnancy. (*Source*: From Thompson J., Moppett I., Wiles M., 2019. *Smith and Aitkenhead's Textbook of Anaesthesia*, 7th edn. Elsevier Ltd., Edinburgh).

where P is the pressure gradient and η the viscosity of the fluid. Flow and peripheral resistance are therefore extremely sensitive to blood vessel radius. A 5% increase in vessel radius increases flow and decreases resistance by 21%. In blood, which is not a Newtonian fluid, viscosity rises markedly when the haematocrit rises above 45%. Such a marked increase in viscosity therefore causes a considerable reduction in blood flow.

Autonomic Nervous System and Blood Pressure Control

Receptors involved in blood pressure control in blood vessels and the heart are shown in Table 10.3. Both cholinergic and α- and β-adrenergic receptors are involved. The major tonic effect is adrenergic vasoconstriction, and vasodilatation is largely achieved by a reduction in vasoconstrictor tone rather than active vasodilatation.

The action of the autonomic system in controlling blood pressure is governed by the cardioinhibitory and vasomotor centres. The cardioinhibitory centre is the dorsal motor nucleus of the vagus nerve. Impulses pass from the cardioinhibitory centre via the vagus nerve to the heart, causing bradycardia and decreasing contractility. These effects reduce cardiac output and therefore blood pressure. The input to the cardioinhibitory centre is from the baroreceptors (see later). An increase in baroreceptor firing rate stimulates the cardioinhibitory centre and so produces reflex slowing of the heart and a reduction in blood pressure. The cardioinhibitory centre also receives inputs from other centres, so that pain and emotion can both increase vagal tone. If the vagal stimulation caused by pain and/or emotion is severe enough, blood pressure is decreased to the point where cerebral perfusion is impaired and the subject faints.

Sympathetic output to the heart and blood vessels is controlled by the vasomotor centre. The input to the vasomotor centre is from the baroreceptors; a *fall* in baroreceptor activity is associated with increased output from the vasomotor centre, thus increasing blood pressure. The vasomotor centre also receives fibres from the aortic carotid body chemoreceptors so that a fall in the P_{O_2} or pH or a rise in the P_{CO_2} will stimulate the vasomotor centre and cause a rise in blood pressure. In addition, baroreceptors in the floor of the fourth ventricle, which are sensitive to cerebrospinal fluid (CSF) pressure, innervate the vasomotor centre. These act so that a rise in CSF pressure causes an equal rise in blood pressure (Cushing reflex). Pain and emotion can also stimulate the vasomotor centre as well as the cardioinhibitory centre. Therefore, these stimuli can cause a rise in blood pressure, as well as a fall in blood pressure.

The carotid sinus baroreceptor is located at the bifurcation of the internal carotid artery. Fibres of the glossopharyngeal nerve carry impulses at frequencies that, within certain limits, are proportional to the instantaneous pressure in the carotid artery. In experimental animals at pressures below 70 mmHg, the receptors do not fire at all. Between 70 and 150 mmHg the receptors fire with increasing frequency as the blood pressure rises. This frequency reaches a maximum at 150 mmHg. Therefore, the carotid sinus baroreceptors can modulate blood pressure between 70 and 150 mmHg, but not outside this range. In patients with hypertension, the baroreceptors adapt and shift upwards the pressures over which they respond.

Local Control of Blood Flow

Metabolites that accumulate during anaerobic metabolism cause vasodilatation. This allows tissues to autoregulate their blood flow; vasodilatation allows an increased blood flow and decreases the tendency for anaerobic metabolism. The metabolites involved are hydrogen ions, potassium, lactate, adenosine (in heart but not skeletal muscle) and carbon dioxide. In addition, hypoxia itself causes vasodilatation.

Another form of autoregulation is the myogenic reflex. If the perfusion pressure in the arteriole decreases, thus tending to decrease local blood flow, the smooth muscle in the arteriole relaxes allowing vasodilatation and an increase in local blood flow. The converse occurs at high perfusion pressures: arteriolar smooth muscle then contracts, causing vasoconstriction, and a reduction in blood flow to offset the high perfusion pressure. Note that these changes induced by the myogenic reflex maintain local blood flow but will exacerbate changes in systemic blood pressure.

Other substances affecting the blood vessels locally are prostaglandins derived enzymatically from fatty acids. The cyclooxygenase pathway creates either prostaglandins or thromboxane from the intermediate phospholipase A2, whereas the lipoxygenase pathway forms leukotrienes. The cyclooxygenases (COX1 and COX2) are located in blood vessels, the kidney and stomach. Technically, prostaglandins are hormones though are rarely classified as such but are known as mediators which have profound physiological effects. Prostaglandins are found in virtually all tissues and act on a variety of cells but most notably endothelium, platelets, uterine and mast cells. Prostaglandin E and prostaglandin A cause a fall in blood pressure by reducing splanchnic vascular resistance. Prostaglandin F causes uterine contraction and bronchoconstriction. Prostacyclin, the levels of which increase considerably in pregnancy and which is produced by blood vessels and the fetoplacental unit, causes a marked vasodilatation, which will cause a fall in blood pressure unless the cardiac output also increases. Thromboxane derived from platelets causes vasoconstriction.

Nitric oxide is an endothelium-derived vasodilator generated from the conversion of L-arginine to L-citrulline by nitric oxide synthase, whilst endothelin is a 21-amino-acid peptide derived from endothelium that is a powerful vasoconstrictor. Another potent vasoconstricting agent is angiotensin II, produced under the influence of renin. Renin is an enzyme largely produced by the juxtaglomerular apparatus of the kidney, but also by the pregnant uterus. It cleaves the peptide bond between the leucine and valine residues of angiotensinogen forming the decapeptide angiotensin I, which itself has no biological activity. The stimuli to renin secretion are β-adrenergic agonists, hyponatraemia, hypovolaemia, whether induced by bleeding or changes in posture, and pregnancy. A similar but smaller rise in renin levels is also seen in patients taking oestrogen-containing contraceptive pills. Angiotensin I is then converted to the intensely vasoconstrictive angiotensin II in the lungs, by angiotensin-converting enzyme (ACE), which removes a further two amino acid residues. Angiotensin II has a number of effects throughout the body other than its vasoconstrictive properties. It has prothrombotic potential due to its adhesion and aggregation of platelets and production of

PAI-1 and PAI-2. It also affects blood volume in a number of ways. Angiotensin II increases thirst sensation, decreases the response to the baroreceptor reflex and increases the desire for salt. It has a direct effect on the proximal tubules of the kidney to increase Na⁺ absorption as well as complex and variable effects on glomerular filtration and renal blood flow. In addition, angiotensin II also stimulates aldosterone production from the zona glomerulosa of the adrenal gland, and this will, in turn, cause a rise in blood volume, and blood pressure over the longer term, by sodium retention. In the luteal phase of the menstrual cycle, elevated plasma angiotensin II levels are responsible for the elevated aldosterone levels found.

All three levels of the renin–angiotensin–aldosterone system (RAAS) are now being targeted by drugs in order to reduce blood pressure. The action of angiotensin II is blocked by angiotensin receptor-blocking drugs (ARBs), whereas the ACE is inhibited by the ACE inhibitors (ACEis) and other similar drugs. Most recently, direct renin inhibitors, such as aliskiren, are now available for use alone or in direct combination with an ACEis or ARB. Unfortunately, ACEis and ARBs are associated with major congenital anomalies of the fetus and should not be taken by the pregnant mother.

BLOOD PRESSURE CHANGES IN PREGNANCY

The marked gestational rise in cardiac output is associated with an initial fall rather than a rise in maternal blood pressure. This can be explained by a decrease in total peripheral vascular resistance, which accommodates the increased blood flow to the uterus, kidney, skin and other organs (see Fig. 10.11).

The decreased peripheral vascular resistance does not always keep strictly in proportion with the increase in cardiac output and a fall in blood pressure if often noted in early pregnancy as peripheral resistance falls by more than cardiac output rises. There is then only a small reduction of 1 mmHg in the median systolic and diastolic blood pressure from 12 to 19 weeks. Blood pressure subsequently rises until term with the median systolic blood pressure increasing by up to 9 mmHg and median diastolic blood pressure by up to 10 mmHg to a maximum in healthy pregnancy of 145/95 mmHg at term. Heart rate typically increases during pregnancy with 10% of healthy pregnant women having a heart rate >100 bpm at 18 weeks' gestation and >105 bpm at 28 weeks' gestation (Fig. 10.12). Other factors affecting blood pressure are posture and uterine contractions, which act via the changes in cardiac output already described. Uterine contractions expel blood from the uterus, increase cardiac output and increase blood pressure. The supine position, by causing vena caval obstruction, decreases cardiac output and will decrease blood pressure.

Endothelium in Pregnancy

The endothelium is a single cell layer that lines the internal surface of all blood vessels and plays a far more important role than that of a barrier between intra- and extravascular spaces. The endothelium controls vascular permeability, it determines vascular tone of the underlying smooth muscle

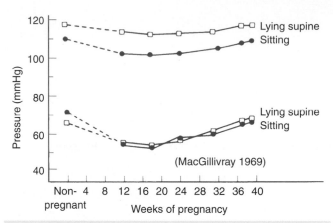

Fig. 10.12 Effect of pregnancy on systolic and diastolic blood pressure as found by MacGillivray. (*Source*: Reproduced with permission from Hytten F, Chamberlain G. *Clinical physiology in obstetrics*. Blackwell Scientific, Oxford.)

and plays a major role in the inflammatory response. In normal pregnancy, the endothelium undergoes many subtle changes in function which contribute to the maintenance of normal cardiovascular function in mother and fetus. The onset of similar cardiovascular changes during the luteal phase of the menstrual cycle suggests that maternal rather than feto-placental factors initiate the vasodilatation associated with early pregnancy. There is now clear evidence that maternal endothelium plays a major role in this adaptation of the cardiovascular system to pregnancy.

ENDOTHELIUM AS A BARRIER

The endothelium provides a passive barrier between blood and extravascular compartments, and prevents easy passage of erythrocytes and leucocytes. Transduction of fluid and small molecules occurs in accordance with the balance of Starling's forces (see p. 12); hydrostatic (blood) pressure favours fluid transfer out of the vessel and plasma oncotic pressure provides the predominant breaking force which limits outward flow. It is also now accepted that an almost invisible layer positioned above the cells in the lumen, the glycocalyx, provides another 'ultrafilter', which contributes to the molecular selectivity of the endothelium. The high incidence of oedema in normal pregnancy is likely to be the result of increased fluid transfer across the endothelium. It is currently uncertain whether the oedema arises from a simple increase in the balance of transcapillary hydrostatic pressure favouring outward fluid transduction or from a combination of this and increased fluid conductivity.

ENDOTHELIUM AS A MODULATOR OF VASCULAR TONE

The endothelium (Fig. 10.13) synthesises a number of potent vasoactive factors that can influence the tone of the underlying vascular smooth muscle. Vasodilators include nitric oxide, prostacyclin and endothelium-derived hyperpolarising factor. Constrictor factors include endothelin, angiotensin and thromboxane. All of these factors are involved in the vasodilatation of healthy pregnancy.

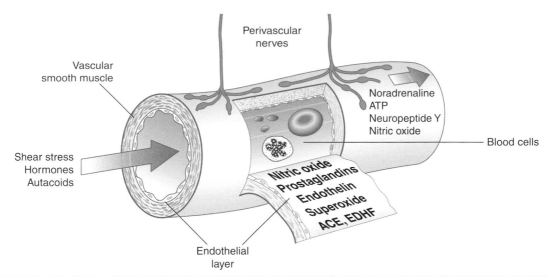

Fig. 10.13 Vascular smooth muscle tone is under the influence of endocrine, autocrine and neuronal factors. The endothelium contributes through the synthesis of locally active vasodilatory factors including nitric oxide, prostaglandin, prostacyclin and the uncharacterised endothelium-derived hyperpolarising factor *(EDHF)*. Under physiological conditions these predominate over the endothelium-derived vasoconstrictors endothelin and the prostanoid, thromboxane. Local activity of angiotensin-converting enzyme *(ACE)* in the endothelial cell may also contribute to vasoconstrictor activity through angiotensin II synthesis, as may the production of superoxide anions, which act by quenching nitric oxide.

Endothelium-Derived Vasodilators

Nitric Oxide. Nitric oxide (NO) is an inorganic molecule synthesised within the endothelium to relax underlying vascular smooth muscle. Endothelial nitric oxide synthase (eNOS) is one of three NOS isoforms that catalyses the conversion of L-arginine to NO and the co-product L-citrulline. Nitric oxide evokes relaxation in vascular smooth muscle through activation of soluble guanylate cyclase and subsequent stimulation of cyclic guanosine monophosphate (cGMP). Increased activity of the L-arginine–NO pathway is evident in healthy human pregnancy but does not appear to be diminished in the vasoconstricted state of pre-eclampsia.

Nitric oxide has a short half-life and cannot easily be measured directly. Other indirect methods have therefore been employed to evaluate its role in pregnancy. In human pregnancy, urinary concentrations of cGMP increase early in pregnancy and remain elevated until term. It is unclear whether plasma cGMP changes during normal pregnancy. A confounding issue is that cGMP is also a second messenger for atrial natriuretic peptide (ANP). However, the circulating concentration of ANP does not rise until the third trimester, long after the increase in urinary cGMP.

In vivo studies provide the most compelling evidence that NO synthase is upregulated in the maternal peripheral circulation during normal pregnancy. Infusion of the NO synthase inhibitor, L-NMMA, into the brachial artery causes a greater reduction of hand and forearm blood flow in pregnancy compared with that in non-pregnant women. Normal pregnancy is also associated with enhanced endothelium-dependent flow-mediated vasodilatation in the brachial artery and isolated vessels. All of these studies support the view that basal and stimulated NOS activity contributes to the fall in peripheral vascular resistance during a healthy pregnancy. Furthermore, circulating levels of an endogenous inhibitor to NOS, asymmetrical dimethylarginine (ADMA), fall during a healthy pregnancy in association with a gestational fall in blood pressure.

Prostacyclin. Prostacyclin (PGI$_2$) is a vasodilator derived from the arachidonic acid pathway after conversion by cyclo-oxygenase. In common with NO, PGI$_2$ has a short half-life and evaluation of PGI$_2$ synthesis depends on the measurement of stable metabolites (e.g. 6-oxo-PGF$_1$). The high circulating concentrations of these metabolites during pregnancy does not necessarily indicate that PGI$_2$ is the predominant vasodilator in pregnancy. This conclusion is upheld by studies in pregnant animals and women in which infusion of the cyclo-oxygenase inhibitor indometacin was shown not to affect blood pressure or peripheral vascular resistance. In sheep, PGI$_2$ biosynthesis seems to be increased preferentially in the uterine circulation during pregnancy, possibly in response to elevated angiotensin II. Pregnancy in the ewe is also associated with a dramatic rise in the expression of COX-1 mRNA and protein in the uterine artery endothelium.

Endothelium-Derived Hyperpolarising Factor. Nitric oxide and prostacyclin do not account for all agonist-induced endothelium-derived vasodilatation. The residual vasodilatation is abolished by potassium channel blockers or by a depolarising concentration of potassium ions, so this factor has become known as endothelium-derived hyperpolarising factor (EDHF). As the name implies, it causes hyperpolarisation of the underlying vascular smooth muscle. Hyperpolarisation, in turn, provokes relaxation. While the existence of an EDHF is indisputable, its variable nature and mechanisms of action has meant that any singular and distinct chemical identification is not possible. For this reason, it is more appropriate to consider EDHF as representing a mechanism of action, rather than a specific factor.

EDHF is most evident in small arteries where it is influential in controlling organ blood flow and blood pressure, especially when NO production is compromised. Intriguingly, there are gender differences with the effects of EDHF. For example, in mice where eNOS and COX-1 have been deleted, blood pressure changes little in females, but males become hypertensive. Due to the nature of its actions, EDHF has not been widely studied in humans. Nitric oxide is, however, undoubtedly the predominant endothelium-derived relaxing factor. Increased synthesis of a vascular EDHF has been described in animal and human pregnancy, and so may play a role in peripheral vasodilatation.

Vascular Endothelial Growth Factor. Vascular endothelial growth factor (VEGF) has potent angiogenic and mitogenic actions. It induces nitric oxide synthase in endothelial cells and is likely to play a part in decreasing vascular tone and blood pressure in healthy pregnancy. The VEGF family of proteins includes VEGF/VEGF-A, VEGF-B, VEGF-C, VEGF-D and VEGF-E. VEGF is a homodimeric 34- to 42-kDa glycoprotein, which in normal tissues is expressed in a number of cell types, including activated macrophages and smooth muscle cells. VEGF-A is expressed in syncytiotrophoblast cells and, along with VEGF-C, is also present in the cytotrophoblast. VEGF interacts through three different receptors: VEGFR-1 (FMS-like tyrosine kinase 1, Flt-1), VEGFR-2 (KDR/Flk-1) and VEGFR-3 (Flt-4), which mediate different functions within endothelial cells. VEGFR 1 and 3 are expressed on invasive cytotrophoblast cells in early pregnancy.

Soluble Flt-1 (sFlt-1) is a soluble form of VEGFR-1 secreted by endothelial cells, monocytes and the placental trophoblast. sFlt-1 can bind, and therefore inactivate, VEGF and placental growth factor (PlGF) thereby mediating an anti-angiogenic effect. sFlt-1 is present in only small concentrations in the serum of non-pregnant females and males. Higher levels are detectable in healthy pregnant women towards term but become pathologically elevated prior to the clinical onset of pre-eclampsia.

There have been conflicting results relating to changes in VEGF levels in pregnancy, as a consequence of difficulties in measuring free as opposed to bound VEGF. Levels appear to be lower in the vasoconstricted state of pre-eclampsia.

Placental Growth Factor. PlGF is a member of the VEGF family and is also distantly related to the platelet-derived growth factor (PDGF) family. PlGF is a 149-amino-acid mature protein with a 21-amino-acid signal sequence and a centrally located PDGF-like domain. It shares a 42% sequence homology with VEGF, and the two are structurally similar. PlGF has angiogenic properties, enhancing survival, growth and migration of endothelial cells *in vitro*, and promotes vessel formation in certain *in-vivo* models. It is thus regarded as a central component in regulating vascular function.

PlGF was first identified in the human placenta and is expressed in greatest quantities under normal conditions. It is important in placental development, as it is present in high concentrations within villous cytotrophoblastic tissue and the syncytiotrophoblast. PlGF concentrations increase throughout pregnancy, peaking during the third trimester, and falling thereafter, probably as a consequence of placental maturation. Low levels of PlGF are evident up to 6 weeks before the clinical onset of pre-eclampsia.

Thromboxane

Human pregnancy is associated with increased synthesis of the vasoconstrictor prostanoid, thromboxane (TXA_2), as assessed by measurement of its stable systemic metabolite 2,3-dinor-TXB_2. Thromboxane is mainly derived from platelets and increases three- to fivefold during pregnancy.

Endothelin

The family of endothelins includes endothelin-1 (ET-1) which plays the predominant physiological role in the control of vascular tone. ET-1 is cleaved from a larger precursor polypeptide, big-endothelin, by the action of membrane-bound enzymes, the endothelin-converting enzymes. The plasma concentration of ET-1 is very low or undetectable in maternal plasma and not affected by healthy pregnancy. Endothelin may however play a role in constriction of the umbilical circulation at birth. Paradoxically, binding of endothelin to a receptor subtype, the ET_B receptor, in the endothelium can lead to vasodilatation through stimulus of nitric oxide release. Studies in rats have suggested that this mechanism may play a role in the increase in renal blood flow in pregnancy.

Angiotensin II

Angiotensin II (AII) was once considered to be synthesised predominantly in the pulmonary circulation, in which ACE activity is high, but it is now known to be widely synthesised in endothelium. In a normal pregnancy, despite a dramatic increase in activity of the renin–angiotensin–aldosterone axis, there is a well-documented blunting of the pressor response to angiotensin II, which may contribute to lowering of peripheral vascular resistance.

OESTROGEN AND THE ENDOTHELIUM

High oestrogen levels have far-reaching systemic effects on pregnant women. They include changes to serum lipoprotein concentrations, coagulation factors, antioxidant activity and vascular tone. Oestrogen has two direct effects on blood vessels: rapid vasodilatation (5 to 20 min after exposure) and chronic (hours to days) protection against vascular injury and atherosclerosis. The rapid vasodilatory effects of oestrogen are non-genomic (i.e. they do not involve changes in gene expression of vasodilator substances). There are two functionally distinct oestrogen receptors (ERs), α and β. ER-α a receptors on the endothelial cell membrane can directly activate NOS. A study of ER knockout mice has confirmed a role for ERs in NO synthesis. The non-genomic mechanism by which oestrogen rapidly activates NOS has not been fully elucidated. Animal studies suggest that involvement of the endothelium in the vasodilatation induced by longer-term exposure to oestrogen is similar to that seen during pregnancy. Enhanced NO-mediated relaxation in the sheep uterine artery induced by oestrogens is associated with greater NOS enzymatic activity.

Clinical evidence that supports a vasodilatory role for oestrogens has mainly come from studies on postmenopausal women given exogenous oestrogen. For example, 17β-oestradiol potentiates endothelium-dependent vasodilatation in the forearm and coronary arteries of postmenopausal women. Oestrogen can also act directly on vascular smooth muscle, independent of the endothelium, by opening calcium-activated potassium channels. Furthermore, 17β-oestradiol may also decrease synthesis of the superoxide free radical, and thereby prolong the half-life of pre-existing NO.

Much less is known about the vascular effects of progesterone. Circulating progesterone levels increase by a similar amount to 17β-oestradiol and may play a role in reducing pressor responsiveness to angiotensin II.

ENDOTHELIUM AND HAEMOSTASIS

In anticipation of haemorrhage at childbirth, normal pregnancy is characterised by low-grade, chronic activation of coagulation within both the maternal and utero-placental circulations. The endothelium is directly involved in promoting a procoagulant state in healthy pregnancy. During the third trimester, plasma levels of endothelium-derived von Willebrand factor are elevated, promoting coagulation and platelet adhesion. Circulating levels of clotting factors, especially fibrinogen, factor V and factor VIII, are increased, while there is a gestational fall in the level of the endogenous anticoagulant, protein S. Furthermore, endothelial production of both plasminogen activator inhibitor (PAI-1) and tissue plasminogen activator (t-PA) are increased during pregnancy, with the effect of both inhibition and promotion of fibrinolysis, respectively. The procoagulant state of the endothelium therefore is to some extent compensated by upregulation of the fibrinolytic system.

ENDOTHELIUM AND INFLAMMATION

A healthy pregnancy stimulates a generalised inflammatory response. Not only do peripheral blood leucocytes develop a more inflammatory phenotype than in non-gravid women, but the expression of leucocyte adhesion molecules on the endothelium also increases. It has recently been shown that these inflammatory changes are even more pronounced during pre-eclampsia. Further details of the complex immune interactions involving many different immune cell types can be found in Chapter 8.

PRE-ECLAMPSIA

Relative to the vasodilated, plasma-expanded state of women in healthy pregnancy, pre-eclampsia is a vasoconstricted, plasma-contracted condition with evidence of intravascular coagulation. Whereas healthy maternal endothelium is crucial for the physiological adaptation to normal pregnancy, the multiple organ failure of severe pre-eclampsia is characterised by widespread endothelial cell dysfunction. The endothelium of women destined to develop pre-eclampsia both fails to adapt properly and can be further damaged during a pre-eclamptic pregnancy. Prior to the onset of clinically identifiable disease, women destined to develop pre-eclampsia show evidence of poor placentation, high uteroplacental resistance and abnormal placental function. Measurement of sFlt-1 and PlGF in mid-pregnancy, in particular the sFlt-1:PlGF ratio can be helpful in the assessment of a woman with suspected pre-eclampsia. A normal ratio is reassuring with a high negative predictive value for pre-eclampsia in the subsequent 1 to 2 weeks. Pre-eclampsia eventuates when reduced placental perfusion is associated with endothelial abnormalities in the mother. Women with risk factors for cardiovascular disease such as hypertension, diabetes mellitus and hyperlipidaemia are predisposed to pre-eclampsia and at risk of these conditions following a pre-eclamptic pregnancy.

Endothelial Dysfunction in Pre-Eclampsia

Damaged endothelial cells in pre-eclampsia (Fig. 10.14) cause increased capillary permeability, platelet thrombosis and increased vascular tone. Evidence of endothelial cell damage prior to clinical manifestation of pre-eclampsia can be demonstrated by the presence of markers of endothelial cell activation. Specifically, levels of fibronectin and factor VIII-related antigen are elevated. Furthermore, women with endothelial cell damage secondary to pre-existing hypertension or other microvascular disease have a higher incidence of pre-eclampsia than normotensive women.

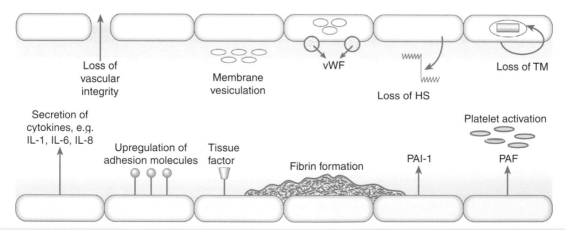

Fig. 10.14 The vascular endothelium in pre-eclampsia shows many of the characteristics of the inflammatory state of 'endothelial cell activation'. Upon stimulation by inflammatory cytokines the endothelium undergoes a series of metabolic changes leading to loss of vascular integrity, prothrombotic changes (*HS*, Loss of heparan sulphate; *TM*, loss of thrombomodulin; *PAI-1*, release of plasminogen activator inhibitor; *PAF*, platelet activating factor; *vWF*, tissue factor and von Willebrand factor), secretion of cytokines and upregulation of leucocyte adhesion molecules. The cell adhesion molecules promote the adhesion and migration of leucocytes across the endothelium and so contribute to the inflammatory process.

Nitric Oxide in Pre-Eclampsia

Nitric oxide synthase activity is competively inhibited by an endogenous guanidino-substituted arginine analogue, $N^G N^G$-dimethylarginine (ADMA). During pre-eclampsia, ADMA levels are significantly higher compared with gestation-matched, normotensive controls. Consequently, endogenous inhibition of NOS by a specific inhibitor is a possible mechanism whereby NO production could be reduced in pre-eclampsia.

In-vivo studies of forearm blood flow have suggested that a reduction in NO is unlikely to be involved in the vasoconstriction characteristic of pre-eclampsia. In contrast, *in-vitro* studies on isolated arteries from women with pre-eclampsia have generally reported reduced endothelium-dependent relaxation, although the role of NOS has not always been identified. One explanation for these differences is that women have a high cardiac output before the onset of clinical pre-eclampsia, suggesting a possible role for increased nitric oxide synthase activity in a hyperdynamic circulation.

Prostanoids in Pre-Eclampsia

In contrast to a normal pregnancy, pre-eclampsia is associated with relative underproduction of the vasodilatory PGI_2 and overabundance of the vasoconstrictor TXA_2. The imbalance between the synthesis of these prostanoids formed the rationale for investigations of 'low-dose aspirin' therapy for prevention of pre-eclampsia. Low-dose aspirin up to 150 mg taken each evening preferentially inhibits synthesis of TXA_2 over PGI_2. This may explain why low-dose aspirin is an effective prophylaxis against early onset pre-eclampsia.

Prothrombotic States

Stimulation of the coagulation cascade in response to endothelial cell damage may be more likely in women who have a predisposition to thrombosis. A number of studies have suggested that patients with inherited thrombophilias are more likely to develop pre-eclampsia compared with women who have normal clotting parameters.

Aetiology of Maternal Endothelial Dysfunction in Pre-Eclampsia

How poor placentation and the resultant poor uterine blood flow with placental ischaemia leads to the maternal syndrome of pre-eclampsia, characterised by widespread endothelial cell damage, remains uncertain. Several factors appear to be important and are likely to be variably important in individual women. Soluble Flt-1, soluble endoglin and possibly angiotensin II type-1 receptor autoantibodies have all been shown to be elevated in women who go on to develop pre-eclampsia. These factors contribute to endothelial dysfunction, inflammation and increased reactive oxygen species. In contrast, PlGF levels are reduced in women who go on to develop pre-eclampsia, also highlighting the imbalance between angiogenic and anti-angiogenic factors in this syndrome. Leucocyte activation, proinflammatory cytokines, trophoblast fragments and prothrombotic states may also increase a woman's risk of pre-eclampsia.

Classical risk factors for cardiovascular disease are evident in women before they develop pre-eclampsia. It is no surprise therefore that women who have had pre-eclampsia have an increased risk of cardiovascular disease in later life. It seems unlikely that the brief time a woman has pre-eclampsia causes irreparable harm to make her vulnerable to future cardiovascular disease.

CONCLUSION

In conclusion, the endothelium plays a central role in the maternal adaptation to a healthy human pregnancy. The peripheral circulation of the healthy mother is vasodilated, prothrombotic and proinflammatory. However, endothelial dysfunction is a characteristic of pre-eclampsia as demonstrated by increased capillary permeability, intravascular coagulation and vasoconstriction leading to multi-organ ischaemia. The ischaemic placenta is the likely source of an imbalance between angiogenic and antiangiogenic factors that perpetuate this cycle of endothelial damage until delivery of the fetus and placenta rescues the situation. Women who have had pre-eclampsia will be at increased risk of cardiovascular disease in the future.

Respiration

THE LUNGS, VENTILATION AND ITS CONTROL

Respiration is the process whereby the body takes in oxygen and eliminates carbon dioxide. This section will consider the action of the lungs and transport of oxygen and carbon dioxide to peripheral tissues.

Gas composition

Table 10.6 shows the partial pressures of dry air, inspired air, alveolar air and expired air at body temperature and normal atmospheric pressure (760 mmHg or 101.1 kPa, where 100 mmHg = 13.3 kPa). Dry air consists of oxygen, nitrogen and a little carbon dioxide. We do not normally breathe completely dry air, and inspired air usually has some water vapour (partial pressure 5.7 mmHg). Alveolar air is fully saturated with water (47 mmHg) and is in equilibrium with pulmonary venous blood. The small difference in the Po_2 between alveolar air (100 mmHg) and pulmonary venous blood (98 mmHg) shows the efficiency of gas exchange in the healthy lung. Expired air is a mixture of alveolar air and inspired air with regard

Table 10.6 Partial Pressures of Gases (mmHg)[a] in a Resting, Healthy Human at Sea Level (Barometric Pressure = 760 mmHg)

	Dry Air	Inspired Air	Alveolar Air	Expired Air
Po_2	159.1 (21%)	158.0	100.0	116.0
Pco_2	0.3 (0.04%)	0.3	40.0	26.8
PH_2O	0.0 (0%)	5.7	47.0	47.0
PN_2[b]	600.6 (79%)	596.0	573.0	569.9
Total	760.0	760.0	760.0	759.7

[a]1 kPa = 7.5 mmHg.
[b]Includes small amounts of rare gases.

to oxygen and carbon dioxide concentrations. As a result of this mixture, the partial pressure of nitrogen is less in expired air (570 mmHg) than in inspired air (596 mmHg). The total volume of alveolar air is about 2 L; alveolar ventilation is about 350 mL for each breath. Alveolar ventilation is therefore a small proportion of total alveolar volume, and the alveolar gas remains relatively constant in composition.

Dead Space

Although the alveolar ventilation is 350 mL/breath, the tidal volume is 500 mL/breath. The difference, 150 mL, is the anatomic dead space: the volume of air between the mouth or nose and the alveoli that does not participate in gas exchange. The anatomic dead space (mL) approximately equals body weight (in pounds avoirdupois) (1 kg = 2.2 lb). In addition, on occasion, some alveoli, particularly in the upper part of the lungs, are well ventilated, but rather poorly perfused, whereas other alveoli in the dependent lower part of the lungs are well perfused, but poorly ventilated. This mismatching of ventilation and perfusion represents a further source of wasted ventilation which, together with the anatomic dead space, makes up the total or physiological dead space. In healthy, supine individuals, the anatomic dead space nearly equals the physiological dead space. In patients who are sick with lung disease, or heart failure, the physiological dead space considerably exceeds the anatomic dead space.

Oxygen Consumption

The normal oxygen consumption at rest is about 250 mL/min. The oxygen capacity of normal blood is about 20 mL/100 mL (200 mL/L). Oxygen consumption of 250 mL/min at rest is achieved by delivering 1 L of oxygen to peripheral tissues (cardiac output, 5 L × 200 mL oxygen per litre = 1 L), of which 25% is extracted and 75% is returned to the heart in venous blood. In extreme exertion, ventilation increases to about 150 L/min. This allows oxygen delivery of 3.2 L/min with a cardiac output of 16 L/min (cardiac output, 16 L/min × oxygen capacity, 200 mL/L = 3.2 L/min). Of this, 75% is extracted and 25% is returned to the heart, giving an oxygen consumption of 2.4 L/min, almost 10 times that at rest.

Lung Volumes

The total lung capacity (Fig. 10.15) is approximately 5 L. Of this, 1.5 L, the residual volume, remains at the end of forced expiration. The volume of gas, 3.5 L, that can be inhaled from forced expiration to forced inspiration is the vital capacity. The normal tidal volume (500 mL) is a small proportion of the maximum 3.5 L that is possible. The tidal volume is situated in the middle of the vital capacity, so that the inspiratory reserve volume is approximately 1.5 L, as is the expiratory reserve volume.

Mechanics of Ventilation

The chest cavity expands by the actions of the intrathoracic musculature, innervated from T1 to T11 and the diaphragm innervated by the phrenic nerve (C3–C5). Thus the cord section below C5 still allows spontaneous ventilation because of the phrenic nerve innervation. Phrenic nerve crush, as used to be performed for the treatment of tuberculosis, still allows spontaneous ventilation because of the

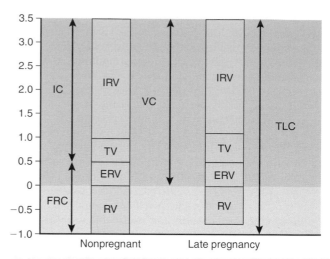

Fig. 10.15 Subdivisions of lung volume and their alterations in pregnancy. (*Source*: From Landon M., Galan H., Jauniaux E. et al, 2021. *Gabbe's Obstetrics: Normal and Problem Pregnancies*, 8th edn. Elsevier Inc., Philadelphia).

action of thoracic musculature. Damage to the spinal cord above the level of C3 needs permanent artificial ventilation since both the phrenic nerve and thoracic innervation are inactivated.

At rest, the pressure in the potential space between the visceral pleura and the parietal pleura is −3 mmHg (i.e. 3 mmHg) less than atmospheric pressure. This pressure can be determined by connecting a balloon catheter with the balloon in the oesophagus at the level of the mediastinum to a pressure transducer. During quiet inspiration, the chest expands and the pressure in the intrapleural space decreases to −6 mmHg. This pressure gradient is sufficient to overcome the elastic recoil of the lung, which therefore expands following the chest wall. In forced inspiration, the pressure in the intrapleural space may fall to as low as 30 mmHg. Expiration is passive; the muscles of the diaphragm and chest wall relax, and the elastic recoil of the lung causes the lung and therefore the chest to contract. Forced expiration may be associated with muscular effort and a positive intrapleural pressure.

Resistance to Air Flow

The rapidity with which expiration occurs depends on the stiffness of the lungs and the resistance of the bronchi. This is measured clinically, by determining the forced expiratory volume in 1 s (FEV_1). Since this volume depends on the vital capacity, it is most easily expressed as FEV_1/FVC (forced vital capacity). In normal individuals this ratio exceeds 75%. The ratio decreases with age. In asthma it may be as low as 25%, and the FEV_1, which in healthy individuals is about 3.0 L, is < 1 L in patients with severe asthma. An alternative measurement of airway resistance is the peak flow rate, which should be between 400 to 700 L/min. Both peak flow rate and FEV_1/FVC depend on large airway calibre and the stiffness of the lung. To measure the stiffness of the lungs independently, it is necessary to use more complicated apparatus and to determine lung compliance.

Oxygen Transfer

Oxygen is transferred across the approximately 500 million alveoli which have a total surface area of about 70 m².

Transfer occurs across the type 1 lining cells; apart from the epithelial cells, mast cells, plasma cells, macrophages and lymphocytes, the alveoli also contain type 2 granular pneumocytes, which make surfactant. The granules that these cells contain are thought to be packages of surfactant. Patients who are deficient in surfactant, such as premature infants or adults suffering from acute respiratory distress syndrome, have type 2 pneumocytes which do not contain granules. Surfactant is necessary to lower the surface tension of alveoli and maintain patency of the alveoli. In the absence of surfactant, the surface tension of the fluid in the alveoli is so high that the alveoli collapse.

Effect of Pregnancy

During pregnancy, ventilation starts to increase during the first trimester, to about 40% above non-pregnancy levels. A similar, but smaller, effect is seen in women taking contraceptive pills containing progestogens, and in the luteal phase of the menstrual cycle. It is therefore thought to be due to progesterone, which acts partly by stimulating the respiratory centre directly, and partly by increasing its sensitivity to carbon dioxide. Some women are aware of the increase in ventilation and feel breathless, others are not. The increase in ventilation is achieved by increasing the tidal volume (i.e. they breathe more deeply) rather than increasing their respiratory rate. This is a more efficient way of increasing ventilation since an increase in respiratory rate involves more work in shifting the dead space more frequently. The tidal volume therefore expands into the expiratory reserve volume and the inspiratory reserve volume (see Fig. 10.15). The consensus of opinion is that the vital capacity does not change. However, the residual volume decreases by about 200 mL, possibly due to the large intra-abdominal swelling. Therefore, the total lung capacity also decreases by about 200 mL. There is no change in FEV_1 or peak flow rate in pregnancy. The increase in ventilation is much greater than the increase in oxygen consumption, which is only about 50 mL extra at term.

The physiological hyperventilation of pregnancy causes a fall in the PCO_2 from a normal value of about 5.3 kPa (40 mmHg) to 4.1 kPa (31 mmHg). Extra bicarbonate is excreted by the kidneys so that plasma levels fall to maintain a normal pH. As bicarbonate levels fall, so too does plasma sodium. There is therefore a decrease in the total number of osmotically active ions and a fall in plasma osmolality of about 10 mosmol/kg. Such a fall in plasma osmolality would normally be associated with profound diuresis, but there is an adaptation of the hypothalamic centres governing vasopressin secretion that permits the reduced osmolality (p. 25).

During pregnancy, bronchodilator stimuli are progesterone (dilates smooth muscle) and prostaglandin E_2. Bronchoconstrictor influences are prostaglandin F_2 and the decrease in resting lung volume, which decreases the overall space available for the airways to occupy. These factors balance each other out so that there is no overall change in airway resistance.

Control of Respiration

Although several respiratory centres with different functions have been described in the midbrain on the basis of experiments performed in decerebrated or anaesthetised animals, it is not clear to what extent such localisation occurs in conscious humans. It is therefore simpler to think of one diffuse medullary respiratory centre. The respiratory centre is responsible for controlling both the depth of respiration and its rhythmicity. Respiratory neurones are of two types: inspiratory and expiratory. When the inspiratory neurones are stimulated at the respiratory centre, the expiratory neurones are inhibited and vice versa. The respiratory centre receives input from higher voluntary centres and pain and emotion will also increase ventilation, but in most healthy patients ventilation is automatic and it is not necessary to be consciously aware of the need to breathe.

The most important input to the respiratory centre comes from chemoreceptors. There are two main groups of these: (1) central chemoreceptors, possibly on the surface of the upper medulla, but separate from the medullary respiratory centre, and (2) peripheral chemoreceptors around the aortic arch and in the carotid body. The aortic arch chemoreceptors are innervated by the vagus nerve and the carotid body chemoreceptors by the glossopharyngeal nerve. The carotid body is highly specialised tissue, which has an exceedingly high blood flow rate. This makes it possible for the chemoreceptors in the carotid body to be sensitive to changes in the PO_2. The carotid body chemoreceptors are the only chemoreceptors sensitive to changes in PO_2. Carotid and aortic body chemoreceptors are also sensitive to changes in PCO_2 and pH. The central chemoreceptors are probably only sensitive to changes in the pH; any effect of a change in the PCO_2 is mediated by the ensuing pH change.

Response to Hypercapnia

If it were not for the activity of the chemoreceptors, a decrease in ventilation would be associated with a rise in the PCO_2 (curve A, Fig. 10.16) and an increase in ventilation would be associated with a decrease in the PCO_2. When the PCO_2 is <5.3 kPa (40 mmHg) this does occur. However, the activity of the respiratory centre is such that any rise in the PCO_2 above 5.3 kPa is associated with a marked increase in ventilation (curve B, Fig. 10.16). The ratio of ventilation observed (b, curve B) to ventilation expected (a, curve A) is the gain of the control system. In normal hyperoxic individuals, this ratio varies between 2 and 5. It is decreased with age and in trained athletes, and it increases in pregnancy to 8,

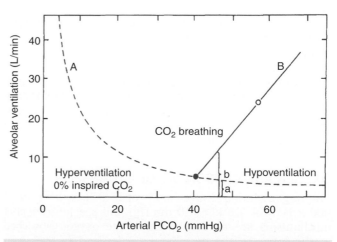

Fig. 10.16 Relations between alveolar ventilation and arterial (alveolar) partial pressure of carbon dioxide (PCO_2) at a constant rate of metabolic carbon dioxide production. See text for information on curves A, B, a, b.

thus increasing the sensitivity of the respiratory centre to carbon dioxide as indicated earlier. Hypoxia also increases respiratory centre sensitivity to carbon dioxide.

Response to Hypoxia

This is more subtle than the response to the Pco_2, since the effect of hypoxia is modulated by the effects of ventilation on the Pco_2, and by changes in the buffering ability of haemoglobin. Any increased ventilation associated with hypoxia will also be associated with a decrease in the Pco_2. A decrease in the Pco_2 will decrease respiratory drive (see Fig. 10.16) and this will therefore decrease the hyperventilation that would otherwise have been caused by falling Po_2; a fall in the Po_2 is also associated with increased quantities of deoxygenated haemoglobin. Deoxygenated haemoglobin is a better buffer than oxygenated haemoglobin, and therefore the patient becomes less acidotic. The stimulus to respiration caused by acidosis is therefore also reduced.

For these reasons, ventilation only shows marked increases when the Po_2 falls below 8 kPa (60 mmHg) (Fig. 10.17). A fall in oxygen saturation of haemoglobin of 1% is associated with an increase in ventilation of 0.6 L/min. The response is blunted by chronic hypoxia, as occurs in patients living at altitude, with cyanotic congenital heart disease or by hypercapnia due to lung disease.

Effect of Changes in Hydrogen Ion Concentration

A rise in hydrogen ion concentration causes an increase in respiration. This is due to peripheral and central stimulation of chemoreceptors. In metabolic acidosis, the increase in ventilation decreases Pco_2, which in turn decreases the hydrogen ion concentration. In metabolic alkalosis, there is a decrease in ventilation which allows the Pco_2 to rise with a consequent compensatory increase in hydrogen ion concentration.

Other inputs to the respiratory centre are from proprioceptors in the chest wall, which sense respiratory movements. An absence of respiratory movements causes stimulation of the respiratory centre. There are irritant receptors in the air passages (J receptors) and lungs which respond to foreign bodies and also stimulate respiration via the respiratory centre. These J receptors are possibly responsible for the increase in ventilation seen in patients with mild respiratory tract infections, where there is no alteration in blood gas composition.

It is not known to what extent the inflation and deflation receptors in the smooth muscle of the airways affect the control of normal respiration.

The baroreceptors have a trivial influence on respiration, in comparison to the profound effect that chemoreceptors have on the circulation. There are also receptors in the pulmonary arteries and coronary circulation, sensitive to *Veratrum* alkaloids, stimulation of which causes decreased respiration and even apnoea. This is the Bezold–Jarisch reflex.

OXYGEN AND CARBON DIOXIDE TRANSPORT

The lungs maintain an alveolar Po_2 of 13.07 kPa (98 mmHg) and a Pco_2 of 5.3 kPa (40 mmHg), but special transport mechanisms are needed to carry the oxygen absorbed at the lungs to the peripheral tissues and to transport carbon dioxide produced by the metabolism from peripheral tissues to the lungs.

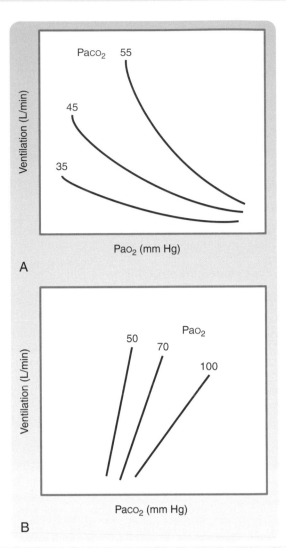

Fig. 10.17 Increase in ventilation due to hypoxia associated with low and high levels of carbon dioxide. (*Source*: From Koeppen B., Stanton B., 2018. *Berne & Levy Physiology*, 7th edn. Elsevier Inc., Philadelphia).

Oxygen Transport

The haemoglobin molecule is specially adapted to transport oxygen. Each molecule has four iron atoms which can combine reversibly with four oxygen atoms. The haemoglobin molecule can alter its shape (quaternary structure) to favour uptake or unloading of oxygen.

However, throughout this molecular adaptation the iron remains in the ferrous state and the association of haemoglobin with oxygen is therefore referred to as oxygenation. If the iron is oxidised to the ferric form, methaemoglobin is formed, which does not act as an oxygen carrier.

Each gram of haemoglobin reacts with 1.34 mL of oxygen. Therefore, 100 mL of blood containing 15 g of haemoglobin can react with 19.5 mL of oxygen. In contrast, 100 mL of blood would only contain 0.3 mL of oxygen in solution at a Po_2 of 13 kPa. Therefore, the presence of haemoglobin increases oxygen-carrying capacity 70-fold. Venous blood at a Pco_2 of 6.1 kPa contains 3.0 mL of carbon dioxide in solution, and 49.7 mL of carbon dioxide as bicarbonate. The formation of bicarbonate (see later) therefore increases carbon dioxide transport 17-fold.

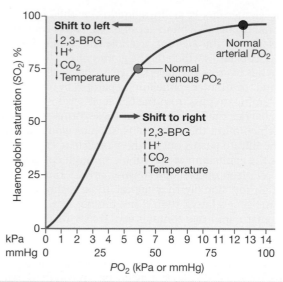

Fig. 10.18 Variations in the haemoglobin *(Hb)* oxygen dissociation curve. (A) Effect of changes in temperature. (B) Effect of changes in blood pH. (C) Hyperbolic curve of 'purified' haemoglobin A *(HbA)* (dialysed to be salt free) similar to curve of myoglobin *(Mb)*. (D) The dissociation curve of fetal blood (but not pure HbF) is to the left of adult blood containing HbA; addition of diphosphoglycerate *(DPG)* shifts curve of blood with HbA to the right and increases P_{50} (decreases affinity of oxygen for Hb and facilitates unloading of oxygen in tissues). (*Source*: From Ralston S., Penman I., Strachan M. et al, 2018. *Davidson's Principles and Practice of Medicine*, 23rd edn. Elsevier Ltd., Edinburgh).

Fig. 10.18 shows that the relationship between the P_{O_2} and oxygen saturation for haemoglobin is hyperbolic. The biggest change in saturation occurs between a P_{O_2} of 5.3 kPa (40 mmHg) and of 9.3 kPa (70 mmHg), and of course this is the change between the P_{O_2} in peripheral tissues and the P_{O_2} in the lungs. There is little change in saturation as the P_{O_2} falls from 13.3 kPa (100 mmHg) to 9.3 kPa (70 mmHg) and, in this way, haemoglobin compensates for any minor falls in the P_{O_2} associated with lung disease or a decrease in inspiratory P_{O_2} which would occur at altitude. However, both acidosis and hyperthermia shift the haemoglobin dissociation curve to the right and decrease the affinity of haemoglobin for oxygen. A fall in the pH to 7.2 or an increase in temperature to 43°C will reduce the oxygen saturation to 90% at a P_{O_2} of 13.2 kPa, and this can have a significant effect in patients who are ill with acidosis or high fever. The presence of methaemoglobin or of other abnormal haemoglobins such as haemoglobin S will also shift the dissociation curve to the right, decreasing affinity and decreasing the uptake of oxygen by haemoglobin.

The shape of the dissociation curve is also beneficial when haemoglobin unloads oxygen in peripheral tissues at a low P_{O_2}. Here acidosis (the Bohr effect) and hyperthermia, both of which will occur in metabolically active tissue, are an advantage. They decrease affinity and help haemoglobin to unload oxygen more easily. The formation of carbamino compounds by the combination of carbon dioxide and haemoglobin (see later) also shifts the curve to the right (Haldane effect) and assists unloading in metabolically active tissue. The position of the haemoglobin dissociation curve can be defined by the P_{50}, the P_{O_2} at which haemoglobin is 50% desaturated.

2,3-Diphosphoglycerate (2,3-DPG) is formed from 3-phosphoglyceraldehyde, a product of glycolysis via the Embden–Meyerhof pathway. It also affects haemoglobin dissociation in red cells and the presence of 2,3-DPG shifts the dissociation curve to the right. 2,3-DPG levels are decreased in acidosis and banked blood, but increased by androgens, thyroxine, growth hormone, anaemia, excrcise and hypoxic conditions (living at altitude and in cardiopulmonary disease). Thus, banked blood does not give up its oxygen very easily, but hypoxic individuals do unload oxygen easily, even if their low haemoglobin affinity is less favourable for oxygen uptake.

The fetus clearly needs high-affinity blood since the P_{O_2} in the fetal umbilical vein is only about 4 kPa (30 mmHg). Different mammalian species have different ways of increasing the affinity of fetal blood. In humans, fetal haemoglobin has a low oxygen affinity, but this is not the mechanism by which fetal red cells increase their affinity for oxygen. Instead, in human fetal red cells the fetal haemoglobin does not interact with 2,3-DPG, and it is this that accounts for the increased affinity of human fetal blood for oxygen.

Carbon Monoxide

Carbon monoxide has 210 times greater affinity for haemoglobin than oxygen. Therefore, if the ratio of carbon monoxide to oxygen in inspired air is 1:210, equivalent to a 0.1% concentration of carbon monoxide in air, haemoglobin will be 50% oxygenated and 50% combined with carbon monoxide (*Note* the oxygen concentration is 21%). This effect alone will reduce the oxygen capacity of haemoglobin by 50% and would be the same as giving the patient a haemoglobin concentration of 7.5 g/100 mL. However, the presence of carboxyhaemoglobin also shifts the haemoglobin dissociation curve of oxygen to the left (increased affinity) so that even the oxygen that is combined with haemoglobin is not liberated in peripheral tissues, and this accounts for the profound tissue hypoxia that occurs in carbon monoxide poisoning. It also explains why such patients are not cyanosed, because the oxygen remains combined with haemoglobin. Cyanosis is not seen until the concentration of deoxygenated haemoglobin in the blood is as low as 5 g/100 mL. The cherry-pink colour that these patients have is due to the presence of carboxyhaemoglobin.

The amount of carboxyhaemoglobin associated with smoking (5% to 8% carboxyhaemoglobin) is sufficient to shift the tissue P_{O_2} from 6 kPa (45 mmHg) to 5.3 kPa (40 mmHg). This may account for the deleterious effect of smoking on ischaemic heart disease, and also for the intrauterine growth restriction seen in the fetuses of women who smoke in pregnancy.

Carbon Dioxide Transport

Carbon dioxide is transported in the plasma, partly in solution, partly by hydration, to form carbonic acid and partly by the formation of carbamino compounds with the N-terminal end of plasma proteins. Hydration is very slow because there is no carbonic anhydrase in the plasma. Hydrogen ions are formed from both reactions, and these are buffered by plasma proteins.

Carbonic anhydrase (red cells only)

$$CO_2 + H_2O \rightleftharpoons H_2CO_3 \rightleftharpoons H^+ + HCO_3^- \quad (1)$$

$$\boxed{Protein} - NH_2 + CO_2 \longrightarrow \boxed{Protein} - N\!\!\!\begin{array}{c} H \\ \\ COOH \end{array}$$

$$\rightleftharpoons \boxed{Protein} - N\!\!\!\begin{array}{c} H \\ \\ COO^- \end{array} + H^+ \quad (2)$$

Carbon dioxide also enters the red cells and is again transported in solution, and by hydration. Hydration occurs rapidly in red cells because of the presence of carbonic anhydrase. The products of the reaction are also dealt with; hydrogen ions are buffered by the relatively high levels of deoxygenated haemoglobin, and bicarbonate ions are able to diffuse out of the red cells, into the plasma which has a relatively lower bicarbonate concentration. To maintain electrical neutrality, the chloride ions diffuse back into the red cells and this process is known as the chloride shift. The process of hydration is associated with a net increase in the total number of ions that are osmotically active, and therefore water also enters the red cells, which swell. The biconcave disc shape of the red cells allows them to swell without bursting.

In addition, carbon dioxide reacts with haemoglobin to form carbamino compounds. The carbamino compounds are fully ionised, giving a further source of hydrogen ions to be buffered by haemoglobin.

The net effect of these reactions is that two-thirds of carbon dioxide is transported in the plasma as bicarbonate, but that the majority of hydrogen ions produced are buffered in the red cells.

Urinary System

The function of the kidney is to contribute to the homeostasis of the internal environment; in particular, the kidney is concerned with salt and water balance and hence blood volume, long-term adjustments in acid–base balance, and the regulation of the blood level of certain ions, such as calcium and phosphate. The kidney is the main pathway for the elimination of nitrogenous waste products, such as urea, and some drugs, such as salicylate and heparin. It also has a major endocrine role in the production of renin, erythropoietin and the final hydroxylation to active vitamin D.

MICROANATOMY

The functional unit of the kidney is the nephron (45 to 65 mm long) (Fig. 10.19). Each healthy human kidney contains approximately 1 million nephrons. Blood is filtered at the glomerulus, which is the beginning of the nephron, and the filtrate is subsequently modified by reabsorption or secretion in its passage through the nephron. Urine is the result of all the modifications to the glomerular filtrate after it has left the nephron at the collecting duct, although some minor alterations in composition may occur in the bladder.

The glomerulus is an invagination at the closed end of the renal tubule (Bowman capsule). Blood is brought to the glomerulus by the afferent arteriole that drains into a network of capillaries which fill the glomerulus. The glomerular filtrate has to cross two layers of cells, the capillary endothelium and the tubular epithelium, separated by an amorphous basal lamina, to pass from the blood vessels to the tubule. It is this barrier that is deranged in those forms of kidney disease which affect the glomerulus, such as glomerulonephritis. The filtrate passes out of the glomerular capillaries and across the epithelium of the tubule through epithelial pores, which electron microscopy suggests are 25 nm in diameter, although functionally they appear to be 8 nm in diameter, since molecules larger than 8 nm are not filtered. Therefore the glomerular filtrate contains no red cells (diameter 7.5 µm) and essentially no protein. In addition, the protein around the capillary pores is negatively charged. Therefore, negatively charged substances such as albumin, whose molecules are less than 8 nm in diameter, may not pass through the capillaries. The capillaries of the glomerulus are a portal system since they drain from the afferent arteriole to the efferent arteriole.

The next portion of the tubule after the glomerulus is the proximal convoluted tubule. Here the majority of the reabsorption of ions and water from the glomerular filtrate occurs. The proximal tubule leads to the loop of Henle, which is largely concerned with salt and water concentration. The loop of Henle then leads to the distal convoluted tubule, which in turn leads to the collecting duct. Between the ascending limb of the loop of Henle and the distal convoluted tubule is a portion of the tubule lined by specialised cells, the macula densa. This portion of the tubule is in close apposition to the efferent and afferent arterioles at the glomerulus, and this region is collectively known as the juxtaglomerular apparatus, which is the site of renin secretion. The loop of Henle differs between the tubules located in the cortex (cortical tubules, 85% of the total) and those located near the medulla (juxtamedullary tubules, 15% of the total). The juxtamedullary tubules have much longer loops of Henle and they alone have a thick portion to the ascending limb of the loop of Henle. This thick portion is thought to be essential for the reabsorption of chloride, an essential part of the mechanism for concentrating urine (see below).

The efferent arteriole leaves the glomerulus to form the blood supply to the tubule. It supplies a network of peritubular capillaries, which then drain into the renal vein. The juxtamedullary nephrons have specialised efferent arterioles, the vasa recta, which supply the loop of Henle (see Fig. 10.19).

RENAL CLEARANCE

Substances such as creatinine or urea which are excreted by the kidney have a lower concentration in the renal vein than the artery; they are therefore said to be cleared by the kidney. But, with few exceptions, most substances are not completely cleared by the kidney. The clearance of a substance such as creatinine is a theoretical concept. Clearance equals the volume of blood that would be totally cleared of creatinine in unit time. Thus, if the creatinine clearance is 120 mL/min and the serum creatinine is 70 µmol/L (0.8 mg/100 mL), the kidney excretes $70 \times 120/1000 = 8.4$ µmol/min (0.1 mg/min). If the renal blood flow is 1.2 L/min, this would reduce the creatinine level by $8.4 \times 1000/1200 = 7.0$ µmol. So a creatinine clearance of

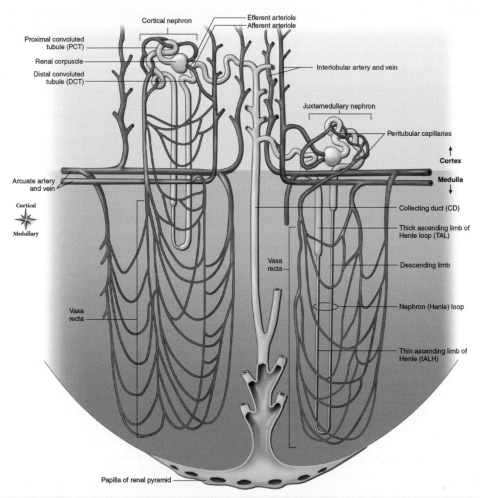

Fig. 10.19 Diagram of nephrons and their blood supply. *AA*, Arcuate artery; *AV*, arcuate vein; *Aa*, afferent arteriole; *Ea*, efferent arteriole; *IA*, interlobular artery; *IV*, interlobular vein; *Ic*, intertubular capillaries; *LH*, loop of Henle; *Vr*, vasa recta; *P*, papilla; *C*, cortex; *OM*, outer medulla; *IM*, inner medulla. (*Source:* From Patton K., 2019. *Anatomy and Physiology*, 10th edn. Elsevier Inc., St Louis).

120 mL/min will maintain a renal vein creatinine level of 70 µmol/L if the renal artery creatinine level is 77 µmol/L.

To calculate the clearance of a substance it is best to work from first principles. For example, let us assume we are told that:

> **Serum creatinine** = 70 µmol/L
>
> **Urine creatinine** = 6 mmol/L   **(1)**
>
> **24h urine volume** = 2 L/24 h

Then:

> **24h urine**
> **creatinine**
> **excretion** = 2 × 6 mmol
> = 2 × 6 × 1000 µmol
>
> **Excretion of**
> **creatinine**   **(2)**
> **in 1 min** = $\dfrac{2 \times 6 \times 1000}{60 \times 24}$ µmol
> = 8.3 µmol

From (1), 1 µmol of creatinine occupies

$$\frac{1000}{70} = 14.3 \text{ mL}$$

From (2), with 8.3 µmol excreted per min, creatinine clearance = 8.3 × 14.3 = 119 mL/min.

GLOMERULAR FILTRATION RATE

The clearance of a substance that is neither reabsorbed from the renal tubule nor secreted into the tubule is equal to the glomerular filtration rate (GFR). The plasma constituent that most closely approaches this is creatinine, and the creatinine clearance is therefore the usual measurement for estimation of the GFR. The normal GFR (both kidneys together) is 120 mL/min. It is proportional to body surface area, but about 10% lower in women than men, even after adjustment for body surface area. Creatinine may be both secreted to and reabsorbed from the renal tubule but has the great advantage that it is endogenously produced and the blood levels do not fluctuate much. For accurate determination of GFR the inulin clearance may be used but inulin has to be infused to maintain a steady plasma level. The clearance of radioactive vitamin B_{12} has also been used for measurement of the GFR, but obviously not in pregnancy.

RENAL BLOOD FLOW

Healthy renal blood flow is normally about 1.2 L/min. It varies with body surface and sex in the same way as the GFR. Since only the plasma is relevant to the excretion of most substance, the term renal plasma flow (RPF) is often used, rather than renal blood flow. If the haematocrit is 45%, the RPF is 660 mL/min when the blood flow is 1.2 L/min: 660 = 1200 ((100–45)/100) mL/min. Renal blood flow could be measured directly by placing flow meters on the renal arteries, but this would be a highly invasive procedure. In practice we measure the clearance of substances such as *p*-aminohippuric acid (PAH), which are not metabolised by the kidney, and are assumed to be almost totally excreted through the kidney. Thus the renal vein concentration of PAH is assumed to be zero. Under these circumstances, the secretion of PAH into the renal tubule, PAH clearance, equals renal blood flow.

The renal blood vessels are innervated by the autonomic nervous system via renal nerves. Stimulation of the renal nerves causes vasoconstriction and a decrease in renal blood flow. This occurs via the vasomotor centre in systemic hypotension and also in severe hypoxia. Renal blood flow is also decreased by the direct action of catecholamines and both neural and humoral mechanisms are likely to be involved in the reduction of renal blood flow associated with exercise.

The filtration fraction is the ratio of GFR to RPF. The normal filtration fraction is 120/660 = 0.18. As the RPF falls in hypotension, the filtration fraction increases, thus maintaining the GFR.

HANDLING OF INDIVIDUAL SUBSTANCES

Glucose and Amino Acids

Glucose and amino acids are reabsorbed by active transport at the proximal tubule. If the filtered load of glucose is too great for the proximal tubule to be able to reabsorb all the filtered glucose, it is excreted in the urine. This usually occurs at blood glucose concentrations ≥10 mmol/L. Glycosuria occurs in patients with hyperglycaemia due to diabetes mellitus. Approximately 10% of pregnant women have glycosuria at lower blood glucose concentrations but this does not necessarily indicate diabetes. Patients with aminoaciduria, as occurs in Fanconi syndrome, have a congenital abnormality of the proximal tubules so that they cannot reabsorb amino acids efficiently.

Sodium and Chloride

The reabsorption of sodium by the renal tubule is a major feat, which consumes considerable energy. The filtered load of sodium presented to the renal tubules is about 200,000 mmol/day. The vast majority of this is reabsorbed, so that the total quantity of sodium excreted varies between 1 and 400 mmol/day, depending on the salt and water balance of the individual. The chief controlling mechanisms accounting for the variation in the sodium reabsorption are: (1) the levels of aldosterone and other mineralocorticoids; (2) GFR; (3) variations in intrarenal pressure, which affects filtration fraction and (4) concomitant changes in potassium and hydrogen ion excretion. In addition, a peptide secreted by the overloaded cardiac atrium, ANP, increases the excretion of sodium through inhibition of the RAAS.

The majority of sodium is reabsorbed actively in the proximal tubule. In addition, sodium is reabsorbed actively in the distal convoluted tubule, collecting duct and bladder under the control of mineralocorticoids. Sodium is also reabsorbed passively in the thick ascending loop of Henle in exchange for chloride ions, which are themselves actively reabsorbed. The anions involved in sodium reabsorption are chloride (80%) and bicarbonate (19%). The remaining 1% of sodium reabsorption takes place in the distal tubule and is accounted for by exchange of potassium (0.5%) and hydrogen (0.5%) ions.

Chloride is usually reabsorbed passively, following sodium and potassium reabsorption in the proximal convoluted tubule. It is also actively reabsorbed in the thick ascending loop of Henle. Chloride reabsorption is decreased when bicarbonate reabsorption is increased, so that the levels of chloride and bicarbonate vary reciprocally in the plasma. Before the measurement of bicarbonate became freely available, it was realised that chloride levels are high in those situations where the bicarbonate level is low (e.g. metabolic acidosis) and much knowledge of acid–base balance was inferred from estimation of the chloride concentration; this is no longer necessary.

Bicarbonate

Bicarbonate is partly reabsorbed passively following sodium reabsorption; it is also reabsorbed by buffering hydrogen ions. Within the renal tubule, hydrogen ions react with bicarbonate to form carbonic acid. The carbonic acid is broken down under the influence of carbonic anhydrase in the brush border of the cells of the proximal convoluted tubule to form carbon dioxide and water. Carbon dioxide is reabsorbed across the tubular cell, and in the proximal tubular cell reacts again with water to form carbonic acid, which subsequently dissociates; bicarbonate is therefore reabsorbed as carbon dioxide, rather than as bicarbonate ions. This mechanism occurs so long as the plasma bicarbonate concentration is less than 28 mmol/L. Once the bicarbonate concentration exceeds this level, bicarbonate appears in the urine, which becomes alkaline.

Potassium

Potassium is reabsorbed actively in the proximal convoluted tubule, in exchange for chloride ions. It is also secreted into the distal convoluted tubule, in exchange for sodium ions, and this is under the control of aldosterone and other mineralocorticoids. High concentrations of aldosterone cause an increase in sodium reabsorption and potassium secretion in the distal tubule, hence the hypokalaemia typical of aldosterone excess, as in Conn syndrome. The kidney is not nearly as efficient in conserving potassium as it is at conserving sodium. When there is hypokalaemia, the obligate excretion of potassium is still about 10 mmol/day, whereas in hypovolaemia the kidney can reduce sodium excretion to 1 mmol/day.

Hydrogen Ions

Hydrogen ions are actively excreted in the proximal and distal tubules in exchange for sodium. In the tubule the hydrogen ions are buffered by bicarbonate, phosphate and ammonia, which keeps the pH of the tubular fluid >4.5, the minimum for hydrogen ion secretion. Ammonia is produced locally in the kidney tubules by deamination of amino acids and is secreted into the tubular fluid at the proximal and distal tubules, and collecting duct.

Water

Of the 170 L of water that is filtered per day, all but 1.5 L is reabsorbed under normal circumstances. However, in extreme hydration the total amount of water excreted may be as high as 50% of the GFR. This control of water reabsorption depends on the level of antidiuretic hormone (ADH), the GFR and the solute load. The bulk of water reabsorption occurs passively in the proximal tubule, where sodium and chloride are reabsorbed, and water is absorbed isotonically. Concentration of the urine occurs because of the high osmotic pressure achieved by reabsorption of chloride followed by sodium in the thick ascending limb of the loop of Henle in the medulla of the kidney. As the filtrate passes down the collecting duct it becomes exposed to this high osmotic pressure and water is reabsorbed. The permeability of the collecting duct is altered by the level of ADH. High levels of ADH increase the permeability of the cells of the collecting duct, therefore allowing more water to be reabsorbed from tubular fluid, and a lower volume of concentrated urine to be finally secreted. Low levels of ADH decrease permeability of the cells of the collecting duct, so that large quantities of dilute urine are excreted.

ADH (arginine vasopressin) is secreted from the posterior pituitary gland, under the influence of the hypothalamus. Its secretion is increased by stress, hypovolaemia and increase in plasma osmolarity, adrenaline and certain drugs such as morphine. Its secretion is decreased by an increase in circulating blood volume, by a fall in plasma osmolarity and by alcohol. During pregnancy, four times as much ADH is produced in order to counteract the effects of placentally derived vasopressinase. A failure of the mother's pituitary to increase vasopressin production to match placental enzymatic degradation will lead to transient (gestational) diabetes insipidus, which resolves following delivery of the placenta.

Urea

Urea accumulates in high concentration in the renal medulla. The kidney tubular cells are freely permeable to urea. When urine flows are low only 10% to 20% of the filtered urea is excreted, while at high urine flow rates 50% to 70% is excreted.

ENDOCRINE FUNCTIONS OF THE KIDNEY

The kidney acts as an endocrine organ to increase production of renin (see above and p. 13), erythropoietin (EPO) and the active hydroxylation of vitamin D. EPO is a circulating glycoprotein consisting of 165 amino acids. It is normally produced by interstitial fibroblasts in the renal cortex, close to peritubular capillaries. The secretion of EPO is stimulated by a widespread system of oxygen-dependent gene expression, specifically hypoxia-inducible transcription factors (HIFs). It is the degradation of HIF associated with an α subunit (HIF-1α and HIF-2α) that is oxygen dependent and determines EPO production. EPO normally stimulates red cell production by binding to EPO receptors on early erythroid progenitor cells. These primitive cells then mature into red blood cells, rather than undergoing apoptosis. In chronic kidney disease there is a failure of EPO production in response to chronic anaemia.

Vitamin D is either produced in the skin by the action of sunlight or ingested in the diet. In the liver it is converted to 25-dihydroxycholecalciferol. In the kidney this is converted to the active metabolite 1,25-dihydroxycholecalciferol. It is this hormone that increases calcium uptake from the gastrointestinal tract and mobilises calcium from bone. Renal rickets is in part due to the failure of the kidney to produce normal quantities of 1,25-hydroxycholecalciferol in renal failure.

EFFECTS OF PREGNANCY

Renal Glomerular Function During Pregnancy

Renal adaptation to pregnancy is anticipated prior to conception, during the luteal phase of each menstrual cycle. Renal blood flow and GFR increase by 10% to 20% before menstruation. If pregnancy is established the corpus luteum persists and these haemodynamic changes continue. By 16 weeks of gestation GFR is 55% above non-pregnant levels (Fig. 10.20). This increment is mediated through an increase in renal blood flow that reaches a maximum of 70% to 80% above non-pregnant levels by the second trimester, before falling to around 45% above non-pregnant levels at term. Elegant human studies have confirmed that, unlike the hyperfiltration that precedes diabetic nephropathy, gestational hyperfiltration is not associated with a damaging rise in glomerular capillary blood pressure.

The changes to renal physiology in healthy pregnancy can both hide and mimic renal disease. The increased GFR of pregnancy leads to a fall in serum creatinine concentration (Scr), so that values considered normal in the non-pregnant state may be abnormal during pregnancy. Serum creatinine levels fall from a non-pregnant mean value of 73 μmol/L (0.82 mg/dL) to 56 μmol/L (0.63 mg/dL), 52 μmol/L (0.59 mg/dL) and 54 μmol/L (0.61 mg/dL) in successive trimesters. A creatinine >77 μmol/L (0.87 mg/dL) in pregnancy is abnormal and should lead to consideration of acute kidney injury or pre-existing chronic kidney disease. Serum creatinine is not, however, linearly correlated with creatinine clearance and is influenced by muscle mass, physical exercise, racial differences and dietary intake of meat. As Scr roughly doubles for every 50% reduction in GFR, a more useful parameter by which to monitor serial changes in renal function is the reciprocal of Scr (1/Scr). Estimates of GFR can be further refined using the Cockcroft–Gault equation, which calculates GFR using Scr, maternal age and pre-pregnancy weight. For women the Cockcroft–Gault equation is:

$$\text{GFR}(\text{mL/min}) = 0.8 \times [140 - \text{age(years)} \times \text{weight (kg)}]/\text{Scr}(\mu\text{mol/L})$$
$$(1\ \text{mg/dL creatinine} = 88.4\ \mu\text{mol/L creatinine})$$

The gestational rise in renal blood flow also causes the kidneys to swell so that bipolar renal length increases by approximately 1 cm. During the third trimester renal blood flow falls, leading to a fall in creatinine clearance and a rise in Scr. Serum urea levels, however, continue to fall in the third trimester due to reduced maternal hepatic urea synthesis. This metabolic adaptation ensures that more nitrogen is available for fetal protein synthesis.

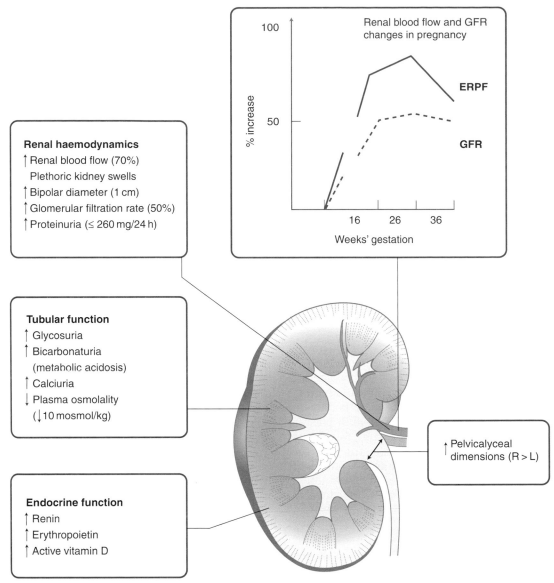

Renal haemodynamics
↑ Renal blood flow (70%)
  Plethoric kidney swells
↑ Bipolar diameter (1 cm)
↑ Glomerular filtration rate (50%)
↑ Proteinuria (≤ 260 mg/24 h)

Tubular function
↑ Glycosuria
↑ Bicarbonaturia
  (metabolic acidosis)
↑ Calciuria
↓ Plasma osmolality
  (↓10 mosmol/kg)

Endocrine function
↑ Renin
↑ Erythropoietin
↑ Active vitamin D

↑ Pelvicalyceal
  dimensions (R > L)

Renal blood flow and GFR
changes in pregnancy

ERPF

GFR

Weeks' gestation

Fig. 10.20 Physiological changes to the kidney during healthy pregnancy. *ERPF*, Effective renal plasma flow; *GFR*, glomerular filtration rate.

The renal pelvicalyceal system and ureters dilate and can appear obstructed to those unaware of these changes, in particular on the right side. The right pelvicalyceal system dilates by a maximum of 0.5 mm each week from 6 to 32 weeks, reaching a maximum diameter of approximately 20 mm (90th centile), which is maintained until term. The left pelvicalyceal system reaches a maximum diameter of 8 mm (90th centile) at 20 weeks of gestation.

Proteinuria increases as pregnancy progresses, but levels over 260 mg/24 hour during the third trimester are above the 95% confidence limit for the normal population. Urine dipsticks are commonly used first line but false positives and false negatives are common. A random urine protein:creatinine ratio is a useful guide to 24-hour urinary protein excretion and has largely replaced 24-hour urine collections in clinical practice. A random urine sample that gives a protein (mg):creatinine (mmol) ratio >0.30 is a good predictor of significant proteinuria (equivalent to >300 mg/24 hours).

Serum albumin levels fall by 5 to 10 g/L, serum cholesterol and triglyceride concentrations increase significantly and dependent oedema affects most pregnancies at term. Normal pregnancy therefore simulates the classic features of nephrotic syndrome.

Renal Tubular Function During Pregnancy

Increased alveolar ventilation causes a respiratory alkalosis to which the kidney responds by increased bicarbonaturia and a compensatory metabolic acidosis. Other renal tubular changes include reduced tubular glucose reabsorption, which leads to glycosuria in approximately 10% of healthy pregnant women, a 250% to 300% increase in urinary calcium excretion and a first trimester increase in urate excretion that decreases towards term, at which time plasma urate levels rise again to non-pregnancy levels.

During healthy pregnancy, a mother gains 6 to 8 kg of fluid, of which approximately 1.2 L is due to an increase in plasma volume. Plasma osmolality falls by 10 mosmol/kg by 5 to 8 weeks of gestation due to a fall in both the threshold for thirst and for the release of antidiuretic hormone (vasopressin). During pregnancy, vasopressin is metabolised by placental vasopressinase, and at term the maternal posterior pituitary produces four times as much vasopressin to maintain physiological concentrations. Failure of the maternal pituitary to keep up with the increased metabolic clearance of vasopressin leads to a transient polyuric state in the third trimester, which is known as transient diabetes insipidus of pregnancy.

Renal Endocrine Function During Pregnancy

The kidney also acts as an endocrine organ that produces EPO, active vitamin D and renin. The production of all three hormones increases during healthy pregnancy, but their effects are masked by other changes. In early pregnancy, peripheral vasodilatation exceeds renin–aldosterone-mediated plasma volume expansion, so diastolic blood pressure falls by 12 weeks. Conversely, plasma volume expansion exceeds the EPO-mediated increase in red cell mass, causing a 'physiological anaemia', which should not normally lead to an Hb concentration <95 g/L. Similarly, extra active vitamin D produced by the placenta circulates at twice non-gravid levels, but concomitant halving of parathyroid hormone levels, hypercalciuria and increased fetal requirements keep plasma ionised calcium levels unchanged.

PHYSIOLOGY OF MICTURITION

Passive Phase

The bladder fills with urine at approximately 1 mL/min. Folds of transitional cell epithelium become flattened and the detrusor muscle fibres passively stretch with very little rise of intravesical pressure.

At the same time, the intraurethral pressure caused by the elastic tissue, the arteriovenous shunts and the tone of the smooth and striated muscle components is maintained at a higher level than the intravesical pressure.

Proprioceptive afferent impulses caused by the stretching of the detrusor fibres pass through the pelvic splanchnic nerves to the sacral roots of S2–S4. As urine volume increases, these impulses pass up the lateral spinothalamic tracts to the thalamus and thence to the cerebral cortex, thus bringing the sensation of bladder filling to a conscious level. The act of micturition is initially subconsciously and later consciously postponed by inhibitory impulses blocking the sacral reflex arc.

Active Phase

At an appropriate time and place, a suitable posture is adopted through the organisation of the frontal lobes of the cerebral cortex and the anterior hypothalamus, and the following sequence of events take place in the act of micturition:

1. The muscles of the pelvic floor are voluntarily relaxed, causing a loss of the posterior urethrovesical angle and funnelling of the bladder neck.
2. At the same time, the voluntary fibres of the external sphincter are relaxed, causing an overall fall of intraurethral pressure by at least 50%.
3. At 5 to 15 s later, the inhibitory activity of the higher centres on the sacral reflex is lifted, allowing a rapid flow of efferent parasympathetic impulses, mainly from S3, to cause the detrusor to contract. As a result the

intravesical pressure rises and can be augmented by the voluntary contraction of the diaphragm and the anterior abdominal wall musculature.
4. Urine flow commences when the intravesical pressure exceeds the intraurethral pressure. The urine flow may also further stimulate the sacral reflex by the conduction of afferent impulses from its lining to S2–S4.
5. At the end of micturition, the flow rate diminishes, the intravesical pressure falls and the striated musculature of the pelvic floor elevates the bladder neck; the external urethral sphincter interrupts the terminal flow in the region of the midurethra and obliterates the urethral lumen. The inhibitory influence of the higher centres is re-established and the bladder becomes passive once more.

Urodynamic Data in the Normal Adult Female

Residual urine	0–10 mL
First sensation of bladder filling	150–200 mL
Voiding volume	220–320 mL
Voiding pressure	45–70 cmH$_2$O
Maximum urine flow rate	20–40 mL/s
Bladder capacity	600 mL
Intravesical pressure rise (0–500 mL)	0–10 cmH$_2$O
	Detrusor contractions do not occur even with rapid filling or at full capacity
Maximal urethral pressure in the absence of micturition	Approx. 50–100 cmH$_2$O, but varies with age and childbearing

Gastrointestinal Tract

MOUTH

Mechanics

Mastication is accomplished by voluntary muscles innervated by the motor branch of the fifth cranial nerve. Pregnancy results in alteration of microflora in the oral cavity favouring acidophilic organisms and predisposing to development of dental caries which may be exacerbated by calcium deficiency.

Digestive Processes

The secretion of saliva is mediated by autonomic nervous stimulation. Salivary mucus provides lubrication for mastication and swallowing. The salivary glands also produce salivary amylase in the mouth which converts starch and glycogen into maltose and maltotriose. The lingual glands produce lingual lipase (Table 10.7) which converts triglycerides into fatty acids and glycerol.

OESOPHAGUS

Mechanics

Swallowing. There are two stages to this process:

1. *Voluntary stage*—food in the form of a bolus is pressed by the tongue upwards and backwards against the soft palate.

Table 10.7   Enzymes in the Mouth

Enzyme	Substrate	Product
Salivary amylase	Starch	Dextrins, maltose, maltotriose
Lingual lipase	Triglycerides	Fatty acids and glycerol

2. *Involuntary stage*—passage of food initially through the pharynx (1 to 2 seconds) and then by peristalsis down the oesophagus (4 to 8 seconds) to the stomach. The process is controlled by the deglutition centre in medulla and lower pons.

The oesophagus is 25 cm long and consists of an outer layer of longitudinal muscle and an inner circular muscle layer. In the upper part of the oesophagus both layers are comprised of striated muscle, and in the lower part both layers are smooth muscle. The pH of the lower oesophagus is 5 to 7. At the gastro-oesophageal junction, the squamous epithelium of the oesophagus is replaced by columnar epithelium.

Gastro-Oesophageal Sphincter

The lower oesophageal sphincter functions as a result of tonic contraction of the circular muscle of the lower end of the oesophagus 2 to 5 cm above the gastro-oesophageal junction. The sphincter remains contracted at all times other than when swallowing, eructating (belching wind) or vomiting. Sphincter function is enhanced as a result of the angulation at the lower end of the oesophagus by the diaphragm. Closure is therefore promoted on raising the intragastric or intra-abdominal pressure, so creating a shutter or flap-valve effect. Closure is further enhanced by virtue of a portion of the oesophagus resting intra-abdominally. Folding of the mucosa within the oesophageal lumen facilitating occlusion and unimpeded gastric emptying is also important in maintaining the competence of the sphincter.

Gastro-Oesophageal Reflux

Gastro-oesophageal reflux occurs in 30% to 50% of all pregnancies and occurs when the lower oesophageal sphincter fails. This results in exposure of the relatively unprotected oesophageal mucosa to the predominantly acidic and irritant peptic contents. In pregnancy, gastric relaxation and delayed emptying may predispose to incompetence of the lower oesophageal sphincter. Additional proposed mechanisms include a role for oestrogen and progesterone in reducing lower oesophageal sphincter pressure. Raised intragastric pressure is a contributory factor in late pregnancy. Simple solutions to reflux in pregnancy include frequent intake of small meals, reduction in fat and alcohol intake and avoidance of manoeuvres that increase intra-abdominal pressure. Drug treatment of gastro-oesophageal reflux is aimed at reducing acid secretion and increasing mucosal resistance to acid.

Gastric pressure and gastric volumes increase in labour and stomach contents are pulmonary irritants if inhaled (aspiration pneumonitis) (e.g. during anaesthesia for emergency caesarean section). Foodstuffs of high osmolarity (e.g. glucose) are especially liable to delay emptying. Women should therefore be advised to drink isotonic drinks in labour which prevent ketosis without a concomitant increase in gastric volume. In addition, women considered at risk of caesarean section should be offered antacids to reduce gastric volume and acidity. Non-particulate antacid suspension gels are preferred and seem to mix more effectively with stomach contents and cause less irritation if inhaled.

STOMACH

Mechanics

Because a meal is eaten more quickly than the digestive enzymes can break it down, the stomach serves as a holding chamber and mixing device. The stomach is the most distensible part of the gastrointestinal tract and storage of food in quantities of up to 1 L is possible. Mixing and maceration of food with secretions generates chyme by a combination of constrictor waves and peristalsis. Peristalsis forces food towards the pyloric sphincter (which is usually closed) and chyme is forced through. Emptying is promoted by:

1. Increased gastric volume causing antral peristalsis.
2. Release of gastrin (Table 10.8) stimulated by food (especially meat) causing acid secretion. This in turn stimulates the pyloric pump (producing H^+) (see later), while at the same time relaxing the pylorus.

Emptying is inhibited by:

1. Enterogastric reflex from the duodenum to pylorus when there is excess of chyme, acid, hyper- or hypotonic fluids, or excess of protein breakdown products.
2. A possible hormonal reflex from the duodenum to pylorus—especially when chyme contains an excess of fats.

During pregnancy, gastric emptying is either unchanged or slowed.

Digestive Processes

Gastric innervation is parasympathetic via the vagus (motor and secretory) and sympathetic via Meissner's and Auerbach's plexus. Blood supply is from the coeliac trunk.

Gastric secretion is initiated reflexively via the vagus and secretions total 3 L/day. Once food has entered the stomach the hormone gastrin is released from the antral portion and is carried in the blood to the parietal (oxyntic) cells of the gastric glands. Parietal cells secrete hydrochloric acid and intrinsic factor. The proton pump actively transports H^+ ions (H^+ ATPase) into the gastric lumen in exchange for K^+ ions. K^+ (and Cl^-) then passively diffuse back into the gastric lumen through their own channels. H^+ ions for this purpose are generated within the parietal cell. Water (H_2O) and carbon dioxide (CO_2) form carbonic acid in a reaction catalysed by carbonic anhydrase, which is abundant in parietal cells. The carbonic acid thus formed then dissociates, generating H^+ (and $HCO3^-$). The $HCO3^-$ product is then exchanged for Cl^- in the interstitial fluid.

Table 10.8 Gastrointestinal Hormones

Hormone	Site of Production	Stimulus for Release	Gastric Acid/ Gastrin Secretion	Gastric Emptying	Other Effect	Changes in Pregnancy
Gastrin	G-cells of gastric antrum	Gastric distension; Amino acids in antrum; Vagal action (inhibited by pH <1.5); Calcium, adrenaline (epinephrine)	↑	↑	Secretion of pepsin and intrinsic factor; Stimulates pancreatic bicarbonate secretion and secretin	Plasma level unchanged
Cholecystokinin (CCK)	Duodenum and jejunum	Intraluminal fat, amino acids, peptides and some cations (Ca^{++}, Mg^{++})	↓	↓	Pancreatic enzyme and bicarbonate secretion; Gall bladder contraction; Satiety	
Secretin	Duodenum and jejunum	Intraluminal acid	↓	↓	Stimulates pancreatic bicarbonate secretion; Stimulates production and increases the water and HCO_3^- content of bile	
Gastric inhibitory peptide (GIP)	Duodenum and jejunum	Glucose, fats and amino acids	↓	↓	Stimulates insulin secretion	
Motilin	Duodenum and jejunum	Acid in small bowel		↑		
Vasoactive intestinal peptide (VIP)	Small intestine	Neural	↓		Inhibits pepsin secretion; Stimulates secretion by intestine and pancreas; Splanchnic vasodilatation	
Pancreatic polypeptide	Pancreas	Protein-rich meal			Relaxes gall bladder; Inhibits pancreatic enzyme secretion	
Somatostatin					Inhibits secretin and actin, most hormones	
Histamine	Histaminocytes in lamina propria		↑	↑		
Glucagon, calcitonin			↓			

Table 10.9 Gastric Enzymes

Enzyme	Type	Substrate	Product
Pepsinogens	Pro-enzyme converted to pepsin by gastric acid in the lumen	Proteins and polypeptides	Peptides
Gastric lipase		Triglycerides	Fatty acids and glycerol

$$H_2O + CO_2 \rightarrow H_2CO_3 \rightarrow H^+ + HCO_3^-$$

Chief cells secrete pepsinogen (Table 10.9)—the only proteolytic enzyme within the stomach. Release of a pro-enzyme (pepsinogen) protects the parietal cell from the proteolytic effect of the enzyme product pepsin. Hydrochloric acid converts pepsinogen into pepsin. Pepsin further acts on pepsinogen in the presence of acid, so enhancing its own production. The low pH (1 to 2) of the stomach has the additional effect of killing many bacteria in food as well as being the optimum pH for function of pepsin. Gastric pH and gastric acid output are unchanged by pregnancy.

Mucus in the stomach comes from glands around the pylorus and protects the mucosa from the extreme acidity. Gastric lipase and amylase are of little quantitative importance. Indeed gastric lipase splits short-chain triglycerides, as found in milk, although this enzyme functions optimally at pH 5 to 6 and so has a limited role in the adult stomach. In infants, rennin (chymosin) causes the milk to curdle, so delaying its emptying from the stomach with subsequent early digestion of casein. Intrinsic factor is a glycoprotein which binds cyanocobalamin (vitamin B_{12}). B_{12} is then absorbed in the terminal ileum and intrinsic factor remains in the lumen. The most common cause of B_{12} deficiency is pernicious anaemia where atrophy of the gastric mucosa leads to failure of intrinsic factor production. Parietal cell antibodies are seen in 90% and intrinsic factor antibodies in 50% of people with pernicious anaemia. Pernicious anaemia is more commonly seen in the elderly and in those with other auto-immune diseases.

GALL BLADDER
Mechanics

The gall bladder stores, concentrates and acidifies bile. Emptying into the duodenum is brought about by the presence of fat in the small intestine causing cholecystokinin–pancreozymin (see Table 10.8) to be released from the mucosa. Cholecystokinin stimulates the gall bladder to contract and the sphincter of Oddi to relax.

Digestive Processes

See under Liver for constituents of bile.

SMALL INTESTINE
Mechanics

Distension is the main stimulus to peristalsis, by autonomic fibres to the myenteric plexus (Fig. 10.21). The parasympathetic fibres stimulate movement; the sympathetic fibres inhibit movement.

The ileocaecal sphincter and valve allows about 750 mL of chyme/day into the caecum. Both ileal peristalsis and gastrin release relax the ileal sphincter, while increased caecal pressure and irritation of the caecum constrict it.

Digestive Processes

Duodenum and Pancreas. Pancreatic juice is an alkaline fluid (pH 8) containing enzymes, pro-enzymes and electrolytes for the digestion of carbohydrates, proteins, fats and nucleic acids; 1200 to 1500 mL/day is secreted from the exocrine acini of epithelial cells, which comprise 98% of the pancreatic mass. The remaining 2% is comprised of the endocrine islets of Langerhans innervated by the coeliac plexus and producing glucagon (alpha cells), insulin (beta cells), somatostatin (delta cells) and pancreatic polypeptide.

Pancreatic juice neutralises gastric juice to provide optimal pH for enzymes to function. Pancreatic enzyme functions are listed in Table 10.10.

Chyme in the duodenum causes the release of the hormone secretin, which induces the pancreas to produce large volumes of fluid rich in bicarbonate but lacking in enzymes. A second hormone, cholecystokinin–pancreozymin, has the effect of releasing pancreatic enzymes and inducing the gall bladder to contract. Nervous stimulation of the pancreas occurs to a limited extent. Most fat digestion occurs in the duodenum as a result of the actions of pancreatic lipase. Activity is facilitated when fats are emulsified. Failure of the exocrine portion of the pancreas results in steatorrhoea (i.e. fatty) clay-coloured stools with an increased fat content. Absorption of the fat-soluble vitamins A, D, E and K is deficient if fat absorption is depressed because of lack of pancreatic enzymes or when bile is prevented from entering the intestine.

Small Intestine. Digestion and absorption of nutrients, salt and water occur in the small intestine. Some 90% of all water absorption occurs here. Most vitamins are absorbed in the upper small intestine (vitamin B_{12} is absorbed in the terminal ileum). The reactions in the small intestine are shown in Table 10.11.

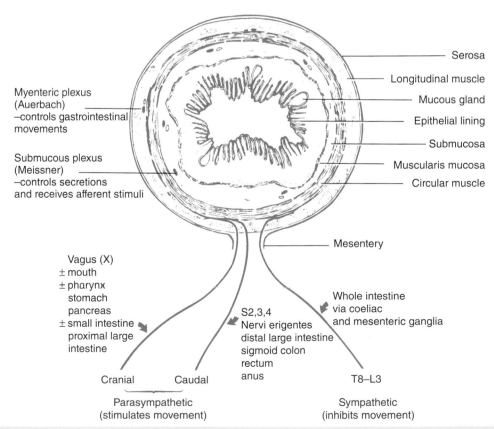

Fig. 10.21 Schematic transverse section of the gut showing nerve supply.

Table 10.10 Pancreatic Enzymes (Exocrine)

Enzyme	Type	Substrate	Product	
Maltase	Enzyme	Maltose	Glucose	
Amylase	Enzyme	Starch	Glucose, maltose and maltotriose	
Lipase	Enzyme	Fats	Free fatty acids and monoglycerides	
Nucleases (ribonuclease and deoxyribonuclease)	Enzyme	RNA and DNA	Nucleotides	
Trypsinogen	Pro-enzyme converted by enteropeptidase to trypsin	Proteins and polypeptides	Polypeptides/peptides	Cleaves peptide bonds on carboxyl-side basic amino acids (arginine and lysine)
Chymotrypsinogen	Pro-enzyme activated by trypsin	Proteins and polypeptides	Polypeptides/peptides	Cleaves peptide bonds on carboxyl-side aromatic amino acids
Pro-aminopeptidase	Pro-enzyme	Proteins and polypeptides	Polypeptides/peptides	
Pro-carboxypeptidase	Pro-enzyme activated by trypsin	Proteins and polypeptides	Polypeptides/peptides	Cleaves carboxyl terminal amino acids that have aromatic or branched aliphatic side chains
Phospholipase	Activated by trypsin	Phospholipids	Fatty acids	

Table 10.11 Small Intestinal Mucosal Enzymes

Enzyme	Substrate	Product	
Aminopeptidases	Polypeptides	Peptides and amino acids	Cleaves terminal amino acid from peptide
Carboxypeptidase	Polypeptides	Peptides	Cleaves carboxyl terminal amino acid from peptide
Enteropeptidase (enterokinase)	Trypsinogen	Trypsin	
Endopeptidase	Polypeptides	Peptides	Cleaves between residues in mid-portion of peptide
Dipeptidase	Dipeptides	Amino acids	
Lactase	Lactose	Glucose and galactose	
Sucrase	Sucrose	Glucose and fructose	
Maltase	Maltose	Glucose	

Small intestinal secretions are mainly induced by reflexes triggered by food stimulating local nerve endings. Brunner's glands secrete mucus, while the crypts of Lieberkühn exude a neutral fluid which is thought to aid absorption of chyle through the epithelial cells of the mucosa, where the constituent substances of chyle are acted on by proteolytic, lipolytic and glycolytic enzymes. Unlike other nutrients, B_{12} and bile salts are not absorbed in the small intestine but have specific receptors in the terminal ileum.

LARGE INTESTINE (CAECUM, COLON, RECTUM AND ANAL CANAL)

Mechanics

In the ascending colon the haustrations propel semi-solid food by combined contractions of circular and longitudinal muscle. In the transverse and sigmoid colon, mass movement drives solid faeces towards the rectum.

Gut transit time is increased in pregnancy. Postulated mechanisms are delayed motility secondary to progesterone or the inhibitory action of motilin.

Digestive Processes

Mucus from the goblet cells is produced under normal conditions by the direct contact of food stimulating local myenteric reflexes. No enzymes are secreted. Bacteria ferment any remaining carbohydrates releasing methane, hydrogen and carbon dioxide which is lost as flatus or dissolves to form organic acids rendering the stool slightly acid (pH 5 to 7). Ammonia is produced and not released if there is liver damage. This may result in raised serum concentrations of ammonia and hepatic encephalopathy. The mucosa of the large intestine facilitates absorption, hence the use of the rectum as a route for administration of drugs. Water, ions and some vitamins are absorbed in the large intestine. Na^+ is actively transported out of the colon and water follows passively along the osmotic gradient generated. Bacteria also decompose bile to give faeces their dark colour. Extreme irritation of the bowel wall (e.g. by infection) will result in the secretion of water and electrolytes, so resulting in diarrhoea. Under conditions of stress, parasympathetic stimulation of the nervi erigentes results in copious mucus secretion, which may also cause frequent bowel actions, but often without any concomitant faecal material.

Defaecation

The rectum is the last 20 cm of the gastrointestinal tract. The terminal 2 to 3 cm is the anal canal. Faeces entering the rectum stimulate reflex parasympathetic stimuli via the nervi erigentes to contract bowel muscle and relax the internal sphincter. If the external sphincter is not voluntarily contracted, defaecation will occur. Constipation affects up to 40% of pregnancies. The decreased physical activity of pregnancy coupled with iron ingestion contributes to the increased incidence which increases with parity and thus implies mechanical problems in the lower gastrointestinal tract have a contributory role. Constipation may be associated with an exacerbation of haemorrhoids and anal fissures.

Liver

ANATOMICAL CONSIDERATIONS

The adult liver weighs around 1.3 kg and contains about 100,000 lobules. The neonatal liver at term weighs around 145 g.

Each liver lobule surrounds a central vein as shown in Fig. 10.22. The central vein drains to the hepatic vein.

The sinusoids are lined by Kupffer cells which, together with the endothelial cells, are powerfully phagocytic. Each sinusoid has a rich lymphatic supply.

METABOLIC FUNCTION

The metabolism of carbohydrate and fat is considered in Chapter 9

Carbohydrate

Glycogen Storage. Glycogen is synthesised from glucose and stored in the liver. The following reactions influence the amount of hepatic glycogen:

1. Glycogen synthetase is activated by high plasma glucose and insulin levels, which thus increase the level of glycogen in the liver and decrease plasma glucose.
2. Phosphorylase is activated by low plasma glucose, adrenaline and glucagon levels, which therefore raise plasma glucose levels by catabolising glycogen.

Galactose and Fructose Conversion. Galactose and fructose are both converted to glucose in the liver by the following reactions:

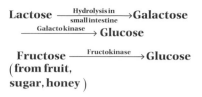

Gluconeogenesis. Depletion of body stores of carbohydrate causes the liver to form glucose from glucogenic amino acids, which are derived from protein, and also from glycerol, which is derived from fat. Metabolic pathways are shown below:

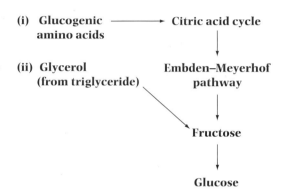

Fat

β-Oxidation and Ketosis. In states of carbohydrate deprivation or type 1 diabetes mellitus, fatty acids are metabolised to ketones as shown below:

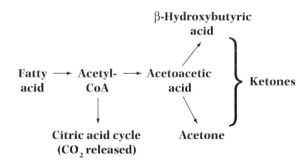

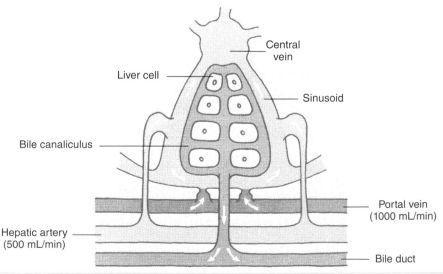

Fig. 10.22 Schematic representation of blood flow through a liver lobule.

Synthesis of Triglyceride (Lipogenesis). The liver is able to synthesise triglyceride from fatty acids and glycerol, which are both derived from dietary carbohydrate. Triglyceride (neutral fat) is mainly concerned with energy expenditure:

$$\left.\begin{array}{c} R_1 \\ R_2 \\ R_3 \end{array}\right\} + \begin{array}{c} CH_2OH \\ | \\ CHOH \\ | \\ CH_2OH \end{array} \quad \underset{\text{Lipolysis}}{\overset{\text{Esterification}}{\rightleftharpoons}} \quad \begin{array}{c} CH_2OR_1 \\ | \\ CHOR_2 \\ | \\ CH_2OR_3 \end{array}$$

3 fatty acids Glycerol   Triglyceride

Synthesis of Lipoproteins. In particular, the liver synthesises very low-density lipoproteins (VLDLs) and pre-β-lipoproteins, which are carrier proteins for plasma lipids.

Synthesis of Phospholipids. There are three types: lecithins, cephalins and sphingomyelins. Phospholipids are essentially structural lipids of body tissues. Lecithin is a powerful surface-active agent, reducing surface tension in the lung alveolae.

Synthesis of Cholesterol. Synthesis is complicated and takes place in several stages whereby acetyl-CoA (CH_3COS–CoA) is built up to form the steroid nucleus and so to cholesterol. About 80% of all cholesterol synthesised is converted into bile acids.

Synthesis of Fats. This may also occur from excess dietary protein through the conversion of amino acids into acetyl-CoA.

Protein

Deamination of Amino Acids and Urea Formation. This occurs by the removal of the amino ($-NH_2$) group from the amino acid. The ammonia produced by deamination is removed by combining it with carbon dioxide to form urea.

Plasma proteins. Virtually all albumin and fibrinogen are synthesised in the liver. Seventy per cent of globulin is synthesised in the liver and the remainder is synthesised in the reticuloendothelial system.

Bile

Volumes of the order 250 to 1100 mL of bile are secreted daily by the liver. The production of bile is increased by stimulation of the vagus nerves and by the hormone secretin. Bile is composed of bile salts, phospholipids, cholesterol, bile pigments (bilirubin and biliverdin) and protein. After reabsorption of the water and electrolytes, the concentrated bile is stored in the gall bladder.

Cholesterol

Cholesterol and triglycerides accumulate in the liver during normal pregnancy. Serum cholesterol levels rise by 25% to 50% and serum triglycerides by 150% from around 20 weeks to their peak at term. This, in association with the enlarged gall bladder and supersaturation of bile with cholesterol, contributes to the increased gallstone formation seen in pregnant women. During routine obstetric ultrasound 2% to 4% of women are found to have asymptomatic gallstones. Symptomatic disease occurs in only 0.5% to 1%.

Bile Acids

Bile acids are transported across hepatocytes by specific transporters. Bile acid concentrations are elevated in intrahepatic cholestasis of pregnancy (ICP; also known as obstetric cholestasis), the cause of which is likely to relate to the interaction between inherited or acquired abnormalities in bile acid transporters and the gestational metabolism of increased concentrations of oestrogen and progesterone. Since bile contains significant quantities of sodium and potassium and the pH is alkaline, it is assumed that the bile acids and the associated conjugates exist in ionised form, hence the term bile salts. Bile salts reduce surface tension and in conjunction with phospholipids and monoglycerides emulsify fats into micelles in preparation for their digestion and absorption in the small intestine. Some 95% of bile salts are re-absorbed from the small intestine. The remainder enter the colon and are converted by the action of intestinal microflora to secondary bile acids. A small fraction of these are then re-absorbed and the remainder lost in faeces.

Bilirubin

Bilirubin is one of the main breakdown products of haemoglobin and is excreted by the liver cells, as shown in Fig. 10.23. Glucuronyl transferase catalyses conjugation of bilirubin with glucuronide rendering it water soluble for excretion. This enzyme is located in the smooth endoplasmic reticulum. Other compounds compete with bilirubin for the enzyme system (e.g. steroids and some drugs). Barbiturates, antihistamines and anticonvulsants cause proliferation of the smooth endoplasmic reticulum and increase glucuronyl transferase activity.

Hyperbilirubinaemia may occur because of excess production (pre-hepatic) or reduced elimination (hepatic or post-hepatic) of bilirubin. In pre-hepatic jaundice the hyperbilirubinaemia is due to excess production or failure of hepatic uptake and thus bilirubin is unconjugated and insoluble. It does not therefore appear in the urine. Examples include haemolysis or congenital hyperbilirubinaemia (Gilbert syndrome). In hepatic jaundice, the hepatocyte is defective. Both conjugated and unconjugated bilirubin appear in the urine (e.g. viral infection (hepatitis A)), drugs (phenothiazines) or cirrhosis. In post-hepatic jaundice, excretion of bilirubin into the biliary system is impaired and conjugated bilirubin in plasma is elevated. Conjugated bilirubin is water soluble and therefore excreted into the urine which is thus dark in colour. Because the bilirubin is not lost to the faeces, the stools are pale. Clinical examples include gallstones, carcinoma of the pancreas, primary biliary cirrhosis or structural abnormalities of the biliary tree.

In the neonate, physiological jaundice results from the inability of the immature liver to conjugate bilirubin. When the unconjugated (fat-soluble) bilirubin level exceeds $350\,\mu mol/L$, it can no longer be tightly bound to the albumin and so penetrates the blood–brain barrier. This may result in kernicterus where bilirubin staining of the brain occurs producing an encephalopathy with seizures, cerebral palsy

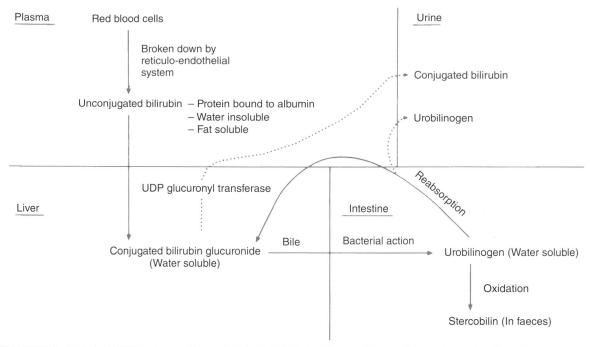

Fig. 10.23 Diagram to illustrate the breakdown and excretion of bilirubin (*UDP*, Uridine 5'-diphospho-glucuronosyltransferase).

and deafness. It is very rare in the term infant but those born prematurely or who are compromised in other ways are at particular risk. Phototherapy alters the shape of the bilirubin molecule in exposed skin, rendering it more water soluble and facilitating secretion.

Cholesterol and alkaline phosphatase (ALP) are excreted in bile, as are adrenocortical and other steroid hormones. Some of the constituents of bile (e.g. bile acids) are re-absorbed in the terminal ileum and then excreted again by the liver (enterohepatic circulation). This may be interrupted by some drugs (e.g. chelating agents: cholestyramine), ileal disease or bacterial overgrowth causing increased de-conjugation. The latter is of particular relevance as it accounts for the reduced efficacy of the combined oral contraceptive pill during periods of gastrointestinal infection or antibiotic use.

TESTING LIVER FUNCTION

Laboratory tests suggestive of impaired synthetic liver function, rather than liver damage, which are widely available for clinical use, are elevated bilirubin (reduced excretion), and low albumin, total protein and glucose (reduced synthesis) and prolonged prothrombin time or international normalised ratio (INR) (reduced synthesis).

Elevated liver transaminases such as alanine aminotransferase (ALT), aspartate aminotransferase (AST) and gamma glutamyl transpeptidase (GGT) reflect hepatocyte damage. Elevated ALP is found in biliary tract disease as well as during the second half of pregnancy, derived from the placenta. Particular patterns of abnormality therefore help determine the site of damage within the liver, with important exceptions in pregnancy.

In pregnancy, serum values for ALT, AST, bilirubin and GGT fall and concentrations are 20% lower than the quoted reference ranges for non-pregnant individuals. Possible mechanisms include a dilutional effect as a result of the expanded plasma volume of pregnancy, an increase in hepatic blood flow or reduced function of the enzymes (and therefore reduced release). Albumin (and total protein) concentrations fall by 20% to 40% in pregnancy as a result of the increased blood volume. This fall does not reflect reduced synthetic function as it might outside pregnancy. ALP concentrations rise in the third trimester of pregnancy as the enzyme is produced and released by the placenta. Individual iso-enzyme assays are available; alternatively the proportion of ALP that is placental in origin can be determined by demonstrating the iso-enzyme's instability on heating. Upper limits of normal for pregnancy have been suggested to be three-fold those of non-pregnant individuals, and concentrations in excess of these may suggest disease.

Liver transaminases may also be affected by mode of delivery; ALT and AST rise after caesarean section and by a smaller degree after vaginal delivery.

An important functional role of the liver is in glucose homeostasis. Hypoglycaemia is evident in acute fatty liver of pregnancy, which is associated with acute liver failure. The liver is also the site of synthesis of blood coagulation substrates such as fibrinogen and prothrombin. It also synthesises clotting factors II, VII, IX and X which all require vitamin K. All are important markers of liver synthetic function. A prolonged prothrombin time (PT/INR), which is dependent on many clotting factors can be an early indicator of severe acute liver damage. A prolonged prothrombin time can be corrected with vitamin K in some disease states (e.g. vitamin K deficiency results if there is obstructed bile flow, as in severe cholestasis) but not in severe hepatitis or chronic liver disease. Clotting factors II, IX and X are raised in normal pregnancies.

MISCELLANEOUS FUNCTIONS

The liver is also concerned in the storage of vitamins, particularly A, D and B_{12}, and in the storage of iron:

$$\text{Apoferritin} + \text{Iron} \rightleftharpoons \text{Ferritin}$$

Many drugs, chemical substances and body compounds are also metabolised and excreted through the liver with bile (e.g. antibiotics (penicillin, sulphonamides, etc.)) steroid hormones (oestrogen, cortisol), alcohol and calcium.

Nervous System

This section outlines the organisation and function of the nervous system.

All integrated neural activity is based on the reflex arc, the process whereby the afferent neurone is stimulated, by either a sense organ or another nerve. The stimulus is transmitted at a synapse to the efferent neurone and conducted either to another neurone or to an effector organ such as muscle cell (Fig. 10.24).

Nervous transmission is an all-or-nothing effect. If there is sufficient depolarisation of the nerve membrane, the impulse will be propagated. If the nerve is not sufficiently depolarised, impulse propagation does not occur. Thus the stimulus from the afferent neurone has to be sufficiently strong to stimulate the efferent neurone. The threshold for nervous transmission at the synapse can be up- or down-regulated by other neurones impinging on the efferent neurone. Somatic neurones innervate somatic, striated muscle; visceral neurones innervate smooth and cardiac musculature as part of the autonomic nervous system.

SOMATIC NERVOUS SYSTEM

Somatic afferent neurones enter the spinal cord via the dorsal roots or cranial nerves, and efferent neurones leave via the ventral roots or the motor cranial nerves.

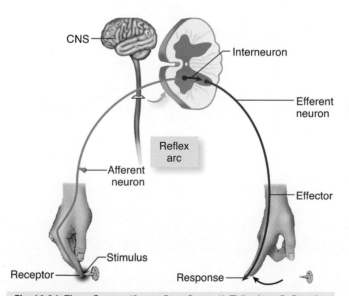

Fig. 10.24 The reflex arc. (*Source*: From Patton K., Thibodeau G., Douglas M., 2012. *Essentials of Anatomy and Physiology*. Elsevier Inc., St. Louis).

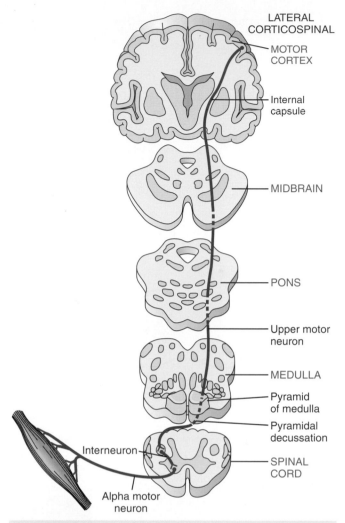

Fig. 10.25 The corticospinal tracts. (*Source*: From Banasik J., 2019. *Pathophysiology*, 6th edn. Elsevier Inc., St. Louis).

The simplest reflex is a monosynaptic reflex of which the only example is the stretch reflex. When a muscle is stretched, the spindles within the muscles are stimulated, which causes a discharge in the afferent neurone. The afferent neurone stimulates the efferent motor neurone at a single synapse in the spinal cord; impulses pass down the motor neurone to the muscle, which then contracts.

Motor System

Most reflexes are polysynaptic with several (often hundreds) of synapses between the sensory receptor and the effector cell. Many different afferent neurones may synapse with each efferent neurone. Thus the motor neurone also receives synapses from nerves originating in the cerebral cortex which allow voluntary control of movement. The motor system is conventionally divided into lower motor neurones, spinal and cranial nerves which directly innervate muscles, and upper motor neurones, those of the brain and spinal cord that innervate lower motor neurones. Lesions of lower motor neurones cause a flaccid paralysis with wasting. Lesions of upper motor neurones often cause a spastic paralysis without initial wasting.

The major innervation from the cortex to somatic muscular cells in humans is via the pyramidal system (Figs. 10.25–10.27). Nerves which have their cell bodies in the

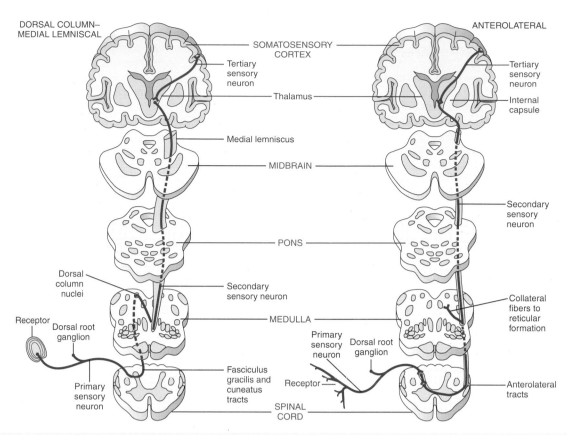

Fig. 10.26 Touch, pressure, pain and proprioception from the trunk and limbs. (*Source*: From Banasik J., 2019. *Pathophysiology*, 6th edn. Elsevier Inc., St. Louis).

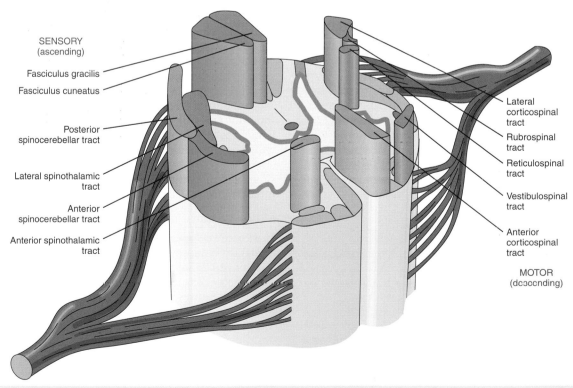

Fig. 10.27 Major spinal pathways. (*Source*: From Banasik J., 2019. *Pathophysiology*, 6th edn. Elsevier Inc., St. Louis).

specialised motor area of the cerebral cortex descend via the internal capsule. About 80% cross the midline in the pyramidal decussation to form the lateral corticospinal tract. The remaining 20% descend the anterior corticospinal tract and cross just before their termination at the spinal lower motor neurone. Current evidence indicates that there are several other areas in the brain which can generate voluntary muscular movement apart from the precentral gyrus, the specialised area where movement of each part of the body is spatially located.

The pyramidal tracts are probably responsible for skilled, fine movement. In addition, the lower motor neurone receives innervation from many other sources. The stretch receptors, acting at a local spinal segmental level, have already been mentioned. The action of these stretch receptors is modulated both by local nervous influences (γ efferent system), which in turn are affected by descending fibres from the cerebrum. The lower motor neurone itself is also innervated from the cerebrum via extrapyramidal tracts, responsible for gross movements and posture, and by fibres from the cerebellum, which are concerned with coordination and control.

Sensory System

Sensation can be divided into the modalities of the special sensory organs—vision, hearing, taste and smell—and the more generalised sensations of pain, touch, temperature and joint position sense. The specialised sensory organs are outside the scope of this book. The organisation and cerebral representation of generalised sensation require further consideration.

Primary afferent fibres from specific receptors enter the spinal cord via the dorsal root. They have their cell bodies in the dorsal root ganglion. Those fibres that come from receptors for proprioception and fine touch ascend in the dorsal columns to the medulla (see Figs. 10.26 and 10.27). There they synapse with second-order neurones in the cuneate and gracile nuclei. The second-order neurones cross the midline, at the level of the medulla, and ascend via the medial lemniscus to the thalamus. Neurones project from the thalamus to at least two areas on the cortex. The most precise localisation is at somatic sensory area I in the postcentral gyrus. Here each part of the body is specifically represented, and within each area are columns of cells which react to specific sensory modalities (e.g. proprioception and fine touch). A second sensory area, somatic sensory area II, is in the wall of the Sylvian fissure. Here, representation of the body is not so complete, nor so specific.

Fibres from pain and temperature receptors and some other touch receptors also enter the spinal cord via the dorsal root, but synapse with nerves in the substantia gelatinosa of the dorsal horn. Fibres from these neurones cross the midline immediately (cf spinothalamic tracts) and then ascend in the anterolateral system of the spinal cord (lateral columns) (see Figs. 10.26 and 10.27). Touch ascends the ventral spinothalamic tract; pain and temperature ascend the lateral spinothalamic tract. These fibres also project to the thalamus and then synapse with other neurones passing to somatic sensory areas I and II. However, the sensations carried by the anterolateral system are not so exclusively represented in the cerebral cortex as those carried by the spinothalamic tracts. Experimental ablation, or observations on patients with spontaneously occurring lesions, show that proprioception and fine touch (spinothalamic tract) are most affected by cortical lesions.

Temperature sensation is less affected and pain sensation (lateral columns) is barely affected at all.

The 'gate' theory accounts for the observation that individuals' perception of pain varies enormously both between individuals and within individuals on different occasions. Many external and internal influences, such as hypnosis, acupuncture and analgesic drugs, can affect pain perception, and probably do so by influencing transmission of impulses from pain receptors at many sites within the central nervous system. One site that has been extensively investigated is in the substantia gelatinosa of the spinal cord (see Fig. 10.27), where pain afferent neurones synapse with fibres that will ascend in the lateral columns. Transmission here can be inhibited by stimulation of other fibres, mediating touch or proprioception in the adjacent spinothalamic tract. Stimulation of these fibres has been used clinically in the relief of pain. The fibres may be stimulated either in the skin (as in the treatment of trigeminal neuralgia using an electrical stimulator) or by implantation of chronic stimulators in the dorsal columns.

RETICULAR ACTIVATING SYSTEM

Apart from the classical projection of sensory input to the cortex, some sensory fibres activate the reticular activating system. This is a diffuse system of nerve fibres in the ventral portion of the midbrain and medulla which appears to be responsible for consciousness and to require sensory input to maintain consciousness (Fig. 10.28). Thus, blunting of sensory input, either experimentally or when, for example, prisoners are 'hooded' for interrogation purposes, is associated with disturbed states of consciousness and hallucinations. Patients with tumours that interrupt the reticular activating system are usually unconscious and, if the tumours are small, may be comatose without any other clinical signs. It appears that the reticular activating system integrates all sensory inputs, and that sensory specificity is therefore not important for its function. The reticular activating system contains the respiratory and cardiovascular centres, and can up- or downregulate sensation, motor

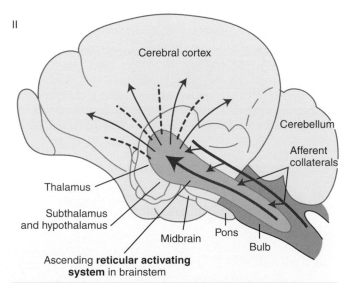

Fig. 10.28 Diagram of ascending reticular activating system. (*Source*: From Daroff R., Jankovic J., Mazziotta J. et al., 2016. *Bradley's Neurology in Clinical Practice*, 7th edn. Elsevier Inc., London).

activity, the electrical activity of the cortex, and many endocrine activities via its hypothalamic connections.

AUTONOMIC NERVOUS SYSTEM

Like the somatic nervous system, the autonomic nervous system has afferent nerves from receptors, central integrating areas (vasomotor centre and respiratory centre) and efferent neurones which run to effector organs. The receptors may be specific to stimuli, such as pressure (carotid sinus baroreceptor) or Po_2 (carotid body chemoreceptor); there are also non-specific receptors in the viscera which respond to pain. Afferents reach the central nervous system via the facial, glossopharyngeal and vagus cranial nerves, and via the dorsal roots from T7 to L2 and from S2 to S4.

The efferent tract of the autonomic nervous system consists of preganglionic fibres followed by postganglionic fibres. The parasympathetic outflow to the visceral structures of the head is via cranial nerves III, VII and IX, to the thorax and upper abdomen via the vagus nerve, and to the pelvis via the sacral outflow, S2 to S4. The preganglionic fibres end in, or very near, the viscus that is innervated. These synapse with short postganglionic fibres that run directly to the effector organ (Fig. 10.29).

By contrast, the sympathetic nervous system is characterised by a chain of ganglia that run outside the spinal cord, but adjacent to it from T1 to L5. The chain is extended towards the head to form three additional cervical ganglia:

the superior, middle and inferior or stellate ganglia. The axons of the preganglionic sympathetic nerves leave the spinal cord in the ventral roots of the spinal nerves and pass via the white rami communicantes to the paravertebral sympathetic ganglion chain. There they synapse with the postganglionic fibres, which run to the viscera. Some postganglionic fibres return to the spinal nerves, via the grey rami communicantes, and then are distributed with the spinal nerves to the autonomic effectors in the appropriate somatic structures innervated by these spinal nerves. Other sympathetic preganglionic fibres do not end in the paravertebral chain but pass through it to collateral ganglia (coeliac ganglions, superior and inferior mesenteric ganglia) near the viscera that they innervate. Short postganglionic fibres then run to each viscus.

The uterus is unusual in that the preganglionic sympathetic fibres run all the way to the uterus and anastomose there with postganglionic fibres. The adrenal medulla is also atypical in that it is innervated by preganglionic sympathetic nerves that pass to it through the coeliac ganglion without synapsing. Alternatively, the adrenal medulla may be considered as a specialised postganglionic nerve that secretes adrenaline, as well as noradrenaline, directly into the bloodstream, rather than secreting noradrenaline at the postganglionic nerve ending.

Chemical Transmission in the Autonomic Nervous System and Autonomic Pharmacology

Parasympathetic Nervous System. Chemical transmission at ganglia and at the ends of postganglionic fibres stimulating smooth muscle and glands is by acetylcholine. The postganglionic effects of acetylcholine are mimicked by the alkaloid muscarine, and these are therefore known as the muscarine actions of acetylcholine. They are blocked by atropine. Transmission at the ganglia is mimicked by nicotine, the nicotinic action of acetylcholine, and this is not blocked by atropine. It is blocked by very high concentrations of acetylcholine. The acetylcholine is metabolised by cholinesterase. Drugs that interfere with cholinesterase activity (e.g. physostigmine) will potentiate transmission at the autonomic ganglia, and at the postganglionic nerve ending (these drugs will also potentiate somatic neuromuscular transmission).

Sympathetic Nervous System. Transmission at the ganglia is by the nicotinic action of acetylcholine. Transmission at most postganglionic nerve endings is by noradrenaline (norepinephrine). Some drugs, such as tyramine or ephedrine, increase sympathetic activity by enhancing noradrenaline release at the postganglionic nerve ending.

Those sympathetic postganglionic neurones which innervate sweat glands are cholinergic (acetylcholine as a transmitter), and so are the sympathetic postganglionic fibres which cause vasodilatation in smooth muscle.

Noradrenaline (norepinephrine) is one of a group of substances, the catecholamines. The other principal catecholamine found outside the central nervous system is adrenaline (epinephrine) secreted by the adrenal medulla. Dopamine is on the metabolic pathway of adrenaline and noradrenaline. So far, it has mainly been studied within the central nervous system and hypothalamopituitary axis, where, for example, dopamine inhibits prolactin release.

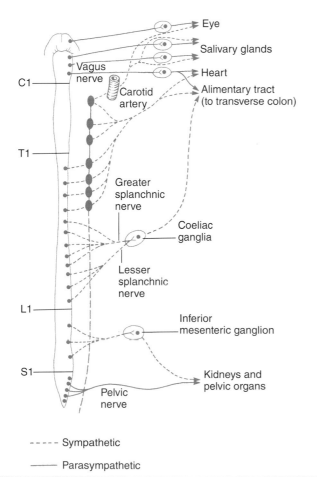

- - - - Sympathetic

——— Parasympathetic

Fig. 10.29 Diagram of the efferent automatic pathways.

The catecholamine receptors are divided into α- and β-receptors on the basis of the drugs which block transmission at the receptor site. α-Receptors, blocked by phentolamine and phenoxybenzamine, can be separated from β-receptors blocked by propranolol.

In general, α-receptors are excitatory (vasoconstriction, pupillary constriction) and β-receptors are inhibitory (bronchodilatation, decreased uterine activity). An important exception is the heart, where β-receptors are excitatory. Not all β-receptors are the same. Some β-adrenergic blocking drugs chiefly affect the heart; these are β_1-adrenergic blocking agents, or cardioselective β-blocking agents, of which the prototype was practolol. Less toxic agents in current clinical usage are metoprolol and atenolol. Other β-receptors are designated as β_2-receptors. These are found in the bronchi and the uterus, and non-selective β-adrenergic blocking agents (e.g. propranolol) block both β_1- and β_2-receptors. The development of specific α-, β_1- and β_2-receptor blocking agents allowed the differentiation of both naturally occurring and synthetic catecholamines into α, β_1 and β_2 agonists. Thus adrenaline and noradrenaline stimulate both α- and β_1-receptors, but adrenaline also stimulates β_2-receptors. Metaraminol and phenylephrine are specific α agonists. Isoprenaline is a specific β agonist which stimulates both β_1- and β_2-receptors. Salbutamol, orciprenaline, terbutaline and ritodrine, all of which have been used for the treatment of premature labour, stimulate β_2-receptors more than β_1 and so cause relaxation of the uterus. In addition, these drugs cause bronchial dilatation, and most have been used and were developed for the treatment of asthma (the exception is ritodrine).

A list of adrenergic (sympathetic) and cholinergic (mainly parasympathetic) activity is given in Table 10.12. Table 10.13 shows some of the drugs that influence autonomic activity.

Blood

IRON METABOLISM

Iron is abundant in most soils and waters of the Earth's surface. It is easily and reversibly oxidised or reduced. It has been incorporated into numerous proteins of critical importance for the sustenance of both plant and animal life.

The total body iron content of a normal adult male is approximately 50 mg/kg, that of an adult woman about 38 mg/kg. This difference merely reflects the high incidence of reduced iron stores in women; there are no fundamental differences in iron metabolism between the sexes.

The iron is distributed in several physiologically and chemically distinct forms (Table 10.14). Haemoglobin iron comprises about 70% of the total body iron and is the largest iron-containing compartment.

Table 10.12 Responses of Organs to Cholinergic and Adrenergic Stimuli

Organ	RESPONSE Adrenergic (α/β)	RESPONSE Cholinergic
Pupil	Constriction (α)	Constriction
	Dilatation (β)	
Salivary glands	Scanty viscid secretion (α)	Copious watery secretion
Blood vessels	Constrictor (α)	Dilator
Heart	Dilator (β_2)	Dilator
Skin	Constrictor (α)	
Muscle	Constrictor (α)	
Pulmonary	Dilator (β_2)	
Kidney	Constrictor (α)	
	Constrictor (α)	
Lung	Relaxation (β_2)	Constriction
Bronchi		Increased secretion
Bronchial glands		
Heart	Increased (β_1)	Decrease
Rate, contractility, conduction velocity		
Kidney	Increased (β_2)	
Renin secretion		
Sweating	Localised (e.g. palms of hands (α))	Generalised
Pregnant uterus	Decreased contraction (β_2)	
	Increased contraction (α)	

Table 10.13 Some Drugs Influencing Autonomic Activity

Site of Action	Agents Decreasing Activity		Agents Increasing Activity	
Sympathetic and parasympathetic ganglia	High concentration of acetylcholine		Acetylcholine	
	Ganglion-blocking agents:		Carbachol	
	Hexamethonium		Nicotine	
	Mecamylamine		Anticholinesterase drugs (e.g. physostigmine)	
	Pentolinium			
	Trimetaphan			
Endings of parasympathetic neurones	Atropine		Anticholinesterase drugs:	
	Scopolamine		Acetylcholine	
	Propantheline		Carbachol	
			Muscarine	
			Pilocarpine	
Sympathetic postganglionic nerve endings	Reserpine		Drugs releasing noradrenaline:	
	Guanethidine		Ephedrine	
			Amphetamines	
			Tyrosine	
β_1-Receptors	Propranolol	Also block β_2-Receptors to a lesser extent	Isoprenaline	
	Atenolol		Adrenaline	
	Metoprolol		Noradrenaline	
	Practolol			
β_2-Receptors	Propranolol		Adrenaline	Also β_1 but mainly β_2
			Isoprenaline	
			Salbutamol	
			Orciprenaline	
			Terbutaline	
			Ritodrine	
α-Receptors	Phenoxybenzamine		Noradrenaline	
	Phentolamine		Adrenaline	
			Metaraminol	
			Methoxamine	
			Phenylephrine	

Table 10.14   Distribution of Iron

Location	Form	Distribution (%)
Haemoglobin iron		70
Tissue iron		30
Storage iron	Haemosiderin	
Essential iron	Ferritin	
	Myoglobin	
	Enzymes	
	Cytochromes	
	Peroxidases	
	Catalases	
Plasma transport iron	Transferrin	0.19

The other haem-containing molecule is myoglobin, a protein present in muscle. It is said to provide a reserve of available oxygen in cases of sudden strenuous exercise.

Storage iron is held available for use as needed in the macrophages of the reticuloendothelial system and is in two forms: ferritin, which is a glycoprotein detectable by chemical analysis, and aggregates of ferritin, which form haemosiderin.

A very small amount of iron is contained in the enzymes—cytochromes, catalases and peroxidases essential for metabolism of all cells in the body.

A minute portion of the total iron (0.19%) is bound to a specific plasma protein—transferrin (see Table 10.14).

The total iron content of the body tends to remain fixed within narrow limits; otherwise iron excess (siderosis) or deficiency occurs. Iron is not excreted in the usual sense of the word; it is lost from the body only when cells are lost, especially epithelial cells from the gastrointestinal tract. Urinary iron amounts to <0.5 mg/day in desquamated cells. In women, menstrual flow constitutes an important additional route of iron loss. Average daily loss has been estimated to be about 1.0 mg/day in normal adult men and non-menstruating women. About twice this amount is lost in menstruating women. In normal situations, these losses are balanced by an equivalent amount of iron absorbed from the diet. Therefore, iron balance is unique in that it is achieved by control of absorption rather than control of excretion.

Iron Absorption

Since the total body iron content depends so greatly on absorption of iron, the mechanisms by which the rate of absorption is regulated are of critical importance.

Iron is absorbed chiefly in portions of the intestine proximal to the jejunum. Maximum absorption occurs in the duodenum.

Two factors are of prime importance in determining absorptive rate:

1. The amount of storage iron. When it is depleted, iron absorption is increased. When it is excessive, iron absorption is decreased.

2. The rate of erythropoiesis. Iron absorption goes up when red cell production rate is increased and down when production is decreased.

Iron absorption takes place in two distinct steps:

1. Mucosal uptake.
2. Transfer of iron from mucosal cell to plasma.

The uptake of iron by the mucosa is influenced by the overall composition of the diet, which determines how much iron is available for absorption (see below).

A normal mixed diet supplies about 14 mg iron each day, of which only 1 to 2 mg is absorbed. The availability in food is quite variable. In most foods, inorganic iron is in the ferric form (Fe^{+++}) and has to be converted to the ferrous form (Fe^{++}) before absorption can take place. In foods derived from grain, iron often forms a stable complex with phytates and only small amounts can be converted to a soluble form. The iron in eggs is poorly absorbed because of binding with phosphates present in the yolk. Milk, particularly cow's milk, is poor in iron content. Tea (tannins) inhibits the absorption of iron. Gastric acid and vitamin C promote reduction of ferric iron (Fe^{+++}) to ferrous iron (Fe^{++}) which is more easily absorbed.

Haem iron derived from haemoglobin and myoglobin of animal origin is more effectively absorbed than non-haem iron. Factors interfering with or promoting the absorption of inorganic iron have no effect on the absorption of haem iron. This puts vegetarians at a disadvantage in terms of iron sufficiency.

Iron Cycle

The metabolism of iron is dominated by its role in haemoglobin synthesis. In this process iron is utilised repeatedly so that the internal movements of iron may be described as a cycle (Fig. 10.30). Central to this cycle is the plasma compartment in which iron is bound to a

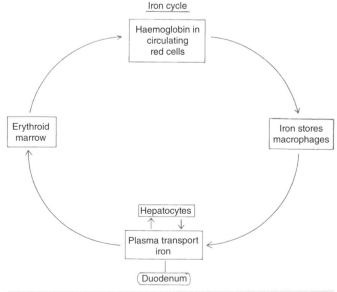

Fig. 10.30 The iron cycle.

transport protein—transferrin. Iron moves from plasma to cells that have the capacity to make haemoglobin. At the end of the red cells' 120-day lifespan, they are ingested by macrophages of the reticuloendothelial system. There, iron is extracted from haemoglobin, delivered to the plasma and bound to transferrin, completing the cycle. A small amount of iron, probably less than 2.0 mg, leaves the plasma each day to enter the hepatic cells and other tissues. Here, the iron is utilised to make tissue haem proteins such as myoglobin and the cytochromes.

HAEMOPOIESIS AND IRON METABOLISM IN PREGNANCY

There is increased erythropoiesis from early pregnancy due to increased EPO production and possibly due to other hormones such as placental lactogen. In spite of this, some degree of anaemia, as judged by normal non-pregnant standards, is manifest by the end of the second trimester. This is due to haemodilution and occurs because the increase in plasma volume (50%) exceeds that of the red cell mass (18% to 25%). The haemoglobin reaches its lowest level at 32 weeks of gestation, when the haemodilution is maximal. The haemodilution is exaggerated in twin pregnancies.

In pregnancy, the demand for iron is increased to meet mainly the needs of the expanded red cell mass and, to a lesser extent, the requirements of the developing fetus and placenta. The fetus derives its iron from the maternal serum by active transport across the placenta. The total requirement of iron is about 700 to 1400 mg. Overall, the requirement is 4 mg/day, but this rises from 2.8 mg/day in the non-pregnant woman to 6.6 mg/day in the last few weeks of pregnancy. This can be met only by mobilising iron stores in addition to achieving maximum absorption of dietary iron.

Iron absorption is increased when there is erythroid hyperplasia (i.e. rapid iron turnover and a high concentration of unsaturated transferrin) both of which are part of the physiological response in the healthy pregnant woman. There is evidence that absorption of dietary iron is enhanced in the latter half of pregnancy, but this still does not provide enough iron for the needs of pregnancy and the puerperium for a woman on a normal mixed diet.

The amount of iron absorbed will depend very much on the extent of the iron stores, the content of the diet and whether or not iron supplements are given.

The commonest haematological problem in pregnancy is anaemia resulting from iron deficiency.

Iron Deficiency in Pregnancy

The changes in blood volume and haemodilution are so variable that the normal range of haemoglobin concentration in healthy pregnancy at 30 weeks of gestation in women who have received parenteral iron is 105 to 145 g/L. Haemoglobin values of less than 105 g/L in the second and third trimesters are likely to reflect non-anaemic iron deficiency.

Red Cell Indices

The appearance of red cells on a stained film is a relatively insensitive gauge of iron status in pregnancy. Electronic counters allow accurate red cell counts to be performed and the size of the red cell (mean cell volume, MCV), its haemoglobin content (mean corpuscular haemoglobin, MCH) and mean corpuscular haemoglobin concentration (MCHC) can be calculated from the red cell count (red blood cell count, RBC), haemoglobin concentration and packed cell volume (PCV).

The earliest effect of iron deficiency on the erythrocyte is a reduction in MCV, and in pregnancy, with the dramatic changes in red cell mass and plasma volume, this is the most sensitive indicator of red cell indices of underlying iron deficiency. Hypochromia and a fall in the MCHC only appear with more severe degrees of iron depletion. However, MCV is elevated in pregnancy, and in B_{12} or folate deficiency and hypothyroidism.

Some women start pregnancy with established iron deficiency or depleted iron stores and quickly develop anaemia with reduced MCV, MCH and MCHC.

Serum Iron and Total Iron-Binding Capacity

The serum iron of a healthy, adult, non-pregnant woman lies between 13 and 27 µmol/L. Serum iron levels vary markedly and even fluctuate from hour to hour. The TIBC in the woman in a non-pregnant state lies between 45 and 72 µmol/L. It is raised in association with iron deficiency and is low in chronic inflammatory states. In the non-anaemic individual, the TIBC is approximately one-third saturated with iron.

In pregnancy, there is a fall in the serum iron and percentage saturation of the TIBC; the fall in serum iron can be prevented by iron supplements. Serum iron, even in combination with the TIBC, is not a reliable indication of iron stores because it fluctuates so widely and is affected by recent ingestion of iron or factors such as infection, which are not directly involved with iron metabolism. With these major reservations, a serum iron of <12 µmol/L and a TIBC saturation of <15% indicates iron deficiency in pregnancy.

Ferritin

Ferritin is a high-molecular-weight glycoprotein, which circulates in the plasma, and is now the first-line test for assessing iron stores in pregnancy. A ferritin of less than 15 µg/L indicates established iron deficiency whilst values of <30µg/L indicate insufficient stores for pregnancy which also warrant treatment. Ferritin levels are stable and not affected by recent ingestion of oral iron. It appears to reflect the iron stores accurately and quantitatively, particularly in the lower range associated with iron deficiency, which is so important in pregnancy. It is however an acute phase reactant and non-specifically rises in acute and chronic inflammatory conditions.

HAEMOSTASIS

Haemostatic mechanisms have two functions:

1. To confine the circulating blood to the vascular bed.
2. To arrest bleeding from injured vessels.

Both of these aspects of haemostasis probably depend on:

- Normal vasculature
- Platelets—number and function

- Coagulation factors
- Healthy fibrinolysis.

HAEMOSTASIS AND PREGNANCY

Normal pregnancy is accompanied by dramatic changes in the coagulation and fibrinolytic systems. There is a marked increase in some of the coagulation factors, particularly fibrinogen. Fibrin is laid down in the uteroplacental vessel walls and fibrinolysis is suppressed. These changes, together with the increased blood volume, help to combat the hazard of haemorrhage at placental separation but play only a secondary role to the unique process of myometrial contraction, which reduces blood flow to the placental site. They also produce a vulnerable state for intravascular clotting and a whole spectrum of disorders involving coagulation which may occur in pregnancy; these fall into two main groups: thromboembolism and bleeding due to disseminated intravascular coagulation (DIC).

A short account of haemostasis during pregnancy and how it differs from non-pregnant haemostasis follows.

Vascular Integrity

It is not known how vascular integrity is normally maintained but it is clear that platelets have a key role. When platelet number is depleted or their function is abnormal, there is a risk of spontaneous capillary haemorrhage. In health, platelets are constantly sealing microdefects of the vasculature with mini-fibrin clots. Unwanted fibrin is then removed by fibrinolysis.

Prostacyclin (PGI_2) is an unstable prostaglandin first discovered in 1976. It is the principal prostanoid synthesised by blood vessels and is a powerful vasodilator and potent inhibitor of platelet aggregation. There is a delicate balance between the production of PGI_2 and thromboxane, a powerful platelet-aggregating agent and vasoconstrictor. Prostacyclin prevents platelet aggregation at much lower concentrations than is needed to prevent adhesion. Therefore, vascular damage leads to platelet adhesion but not necessarily to aggregation and thrombus formation.

When the injury is minor, small platelet thrombi form and are washed away by the circulation as described earlier, but the extent of the injury is an important determinant of the size of the thrombus and whether or not platelet aggregation is stimulated. Prostacyclin synthetase is abundant in the endothelium and progressively decreases in concentration from the intima to the adventitia. In contrast the pro-aggregating elements increase in concentration from the subendothelium to the adventitia. It follows that severe vessel damage or physical detachment of the endothelium will lead to the development of a large thrombus rather than simple platelet adherence.

The platelet count gradually falls during healthy uncomplicated pregnancy. At term approximately 10% of women with uncomplicated pregnancies have a platelet count $<150 \times 10^9$/L, and 1% have a platelet count $<100 \times 10^9$/L. Platelet count falls in pregnancies complicated by pre-eclampsia. There is no evidence of changes in platelet function, or differences in platelet lifespan, between healthy non-pregnant and pregnant women, although the lifespan is shortened significantly when pre-eclampsia is present.

Arrest of Bleeding After Trauma

An essential function of the haemostatic system is a rapid reaction to injury, which remains confined to the area of damage. This requires control mechanisms which will stimulate coagulation after trauma and limit the extent of the response. The substances involved in the formation of the haemostatic plug normally circulate in an inert form until activated at the site of injury or by some factor released into the circulation which will trigger off intravascular coagulation.

Local Response

Platelets adhere to collagen on the injured basement membrane. This initiates a series of changes in the platelets themselves, including a change in their shape and release of ADP (adenosine diphosphate) and other substances. ADP release stimulates further aggregation of platelets, the coagulation cascade is triggered off and the action of thrombin leads to the formation of fibrin, which converts the loose platelet plug into a firm, stable wound seal. The role of platelets is of less importance in injury involving large vessels because platelet aggregates are of insufficient size and strength to breach the defect. The coagulation mechanism is of major importance here, together with vascular contraction.

Coagulation System

The end result of blood coagulation is the formation of an insoluble fibrin clot from the soluble precursor fibrinogen in the plasma. This involves a complex interaction of clotting factors and a sequential activation of a series of pro-enzymes, which has been termed the coagulation cascade (Fig. 10.31). When a blood vessel is injured, blood coagulation is initiated by activation of factor XII by collagen (intrinsic mechanism) and activation of factor VII by thromboplastin release (extrinsic mechanism from the damaged tissue). But the intrinsic and extrinsic mechanisms are activated by components of the vessel wall and both are required for normal haemostasis.

Strict divisions between the two pathways do not exist and interactions between activated factors in both pathways have been shown. They share a common pathway following activation of factor X.

The intrinsic pathway, or contact system, proceeds spontaneously and is relatively slow, requiring 5 to 20 minutes for visible fibrin formation. All tissues contain a specific lipoprotein, thromboplastin, which markedly increases the rate at which blood clots. It is particularly concentrated in the lung and brain. The placenta is also very rich in tissue factor, which will produce fibrin formation within 12 seconds, the acceleration of coagulation being brought about by bypassing the reactions involving the contact (intrinsic) system.

Blood coagulation is strictly confined to the site of tissue injury in normal circumstances. Powerful control mechanisms must act to prevent dissemination of coagulation beyond the site of trauma.

The action of thrombin in vivo is controlled by a number of mechanisms, particularly its absorption onto the locally formed fibrin, and the presence of a potent inhibitor, antithrombin, and α_2-globulin, which destroys thrombin activity. Heparin, which potentiates the action of anti-X_a, may be similar to antithrombin. This is the rationale for low-dose heparin therapy as prophylaxis in patients at risk of

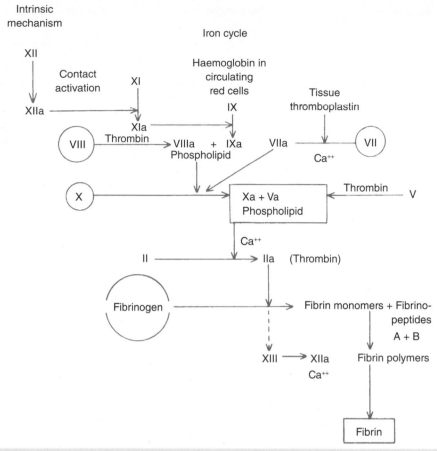

Fig. 10.31 The factors involved in blood coagulation and their interactions. The circled factors show significant increases in pregnancy. (*Source*: Reproduced with permission from Hytten F, Chamberlain G. *Clinical physiology in obstetrics*. Blackwell Scientific, Oxford.)

thromboembolic phenomena postoperatively, and in pregnancy and the puerperium.

Normal pregnancy is accompanied by major changes in the coagulation system with increases in the levels of factors VII, VIII and X, and a particularly marked increase in the level of plasma fibrinogen (see Fig. 10.31). The increased fibrinogen concentration is probably the chief cause of the accelerated erythrocyte sedimentation rate observed during pregnancy.

The effect of pregnancy on the coagulation factors can be detected from about the third month of gestation. In late pregnancy, the fibrinogen concentration is at least double that of the non-pregnant state.

Fibrinolysis

Fibrinolytic activity is an essential part of the dynamic haemostatic system and is dependent on plasminogen activator in the blood (Fig. 10.32). Fibrin and fibrinogen are digested by plasmin, a proenzyme derived from an inactive plasma precursor, plasminogen.

Increased amounts of activator are found in the plasma after strenuous exercise, emotional stress, surgical operations and other trauma.

Tissue activator can be extracted from most human organs with the exception of the placenta. Tissues especially rich in activator include the uterus, ovaries, prostate, heart, lungs, thyroid, adrenal glands and lymph nodes. Activity in tissues is concentrated mainly around blood vessels, veins showing greater activity than arteries. Venous occlusion of the limbs will stimulate fibrinolytic activity, a fact which should be remembered if tourniquets are applied for any length of time before blood is drawn for measurement of fibrin degradation products (FDPs).

The inhibitors of fibrinolytic activity are of two types: anti-activators (anti-plasminogens) and the antiplasmins.

Anti-plasminogens include ε-aminocaproic acid (EACA) and tranexamic acid (AMCA). Aprotinin (Trasylol) is another anti-plasminogen commercially prepared from bovine lung.

Platelets, plasma and serum exert a strong inhibitory action on plasmin. Normally, plasma antiplasmin levels exceed levels of plasminogen, and hence the levels of potential plasmin; otherwise, we would dissolve away our connecting cement! Plasma fibrinolytic activity is decreased during pregnancy, remains low during labour and delivery, and returns to normal within 1 hour of placental delivery. The rapid return of systemic fibrinolytic activity to normal following delivery of the placenta, and the fact that the placenta has been shown to contain inhibitors which block fibrinolysis, suggest that inhibition of fibrinolysis during pregnancy is mediated through the placenta. When fibrinogen, soluble fibrin or cross-linked fibrin is broken down by plasmin, FDPs are formed. The

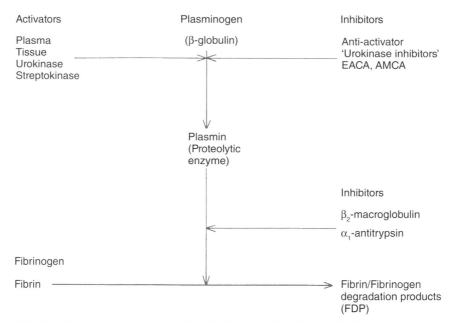

Fig. 10.32 Components of the fibrinolytic system. *AMCA*, Tranexamic acid; *EACA*, ε-aminocaproic acid. (*Source*: Reproduced with permission from F. Hytten F, Chamberlain G. *Clinical physiology in obstetrics*. Blackwell Scientific, Oxford.)

most commonly measured FDP in clinical practice is the D-dimer, with elevated levels seen in conditions such as DIC and thromboembolism. D-dimers are formed when fibrin is cross-linked by thrombin-activated factor XIIIa to make an insoluble protein with a D-D neoepitope which plasmin then proteolyses to release the soluble D-dimer. As such the D-dimer reflects activation of coagulation (thrombin) and fibrinolysis (plasmin) pathways, in contrast to other FDPs which are only indicative of plasmin activity. D-dimer levels increase in normal pregnancy with the highest levels seen at term.

Summary of Changes in Haemostasis in Pregnancy

The changes in the coagulation system in normal pregnancy are consistent with a continuing low-grade process of pro-coagulant activity. Using electron microscopy, fibrin deposition can be demonstrated in the intervillous space of the placenta and in all the walls of the spiral arteries supplying the placenta. As pregnancy advances, the elastic lamina and smooth muscle of these spiral arteries are replaced by a matrix containing fibrin. This allows expansion of the lumen to accommodate an increasing blood flow and reduces the pressure in arterial blood flowing to the placenta. At placental separation, a blood flow of 500 to 800 mL/min has to be staunched within seconds, or serious haemorrhage occurs. Myometrial contraction plays a vital role in securing haemostasis by reducing the blood flow to the placental site. Rapid closure of the terminal part of the spiral arteries will be further facilitated by the structural changes within their walls.

The placental site is rapidly covered by a fibrin mesh following delivery. The increased levels of fibrinogen and other coagulation factors will meet the sudden demand for haemostatic components at placental separation.

Thromboembolism

The dramatic changes described above facilitate arrest of bleeding from the placental site at delivery but carry with them an increased risk of thromboembolism. The rise in D-dimers during normal pregnancy negates its use as a screening tool for thromboembolism in low-risk pregnant women. Pregnant women have a 5-fold increased risk of thromboembolic disease, rising to 10-fold in the puerperium. The increased risk of thromboembolism starts in the first trimester and is steady throughout gestation. The 2016–2018 MBRRACE report showed, as in previous reports, that thromboembolism remains the leading 'direct' cause of maternal mortality in the UK.

Disseminated Intravascular Coagulation

The changes in the haemostatic system during pregnancy and the local activation of the clotting system during parturition carry with them a risk, not only of thromboembolism, but of DIC, consumption of clotting factors and platelets leading to severe bleeding—particularly uterine and sometimes generalised. Despite the advances in obstetric care and highly developed blood transfusion services, haemorrhage still constitutes a major factor in maternal mortality and morbidity.

The first problem with DIC is its definition. It is never primary, but always secondary to some general stimulation of coagulation activity by release of procoagulant substances into the blood (Fig. 10.33). Potential triggers of this process in pregnancy include the leaking of placental tissue fragments, amniotic fluid, incompatible red cells or bacterial products into the maternal circulation. There is a great spectrum of manifestations of the process of DIC, ranging from a compensated state with no clinical manifestation, but evidence of increased production and breakdown of coagulation factors, to the condition of massive

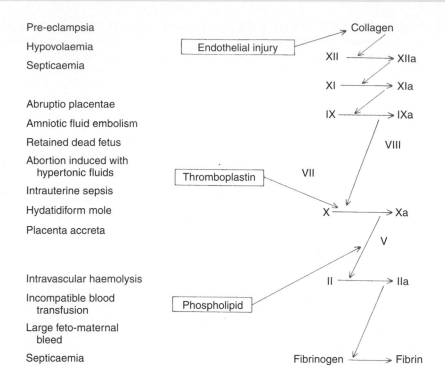

Pre-eclampsia
Hypovolaemia
Septicaemia

Abruptio placentae
Amniotic fluid embolism
Retained dead fetus
Abortion induced with
    hypertonic fluids
Intrauterine sepsis
Hydatidiform mole
Placenta accreta

Intravascular haemolysis
Incompatible blood
    transfusion
Large feto-maternal
    bleed
Septicaemia

Interactions of the trigger mechanisms
occur in many of these obstetric
complications

Fig. 10.33 Trigger mechanisms of disseminated intravascular coagulation in pregnancy. (*Source*: Reproduced with permission from de Swiet M. *Medical disorders in pregnancy*. Blackwell Scientific, Oxford.)

uncontrollable haemorrhage with very low concentrations of plasma fibrinogen, pathological raised levels of FDPs and variable degrees of thrombocytopenia.

Fibrinolysis is stimulated by DIC and FDPs resulting from the process interfering with the formation of firm fibrin clots. A vicious circle is established, which results in further severe bleeding.

Obstetric conditions classically associated with DIC include: placental abruption, amniotic fluid embolism, septic abortion and other intrauterine infection, retained dead fetus, hydatidiform mole, placenta accreta, pre-eclampsia, and prolonged shock from any cause (see Fig. 10.33).

RHESUS INCOMPATIBILITY

In the late 1930s, it was discovered that red cells from Rhesus monkeys injected into guineapigs and rabbits produced an antibody in the animals' sera which reacted strongly with the red cells of 85% of Caucasians. Those individuals whose red cells were agglutinated strongly with the Rhesus (Rh) antibody were called Rh-positive and the remaining 15% were termed Rh-negative.

Soon after the recognition of the Rh factor, it was shown that this antigen had important clinical significance in terms of haemolytic disease of the newborn (HDN) and transfusion reactions.

The Rh-negative recipients of Rh-positive transfusions could suffer haemolytic transfusion reactions and

Rh-positive babies carried by Rh-negative mothers were frequently affected by haemolytic anaemia *in utero* and in the postnatal period.

An immediate recommendation was that Rh-negative female recipients in or below childbearing years should be transfused with Rh-negative blood.

However, there were differences in the specificities of the antibodies produced by the sensitised Rh-negative mothers, and it became clear that the Rh factor was complex and it would be more reasonable to use the term 'Rh blood group system'.

For a basic understanding of the Rh system, only five of the 26 or more recognised antigens need to be considered: C, $\bar{c}$, D, E, $\bar{e}$. The Rh blood group antigens are carried by a series of at least three homologous but distinct red cell membrane associated proteins. Two of these proteins have immunologically distinguishable isoforms designated C, $\bar{c}$ and E, $\bar{e}$. The principal protein, D, has no immunologically detectable isoform d. The RH gene locus (on chromosome 1p34 to p36) consists, in RhD-positive individuals, of two similar genes designated C$\bar{c}$ E$\bar{e}$ and D. The first gene, C/$\bar{c}$ E$\bar{e}$, encodes both the C/$\bar{c}$ and E/$\bar{e}$ proteins, by alternative splicing of a primary transcript. The second gene, D, encodes the major antigen RhD and is absent in RhD-negative individuals. Therefore, the presence or absence of the D gene in the genome determines the genetic basis of the Rh-positive/Rh-negative blood group polymorphism, which explains the absence of a detectable isoform of the D antigen (d) at the red cell surface of Rh-negative individuals. Although haematologists will refer to an individual as DD, Dd or dd, the designation 'd' indicates the absence of the 'D' antigen. In the case of C$\overline{\text{c}}$ and E$\overline{\text{e}}$, both the upper- and lower-case letters indicate the presence of a serologically definable antigen.

The genes encoding the three major sets of antigens are inherited together so that specific sets of antigens are inherited together rather than random inheritance of each of the C/$\overline{\text{c}}$, D/d, E/$\overline{\text{e}}$ antigens. This suggested to earlier investigators that there would be either one single gene encoding all the C/$\overline{\text{c}}$, D/d, E/$\overline{\text{e}}$ epitopes, or three genes closely linked on the chromosome so that recombination rarely takes place between them. Whether from Rh-positive or Rh-negative individuals, virtually all normal erythrocytes carry the antithetical antigens C and/or $\overline{\text{c}}$ and E and/or $\overline{\text{e}}$. The erythrocytes of very rare individuals who lack all these antigens have multiple membrane abnormalities, suggesting that the Rh antigens are of major physiological importance. The RhD-negative phenotype is a trait of Caucasians in whom the incidence is 15%. In Basques, 35% are RhD-negative, while only 1% of North American Indians and 7% of African-Americans are RhD negative. The incidence in Asiatic Chinese and Japanese is almost zero.

It is the D antigens that are the major cause of HDN. In Caucasian populations, 56% of RhD-positive individuals are heterozygous for the D antigen. If a RhD-negative woman has a RhD-positive partner there is therefore an approximately 50% chance that he will be a homozygote, in which case all of their children will be RhD positive (all being heterozygotes), and an approximately 50% chance that he will be a heterozygote, in which case half of their children will be heterozygote RhD positive and half will be RhD negative.

D^{u} antigen. A few individuals have antigens on their cells which react weakly and variably with the various forms of anti-D antisera—these are termed group D^{u}. For transfusion purposes an individual with the blood group D^{u} should be regarded as Rh(D) negative when receiving blood but as Rh(D) positive when donating blood.

Haemolytic Disease of the Newborn

HDN is a condition in which the lifespan of the infant's red cells is shortened by the action of specific antibodies derived from the mother. The immune antibodies in the maternal plasma are small molecular immunoglobulins of the IgG subclass and therefore, unlike the large molecule, naturally occurring antibodies of the ABO blood group systems (IgM) are able to cross the placenta.

Although HDN can occur in several situations where the mother lacks an antigen which her baby carries on its red cells, there is no doubt that, prior to the introduction of the specific immunoglobulin for the prevention of Rh(D) haemolytic disease, Rh(D) HDN was by far the most important form of HDN in terms of clinical severity and frequency in Caucasian populations. Other Rh antibodies which can cause HDN are anti-E and anti-c, in which case the mother is usually Rh(D) positive.

Outside the Rh blood group system, the most frequently observed immune-induced antibody is anti-Kell. This is usually more transfusion provoked, 95% of the Caucasian population being Kell negative. Occasionally, this antibody can cause severe HDN where the father is Kell positive (heterozygous or homozygous) and he has transmitted the Kell positive gene to his offspring.

HDN begins in intrauterine life and may result in death *in utero*. In liveborn infants the haemolytic process is maximal at the time of birth and thereafter diminishes as the concentration of maternal antibody in the infant's circulation declines.

During pregnancy, the fetal and maternal circulations are separate. Red cells are not thought to cross the placental barrier in significant numbers in normal circumstances. Oxygen, nutrient and waste exchange takes place by diffusion across the intervillous space. IgG antibodies cross the placenta freely, carrying protection (passive immunity) for the fetus against infective agents to which the mother has had a healthy immune response.

Following delivery and placental separation, rupture of the placental villi and connective tissue allows escape of fetal blood cells into the maternal circulation, prior to constriction of the open maternal vessels. This is when sensitisation takes place in the majority of cases unless prevented via the administration of anti-D immunoglobulin derived from pooled plasma from multiple donors.

The incompatible Rh(D) fetal cells enter the maternal spleen and the foreign antigen on the fetal red cell triggers off an immune response causing production of antibody.

In a subsequent pregnancy with an Rh(D)-positive fetus, the immune IgG anti-D maternal antibody will cross the placenta and attach to the specific D antigen sites on the fetal red cell. IgG-coated red cells do not have a normal lifespan. They are particularly sensitive to cells of the reticuloendothelial system and are removed from the circulation prematurely. Progressive anaemia *in utero* occurs from about the fourth month of pregnancy and, in the most severe cases, intrauterine death has been recorded from the 20th week of pregnancy, although it is uncommon before the 24th week. Many of the stillborn infants are grossly oedematous and are then described as having hydrops fetalis. Hydropic infants are occasionally born alive and are found to be severely anaemic with cord haemoglobin as low as 35 g/L. There is a great increase in the number of nucleated red cells in the circulating blood, hence the term erythroblastosis fetalis is sometimes used to describe the haematological condition.

Jaundice does not occur before delivery because bilirubin produced by the breakdown of cells in the fetal spleen passes via the placenta to the maternal circulation. Albumin transports the fetal bilirubin to the maternal liver where glucuronyl transferase converts it to excretable, direct-reacting bilirubin. The liver of the neonate does not produce glucuronyl transferase and cannot convert bilirubin to an excretable form. Consequently, bilirubin accumulates and if not removed (by exchange transfusion) will collect in the tissues causing jaundice and brain damage. Deeply jaundiced infants often exhibit signs of damage to the central nervous system. These signs usually develop after the age of 36 hour.

It has been shown that the brain contains lipid which takes up the unconjugated bilirubin but does not take up conjugated bilirubin. In kernicterus, the yellow-staining material has been shown to be unconjugated bilirubin.

Assessment of Rhesus Status

Non-invasive pre-natal testing of fetal RhD status now exists through analysis of cell free DNA in maternal blood—small fragments of extracellular fetal DNA shed by the placenta which can be extracted from the mother's peripheral blood. The presence of a RhD genotype in the singleton pregnancy of a RhD negative woman indicates that the fetus is RhD positive. If she is carrying twins or higher multiples it indicates that at least one fetus is RhD positive. If there is feto-maternal discordance in RhD status then anti-D immunoglobulin can be administered to the RhD negative mother at birth and during any potentially sensitising event (e.g. external cephalic version of a breach infant, invasive antenatal procedures, miscarriage). If both mother and fetus are RhD negative then anti-D is not required. By limiting exposure to anti-D immunoglobulin we protect a finite resource and limit the risks of blood products including reactions and the potential of future unknown transmissible diseases such as blood borne viruses and prion diseases.

Detection of Rhesus Anti-D Antibody

Direct Antiglobulin (Coombs) Test (Baby's Red Blood Cells, One-Stage Test). When a neonate suffers from HDN the red cells are coated with immune IgG antibody. This is known as incomplete antibody. These cells do not agglutinate but if an anti-IgG antiserum is added to a mixture of sensitised cells the gap is bridged between antibody on individual red cells and visible agglutination occurs. This is known as a positive direct Coombs test.

Indirect Antiglobulin (Coombs) Test (Maternal Serum, Two-Stage Test). The mother produces antibody against the Rh(D)-positive fetal cells. The antibody is free in her serum because her Rh(D)-negative red cells do not carry the appropriate antigen. If her serum is incubated with Rh(D)-positive cells the antibodies will attach to them but, as it is an IgG, agglutination does not occur. However, if anti-IgG antiserum is then added to the sensitised cells (cf direct Coombs test), visible agglutination will occur. This is known as the 'indirect Coombs test' and is used routinely to detect the presence of anti-Rh and other immune antibodies in maternal serum during pregnancy. By serial dilution of maternal serum and reporting the weakest dilution of the serum at which a reaction with the Rh(D)-positive red cell takes place, a crude estimation of the concentration of the antibody can be made. Serial estimations will give an indication of the rate of increase of antibody in a particular pregnancy.

With the advent of automation in blood transfusion laboratories, it has now become routine in large centres to estimate the Rh(D) antibody in international units based on an automated system using the Coombs test principle.

Amniocentesis

Although measurement of antenatal anti-D concentration has become more exact, correlation between antibody levels and severity of the haemolytic process in the fetus is not sufficient to plan management during pregnancy; however, maternal titres <15 IU/mL are unlikely to cause fetal complications.

By estimation of the bilirubin concentration in the amniotic fluid, the degree of haemolysis of the infant's red cells can be predicted with greater accuracy.

Several methods are in current usage but the most popular is the spectrophotometric measurement of the bilirubin 'bulge' at a wavelength of 450 to 460 nm (Liley curve). A decision can then be taken on the need for intrauterine transfusion. Donor blood should be compatible with mother and fetus and it should be remembered that the donor RBC will decline by 2% a day. Amniocentesis is only reliable from 27 weeks of gestation onwards.

Fetal Doppler assessment of the middle cerebral artery with hyperdynamic flow seen in anaemic fetuses is now a more widely practiced assessment tool.

References

Banasik J 2019 Pathophysiology 6th edn Elsevier Inc, St Louis.

Campos O 1996 Doppler echocardiography during pregnancy: physiological and abnormal findings. Echocardiography 13:135–146.

Daroff R, Jankovic J, Mazziotta J et al 2016 Bradley's Neurology in Clinical Practice 7th edn Elsevier Inc, London.

Evans J, Newby DE, Horton-Szar D 2012 Crash Course: Cardiovascular System 4th edn Elsevier Ltd, Oxford.

Kacmarek R, Stoller J, Heuer A 2021 Egan's Fundamentals of Respiratory Care 12th edn Elsevier Inc, St. Louis.

Khurana I, Khurana A, 2015 Textbook of Medical Physiology 2nd edn Elsevier India, New Delhi.

Koeppen B, Stanton B, 2018 Berne & Levy Physiology 7th edn Elsevier Inc, Philadelphia.

Kumar P, Clark M, 2011 Kumar & Clark's Medical Management and Therapeutics Elsevier Ltd, Edinburgh.

Landon M, Galan H, Jauniaux E et al 2021 Gabbe's Obstetrics: Normal and Problem Pregnancies 8th edn Elsevier Inc, Philadelphia.

Ralston S, Penman I, Strachan M et al 2018 Davidson's Principles and Practice of Medicine 23rd edn Elsevier Ltd, Edinburgh.

Rankin J 2017 Physiology in Childbearing: With Anatomy and Related Biosciences 4th edn Elsevier Ltd, Oxford.

Patton K 2019 Anatomy and Physiology 10th edn Elsevier Inc, St Louis.

Patton K, Thibodeau G, Douglas M, 2012 Essentials of Anatomy and Physiology Elsevier Inc, St. Louis.

Thompson J, Moppett I, Wiles M, 2019 Smith and Aitkenhead's Textbook of Anaesthesia 7th edn Elsevier Ltd, Edinburgh.

11

Endocrinology

SHEBA JARVIS AND MARK R. JOHNSON

Introduction

In this chapter, the endocrine system is introduced by describing mechanisms of hormone action and the types of hormones. Six groups of hormones and/or endocrine systems will then be discussed, which include: (1) hypothalamus, pituitary and pineal glands; (2) reproduction (puberty, menstrual cycle, pregnancy, lactation and menopause); (3) growth; (4) metabolism and the pancreas; (5) thyroid; (6) adrenal.

Mechanisms of Hormone Action and Second Messenger Systems

CELL SURFACE RECEPTORS

Hormones may act in an autocrine (acting upon the cells that produced them), paracrine (acting on neighbouring cells) or endocrine manner (acting on cells at a distant site having been transported to that site in the blood or lymphatic system). In the circulation, some hormones such as steroids, insulin-related growth factors (IGFs) and thyroid hormones are bound to carrier proteins. Only the free hormone, the fraction of the total hormone level that is unbound, is active and available to bind to specific receptors to induce its effects. These receptors may be on the cell surface and have associated secondary messenger systems or may be nuclear with effects directly on the deoxyribonucleic acid (DNA) to alter messenger RNA (mRNA) levels (i.e. gene expression). At each receptor, a hormone may function as an agonist, a partial agonist or an antagonist. Furthermore, there is some 'promiscuity', with various hormones acting at multiple receptor types, as well as the complexity of hormone receptor crosstalk, which is beyond the scope of this chapter.

Peptide hormones and neurotransmitters act predominantly through cell surface receptors. These are divided into four main groups: (1) seven-transmembrane domain (luteinising hormone (LH), follicle stimulating hormone (FSH), thyroid-stimulating hormone (TSH), β-adrenergic, typically linked to G-protein second messenger system); (2) single transmembrane domain growth factor receptors (insulin, IGFs, linked to tyrosine kinase second messenger system); (3) cytokine receptors (cytokines, growth hormone (GH), prolactin); (4) guanylyl cyclase-linked receptors (natriuretic peptides related to guanyl cyclase second messenger system).

The seven-transmembrane receptors, as their name implies, loop in and out of the cytoplasm (Fig. 11.1). The amino (-NH₃) terminus has the hormone binding domain and the carboxy terminus (-COOH), the G-protein transducer. There are multiple types of G-protein, which are heterotrimers made up of an α-, β- and γ-subunit (Fig. 11.2). Each type (determined by the α-subunit) may relate to different receptors and be linked to different second messenger systems. For example, the β-adrenergic system is linked to the $α_s$ G-protein, which in turn is linked to adenylyl cyclase. β-adrenergic activation is thus associated with an increase in intracellular cyclic adenosine monophosphate (cAMP) (see Fig. 11.2). Each G-protein is made up of a guanosine diphosphate–guanosine triphosphate (GDP–GTP) binding domain (the α-subunit), and a β- and γ-subunit. In the absence of stimulation, the G-protein is bound to GDP. With

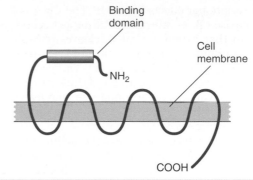

Fig. 11.1 Seven-transmembrane receptor.

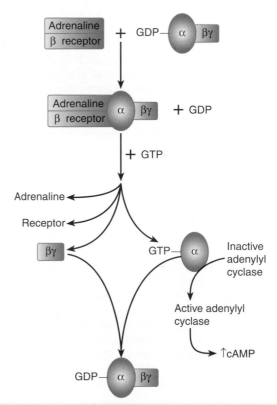

Fig. 11.2 G-protein receptor activation represented by a β-adrenergic receptor.

receptor activation, the α-subunit binds to the receptor and dissociates from the GDP and the β- and γ-subunit. GTP then binds to the receptor-linked α-subunit, initiating its dissociation from the hormone–receptor complex. The activated G-protein then activates its second messenger system (e.g. adenylyl cyclase). The deactivated GDP–α-subunit complex re-associates with the β- and γ-subunit (see Fig. 11.2). The G-protein system can be manipulated experimentally by using agents such as cholera toxin, which prolongs activity of the α-subunit–GTP complex, or using the pertussis toxin, which uncouples the G-protein system and inhibits its activity.

As described earlier, adenylyl cyclase activation generates cAMP, which activates protein kinase A (PKA), leading to phosphorylation and activation of other intracellular proteins, such as the cyclic AMP response element binding protein (CREB). This protein mediates many of the transcriptional effects of cAMP. The Gα q is linked to phospholipase Cβ, an initiator of another second messenger system that, when activated, cleaves phosphoinositol 4,5-bisphosphonate, generating inositol 1,4,5-triphosphate (IP₃) and diacylglycerol (DAG). IP₃ acts via specific receptors to increase intracellular calcium and DAG activates protein kinase C. Activation of phospholipase A releases arachidonic acid, which is a precursor molecule for prostaglandins and leukotrienes.

Growth factor receptors span the cellular membrane once and are linked to tyrosine kinase. For instance, binding to the GH receptor initiates phosphorylation of the receptor itself and of tyrosines in other molecules, triggering a cascade of intracellular responses. The cytokine receptors, like the growth factor receptors, cross the cell membrane once; they are linked to the Janus Kinase/ Signal Transducers and Activators of Transcription (JAK/ STAT) pathway. Binding of a cytokine to its receptor activates JAK, which in turn activates docking sites for STAT that is activated and translocates to the nucleus where it alters gene expression. The pathway is controlled by a negative feedback loop involving Supressors of Cytokine Signalling (SOCs).

The guanylyl cyclase-linked receptors can be activated in three ways:

1. They may be activated by nitric oxide (NO) produced by nitric oxide synthase (NOS). NOS exists in either constitutive (endothelial (eNOS) or neuronal (nNOS)) or inducible (iNOS) forms. In the vasculature, agents such as acetylcholine or bradykinin bind to endothelial cell surface receptors and increase intracellular calcium, which enhances eNOS activity and increases NO production. Increased NO levels diffuse into the smooth muscle cell and activate soluble guanylyl cyclase; this in turn produces cyclic guanosine monophosphate (cGMP), which stimulates relaxation of the smooth muscle.
2. iNOS is present predominantly in immune cells but is also found in vascular smooth muscle cells. As its name implies, it can be induced by various hormones, leading to an increase in NO production and cGMP levels.
3. Guanylyl cyclase is also linked to peptide receptors and the ligand–receptor interaction activates it directly.

Peptide hormones also affect the transcription of genes through the activation of c-jun and c-fos (via kinases and phosphatases). These are nuclear transcription factors that bind to specific sites on the DNA to alter gene expression. cAMP activates PKA, which, as mentioned above, phosphorylates a number of proteins including the transcription factor CREB, which alters gene expression.

NUCLEAR RECEPTORS

The nuclear receptor superfamily has a critical role in development, general physiology, fertility and disease. Several hormones act through nuclear receptors. These include steroid hormones (progesterone, oestrogen and androgens), thyroid hormones, retinoic acid and vitamin D. Some of the receptors exist principally in the cytoplasm (the 'steroid' family includes glucocorticoid, mineralocorticoid, androgen and progesterone receptors) or nucleus (the 'thyroid' family that includes oestrogen, retinoic acid and vitamin D

receptors). However, independent of their location, when these hormones bind to their receptors, most will act in the nucleus to alter gene expression, though in recent years non-genomic effects of activation of nuclear receptors have been recognised. While this is worth noting , it is beyond the scope of this chapter. The different receptor groups are shown as an example in Fig. 11.3.

Regarding the steroid family of NRs, these tend to exist in the cytoplasm as a complex with multiple protein coregulators, as well as heat shock protein (HSP). When the ligand binds with the receptor, HSP dissociates, revealing a nuclear translocation signal that initiates the transport of the hormone–receptor complex to the nucleus where it binds to the hormone response element to exert its effect (see Fig. 11.3). The DNA binding region has two zinc 'fingers'; between the two zinc molecules lies the amino acid sequence which binds to the DNA. The thyroid family of nuclear receptors exists in the nucleus and, except for the oestrogen receptor, does not associate with HSP. They bind to DNA as dimers; for oestrogen this is a homodimer (i.e. two oestrogen receptor molecules) and for the other members of the family, as heterodimers formed between the receptor molecule and a retinoid X receptor.

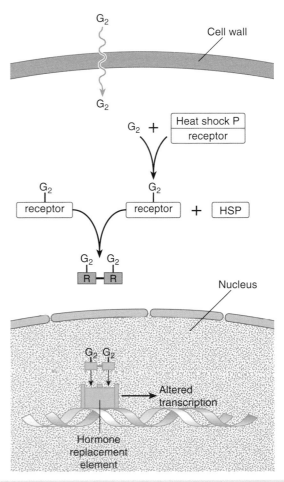

Fig. 11.3 Nuclear receptor activation by ligand G2, which passes through the cell wall and binds to its receptor in the cytoplasm before passing into the nucleus to bind to its response element on deoxyribonucleic acid. *HSP*, Heat shock protein.

Hormone Types

PEPTIDE HORMONES

Most hormones are peptides, and a peptide is made up of a chain of a variable number of amino acids. The precise sequence is determined by the DNA encoding the peptide. Therefore, peptide synthesis is initiated by the transcription of DNA into a specific mRNA. This passes from the nucleus into the cytoplasm, where it binds to ribosomes in the rough endoplasmic reticulum (RER) and is translated into the peptide sequence (illustrated by insulin in Fig. 11.4). This is usually in the form of a pre-pro-hormone, which is then cleaved to first form a pro-hormone and then the hormone itself. Some peptides are secreted immediately, while others are stored in secretory granules.

STEROID HORMONES

In terms of reproduction, this is the most important group of hormones. Steroid hormones are synthesised from cholesterol and all have the same basic ring structure consisting of 17 carbon atoms with different numbers of carbon atoms added. Glucocorticoids (stress and metabolism), aldosterone (fluid balance) and progesterone (reproduction) have 21 carbon atoms; testosterone and other androgens have 19 carbon atoms, while oestrogens have 18 (Fig. 11.5). The synthetic pathways are the same in the ovary, testis and adrenal, but the dominant product varies from tissue to tissue (Fig. 11.6). The pathway always starts from cholesterol, which is derived either from circulating LDL or from intracellular cholesterol esters.

Ovary

Ovarian steroid production varies during the cycle. Overall, the ovary is the main source of circulating oestrogens, although peripheral conversion of androgens also makes a significant contribution in some situations. During the follicular phase of the cycle, the ovary produces oestrogens predominantly, and both oestrogen and progesterone in the luteal phase.

Adrenal

The adrenal cortex is divided into three zones, which can be remembered using the acronym GFR: (1) the outer zona glomerulosa (zG); (2) the middle zona fasciculata (zF), which consists of cells full of cholesterol and (3) the inner zona reticularis (zR). The zG is the site of aldosterone secretion. It is regulated by the control of the renin–angiotensin pathway, whereas last two are controlled by adrenocorticotrophic hormone (ACTH) and are concerned primarily with the secretion of cortisol and, to a lesser extent, adrenal androgens. More details will be given about each in their relevant sections.

Testis

The Leydig cells of the testis produce testosterone in response to LH. This circulates predominantly bound (97%) to sex hormone binding globulin (SHBG) and, to a lesser extent, to albumin. In some tissues, testosterone is active, but in others it has to be converted to dihydrotestosterone (DHT) by the enzyme 5α-reductase. Both testosterone and DHT bind to a cytoplasmic receptor before passing into the cell nucleus to bind to specific areas of DNA to produce their effect.

Placenta

During pregnancy, the placenta synthesises and releases large amounts of progesterone into the maternal circulation. Pregnenolone is also released into the fetal circulation to be converted by the fetal adrenal into androgens, which pass back to the placenta to be aromatised to oestrogens and released into the maternal circulation (Fig. 11.7).

Steroid Binding and Metabolism

In the circulation, all steroid hormones circulate bound to various proteins (Table 11.1). Steroid hormone metabolism occurs in the liver. For example, oestradiol is converted to oestrone, which may re-enter the circulation, be further metabolised to oestrogens or conjugated to form oestrone sulphate, and excreted. Progesterone is converted to pregnanediol and conjugated to glucuronic acid, after which it is excreted as pregnanediol glucuronide. Androgens are metabolised and excreted predominantly as 17-oxosteroids (which used to be measured to assess androgen synthesis). Cortisol is mainly conjugated to glucuronide and excreted. Its metabolites can be measured in the urine in the form of 17-oxogenic steroids (not to be confused with the androgen metabolites, 17-oxosteroids), but this is rarely measured now, as cortisol can be measured in the urine directly.

AMINO ACID HORMONES

Several hormones, thyroid (tyrosine), catecholamines (tyrosine) and melatonin (tryptophan) are derived from amino acids, and all are stored in granules. Their activities are regulated by their release and by the expression of the enzymes necessary for their synthesis.

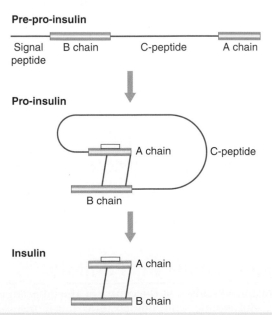

Pre-pro-insulin

Signal peptide   B chain   C-peptide   A chain

Pro-insulin

A chain   C-peptide   B chain

Insulin

A chain   B chain

Fig. 11.4 Synthesis of insulin.

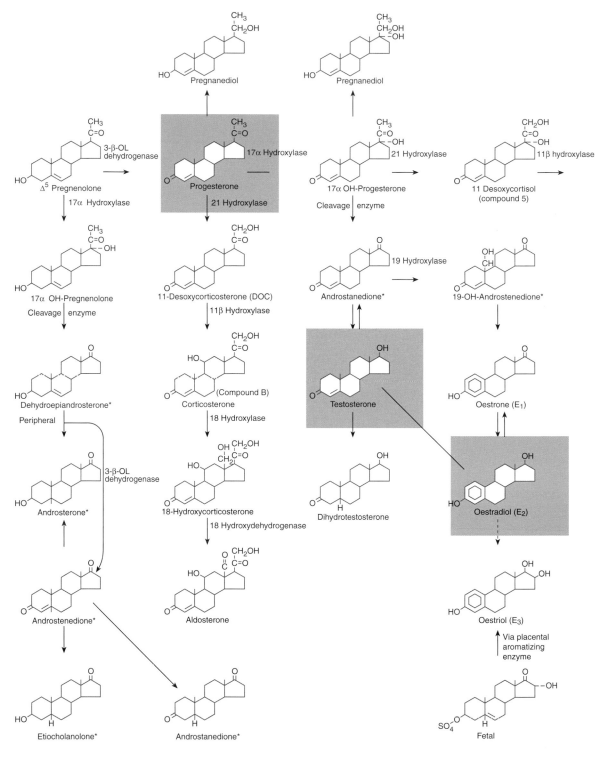

Fig. 11.5 The synthesis of the key reproductive steroids (highlighted).

PROSTAGLANDINS AND LEUKOTRIENES

Collectively known as the eicosanoids, these hormones are derived from arachidonic acid. Synthesis occurs in the cell wall and the hormones pass either into the cell cytoplasm or out of the cell (Fig. 11.8).

Hypothalamus and Pituitary

The hypothalamus is at the centre of the different endocrine, autonomic and homeostatic mechanisms that maintain the body and allow it to reproduce. It directly controls the pituitary, which in turn controls the

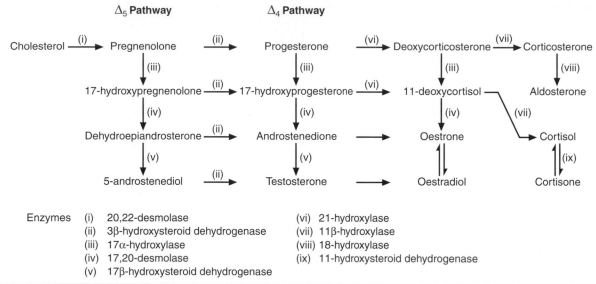

Δ₅ Pathway   **Δ₄ Pathway**

Enzymes (i) 20,22-desmolase   (vi) 21-hydroxylase
         (ii) 3β-hydroxysteroid dehydrogenase   (vii) 11β-hydroxylase
         (iii) 17α-hydroxylase   (viii) 18-hydroxylase
         (iv) 17,20-desmolase   (ix) 11-hydroxysteroid dehydrogenase
         (v) 17β-hydroxysteroid dehydrogenase

Fig. 11.6 Steroid hormone synthesis.

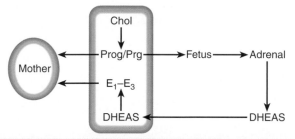

Fig. 11.7 Feto-placental oestrogen production. The fetus lacks sulphatases, 3β-hydroxysteroid dehydrogenase (3βHSD) and aromatase, and therefore produces dehydroepiandrosterone sulphate *(DHEAS)*, which it exports to the placenta, which possesses these enzymes and produces oestrone (E₁), oestradiol (E₂) and oestriol (E₃). *Chol*, Cholesterol; *Prog*, progesterone; *Prg*, pregnenolone.

Table 11.1 Steroid Binding Profiles

Hormone	Plasma Conc. (nmol/L)	Free (%)	SHBG (%)	CBG (%)	Albumin (%)
Oestradiol	0.29	1.8	37.3	0.1	60.8
Oestrone	0.23	3.6	16.3	0.1	80.1
Progesterone	0.65	2.4	0.6	17.7	79.3
Testosterone	1.3	1.4	66	2.3	30.4
Androstenedione	5.4	7.5	6.6	1.4	84.5
Cortisol	400	3.8	0.2	89.7	6.3

CBG, Cortisol binding globulin; *SHBG*, sex hormone binding globulin.

reproductive axis, lactation, growth, the thyroid, and adrenal glands.

EMBRYOLOGY

The thalamus and the hypothalamus develop from the diencephalon, which with the telencephalon (which forms the cerebral hemispheres) forms the prosencephalon. Both the thalamus and the hypothalamus develop in the lateral walls of the diencephalon, the cavity that becomes the third ventricle (Fig. 11.9).

The pituitary develops in close association with the hypothalamus and is made up of two parts: (1) the anterior or adenohypophysis and (2) the posterior or neurohypophysis. The anterior pituitary is formed from the ventral ridges of the primitive neural tube, which are pushed forward by the developing Rathke's pouch (Fig. 11.10A–C). By 7 weeks, the sella floor has formed and the pituitary starts to develop under the influence of the hypothalamus. The posterior pituitary is formed by a downward evagination of the diencephalon called the infundibulum. Thus, the neurohypophysis is in direct contact with the hypothalamus, while the anterior pituitary is connected to the hypothalamus via the richly vascular portal system. The portal system carries all the hypothalamic hormones that regulate the function of the anterior pituitary (Fig. 11.11). A small part of the anterior pituitary immediately opposed to the neurohypophysis becomes the intermediate lobe (Fig. 11.12).

ANATOMY

Boundaries

The thalamus lies superior to the hypothalamus, separated from it by the hypothalamic sulcus. Medially the third ventricle, superiorly the thalamus and inferiorly the pituitary stalk provides anatomical limits for the hypothalamus; the hypothalamus is without distinct boundaries anteriorly, posteriorly and laterally.

The pituitary lies within the sella turcica; the sphenoid sinus lies anteriorly and inferiorly, the cavernous sinus laterally (containing internal carotid arteries, and sixth cranial nerve), the clinoid processes posteriorly of the sphenoid bone (often eroded on skull x-rays in the presence of a pituitary tumour), and the pituitary stalk superiorly, which merges into the hypothalamus (see Fig. 11.12). The optic chiasma lies anterior to the pituitary stalk,

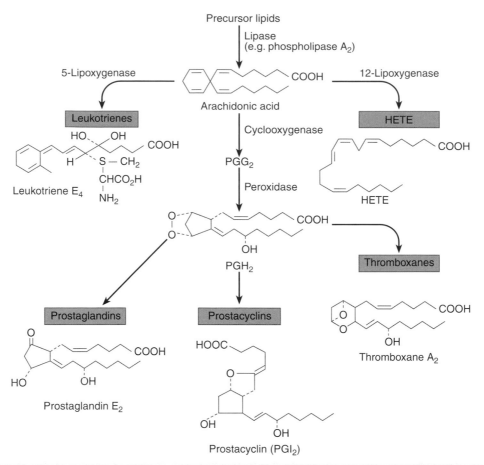

Fig. 11.8 Prostaglandin and leukotriene synthesis from arachidonic acid (*HETE*, Hydroxyeicosatetraenoic acid). (Reproduced with permission from Greenspan FS, Strewler GJ 1997 Basic and clinical endocrinology, 5th edn. Appleton and Lange, London.)

which may be compressed by an expanding pituitary tumour, giving the typical presentation of bi-temporal hemianopia.

Blood Supply

The hypothalamus, pituitary stalk and the pituitary are supplied by the carotid arteries via the superior and inferior hypophyseal arteries (see Fig. 11.11). The superior hypophyseal arteries form a primary plexus in the base of the hypothalamus in a region called the median eminence. The plexus forms into the portal vessels that pass on either side of the pituitary stalk to the anterior pituitary, where they form a secondary plexus. The nerves from the hypothalamic nuclei, which regulate anterior pituitary function, end close to primary plexus and release their regulatory hormones, which are taken up and carried via the portal vessels to the anterior pituitary. The posterior pituitary is supplied by the inferior hypophyseal artery.

Structure

The hypothalamus is made up of a series of nuclei arranged around the third ventricle. The nuclei consist of the cell bodies of neurones. In the case of the nuclei, which regulate the anterior pituitary, the axons pass to the area of the median eminence (see earlier). The axons of the paraventricular (situated in the lateral wall of the third ventricle) and the supraoptic nuclei (situated above the optic tract) pass down the pituitary stalk to the posterior pituitary. Both synthesise and release oxytocin and vasopressin (Fig. 11.13).

The pituitary gland develops from two parts. The anterior pituitary is made up of a mixture of cells with different secretory properties divided into three groups, based on their staining with Haematoxylin and Eosin. The chromophobes (which do not stain) are thought to be resting cells, but chromophobe adenomas have been shown to secrete gonadotrophin subunits. The acidophils synthesise prolactin, GH and the basophils, which secrete the gonadotrophins, TSH and ACTH. The posterior pituitary is pale and consists of the nerve terminals of the paraventricular and the supraoptic nuclei. The axons are surrounded by glial cells called pituicytes, which regulate the rate of transmission and the crosstalk between neurones.

HYPOTHALAMIC PRODUCTS

Table 11.2 summarises the hormones produced by the hypothalamus that regulate anterior pituitary function. More details are provided in the relevant sections further in this chapter.

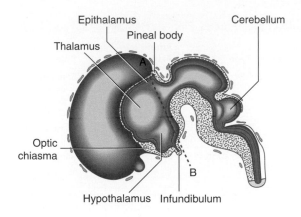

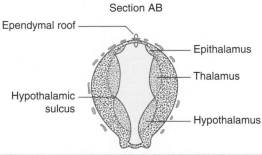

Fig. 11.9 Embryonic development of the hypothalamus. (Reproduced with permission from Moore KL 1993 The developing human—clinically oriented embryology, 5th edn. WB Saunders, Philadelphia.)

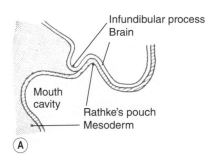

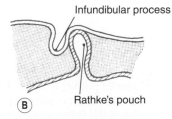

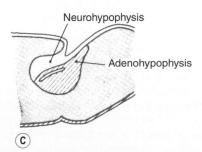

Fig. 11.10 The development of the pituitary.

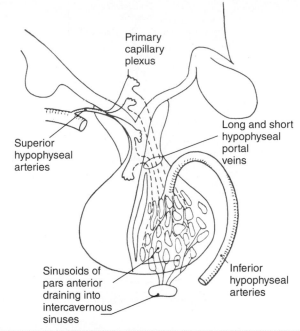

Fig. 11.11 The pituitary portal system and its connections.

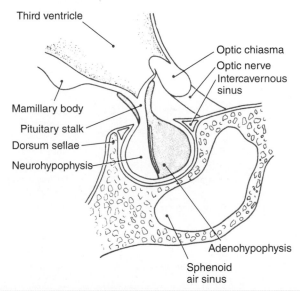

Fig. 11.12 Relations of the pituitary.

PITUITARY GLAND PRODUCTS

Tables 11.3A and B summarise the hormones produced by the anterior and posterior parts of the pituitary gland, respectively. Further details are given in the upcoming sections of this chapter.

Pineal Gland

The pineal gland lies in the roof of the third ventricle at the posterior end and it produces melatonin, with roles in the regulation of the 'body clock' and puberty. Pineal gland tumours are associated with symptoms and signs of a space-occupying lesion with deficiency of hypothalamic

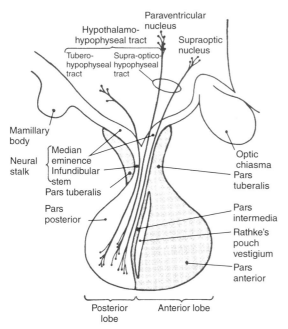

Fig. 11.13 Diagrammatic representation of the hypothalamus and pituitary. The connections of the posterior lobe of the gland with the hypothalamus are indicated. (Figs. 11.10–11.13 courtesy of Passmore R, Robson J (eds). Companion to medical studies. Blackwell Scientific, Oxford.)

Table 11.2   Regulators of Anterior Pituitary Function

Hormone	Source	Amino Acids	Role
GnRH	Pre-optic area	10	Stimulates LH and FSH release
GHRH	Anterior paraventricular nucleus	41	Stimulates ACTH release
GRH	Arcuate nucleus	44	Stimulates GH release
Somatostatin	Periventricular area	14	Inhibits GH release
TRH	Medial paraventricular nucleus	3	Stimulates TSH release
Dopamine	Arcuate nucleus		Inhibits prolactin release

ACTH, Adrenocorticotrophic hormone; *CRH*, corticotrophin-releasing hormone; *FSH*, follicle stimulating hormone; *GH*, growth hormone; *GHRH*, growth-hormone-releasing hormone; *GnRH*, Gonadotrophin-releasing hormone; *LH*, luteinising hormone; *TRH*, thyrotropin releasing hormone; *TSH*, thyroid-stimulating hormone.

hormones or occasionally with precocious puberty. With age, the pineal gland calcifies and may be visible on an x-ray of the skull.

Reproductive Hormones

The reproductive axis is made up of the hypothalamus, pituitary and gonads. The embryology and anatomy of the reproductive tract are discussed elsewhere. The endocrine aspects are considered here.

Table 11.3A   Anterior Pituitary Hormones

Hormone	Type	Amino Acids	Size	Role
LH	Glycoprotein	204	30,000	Stimulates ovarian hormone synthesis and oocyte release
FSH	Glycoprotein	204	30,000	Stimulates follicle maturation
TSH	Glycoprotein	201	28,000	Stimulates thyroid hormone release
ACTH	Protein	39	4500	Stimulates cortisol synthesis in the adrenal
GH	Protein	191	21,500	Stimulates hepatic IGF-II synthesis and release
Prolactin	Protein	198	22,000	Stimulates lactation

ACTH, Adrenocorticotrophic hormone; *FSH*, follicle stimulating hormone; *GH*, growth hormone; *IGF*, insulin-related growth factors; *LH*, luteinising hormone; *TSH*, thyroid-stimulating hormone.

Table 11.3B   Posterior Pituitary Hormones

Hormone	Source	Amino Acids	Role
Oxytocin	Lateral and superior paraventricular and supraoptic nuclei	9	Stimulates contraction of the myoepithelial cells of the breast causing milk let-down, and of the uterine myocytes in labour
Vasopressin	Lateral and superior paraventricular and supraoptic nuclei	9	Retains water by altering the permeability of the collecting ducts in the kidney; cardiovascular regulation; enhances CRH-stimulated ACTH release

ACTH, Adrenocorticotrophic hormone; *CRH*, corticotrophin-releasing hormone.

FUNCTION

Gonadotrophin-releasing hormone (GnRH) is synthesised in the pre-optic area of the hypothalamus and passes via the median eminence and the portal vessels to the anterior pituitary, where it stimulates the gonadotrophs to synthesise and release LH and FSH. It is released in a pulsatile manner. In females, the pulsatile release of GnRH varies with the phase of the cycle; it is released every 60 minutes during the follicular phase and every 90 minutes during the luteal phase. GnRH is synthesised from a 92-amino-acid pro-hormone, which is split into GnRH and a 56-amino-acid GnRH-associated peptide (GAP). The physiological role of GAP is unknown, but it has been shown to inhibit prolactin secretion.

The release of GnRH is modulated by opioid and catecholamine inputs. In recent years, the critical importance of the kisspeptin system has been shown to be key for normal GnRH secretion, and acts as an salient gatekeeper in the initiation of puberty, as well as the regulation of roles in reproductive function. The *KISS1* gene, which encodes Kisspeptin, is highly expressed in the brain and other organs, including the placenta and kisspeptin signals via the G protein coupled receptor GPR54, which is expressed in multiple sites of the body (Fig. 11.14).

LH and FSH are glycoproteins from the family that includes TSH and human chorionic gonadotrophin (hCG). These hormones consist of a common α-subunit and specific β-subunit. All are glycosylated, which determines their bioactivity and half-life. Both LH and FSH act on the gonads to stimulate gametogenesis and hormone synthesis

(see later). The levels of the gonadotrophins vary with age. Before puberty they are low; they rise at puberty, initially at night in both sexes, then continuously in the male and cyclically in the female. With the menopause, the levels of both rise markedly.

During the follicular phase, FSH and LH stimulate oestrogen synthesis by the developing follicle. This initially feeds back to the level of the hypothalamus and possibly to the pituitary to inhibit the release of FSH and LH. Negative feedback occurs in a short and ultrashort manner too, in that LH and FSH feed back to the hypothalamus to reduce further GnRH; GnRH also feeds back to inhibit its own release.

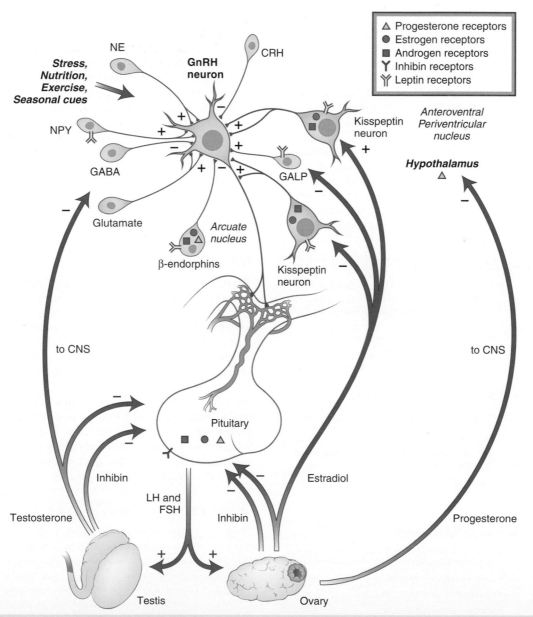

Fig. 11.14 Regulation of the hypothalamic-pituitary-gonadal axis. Schematic diagram of the hypothalamic-pituitary-gonadal axis showing neural systems that regulate gonadotropin-releasing hormone (GnRH) secretion and feedback of gonadal steroid hormones at the level of the hypothalamus and pituitary. *CNS,* Central nervous system; *CRH,* corticotropin-releasing hormone; *FSH,* follicle-stimulating hormone; *GABA,* γ-aminobutyric acid; *GALP,* galanin-like peptide; *LH,* luteinising hormone; *NE,* norepinephrine; *NPY,* neuropeptide Y. (Reproduced with permission from Melmed S et al 2020 Williams textbook of endocrinology, 14th edn. Elsevier Inc, Philadelphia.)

Positive feedback also occurs at mid-cycle. Oestrogens rise to such a point that their usual negative feedback is reversed, leading to a marked positive effect. GnRH release increases and results in an LH and, to a lesser extent, FSH peak. The former, but not the latter, is responsible for ovulation and initiation of luteinisation of the follicle.

Oestrogen and Progesterone

Oestrogens have a number of important general effects (Table 11.4), but during the menstrual cycle their most important role is to stimulate endometrial growth. Following ovulation, the corpus luteum continues to synthesise and release oestrogens and progesterone. Their production peaks 7 days after ovulation and thereafter declines, unless conception and implantation occur, when the developing embryo releases hCG into the maternal circulation that maintains corpus luteum function. Progesterone also has several effects (Table 11.5), but during the luteal phase it regulates endometrial receptivity.

Androgens

In the female, androgens are synthesised in both the ovary and adrenal glands. Of the circulating testosterone, 25% is produced in the ovary. The remainder is derived either directly from the adrenal (25%), or indirectly through the peripheral conversion predominantly of androstenedione (50% from the ovary and 50% from the adrenal) and, to a much lesser extent, of dihydroepiandrostenedione (DHEA, derived mainly from the adrenal glands). In the female, androgens are probably responsible for the maintenance of pubic and axillary hair, as well as controlling libido.

Table 11.4 Properties of Oestrogen

Structure	Stimulates endometrial growth, maintenance of vessels and skin, reduces bone resorption, increases bone formation, increases uterine growth
Protein synthesis	Increases hepatic synthesis of binding proteins
Coagulation	Increases circulating levels of factors II, VII, IX, X, antithrombin III and plasminogen; increases platelet adhesiveness
Lipid	Increases HDL and reduces LDL, increases triglycerides, reduces ketone formation, increases fat deposition
Fluid balance	Salt and water retention
Gastrointestinal	Reduces bowel motility, increases cholesterol in bile

HDH, High density lipoproteins; *LDL,* low density lipoproteins.

Table 11.5 Properties of Progesterone

Structure	Enhances endometrial receptivity, maintains myometrial quiescence, breast development
Respiration	Increases respiratory drive
Lipid	Reduces HDL and increases LDL
Fluid balance	Promotes sodium exertion
Bowel	Reduces bowel motility
Metabolism	Increases body temperature

SEX DIFFERENTIATION *IN UTERO*

In the absence of any stimulation, the default phenotype is female. The male phenotype is determined by the sex determining region Y (*SRY*) gene found on the short arm of the Y chromosome, which regulated another key transcription factor *SOX9*. Both the *SRY* and *SOX9*, expressed by the support cells of the embryonic testis, develop into Sertoli cells. It also stimulates the germ cells to become spermatogonia, the steroid secreting cells to become Leydig cells and the connective tissue cells to be peritubular cells. In the absence of *SRY*, the four cell lineages develop into the granulosa cells, oogonia, thecal cells and stromal cells of the ovary.

The Wolffian and Müllerian systems initially develop in parallel. The secretion of Anti-Müllerian hormone (also known as Müllerian inhibitory substance) by the Sertoli cells leads to regression of the Müllerian system. Further sex differentiation occurs with the secretion of testosterone by the testis. Testosterone promotes the development of the Wolffian ducts into the vas deferens, seminal vesicles and epididymis, as well as the external male genitalia. The development of the external male genitalia (penis, scrotum and prostate) is promoted by the action of DHT converted from the testosterone secreted by the Leydig cells of the testis. This conversion from testosterone to DHT is by the action of 5α-reductase. The absence of testosterone (and thus of DHT) leads to disorder of sexual differentiation (DSDs) with poor virilisation in the case of defects in 5α-reductase.

Puberty

FEMALE

There is variation in the timing and order of the events of puberty with differences in timing between the sexes. In the female, breast growth and the growth spurt usually occur first, followed by the appearance of pubic hair, then axillary hair, and then menstruation (Tables 11.6 and 11.7). The increase in height prior to puberty is about 5 cm per year. This increases to 8 to 9 cm per year during the growth spurt, which lasts between 2 and 3 years. Peak growth velocity usually occurs at around 12 years. Breast growth usually begins between 9 and 13 years. The average time to develop from stage II to V (see Table 11.6) is 4 years (range, 1.5 to 9 years); for pubic hair the average is 3 years (range, 2 to 5 years). The first menstrual period usually occurs at the age

Table 11.6 Stages of Breast Growth

Stage I	The prepubertal stage. No development has occurred yet
Stage II	The breast bud begins to grow beneath the nipple
Stage III	The breast is more rounded and begins to resemble the adult breast in appearance, but is much smaller
Stage IV	Greater development has taken place, and the breast is larger than at stage III. In addition, the nipple and areola project forward in front of the contour of the breast as a secondary mound
Stage V	Full adult breast size and form has been achieved

Table 11.7   Stages of Pubic Hair Development

Stage I	Prepubertal stage. No terminal hair is visible
Stage II	Terminal hair appears on the vulva and in the midline of the mons
Stage III	The narrow triangular area of the pubis shows darker hair, which is still sparse in amount
Stage IV	A wider triangular area of the pubis is covered, and the density is greater. The lateral angles of the triangle still have to be filled in
Stage V	The adult stage has been achieved

of 13 years (range, 11 to 15 years). In affluent societies, better nutrition and health mean that the age of menarche is decreasing.

Structurally, the reproductive organs change markedly with puberty. The ovaries elongate and become oval due to follicular development and an increase in stroma. Before puberty, the cervix makes up two-thirds of the uterus; with puberty this changes so that at menarche it makes up half and within 2 years only one-third. This is due to the increased size of the body of the uterus. The vagina changes from having a thin epithelium, to a thicker stratified multi-layered squamous epithelium, rich in glycogen.

MALE

The first sign of puberty in boys is an increase in the size of the testis, secondary to an FSH-induced increase in the seminiferous tubules. This is defined as stage II. At stage III, the scrotum reddens, and the penis starts to increase in length. At stage IV the process continues with a more marked increase in the size of the penis, testes and scrotum. Stage V is reached when the testes are approximately 5 cm in length, the scrotum is pigmented and thickened and the penis is of adult size and proportions. Pubic hair starts to appear at stage III and is of an adult pattern at stage V. The growth spurt starts 12 months after the increase in testicular volume is noted.

ENDOCRINOLOGY OF PUBERTY

The factors controlling the time of onset of puberty are uncertain. It is thought that the hypothalamus in childhood is highly sensitive to sex steroid inhibition of GnRH secretion and that, as puberty approaches, this inhibition reduces, resulting in an increased secretion of GnRH and consequently of the gonadotrophins. However, in children without gonads, there is still inhibition of gonadotrophin secretion, implying the existence of another mechanism. This may involve leptin (see later), the hormone produced by fat tissue. Once the hypothalamic inhibition is overcome, and/or the inhibition from other factors is released, then, in females, the initial endocrine change is an increase in the nocturnal pulse frequency of GnRH. This stimulates FSH secretion and results in a multi-cystic appearance in the ovaries (also seen in the recovery phase of anorexia nervosa or exercise-induced amenorrhoea) and in oestrogen secretion. Later in puberty, the levels of LH also increase. As puberty advances, the peaks in gonadotrophins occur during the day as well as at night and, finally, in late puberty the secretion of gonadotrophins loses its diurnal pattern and the levels remain elevated. The next step is the onset

of positive feedback of oestrogen on GnRH release, resulting in the LH surge, ovulation and menstruation (see later). Of the initial cycles, 90% are anovulatory. With time, the number falls, so that 4 to 5 years after menarche, less than 20% of cycles are anovulatory. The increasing levels of oestrogen stimulate the maturation of the female genital tract, breasts, the initial growth spurt followed by fusion of the epiphyses and the redistribution of body fat. Fusion of the epiphyses limits growth. Therefore, high levels of oestrogen (endogenous or exogenous) in early life are one cause of stunted growth (see later).

Independent of the changes in gonadotrophins and oestrogen, the adrenal gland is increasingly active early in puberty, as shown by the higher circulating levels of dihydroepiandrostenedione sulphate (DHEAS). The factors controlling the onset of adrenal activity (adrenarche) are uncertain.

Leptin

Leptin is the 167-amino-acid product of the *Ob*-gene in white adipocytes. It is a helical molecule and a member of the tumour necrosis factor group of cytokines. It was discovered in the *Ob/Ob* mouse, where a mutation of the *Ob*-gene resulted in obesity and hypogonadotropic infertility. Replacement with leptin resulted in weight loss and the restoration of fertility, probably by increasing GnRH levels. Leptin expression is increased by insulin, glucocorticoids, noradrenaline and food. Circulating levels are reduced in weight-related amenorrhoea. Leptin is the probable link between body weight and menstruation.

MENSTRUAL CYCLE

At the time of puberty, the ovary contains between 300,000 and 600,000 primordial follicles. These consist of an oocyte (<25 μm) and its associated granulosa cells. Maturation from a primordial follicle is independent of gonadotrophins until the follicle reaches secondary follicle stage, when further maturation is dependent on FSH (Fig. 11.15). The tertiary follicle contains a steroid-rich, fluid-filled antrum and rapidly grows to become a pre-ovulatory, or graafian follicle (2.0 to 2.5 cm). In each cycle, around 10 secondary follicles are recruited. Eventually, one becomes the dominant follicle and the remainder become atretic. Following ovulation, the granulosa cells luteinise and vessels from the theca invade as the remnant of the follicle becomes the corpus luteum.

Oestrogen synthesis by the developing follicle is controlled by FSH, which stimulates the production of aromatase by the granulosa cells. Androgens, synthesised by thecal cells in response to LH, pass across the basement membrane to granulosa cells to be converted by aromatase to oestrogens. This, the 'two-cell' theory of oestrogen synthesis, developed from observations that granulosa cells do not possess the enzymes to be able to synthesise oestrogen from pregnenolone and progesterone themselves. However, thecal cells can also produce oestrogens, and it has been suggested that the thecal cell oestrogen production determines the circulating level of oestradiol, while the follicular fluid oestrogen is granulosa cell derived. Circulating oestrogen levels rise through the follicular phase of the cycle, peaking between days 12 and 14 (Fig. 11.16). The increasing levels trigger

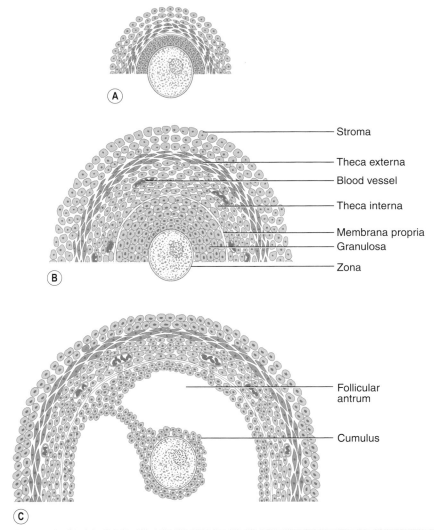

Stroma

Theca externa

Blood vessel

Theca interna

Membrana propria
Granulosa

Zona

Follicular
antrum

Cumulus

Fig. 11.15 Follicular maturation form (A) 1° to (B) 2° to the mature 3° (C) graafian follicle. (Reproduced with permission from Johnston MH 1988 Essential reproduction, 3rd edn. Blackwell Scientific, Oxford.)

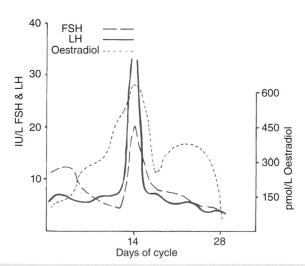

Fig. 11.16 Diagrammatic representation of changes in hormone levels during the menstrual cycle. The luteinising hormone *(LH)* peak is left open because it is subject to great variation. *FSH*, Follicle stimulating hormone.

the LH surge, which stimulates ovulation. Progesterone levels increase slightly towards the end of the follicular phase and may also play a role in the LH surge.

After ovulation, the follicle remnant becomes the corpus luteum and produces oestrogen and progesterone. It also produces relaxin, inhibin-A and inhibin-B. The role of relaxin is uncertain during both the menstrual cycle and pregnancy. Inhibin has been suggested to feed back to the pituitary to inhibit FSH release in both the male and female (see below). If pregnancy occurs, increasing levels of hCG maintains the corpus luteum and its production of oestrogen and progesterone until 8 to 9 weeks of pregnancy. Thereafter, the placenta becomes the main source of oestrogen and progesterone. The corpus luteum continues to produce relaxin throughout pregnancy.

Inhibin and Activin

Inhibin and activin belong to the same family. Inhibin is a heterodimer made up of an α and β subunit. There are two β-subunits, A and B. Inhibin may thus exist as either inhibin-A or inhibin-B. Activin is a homodimer of the

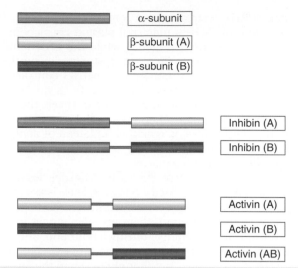

Fig. 11.17 The subunits forming activin and inhibin.

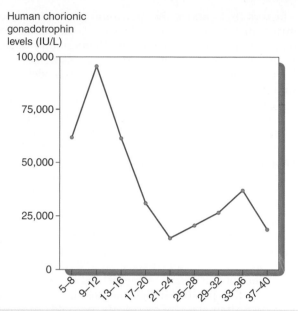

Fig. 11.18 Levels of human chorionic gonadotrophin during pregnancy.

β-subunit, and thus may exist as activin-A, activin-B or activin-AB (Fig. 11.17). During the menstrual cycle, activin is undetectable or present at very low levels. Inhibin-A and -B are present in the circulation and are derived from the ovary. Inhibin is known to inhibit FSH release while activin stimulates it, but as both inhibin and activin are synthesised in the pituitary, they may act in a paracrine manner to inhibit or stimulate FSH synthesis and release. During pregnancy, circulating levels of inhibin-A and activin-A are derived from the feto-placental unit. Circulating levels of inhibin-A peak in early pregnancy and rise again at the end; those of activin increase gradually with gestation. A further marked increase in activin-A levels occurs with the onset of labour and in pregnancies complicated by pre-eclampsia. No changes have been reported in the circulating levels of inhibin-A with the onset of labour but marked increases have also been reported in pregnancies complicated by pre-eclampsia. The roles of activin and inhibin during pregnancy are uncertain, but activin has been linked with embryo implantation and higher levels of inhibin have been linked with adverse pregnancy outcomes.

Pregnancy

The placenta becomes the dominant source of circulating oestrogen and progesterone from 8 to 9 weeks of gestation. In addition, the placenta produces several peptides (hCG, human placental lactogen (HPL)) and virtually all the hypothalamic-releasing hormones. hCG is structurally similar to LH but has an additional 30 amino acids. It is detectable in the maternal circulation approximately 10 days after ovulation. The level rises and peaks at 10 to 12 weeks' gestation (Fig. 11.18). While hCG prevents corpus luteum involution, it may also stimulate the maternal thyroid and be responsible for hyperemesis gravidarum. It is produced in excessive amounts by placental tumours and is used as a marker of therapeutic response.

During pregnancy, progesterone acts to maintain myometrial quiescence. Its importance is confirmed by the efficacy of progesterone antagonists in the induction of abortion in early pregnancy or labour in late pregnancy. In addition, it inhibits other smooth muscles of the body (the GI tract and urinary tract) and stimulates the appetite, fat storage and the respiratory centres (see Table 11.5). The role of the three dominant oestrogens, oestrone (E_1), oestradiol (E_2) and oestriol (E_3), during pregnancy is not entirely clear. They may promote uterine blood flow, myometrial growth, stimulate breast growth and, at term, promote cervical softening and the expression of myometrial oxytocin receptors (see Table 11.4).

HPL is a member of the GH–prolactin family. It antagonises the effect of insulin and so promotes lipolysis, reduces glucose utilisation and enhances amino acid transfer across the placenta. These effects may be designed to increase nutrient supply to the fetus. Prolactin levels rise throughout pregnancy probably from both pituitary and decidual sources. It promotes breast development, regulates fat metabolism and may contribute to the maternal immune suppression.

BIOCHEMISTRY OF HUMAN LABOUR

During pregnancy, the uterus expands to accommodate the growing fetus and placenta, without increasing contractility, while the cervix remains firm and closed. Throughout pregnancy 'pro-pregnancy' factors operate to inhibit myometrial contractility and allow myometrial hypertrophy until, near to term, 'pro-labour' factors begin to operate to mediate remodelling of the cervix. These factors allow the cervix to efface and dilate and stimulate the uterus to begin coordinated contractions. Labour is the result of the activation of a 'cassette of contraction-associated proteins' which act to convert the myometrium from a state of quiescence to a state of contractility. These include gap junction proteins, oxytocin and prostaglandin receptors, enzymes for the synthesis of prostaglandins or cytokines, and components of cell-signalling mechanisms, which affect the way in which the uterus responds to receptor activation. It is likely that the factors that control the activation of the 'cassette of contraction-associated proteins' also activate factors in the fetal membranes that lead to the production of prostaglandins and cytokines associated with labour, as well as factors within the cervix, which lead to cervical remodelling and ripening.

Pregnancy can be divided into four parturitional phases. The first phase, during the first and second trimesters, is dominated by 'pro-pregnancy factors' and is the period of myometrial growth and quiescence. The second phase, during the early and mid-third trimester, is also a phase of myometrial quiescence, but during which preparation for labour is made by upregulation of myometrial, cervical and fetal membrane proteins, which will be needed for labour. The third phase is the phase of labour and has the character of an inflammatory reaction. During this phase of pregnancy, the 'brake' on myometrial contractility caused by 'pro-pregnancy' factors is released and the spontaneous contractility of the uterus is augmented by oxytocic compounds, such as prostaglandins and possibly oxytocin. The fourth parturitional phase represents the state of the intra-uterine tissues after the process of labour.

Pro-Pregnancy Factors

Progesterone is the principal pro-pregnancy factor. It has a negative regulatory effect upon many of the 'contraction-associated proteins' associated with the formation of myometrial gap junctions (connexins) and the modulation of cervical ripening (interleukin-8). It also decreases uterine sensitivity to oxytocin. In many species, a withdrawal of progesterone immediately precedes the onset of labour, either through regression of the corpus luteum (e.g. in rodents) or through changes in placental steroidogenesis (e.g. in sheep). There is no obvious systemic withdrawal of progesterone prior to labour in the human or other primates. However, inhibition of progesterone, using mifepristone (RU486), causes cervical ripening and increases myometrial contractility. It is possible that there is no actual or functional withdrawal of progesterone prior to labour in humans; rather, its 'pro-pregnancy' action is simply overwhelmed by 'pro-labour' factors. Alternative hypotheses are that there is a reduction in free, active progesterone, that progesterone withdrawal is a local event seen only within the fetal membranes, or that functional progesterone withdrawal occurs because of a switch from expression from being type B dominated to type A dominated. A represses the progestational effect of progesterone, which is mediated through the type B receptor within the uterus near to term. It has also been suggested that functional progesterone withdrawal may occur because of competition between progesterone and increased concentrations of cortisol, which compete for binding to the same receptor.

In some species, the rabbit for example, NO synthesis in the endometrium also mediates myometrial quiescence and there is abrupt withdrawal just before labour. This is not seen in primates. Although the human uterus will relax if exposed to high concentrations of NO, there is no evidence for any physiological role for NO in human labour.

Placental Clock

The timing of human labour is probably controlled by increased placental release of corticotrophin-releasing hormone (CRH), oestrogens or a combination of both. The concentration of CRH in maternal plasma rises about 90 days prior to the onset of labour while the CRH binding protein falls. CRH acts to increase prostaglandin synthesis and may also directly stimulate myometrial contractility. Although maternal oestrogen concentrations do not rise acutely before human labour, as they do in sheep, there is a gradual rise in both oestriol and oestradiol concentrations during the third trimester, reaching a plateau at about 38 weeks. Oestradiol upregulates oxytocin receptors and oxytocin synthesis within the uterus.

The role of oxytocin probably varies from species to species. In the monkey, increased oxytocin release is associated with the switch from pre-labour contractures to labour contractions. In the human, there are no changes in oxytocin concentrations before or during labour and, although the density of myometrial oxytocin receptors does increase towards term, oxytocin is not thought to signal the onset of human labour.

Labour: An Inflammatory Reaction

Labour is associated with increased prostaglandin synthesis within the uterus, especially within the fetal membranes. This increase is associated with increased activity of the pro-inflammatory prostaglandin synthetic enzyme cyclooxygenase type 2. Prostaglandins mediate cervical ripening and stimulate uterine contractions. They also act indirectly to increase fundally dominant myometrial contractility, by upregulation of oxytocin receptors and synchronisation of contractions. There is also an increase in the production of inflammatory cytokines, such as interleukin-1β and of chemokines such as interleukin-8. These are involved in complex feed-forward and feed-back mechanisms, which further increase cytokine and prostaglandin synthesis. At term, near to labour, the collagen of the cervix changes, undergoing collagenolysis. The fibrils become dissociated from their tightly organised bundles and are more widely scattered in an increased amount of ground substance; there is also a loosening of the collagen bundles in the cervical stroma. There is an accumulation of neutrophils that release collagenase into the cervix. Cervical ripening therefore resembles an inflammatory reaction. It is currently thought that neutrophils are attracted into the cervix at term by the combination of increased prostaglandin synthesis and the 'neutrophil attractant peptide' interleukin-8.

A Unified Hypothesis of the Onset of Labour in Humans

How each of these various factors that are associated with the control of the length of human pregnancy and the onset of labour are linked is currently not understood. A current hypothesis is that during the first parturitional phase, the uterus is under strong progesterone repression. During the second phase, rising oestrogen and CRH concentrations activate proteins, such as cell surface receptors and gap junctions, which will be needed for labour. CRH also increases the expression of inflammatory cytokines and of type 2 cyclooxygenase.

Labour arises because a relatively rapid increase in synthesis of inflammatory mediators and the influx of inflammatory cells leads to cervical ripening and uterine contractions. It is probable that the transition from parturitional phase two to phase three occurs once a certain threshold of CRH, or of cytokines stimulated by CRH, is reached. In addition, the fetus may signal its maturity, either through increased cortisol release, which stimulates placental CRH synthesis, and/or through release of platelet-activating factor from the lungs, which also stimulates prostaglandin and cytokine synthesis. Once phase three is entered, there are multiple positive feedback mechanisms that accelerate the processes of labour, which only stops once delivery is complete.

LACTATION

During pregnancy, several hormones stimulate breast growth (oestrogen, progesterone, HPL, prolactin, cortisol and insulin). However, the high concentrations of oestrogens inhibit lactation. After delivery, with the fall in oestrogen levels, lactation is initiated by the continuing prolactin stimulation. Prolactin is released from the anterior pituitary under the control of dopamine (inhibitory) and TRH (stimulatory). Prolactin continues to be released in response to suckling and promotes milk formation. The milk let-down reflex involves the release of oxytocin from the posterior pituitary, which stimulates the smooth muscle surrounding the acini to contract and cause milk ejection.

Menopause

Menopause is a retrospective diagnosis made after the absence of periods for 1 year. The average age for the onset of menopause in the UK is 50 years. It occurs because the ovary has run out of recruitable follicles. *In utero*, the peak number of oocytes is 7 million. By birth, this has fallen to 2 million and by the time of puberty only 3 to 600,000 remain. The factors that determine the initial number of oocytes and their rate of loss are unknown, but premature menopause is associated with deletions of the X chromosome, smoking and galactosaemia. In the absence of sex steroids and probably of inhibin, gonadotrophin levels rise and remain elevated for 10 years or more. The ovaries become atrophic, as does the uterus (which reverts to a 1:1 ratio of body to cervix) and the vagina. The lack of oestrogen induces a series of vasomotor changes that include hot flushes, night sweats and palpitations. Depression is also more common during menopause and all these symptoms may be helped by hormone replacement therapy (HRT). Other structurally significant changes occur in the heart, which becomes more susceptible to ischaemic heart disease (probably due to changes in the structure of the vessel wall and reductions in HDL and increases in LDL levels), and in the bones where bone resorption increases and formation reduces, together resulting in osteoporosis.

Growth

Growth *in utero* seems to be determined primarily by the maternal environment rather than any genetic influence. By the first birthday, there is a closer relationship between the current size and the child's final height. Whether a child will fulfil its genetic potential or not will depend on nutrition, health and the expression of the correct GHs. Growth is at its most rapid *in utero* and immediately after birth; thereafter a second peak occurs before puberty, but during puberty itself the increased levels of oestrogen and testosterone result in epiphyseal fusion and the cessation of longitudinal growth.

PHYSIOLOGY

GH is a 191-amino-acid peptide secreted from the somatotrophs of the anterior pituitary. It has some homology with prolactin and HPL and its synthesis is increased in response to the GH releasing hormone (GHRH) and reduced by somatostatin. Both GHRH and somatostatin are synthesised in the hypothalamus and carried to the anterior pituitary in the portal blood system. GH stimulates the synthesis of the insulin-related growth factors (IGF-I and IGF-II) predominantly in the liver, but also in the chondrocytes, fat and muscle. It promotes lipolysis in fat and gluconeogenesis in the muscle. Plasma levels of the IGFs are highest in childhood and fall with age. They act in both a paracrine and endocrine manner to promote bone growth, protein synthesis in muscle and lipolysis in fat cells. GH release is also stimulated by exercise and hypoglycaemia.

Other hormones are important in growth. These include those that: (1) control the availability of materials for growth, such as parathyroid hormone (PTH) (calcium) and insulin (fats, carbohydrates and amino acids); (2) inhibit GH release, such as cortisol; and (3) have effects on cell growth and differentiation, such as insulin, thyroid hormones, as well as oestrogen and progesterone.

DYSFUNCTION

GH deficiency leads to short stature in children and weight loss, lethargy and impaired physical performance in adults. Excess GH leads to gigantism in children and acromegaly in adults. The latter is characterised by excessive growth of soft tissues (tongue, liver, heart) and bones (hand, feet and jaw), as well as diabetes mellitus and hypertension.

Pancreas

Glycaemic control requires cooperation of the various hormones produced in the pancreas, working in concert with the liver, which acts as a glycogen store. Excess glucose is stored in the liver and muscle as glycogen and in adipose tissue as fat. At times of fasting, these stores are broken down to provide glucose and fatty acids as sources of energy. Insulin acts to lower blood glucose levels. Several other hormones act to increase blood glucose; these include glucagon, adrenaline, GH and cortisol. Both insulin and glucagon are synthesised and released in the beta islet cells and alpha islet cells of the pancreas, respectively

EMBRYOLOGY

The pancreas develops between the layers of ventral mesentery from endodermal buds (ventral and dorsal), which originate from the caudal part of the foregut. The ventral bud forms the uncinate process and some of the head of the pancreas, but the majority of the pancreas is derived from the dorsal bud. The main pancreatic duct is derived from the ventral bud; this usually fuses with the dorsal bud duct, but the dorsal bud duct occasionally persists and opens into the duodenum independently.

ANATOMY

The pancreas weighs approximately 80 g and is divided into the head (including the uncinate process), neck, body and tail. It is retroperitoneal, the head lying within the curve of the duodenum and the neck, body and tail extending in front of the vena cava and aorta to the spleen. The stomach lies anterior to the body and tail. The pancreas is made up of glandular acini (which secrete enzymes and bicarbonate) and the islets of Langerhans (1% to 2% of the pancreas) which synthesise glucagon (α cells), insulin (β cells), somatostatin (δ cells) and pancreatic polypeptide (PP).

FUNCTION

Insulin is made up of 51 amino acids and comprised of two chains (A and B). It is synthesised as a pre-prohormone and cleaved to pro-insulin and finally to insulin and C-peptide, which are released in equal amounts (see Fig. 11.4). Its release is stimulated by glucose (oral stimulus is greater than intravenous due to the involvement of the intestinal hormones), basic amino acids, ketones and free fatty acids. Insulin release is further potentiated by glucagon, GH and gut hormones, and inhibited by hypocalcaemia, adrenaline and somatostatin. The release profile of insulin is divided into two phases; the first is a burst lasting less than 1 minute, and the second is more prolonged, persisting as long as the stimulus to insulin secretion. Insulin promotes the transport of glucose and amino acids across the cell membrane in muscle and adipose tissues. It inhibits lipolysis in adipose tissue, and increases glucose uptake and glycogen formation in the liver. Insulin is metabolised by the liver and kidney and has a half-life of approximately 10 to 15 minutes.

Glucagon (molecular weight 3485, 29 amino acids) is released in response to hypoglycaemia, basic amino acids, gut hormones, exercise and adrenaline. Its release is inhibited by increasing blood glucose, ketones, free fatty acids, insulin and somatostatin. It generally inhibits the uptake of glucose and amino acids, promotes lipolysis and hepatic glycogenolysis, gluconeogenesis and ketone generation.

Pancreatic somatostatin regulates stomach motility and the secretion of gut hormone and PP may have a role in the regulation of digestion.

DYSFUNCTION

Insulin deficiency results in hyperglycaemia. The effects of hyperglycaemia are salt and water depletion due to an osmotic diuresis, weight loss, tiredness, vomiting, hypotension, infections, hyperventilation (due to ketoacidosis), as well as an impaired conscious level and coma. Chronic hyperglycaemia results in microangiopathy (affecting the kidney, nerves and retina) and macroangiopathy (causing peripheral, coronary and cerebral vascular disease).

Hypoglycaemia (defined as a blood sugar of <2.5 mmol/L) is usually a complication of insulin treatment and rarely the presenting symptom of liver disease, hypoadrenalism or insulinoma. In the early stages of hypoglycaemia, patients are pale, sweaty and tachycardic; they may complain of hunger and palpitations, and may later become confused. If left untreated, it can lead to seizures and death.

Thyroid

EMBRYOLOGY

The thyroid is the first endocrine gland to appear, beginning development at 24 days after fertilisation and becoming active in terms of thyroid hormone secretion at about 11 weeks of pregnancy. It is derived from the floor of the primitive pharynx in the form of the 'thyroid diverticulum'. As the embryo grows, the thyroid descends to lie below the hyoid bone in front of the developing tracheal rings. During development, the thyroid is connected to the tongue via the thyroglossal duct, a remnant of which may give rise to a thyroglossal cyst. The thyroid diverticulum divides into the left and right lobes and is connected by the isthmus (Fig. 11.19).

ANATOMY

The thyroid weighs about 20 g and each lateral lobe is about 4 cm long. Its blood supply is from the superior thyroid artery (external carotid) and the inferior thyroid artery (subclavian artery), and the superior and middle thyroid veins drain into the internal jugular and the inferior into the brachiocephalic vein (see Fig. 11.19). The four parathyroid glands lie on its posterior aspect. Microscopically, the thyroid is seen to consist of 1 million or more follicles. Each has a layer of follicular cells surrounding a central colloid. The follicular cells secrete thyroxine (T_4) and tri-iodothyronine (T_3) into the colloid, which are then stored and bound to thyroglobulin. Parafollicular cells (C-cells) synthesise and secrete calcitonin.

THYROID HORMONE SYNTHESIS

Thyroid hormones are iodinated metabolites of tyrosine (T_3 has three iodine molecules and T_4, four). The process of thyroid hormone synthesis (Fig. 11.20) is split into several steps: (1) iodide is actively taken up into the follicular cells by the iodide pump against the concentration gradient (iodide trapping); (2) it is converted to iodine (iodide oxidation); (3) tyrosine is incorporated to form pre-thyroglobulin; (4) pre-thyroglobulin is iodinated to form iodoprethyroglobulin (contains 134 tyrosine residues, of which only 25 to 30 can be iodinated and 6 to 8 coupled into hormone residues) (Fig. 11.21); (5) coupling of T_1 and T_2 to form T_3 and of T_2 and T_2 to form T_4, both of which are stored in the colloid in the form of iodothyroglobulin; (6) iodothyroglobulin is taken up by the follicular cells and broken down into free T_3 and T_4,

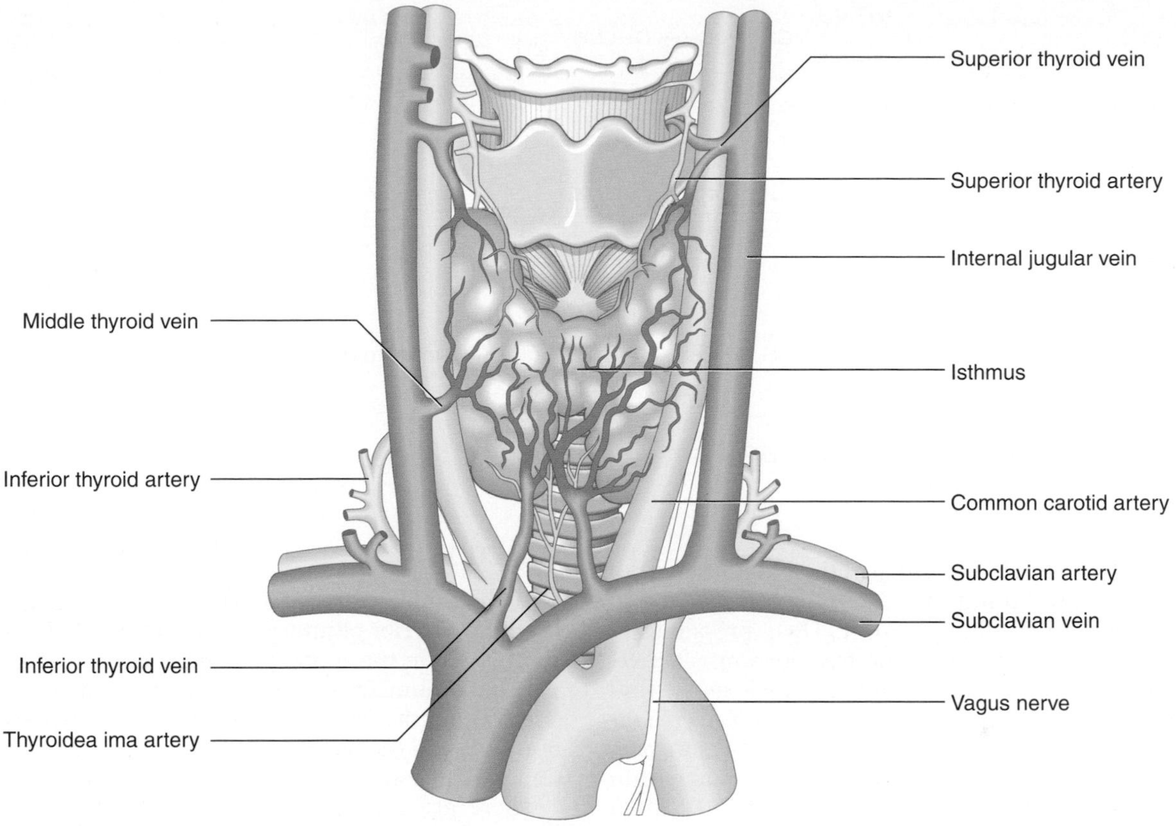
Superior thyroid vein
Superior thyroid artery
Internal jugular vein
Middle thyroid vein
Isthmus
Inferior thyroid artery
Common carotid artery
Subclavian artery
Subclavian vein
Inferior thyroid vein
Vagus nerve
Thyroidea ima artery

Fig. 11.19 The vascular supply of the thyroid gland.

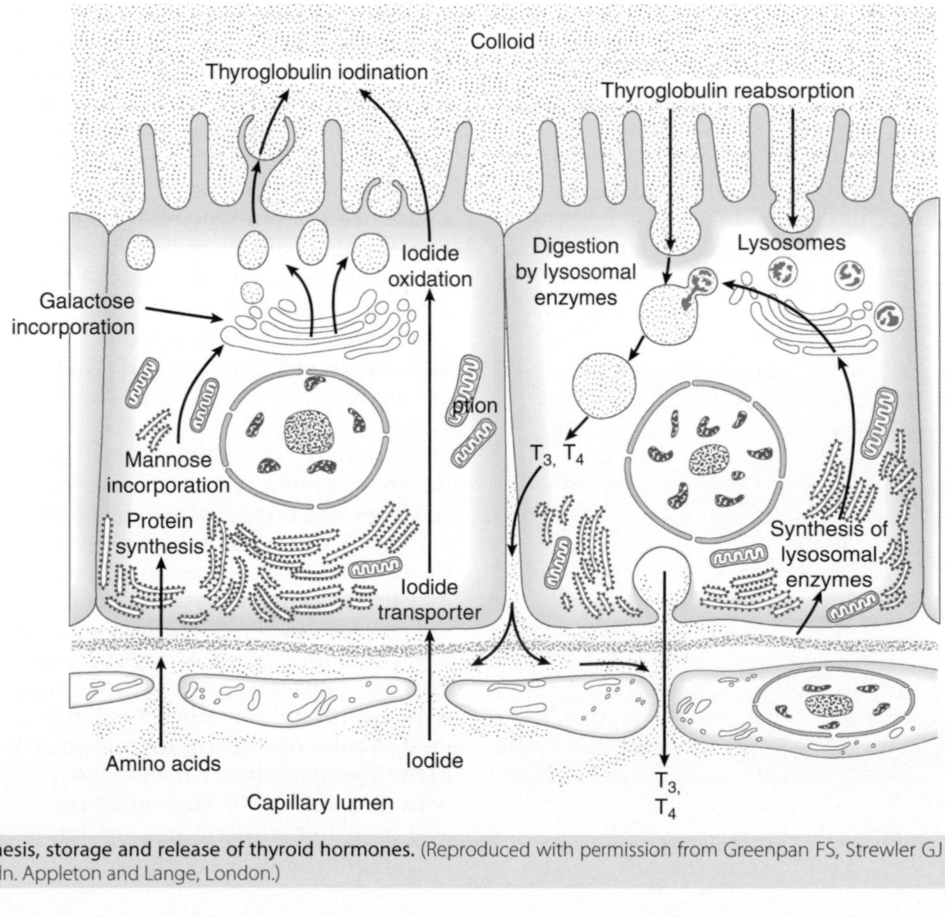
Colloid
Thyroglobulin iodination
Thyroglobulin reabsorption
Iodide oxidation
Digestion by lysosomal enzymes
Lysosomes
Galactose incorporation
Mannose incorporation
Protein synthesis
Iodide transporter
T_3, T_4
Synthesis of lysosomal enzymes
Amino acids
Iodide
Capillary lumen
T_3, T_4

Fig. 11.20 The synthesis, storage and release of thyroid hormones. (Reproduced with permission from Greenpan FS, Strewler GJ 1997 Basic and clinical endocrinology, 5th edn. Appleton and Lange, London.)

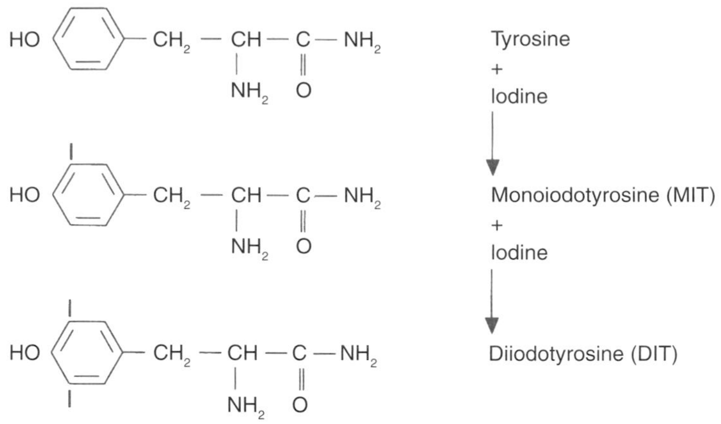

Fig. 11.21 The structure of monoiodotyrosine and diiodotyrosine.

which diffuse into the blood. Once in the circulation, thyroid hormones are bound (T_4, 99.96% and T_3, 99.4%) either to thyroxine binding globulin (TBG), pre-albumin or albumin (Table 11.8); only the free portion is active. The circulating levels of T_4 are higher than T_3 as the thyroid secretes more T_4 than T_3 and T_4 has a longer half-life. However, T_4 is less active than T_3 and acts more as a storage form. It is also converted peripherally and within cells to T_3. T_4 can be converted to T_3 and to rT_3 (an inactive form). The relative balance in this conversion varies and more T_4 is converted to rT_3 during illness. Also during illness, the feedback effects of thyroid hormones seem to be lost so that, although the peripheral concentrations are low, the pituitary response seems to be reduced and TSH levels are not elevated, giving rise to the 'sick-euthyroid' picture. T_3 is inactivated by further deiodination or conjugation in the liver. The fetus and neonate also have relatively high levels of rT_3.

The recommended daily intake of iodine, found in, is 140–150 micrograms. Thyroid uptake of iodine is enhanced by TSH and iodine deficiency but reduced by an excess of iodine and digoxin. Most iodine is excreted via the kidneys (Fig. 11.22).

Table 11.8 Relative Binding of T_4 and T_3 to Plasma Proteins and Its Effect on Their Activities

	T_4	T_3
Total in serum (nmol/L)	50	1
Fraction bound (%)	85	75
• TBG[a]	14	0
• TBPA[b]	0.95	24.5
• Albumin		
Fraction free (%)	0.05	0.5
Total free (pmol/L)	25	5
Potency[c] of free hormone	1	8
Activity (total free × potency)	25	40

[a]TBG, thyroxine-binding globulin.
[b]TBPA, thyroxine-binding prealbumin.
[c]Potency, calorigenic effect and prevention of goitre in propylthiouracil-treated animals.

FUNCTION

TSH (molecular weight 28,000, 204 amino acids) is released from the anterior pituitary in response to TRH, a tripeptide synthesised in the supraoptic and supraventricular nuclei. TSH has a number of effects on the thyroid: it increases its size, vascularity, iodine uptake, protein synthesis, storage of colloid and the secretion of T_3 and T_4. Thyroid hormones feed back to both the hypothalamus and pituitary.

There are several thyroid receptors that bind to the thyroid hormone response element on DNA. The transcriptional effects of T_3 take hours or days to occur (such as tissue growth, brain maturation, increased heat production and oxygen consumption). Other non-genomic effects are more immediate; these include an increase in glucose and amino acid transport. T_4 and T_3 are essential for normal fetal development. In their absence, brain development and musculoskeletal maturation are markedly impaired, resulting in 'cretinism'. Thyroid hormones maintain the normal hypoxic and hypercapnic drives to the respiratory centre and this may account for the occasional need to ventilate patients with severe hypothyroidism. Metabolically, T_4 and T_3 stimulate lipolysis, glycolysis, gluconeogenesis, the absorption of glucose and the metabolism of insulin and cortisol.

In excess, thyroid hormones increase O_2 consumption and heat production by stimulation of Na^+-K^+ ATPase and are positively inotropic and chronotropic on the heart. Part of their cardiovascular effects is mediated through an increase in the expression of β-receptors in the heart, and they have similar effects in skeletal muscle and adipose tissue. Thyroid hormones increase gut motility and thus cause diarrhoea. They also increase bone resorption and thyrotoxicosis or excess thyroxine replacement therapy, which may be associated with osteopenia.

Thyroid function in pregnancy is altered in two ways. The circulating levels of thyroid binding proteins notably TBG are increased secondary to estrogenic stimulation and reduced hepatic clearance, resulting in an increase in the total circulating levels of thyroid hormones (but a slight fall in the free component). In addition, pregnancy is associated with stimulation of thyroid hormone production, probably by a direct effect of hCG on the thyroid so that in some normal pregnancies TSH may be suppressed. This effect is

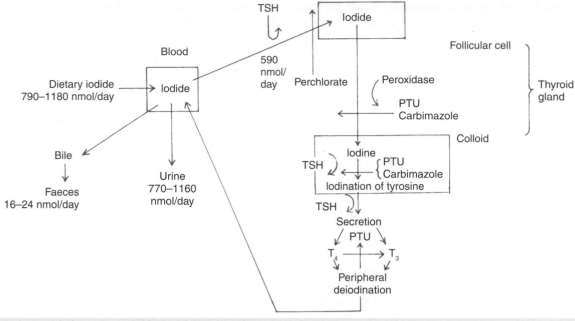

Fig. 11.22 Iodine metabolism. *PTU*, Propylthiouracil; *TSH*, thyroid-stimulating hormone.

particularly marked in hyperemesis gravidarum, where the TSH is usually suppressed, raising the question of thyrotoxicosis. Also, during pregnancy, maternal thyroid disease can affect the fetus in two ways: (1) the maternal antibodies causing thyrotoxicosis or hypothyroidism may cross the placenta and cause a similar self-limiting problem in the fetus and (2) the therapy used in the treatment of thyrotoxicosis may cross the placenta and cause fetal hypothyroidism.

DYSFUNCTION

The effects of thyroid hormone deficiency and excess are shown in Table 11.9.

THERAPY FOR THYROID DISEASE

The management of thyrotoxicosis due to Graves disease is usually with antithyroid drugs, the most common of which are carbimazole and propylthiouracil (PTU). Both act to inhibit the conversion of iodide to iodine, the iodination of tyrosine and the release of both T_4 and T_3; in addition,

PTU prevents the deiodination of T_4. The dose of antithyroid drugs used during pregnancy should be determined by the maternal free thyroxine and TSH levels. As these drugs readily cross the placenta while a relatively smaller proportion of the maternal thyroid hormones cross the placenta, a block and replace approach is not appropriate. Although both drugs are present in breast milk, the amount of PTU is relatively less.

In women with hypothyroidism, the replacement dosage of thyroxine should also be titrated to the TSH and for maternal free thyroxine levels using normal ranges for pregnancy.

Adrenal Gland

EMBRYOLOGY

The cortex of the adrenal gland develops from mesoderm (the mesothelium of the posterior abdominal wall) and the medulla from neural crest cells. The latter is essentially part of the sympathetic nervous system. Differentiation of the cortex begins in late fetal life, but the zones are not recognisable until 3 years of age. At birth, the adrenal cortex is large, due to the presence of the fetal cortex, which produces DHEAS as a substrate for placental oestrogen synthesis. This regresses over the first year of life.

ANATOMY

The adrenal glands weigh approximately 4 to 5 g, are retroperitoneal, lying on top of the kidneys. The yellowish cortex accounts for 90% of the gland weight and the medulla, the remainder. The adrenals are supplied with blood by branches of the aorta, renal and inferior phrenic arteries. Each gland has one vein, which drains on the right into the inferior vena cava and on the left into the renal vein.

Table 11.9 Effects of Thyroid Excess and Deficiency

Process	Thyrotoxicosis	Hypothyroidism
Metabolism	High	Low
	Weight loss	Weight gain
Heat production	Increased	Reduced
	Heat intolerance	Cold intolerance
Gut	Increased motility	Reduced motility
	Diarrhoea	Constipation
Heart	Fast heart rate, palpitations	Slow heart rate
General	Sweating, tremor, anxiety	Dry skin, depression, lethargy

The cortex is divided into three layers. The outer, zG, produces aldosterone (it lacks 17α-hydroxylase and so cannot produce cortisol or androgens); the middle, zF, which is the thickest layer and produces androgens and cortisol; and the inner, zR, which also produces androgens and cortisol. Both of the inner zones are controlled by ACTH.

ADRENAL CORTISOL SYNTHESIS

ACTH controls the synthesis of cortisol (and androgens) by the zF and zR. ACTH is controlled by the hypothalamic hormones CRH and vasopressin. ACTH stimulation of the adrenal results in an immediate increase in the circulating levels of cortisol; it also increases the availability of cholesterol.

ACTH is released in a circadian rhythm, so that cortisol is lowest in the evening and highest in the early hours of the morning. This pattern is lost during illness, stress, Cushing syndrome and alcoholism. Acute stress, physical or otherwise, results in an increase in ACTH and cortisol levels. Cortisol feeds back at the level of the hypothalamus and the pituitary. At the level of the pituitary, cortisol reduces ACTH release acutely within minutes, and chronically by reducing synthesis of its precursor, pro-opiomelanocortin.

Once released, 95% of cortisol circulates bound to cortisol binding protein (80%) and albumin (15%). Most is metabolised in the liver and a small amount is excreted unchanged in the urine (24-hour urine collection and cortisol measurement are used as an initial estimation of cortisol production).

FUNCTION

Cortisol, like the other steroid hormones, enters the cell, binds to its receptor and then directly interacts with a response element on DNA to alter gene expression. It is important metabolically and in the management of 'stress'.

Metabolism

Cortisol stimulates gluconeogenesis and lipolysis (increasing glycerol and free fatty acid levels) but inhibits peripheral glucose usage. Its overall effect is to maintain glucose levels.

Connective Tissue

Fibroblasts are inhibited and collagen is lost, resulting in thin skin that bruises easily and poor healing of wounds. Bone resorption is enhanced and formation inhibited, resulting in bone loss, both through a direct effect on bone and indirectly by (1) enhancing the activity of PTH and vitamin D, and (2) increasing urinary calcium excretion and reducing calcium absorption in the gut. In the adult, this results in bone loss, and in children this may contribute to the observed reduction in growth.

Haematology and Immunology

Cortisol has little effect on haematopoiesis, but it increases the circulating neutrophil count by increasing their production and half-life and reducing their movement out of the circulation. Circulating numbers of lymphocytes, eosinophils and monocytes are reduced by increasing their movement out of the circulation. Glucocorticoid steroids are generally immunosuppressive.

Cardiovascular and Renal Effects

Cardiac output is increased, as is peripheral resistance. The combination results in an increase in blood pressure. This effect is augmented by salt and water retention (potassium excretion), which is induced by stimulation of the mineralocorticoid receptors.

Miscellaneous Effects

Corticosteroids may cause a change in emotions, resulting in euphoria; other psychiatric states may also be observed. Gonadal function may be suppressed.

DYSFUNCTION

The typical pictures of Cushing syndrome (cortisol excess) and Addison disease (cortisol deficiency) are shown in Table 11.10.

ADRENAL ANDROGENS

Adrenal androgen synthesis occurs predominantly in the zR, is controlled by ACTH and starts between 7 and 9 years of age (adrenarche). DHEA and androstenedione, as well as testosterone, to a lesser extent, are synthesised and account for 50% of testosterone in the female and 5% in the male. Excessive secretion results in hirsutism and virilism in the female.

ADRENAL MEDULLA

The adrenal medulla is essentially part of the sympathetic nervous system from which it receives a rich nerve supply. Sympathetic stimulation results in the release of adrenaline and noradrenaline (both synthesised from the amino acid tyrosine) into the blood, where they circulate bound to albumin until metabolised in the liver (by catecholamine-O-methyl transferase and monoamine oxidase into vanillylmandelic acid, VMA). The effects of adrenaline and noradrenaline are mediated through G-protein-linked surface receptors, which are classified generally into α

Table 11.10 Features of Cortisol Excess and Deficiency

Process	Cushing Syndrome	Addison Disease
Metabolic	Increased glucose and free fatty acids, central fat deposition	Hypoglycaemia
Connective tissue	Collagen loss causing thin skin, muscle wastage, osteoporosis	
Haematology and immunology	Increased neutrophils Reduced lymphocytes	Reduced neutrophils, increased lymphocytes
Psychiatric	Euphoria and other psychiatric disturbances	Lethargy
Cardiovascular and renal effects	Hypertension, fluid retention and hypokalaemia	Hypotension, hyponatraemia and hyperkalaemia

Table 11.11 Effects of Sympathetic Activation

Organ/System	Effect
CVS	Tachycardia, hypertension
Skin	Sweating and vasoconstriction
Muscle	Vasodilatation
Liver	Increased gluconeogenesis
Pancreas	Reduced insulin and increased glucagon release
Adrenal gland	Increased cortisol release
Fat	Increased lipolysis
CNS	Dilated pupils, increased level of alertness

CNS, Central nervous system; *CVS*, cardiovascular system.

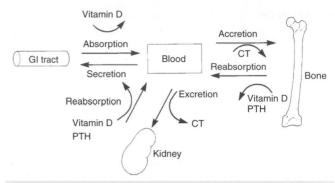

Fig. 11.23 Calcium: secretion into an excretion from the blood to the gastrointestinal tract, bone and kidney. The influences of vitamin D, parathyroid hormone and calcitonin. *CT*, Computed tomography; *GI*, gastrointestinal; *PTH*, parathyroid hormone.

and β. Their activation produces the typical 'flight or fight response' (Table 11.11).

In excess, as seen in a phaeochromocytoma, adrenaline causes marked hypertension and anxiety. It may also be associated with sweating, pallor and tremor, as expected from its effects listed in Table 11.11. It is possible to measure the circulating levels of catecholamines to make the diagnosis of a phaeochromocytoma using the plasma free metanephrine test, but many units still use 24-hour urinary excretion of catecholamine metabolites include metanephrine, normetanephrine, dopamine, or vanillylmandelic acid (VMA). If either is elevated, further investigation involves visualisation of the adrenals.

Calcium Homeostasis

Calcium is essential for many of the body's processes. It is a key intracellular messenger necessary for the maintenance of cell membrane potential in excitable cells (nerve, cardiac), muscle contraction, enzyme action and inhibition and hormone release; it also is important in bone formation and clotting factor activity. It is not surprising, therefore, that there is a complex mechanism to ensure that its levels are tightly regulated. The key components are PTH, vitamin D and calcitonin, which act on the bone (which contains most of the body's calcium), kidney and gut (Fig. 11.23). The calcium concentration in plasma is 2.5 mmol/L; approximately 45% is protein bound (albumin) and the remainder is either free (47%) and therefore active, or complexed with other compounds.

PARATHYROID HORMONE

Parathyroid Hormone Anatomy and Embryology

There are four parathyroid glands that develop from the pharyngeal pouches: the superior glands from the dorsal portion of the third pouch and the inferior glands from the superior portion of the fourth pouch. They are oval shaped, about 0.5 cm in size, 40 milligrams in weight and embedded beneath the capsule in the posterior aspect of the thyroid gland. Their blood supply is derived from the thyroid arteries. They contain two sorts of cell: the chief cells that synthesise, store and secrete PTH, and the oxyphil cells of unknown function.

Parathyroid Hormone Synthesis

The gene for PTH is located on chromosome 11. It is synthesised as a pre-pro-hormone; the signal peptide is removed to form pro-PTH, which is converted to PTH by the removal of the pro-sequence in the Golgi apparatus prior to storage in the cell cytoplasm. It is an 84-amino-acid peptide with a molecular weight of 9300. Low plasma calcium levels stimulates its release, which is suppressed by increased plasma calcium levels.

Parathyroid Hormone Function

PTH acts via G-protein-linked cell surface receptors in bone and in the kidney. In the kidney, it acts on the renal tubule to enhance phosphate and bicarbonate excretion (proximal), and calcium and hydrogen ion reabsorption (distal); it also enhances the renal 1α-hydroxylation of vitamin D, thus increasing vitamin D activity. PTH acts indirectly on the gut through increased vitamin D activity to enhance calcium and phosphate absorption. In the bone, PTH reduces osteoblast collagen synthesis and enhances osteoclast activity, which results in increased osteolysis and the release of collagenase and hydrogen ions; the last two enhance bone resorption. The overall effect of PTH is to increase circulating calcium and phosphate.

Parathyroid Hormone Dysfunction

A deficiency of PTH results in hypocalcaemia and the clinical picture of brisk reflexes – Chvostek sign, (tapping over the facial nerve causes a facial twitch), numbness and paraesthesia, tetany carpopedal spasm (Trousseau sign, induced by inflating a blood pressure cuff), and a prolonged QT interval on ECG. An excess causes hypercalcaemia and the clinical picture of 'bones, stones moans, and groans':

1. *Bones* are painful and fragile due to excessive resorption.
2. Renal *stones* are due to increased urinary calcium levels and ectopic calcification secondary to hypercalcaemia in the heart, pancreas, uterus and liver.
3. *Groans* include headache, abdominal pain, anorexia and constipation.
4. *Moans* include weakness and tiredness. Reflexes are sluggish and there is polyuria, dehydration, renal failure, confusion and coma. On ECG, the QT interval is short and cardiac arrhythmias may be seen.

VITAMIN D

Vitamin D Synthesis

Vitamin D is a sterol hormone (synthesised from cholesterol). It is either synthesised in the skin by photo-isomerisation (90%, action of UV light) or absorbed in the diet (10%, fish and eggs). It is activated in the liver and kidney. In the liver, vitamin D is 25-hydroxylated and then stored in body fat. It is transported to the kidney where it is 1-hydroxylated in the proximal tubules. The 1α-hydroxylation is controlled by PTH (see earlier), calcium and phosphate levels, GH, cortisol, oestrogens and prolactin.

Vitamin D Function

Vitamin D promotes calcium absorption at various sites (gut, kidney and bone). It does this by binding to a nuclear receptor (VDR) that has a DNA binding domain. Once vitamin D has bound, the complex (vitamin D–VDR) has to bind with a retinoic acid receptor to form a heterodimer to be able to bind to DNA and to exert its genomic effects. In the gut, vitamin D increases calcium and phosphate absorption in the jejunum and ileum. There are several possible mechanisms: (1) opening of calcium channels; (2) the increased synthesis of two calcium binding proteins (calbindins), which promote the passage of calcium across the cell into the blood and (3) the promotion of mucosal cell division and growth. In the bone, it increases calcium and phosphate release by enhancing osteoclast activity; this effect is indirect as osteoclasts lack VDR. In addition, osteoblast synthesis of osteocalcin is increased. Thus, in the bone, vitamin D has effects that promote formation and resorption. Still, its overall effects remain uncertain (see later). In the kidney, vitamin D increases tubular calcium and phosphate reabsorption.

Vitamin D Dysfunction

A deficiency of vitamin D has varying effects, depending on the age of the subject. In children, deficiency results in rickets with bowed legs, chest deformity and hypocalcaemia. In adults, deficiency results in osteomalacia with bone pain, fractures, hypocalcaemia. Additionally, pseudofractures can be seen on x-ray (Looser's zones). The effects of vitamin D deficiency relate to impaired gut absorption of calcium, which results in hypocalcaemia. This increases serum PTH, which stimulates bone resorption and causes the picture of bone demineralisation. Vitamin D-resistant rickets rarely occurs and is an X-linked dominant condition, which is the result of an abnormal vitamin D receptor. Vitamin D excess results in hypercalcaemia, the features of which have been described earlier in the section on PTH.

Vitamin D deficiency may arise in a variety of ways: (1) dietary deficiency; (2) malabsorption due either to obstruction of the bile duct or bowel disease as seen in coeliac or Crohn disease; (3) liver disease that may result in reduced 25-hydroxylation and (4) renal disease that may result in reduced 1α-hydroxylation.

CALCITONIN

Calcitonin is synthesised by the parafollicular C-cells of the thyroid. These are neuroendocrine cells derived from the neural crest, which make up less than 0.1% of the mass of the thyroid.

Calcitonin Synthesis

Calcitonin is 32 amino acids in length and its synthesis is regulated by circulating calcium levels, increasing when the levels are higher and reducing when they are lower. The gene encodes two different peptides that are formed by alternative splicing. The first is calcitonin and the second calcitonin gene-related peptide (CGRP). CGRP is a 37-amino-acid peptide with potent vasodilator properties that are thought to be, at least in part, responsible for the marked vasodilatation of pregnancy.

Calcitonin Function

Calcitonin acts via a G-protein-linked receptor that is linked to adenyl cyclase. Its primary site of action is the bone, where it reduces osteoclast activity, although it also acts in the renal tubule to reduce phosphate reabsorption and to a lesser extent calcium. The importance of calcitonin in calcium homeostasis is uncertain (see later).

Calcitonin Dysfunction

Medullary tumours of the thyroid secrete calcitonin and result in high circulating levels. Despite this, calcium levels are unaltered. Calcium levels are also not altered by a total thyroidectomy, which removes the only source of calcitonin. In the human it is thus uncertain whether calcitonin has any role in calcium homeostasis. Nevertheless, therapeutically, calcitonin is useful for the treatment of Paget disease of bone and as an inhibitor of osteoclast activity.

OSTEOPOROSIS

In contrast to osteomalacia, osteoporosis occurs when there is insufficient protein synthesis (i.e. a deficiency of bone trophic hormones) but mineralisation is normal. The most common example is in postmenopausal women, although hypogonadal men have the same problem. Peak bone mass is typically reached between 25 and 30 years and declines thereafter at an annual rate of 2% to 5% in women and 0.3% to 0.5% in men. Bone loss may be prevented or reduced through a number of approaches: (1) HRT; (2) calcium supplements in combination with vitamin D; (3) calcitonin (inhibitors of osteoclast activity such as the bisphosphonate) and (4) weight-bearing exercises.

12

Drugs and Drug Therapy

AMANDA ALI, MARIANE SILVA EDGE AND HASSAN SHEHATA

Introduction

A drug is broadly defined as any chemical agent that affects living protoplasm. About one-third of women in the UK take drugs at least once during pregnancy, but only 6% take a drug during the first trimester. In the puerperium, the use of drugs increases substantially with no difference in the pattern of prescribing between mothers who breastfeed and those who bottle-feed.

Possible effects of drugs in pregnancy include:

- Teratogenicity (e.g. thalidomide)
- Long-term latency (e.g. diethylstilbestrol (DES) – increased risk of vaginal adenocarcinoma after puberty, or abnormalities in testicular function and semen production)
- Impaired intellectual or social development (e.g. phenobarbital or sodium valproate).

Language of Clinical Pharmacy

Prodrugs are pharmacologically inactive derivatives of active drugs. They are designed to maximise the amount of active drug that reaches its site of action through manipulation of the physicochemical, biopharmaceutical or pharmacokinetic properties of the drug. Prodrugs are converted into the active drug within the body through enzymatic or non-enzymatic reactions.

Distribution volume is a hypothetical concept that is defined as the volume that a drug would occupy if the concentration throughout the body were equal to that in plasma. The distribution volume depends on factors like lipid solubility and protein binding.

Clearance is the volume of plasma cleared of the drug in unit time. It determines what dose of drug is necessary to maintain a certain plasma concentration but does not indicate how rapidly the drug disappears when treatment is stopped. Patients with abnormal renal or liver function can have increased clearance times.

A receptor is any cellular molecule to which a drug binds to initiate its effects. Receptors can be proteins (hormones, growth factors and neurotransmitters) or nucleic acids (cancer chemotherapeutic agents). An agonist binds to a physiological receptor and often mimics the regulatory effects of endogenous signalling compounds. An antagonist binds to receptors without regulatory effects and blocks the endogenous agonist. Drugs that stabilise the receptor in its inactive form are called inverse antagonists. Receptors of relevance to clinical practice are summarised in Table 12.1.

pKa is the pH at which half the drug is in its ionised form.

Henderson–Hasselbalch equation is used to calculate the ratio of ionised to non-ionised drug at each pH.

Absorption is the rate at which a drug leaves its site of administration and the extent to which this occurs.

Bioavailability is the term used to indicate the fractional extent to which a dose of drug reaches its site of action or a biological fluid from which the drug has access to its site of action.

Half-life (t½) is the time taken for the plasma concentration, or the amount of the drug in the body, to be reduced by 50%. The half-life of a drug depends on its rate of clearance and volume of distribution. Highly lipophilic drugs may have an increased clearance but prolonged half-life.

Table 12.1 Some Receptors Involved in the Action of Commonly Used Drugs

Receptor	Subtype	Main Actions of Natural Agonist	Drug Agonist	Drug Antagonist
Adrenoceptor	α_1	Vasoconstriction		Prazosin
	α_2	Hypotension, sedation	Clonidine	
	β_1	↑ Heart rate	Dopamine	Atenolol
			Dobutamine	Metoprolol
	β_2	Bronchodilation; vasodilation	Salbutamol, terbutaline	
		Uterine relaxation	Ritodrine	
Cholinergic	Muscarinic	↓ Heart rate		Atropine
		↑ Secretion		Benztropine
		↑ Gut motility		Orphenadrine
		Bronchoconstriction		Ipratropium
	Nicotinic	Contraction of striated muscle		Suxamethonium
				Tubocurarine
Histamine	H_1	Bronchoconstriction		Chlorpheniramine
		Capillary dilation		Terfenadine
	H_2	↑ Gastric acid		Cimetidine
				Ranitidine
Dopamine		CNS neurotransmitter	Bromocriptine	Chlorpromazine
				Haloperidol
				Thioridazine
Opioid		CNS neurotransmitter	Morphine, pethidine, etc.	Naloxone

CNS, Central nervous system.

Steady-state concentration is reached when drug elimination is equal to availability with repeated equal doses. It takes repeated dosing for about five half-lives to achieve steady state.

TERATOGENESIS

This is defined as structural or functional (e.g. renal failure) dysgenesis of the fetal organs. Typical manifestations of teratogenesis include congenital malformations with varying severity, fetal growth restriction (FGR), carcinogenesis and fetal demise. Lack of understanding of the mechanisms of teratogenicity makes it difficult to predict on pharmacological grounds that a particular drug will produce congenital malformations. The period of highest sensitivity to teratogens is early organogenesis. Later in fetal development, exposure to a teratogen is far less likely to be the cause of a structural defect, but can cause serious functional abnormalities, notably of the neuro behavioural type.

ORGANOGENESIS

The major body structures are formed in the first 12 weeks after conception (Fig. 12.1). Interference in this process causes a teratogenic effect. If a drug is given after this time, it will not produce a major anatomical defect, but possibly a functional one. The overall incidence of major congenital malformations is around 2% to 3% of all births, and of minor malformations, 9%. The part played by drugs is probably small. It has been estimated that 25% of congenital malformations are due to genetic or chromosomal abnormalities, 10% due to environmental causes including drugs and 65% are of unknown aetiology. Even known teratogens do not invariably cause anatomical defects and the mechanism of drug-induced teratogenicity remains unclear. The genetic composition of the fetus, the timing of the insult, maternal age, nutritional condition, disease status and the dose of the drug may play a role. The critical time for drug-induced congenital malformations is usually the period of organogenesis. This occurs approximately

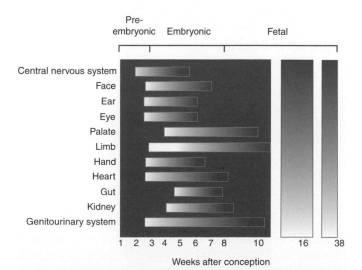

Fig. 12.1 Timing of the development of major body structures in the embryo and fetus. (From Whittle MJ, Hanretty KP. Prescribing in pregnancy. Identifying abnormalities. *Br Med J (Clin Res Ed)*. 1986;293(6560): 1485-1488., with permission of BMJ Publishing.)

20 to 55 days after conception, that is, 34 to 69 days (7 to 10 weeks) after the first day of the last menstrual period (see Fig. 12.1).

PHARMACOKINETICS

Pharmacokinetics is the mathematical description of the rate and extent of uptake, distribution and elimination of drugs in the body. It mainly concerns time. Pharmacokinetics is important for drugs that are given for more than an isolated dose, and those whose margin of safety is narrow. The pharmacokinetics of a drug depends upon its concentration, structure, degree of ionisation, relative lipid solubility and binding to tissue proteins.

Oral absorption is unpredictable and is dependent on various factors such as gastric emptying time, surface area of absorption, blood flow, lipid solubility and physical state of the drug. Venous drainage from the oral mucosa is to the superior vena cava and hence bypasses first-pass metabolism. Rectal administration causes erratic absorption and irritation of the rectal mucosa but 50% of the dose will bypass the liver. Absorption after subcutaneous or intramuscular injection occurs by simple diffusion.

Distribution occurs in two phases: an initial rapid phase to the liver, kidney and brain followed by a slow phase to the muscles, viscera, skin and fat. The distribution of a drug is determined by its lipid solubility and the pH gradient between the intracellular and extracellular fluids.

- Acidic drugs bind to albumin (e.g. salicylates, warfarin, anticonvulsants, non-steroidal anti-inflammatory drugs (NSAIDs))
- Basic drugs bind to α_1-acid glycoprotein (e.g. β-blockers, opioid analgesics, local anaesthetics)
- Covalent bonding can occur with reactive drugs (e.g. alkylating agents).

Hypoalbuminaemia due to liver disease or nephrotic syndrome results in reduced binding and an increase in the unbound fraction of acidic drugs. An acute-phase response leads to an elevation of α_1-acid glycoprotein levels and therefore to reduced availability of basic drugs. Fig. 12.2 summarises the different compartments in which drugs can be distributed in the materno-fetal unit.

Drugs Can Undergo Different Types of Transport

Transcapillary movement: this is transfer of the drug with bulk transfer of water due to hydrostatic or osmotic pressure differences and accounts for the majority of unbound drug transfer.

Paracellular transport: this occurs between cell junctions and is the principal mechanism of excretion of drugs by the kidney.

Passive transport: this is diffusion of the drug through the cell membrane along a concentration gradient by virtue of its lipid solubility.

Active transport: this is characterised by a requirement for energy and involves the movement of a drug against an electrochemical gradient.

Facilitated diffusion: this is a carrier-mediated transport process in which there is no input of energy. Enhanced movement is down an electrochemical gradient.

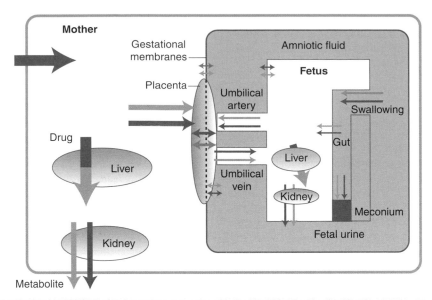

Fig. 12.2 Drug disposition in the maternal–fetal unit.

Table 12.2 The Principal Factors That Influence Maternal, Fetal and Placental Pharmacokinetics in Normal Pregnancy

Maternal Pharmacokinetics	Fetal Pharmacokinetics	Placental Pharmacokinetics
Changes in body fluid volume	Plasma binding proteins differ from maternal so free fractions of basic drugs are elevated	Blood flow through the placenta (maternal side) increases during gestation (i.e. from 50 mL/min at 10 weeks of pregnancy to 600 mL/min at 38 weeks)
Changes in CVS parameters		
Changes in pulmonary function		
Alterations in gastric activity	Liver expresses metabolising enzymes, but capacity less than in mother	
Changes in serum binding protein concentrations and occupancy	Drugs transferred across the placenta undergo first pass through the fetal liver	Transfer of flow-limited drugs is affected by placental flow
Alterations in kidney function	The fetal kidney is immature	Compounds that alter blood flow alter maternal drug disposition and placental transfer
	Fetal urine enters amniotic fluid which may be swallowed by the fetus	Placental metabolism (dealkylation, hydroxylation, demethylation) affects drug transfer across the placenta
		At term, the surface area of the placenta is at its maximum and nearly all substances can reach the fetus

CVS, Chorionic villus sampling.

Drugs that are lipid soluble are less likely to be excreted and polar compounds are likely to be excreted more quickly. The kidneys excrete drugs by filtration, tubular secretion and tubular re-absorption. Changes in renal function affect all three functions and are impaired in the elderly, as adult renal function decreases by 1% per year. Unbound drugs are excreted by filtration. P glycoprotein and multidrug resistance associated protein type 2 secrete ions and conjugated metabolites, respectively, into the tubules. Some of the ways that pregnancy influences pharmacokinetics are summarised in Table 12.2.

PHARMACODYNAMICS

Pharmacodynamics is the study of biochemical and physiological effects of drugs on the body and their mechanism of action. The majority of the drugs pass through cells rather than between them. Broadly speaking, drugs act on four different targets: receptors, enzymes, membrane ion channels and metabolic processes. Drugs commonly act on electrical or chemical signalling pathways and drug action commonly involves a signal transduction pathway, which consists of receptor, cellular target and intermediary molecules.

Factors That Influence Drug Action

DRUG METABOLISM

Drug metabolism will influence the duration and potency of the effect of specific drugs. Drugs are commonly converted to more polar metabolites to facilitate their excretion. This is frequently catalysed by enzymic reactions. While the majority of drug metabolism results in less toxic metabolites, occasionally it can result in the formation of more toxic compounds. A large number of drugs are metabolised by hepatic phase I and II reactions.

Phase I metabolism occurs in the endoplasmic reticulum and involves the formation of more polar metabolites of the original compound. These reactions can involve oxidation (catalysed by cytochrome P450 enzymes), hydrolysis, reduction, cyclisation or decyclisation. The polar metabolites may be directly excreted, usually in the urine, or may be converted further by phase II reactions.

Phase II reactions occur in the cytoplasm and commonly involve conjugation with sulphates, glucuronides, glutathione or amino acids and result in the formation of metabolites that are usually less toxic and more easily excreted.

Table 12.3 Common Drugs That Influence Microsomal Enzyme Induction and Inhibition

Microsomal Induction (Cytochrome P450)	Microsomal Inhibition
Smoking	Oestrogen
Anticonvulsants	Ciprofloxacin
Progestogen	Fluconazole
Rifampicin	Omeprazole
Theophylline	Quinidine
Ethanol	Erythromycin, sulphonamide
Griseofulvin	Grapefruit juice, metronidazole

The metabolism of a drug can be affected by enzyme induction, protein binding and the liver extraction ratio. Table 12.3 summarises the common drugs that influence the activity of the liver microsomal enzymes.

DRUG INTERACTIONS

Drugs that are likely to precipitate drug interactions are those that are highly protein bound, alter metabolism of other drugs or alter renal or hepatic metabolism. Drugs that are affected by drug interactions are those that have a steep dose–response curve and those that have a low toxic : therapeutic ratio (e.g. aminoglycosides, anticoagulants, anticonvulsants, antihypertensives, cardiac glycosides, cytotoxic drugs, oral contraceptives).

Pharmacokinetic interactions can be related to:

- Absorption
  - Drugs that decrease gastric emptying (e.g. morphine, anticholinergics)
  - Chelation of calcium, aluminium, magnesium salts by tetracycline
  - Binding of warfarin and digoxin by cholestyramine
- Protein-binding displacement interactions
  - For example, warfarin and phenytoin are displaced by sulphonamides, salicylates, phenylbutazone and valproate
- Metabolism interactions with induction or inhibition of cytochrome P450 or phase I functionalisation reactions (e.g. oral contraceptives decrease anticoagulant effect of warfarin). Table 12.3 summarises drugs that commonly influence microsomal enzymes
- Excretion interactions
  - Probenecid and penicillin at the renal tubules
  - Quinidine doubles digoxin levels
  - Diuretics causing lithium retention

Pharmacodynamic interactions could be antagonism at same site (e.g. pethidine/naloxone), synergism at same site (e.g. verapamil/β-blockers increase arrhythmias) or indirect, for example when alterations in coagulation, fluid and electrolyte balance affect drug action.

IMPAIRED LIVER FUNCTION

Liver disease can lead to impaired drug metabolism. The severity of the liver damage reflects the extent of the reduced metabolism, but clinical liver enzymes are of little value in predicting this. Drugs with high hepatic first-pass metabolism are most severely affected.

Physiological Changes That Affect Drug Metabolism in Pregnancy

- The distribution volume for all drugs increases
- There is delayed gastric emptying, resulting in slow peak levels of readily absorbed drugs (e.g. paracetamol) and increased bioavailability of slowly absorbed drugs (e.g. digoxin)
- Nausea and vomiting in early pregnancy increases the clearance time affecting the dosage of drugs (e.g. anti-epileptics)
- Increased body fat increases clearance of lipophilic drugs (e.g. thiopental) even though the plasma half-life is prolonged
- Decreased albumin and raised free fatty acids lead to increase in free levels of albumin-bound drugs. Therefore measurement of these drugs may not reflect the actual concentration and saliva monitoring may be needed
- Increased alveolar ventilation and cardiac output seen in normal pregnancy may lead to enhanced alveolar and intramuscular drug absorption
- Renal blood flow increases and glomerular filtration rate (GFR) increases by 50% leading to enhanced renal clearance of many medications
- α_1-Acid glycoprotein levels do not change, but there is a large transplacental concentration gradient that affects transfer of drugs
- Maternal albumin concentrations progressively decrease during pregnancy and fetal albumin concentrations progressively increase. They achieve equivalence at around week 30 of gestation. Albumin-bound drugs may be transferred to the fetus in a higher concentration. The placenta has cytochrome P450 sulphating and acetylating enzymes that can metabolise drugs.

The Placental Barrier

Virtually all drugs cross the placenta and achieve equal concentrations on either side over repeated administration. Most drugs have a molecular weight below 1000 daltons (Da), and molecules of this size cross the placenta (<600 Da cross easily). Lipid-soluble drugs are readily transferred across the placenta. Diffusion is the most important mode of transfer of drugs through the placenta. Fetal plasma is more acidic and leads to ion trapping of basic drugs.

Some Commonly Used Drugs

ADRENOCORTICAL STEROIDS

The adrenal cortex synthesises two classes of steroid: the corticosteroids (glucocorticoids and mineralocorticoids), which have 21 carbon atoms, and the androgens, which have 19. Cortisone is the main glucocorticoid and aldosterone is the main mineralocorticoid. Cortisol is produced at a rate of 10 mg/day.

Corticosteroids act with specific receptor proteins in target tissues to modulate proteins synthesised by various target tissues. Hence, most effects of corticosteroids are not immediate but become apparent after several hours. The receptors are members of the nuclear receptor family. The glucocorticoid receptor is predominantly in the cytoplasm in an inactive form until it binds to glucocorticoids. Steroid binding results in receptor activation and translocation to the nucleus. The activated receptor interacts with specific DNA sequences in the regulatory regions of genes called glucocorticoid response elements (GREs) and these provide specificity to the induction of gene transcription.

Mineralocorticoids act similarly though the exact mechanism is unclear.

Hydrocortisone and numerous congeners including the synthetic analogues are orally effective. They can be administered intravenously to achieve high concentrations. Absorption from the skin is low but, if they are applied to a large area or on an occlusive dressing, the absorption may be sufficient to cause systemic effects. After absorption, >90% of cortisol is reversibly bound to protein. Two plasma proteins account for almost all of the steroid-binding capacity: corticosteroid-binding globulin (CBG) and albumin. A state of physiological hypercortisolism occurs during pregnancy. The elevated circulating oestrogens induce CBG production, and CBG and total plasma cortisol increase several-fold.

Glucocorticoids are administered in multiple formulations for disorders that share an inflammatory or immunological basis. With the exception of patients receiving replacement therapy for adrenal insufficiency, glucocorticoids are neither specific nor curative, but rather are palliative because of their anti-inflammatory and immunosuppressive actions.

Prednisolone is the biologically active form of prednisone. The placenta can oxidise prednisolone to inactive prednisone or even less active cortisone. Only 10% of the maternal prednisolone dose crosses the placenta. Four large epidemiological studies including steroids that readily cross the placenta (betamethasone and dexamethasone) have looked at the use of corticosteroids in first trimester and found an association with non-syndromic orofacial clefts. However, the overall risk is low. The Michigan Medicaid surveillance study looked at 229,101 patients exposed to prednisolone, prednisone and methylprednisolone during the first trimester; the data did not support an association between these agents and congenital defects. There are isolated reports of cataracts in the newborn if prednisolone was used throughout the pregnancy. During lactation, the infant is exposed to minimal amounts of steroid through the breast milk. At higher doses (>20 mg), it is recommended to wait at least 4 hours after a dose before nursing the baby.

Betamethasone administration to women with threatened preterm labour is associated with a decrease in respiratory distress syndrome, periventricular leukomalacia and intraventricular haemorrhage in pre-term infants. It can induce hyperglycaemia and may rarely precipitate myasthenic crisis or hypertensive crisis in the mother. Approximately 80% of the maternal betamethasone dose crosses the placenta. Single courses of betamethasone have no effects on the fetus but multiple courses have been associated with lower birth weights and reduced head circumference at birth. Follow-up studies have not shown any differences in cognitive and psychosocial development when compared with controls.

Hydrocortisone and its inactive precursor, cortisone, appear to present a small risk to the human fetus.

Approximately 50% of the maternal dose of hydrocortisone crosses the placenta. These corticosteroids produce dose-related teratogenic and toxic effects in genetically susceptible experimental animals consisting of cleft palate, cataracts, spontaneous abortion, IUGR and polycystic kidney disease. However, there are no data to support these effects in the great majority of human pregnancies, although the small increase in incidence of cleft lip with or without cleft palate is supported by large epidemiological studies.

It is important to remember that in some women the benefits of corticosteroids can far outweigh the fetal risks when used to treat maternal inflammatory and autoimmune disease, and these agents should not be withheld if the mother's condition requires their use.

ANAESTHETIC AGENTS

General Anaesthetics

General anaesthetics act by increasing the sensitivity of the γ-aminobutyric acid (GABA) A receptor to GABA thus enhancing inhibitory neurotransmission and depressing nervous system activity. Glycine receptor-mediated activation of chloride channels is responsible for inhibition of neurotransmission in the spinal cord and brain stem. Ketamine, nitrous oxide and xenon act via N-methyl-D-aspartate (NMDA) receptors and cause long-term modulation of synaptic responses.

Intravenous Anaesthetics

Intravenous (i.v.) anaesthetics are unique drugs that induce anaesthesia rapidly as they quickly achieve high concentrations in the central nervous system (CNS). Intravenous anaesthetics affect synaptic function by inhibiting excitatory synapses and enhancing inhibitory synapses their pharmacological effects are terminated by redistribution to tissues with low blood flow. Commonly used drugs are thiopental and propofol for induction of anaesthesia. Thiopental is an ultrashort-acting agent that has quick entry into the CNS followed by quick redistribution of the drug. After i.v. administration, it causes unconsciousness with amnesia without analgesia or muscle relaxation. It is used mainly as an induction agent and by infusion during short procedures. It is also used to control convulsions in status epilepticus and eclamptic convulsions not responding to magnesium sulphate.

Inhalational Anaesthetics

Inhalational anaesthetics can hyperpolarise neurones and hence reduce both pacemaker neurone and postsynaptic neurone action potentials. *Halothane* is commonly used. Due to its high lipid solubility and increased clearance from lungs, induction is slow and speed of recovery is also lengthened. Some 80% is excreted unchanged and 20% is metabolised by cytochrome P450 enzymes to trifluoroacetylate, which can bind to several liver proteins. Hypersensitivity to these proteins leads to halothane-induced hepatotoxicity.

A side effect of the drug is uterine smooth muscle relaxation and this can be helpful for manipulation of fetus (version) and for manual removal of placenta. It can also lead to an increased risk of postpartum haemorrhage. It is a triggering agent for malignant hyperthermia.

Nitric oxide (NO) is very insoluble in blood and other tissues. Due to its high insolubility, rapid induction and rapid emergence occurs during anaesthesia. On discontinuation of nitrous oxide it can diffuse from blood to alveoli and decrease the concentration of oxygen in alveoli (diffusional hypoxia). Hence 100% oxygen should be administered during recovery from NO. NO is a weak anaesthetic and analgesic at 20%, and is a sedative. A 50% concentration is frequently used to provide analgesia in labour and outpatient dentistry.

A collaborative perinatal project showed no embryonic or fetal effects of NO. Its use during delivery may lead to neonatal depression and fetal accumulation of nitrous oxide, which increases over time; hence, it is safer to keep the induction to delivery time as short as possible.

Neuromuscular Blocking Agents

These agents are used as an adjunct to anaesthetics to provide muscle relaxation. Based on their mechanism of action they are divided into depolarising (e.g. succinylcholine) and non-depolarising (e.g. pancuronium). The actions of neuromuscular blocking agents are reversed by acetylcholine esterase inhibitors (e.g. neostigmine) and muscarinic receptor antagonists (e.g. glycopyrrolate). The only depolarising agent in use is succinyl choline, which acts by depolarising the membrane by opening sodium channels. A series of repetitive excitation followed by block transmission and neuromuscular paralysis occurs. Competitive antagonists act by decreasing the frequency of channel opening events that result in an action potential. At increasing doses the drug binds to the channels in a non-competitive manner.

Depolarising muscle relaxants (e.g. suxamethonium and succinylcholine) can cause histamine release and hyperkalaemia (and therefore should be avoided in patients with heart disease, trauma and burns). Malignant hyperthermia occurs due to calcium release from the sarcoplasmic reticulum of the skeletal muscle. Clinical features include contracture, rigidity and heat production resulting in hyperthermia-accelerated muscle metabolism and acidosis. Malignant hyperthermia is treated with dantrolene which inhibits calcium release.

LOCAL ANAESTHETICS

Local anaesthetics cause a reversible block in the action potential responsible for nerve conduction. They decrease the permeability of the nerve to sodium and block propagation of electrical impulses. Combination with adrenaline (epinephrine) doubles their duration of action. Excessive administration can cause cerebral irritation and convulsions.

ANTICOAGULANTS

Warfarin

Warfarin interferes with cyclic conversion of vitamin K to its active metabolite, which is essential in carboxylation of glutamic acid residues of vitamin K-dependent coagulation factors (II, VII, IX, X). Carboxylation is necessary for binding of these factors to calcium and phospholipids. As protein S levels are also dependent on vitamin K activity, warfarin administration causes a prothrombotic state prior to the onset of an anticoagulant effect. It causes embryopathy

in 5% to 10% of pregnancies where there is first-trimester exposure. The clinical features are similar to those of chondromalacia punctata (stippled epiphysis, nasal and limb hypoplasia). The embryopathy is secondary to vitamin K involvement in the post-translational modification of proteins enabling them to bind calcium. The use of warfarin in the second and third trimester is associated with recurrent micro-haemorrhages in the brain leading to optic atrophy, dorsal midline dysplasia and mental retardation. It is avoided after 36 weeks to prevent maternal and neonatal complications related to delivery.

Heparin

Heparin is the anticoagulant of choice from the fetal perspective as it does not cross the placenta. It is a glycosaminoglycan and acts through interaction with antithrombin III. Antithrombin III inactivates thrombin, factor Xa and factor IXa. Two major side effects that can occur with heparin treatment are heparin-induced thrombocytopenia and osteoporosis. There are two types of thrombocytopenia that occur in association with heparin treatment. Non-immune heparin-associated thrombocytopenia is associated with a mild reduction in platelet count and occurs 2 to 5 days after heparin injection. Immune thrombocytopenia occurs due to IgG antiplatelet antibodies, 3 to 4 weeks after therapy, and increases the risk of thrombus formation.

Direct Oral Anticoagulants

These are oral anticoagulants that specifically inhibit factors IIa or Xa. They are also known as new oral anticoagulants (NOACs). Factor Xa is a clotting factor in the coagulation pathway that leads to thrombin generation and clot formation. They act by inhibition of prothrombinase complex-bound and clot-associated factor Xa, resulting in a reduction of thrombin in the coagulation cascade. The main advantage of direct oral anticoagulants (DOACs) is the oral administration and that they do not need drug monitoring or dose adjustments. Examples are Rivaroxaban and Apixaban.

All DOACs can cross the placenta and although no specific embryopathy pattern has been established, they are contraindicated in pregnancy and breastfeeding.

ANTICONVULSANTS

The pharmacokinetics of all antiepileptics is altered in pregnancy and therapeutic drug monitoring can be of benefit. Phenytoin, primidone, phenobarbital, carbamazepine and sodium valproate all cross the placenta and are teratogenic. Major abnormalities produced by anticonvulsants are neural tube, orofacial and congenital heart defects. Fetal hydantoin syndrome includes prenatal and postnatal growth restriction, motor or mental deficiency, short nose with broad nasal bridge, microcephaly, hypertelorism, strabismus, low-set or abnormally formed ears, limb and positional deformities. Sodium valproate and carbamazepine mainly cause neural tube defects and spina bifida (always lumbar). Valproate is no longer prescribed to women of childbearing age due to its significant association with neural tube defects and neurodevelopmental delay. Phenobarbital appears to be safer than phenytoin. The risk of teratogenicity rises with the use of more than one drug. The newer anticonvulsants are often prescribed along with other drugs, and it is difficult to ascertain teratogenic risk of these drugs in isolation.

Altered pharmacokinetics in pregnancy may lead to changes in drug levels and for most drugs the concentration of the free drug falls. If a woman is fit free, there is usually no need to measure serial drug levels or adjust the dose for most anticonvulsants. An exception is lamotrigine as levels of this drug invariably fall in pregnancy. In women who have regular seizures, and who are dependent on critical drug levels, it is worth monitoring drug levels and increasing dosages of anticonvulsants should be guided by serum concentrations. Vitamin K is given in the last 4 weeks of pregnancy to prevent haemorrhagic disease of the newborn. Carbamazepine, phenytoin and valproic acid are safe in breastfeeding. Succinimides (e.g. ethosuximide) are commonly used to treat petit mal epilepsy and are thought to have a low or no teratogenic potential.

ANTIEMETICS

Antiemetics are classified according to the predominant receptor on which they act.

Serotonin Receptor Antagonists

Serotonin (5-HT3) receptors are present in multiple places involved in emesis, such as the vagal nerve, the solitary tract nucleus and the area postrema (located at the bottom of the fourth ventricle and contains the chemoreceptor trigger zone). Serotonin is released by the entero-chromaffin cells of the small intestine and may stimulate vagal afferents to initiate the vomiting reflex. 5-HT3 agents (i.e. Ondansetron) are widely used and effective against chemotherapy-induced nausea and hyperemesis gravidarum. Common adverse effects of these drugs include constipation or diarrhoea, headache and light-headedness. Ondansetron can be safely used in pregnancy and lactation. Early concerns regarding teratogenicity of this drug have not been confirmed by recent trials.

Dopamine Receptor Antagonists

Phenothiazines (prochlorperazine, chlorpromazine) and Benzamides (metoclopramide, domperidone) antagonise dopamine receptor (D2) at the chemoreceptor trigger zone at the area postrema. In addition, these drugs also have antihistaminic and anticholinergic effects. Side effects include orthostatic hypotension, peripheral anticholinergic effects (i.e. dry mouth, blurred vision, constipation, urinary retention), central anticholinergic effects (i.e. agitation, delirium, hallucinations, seizures and coma) and extrapyramidal effects, such as oculogyric crisis and parkinsonism. Dopamine receptor antagonists are not teratogenic and can be used in pregnancy and breastfeeding.

Antihistamines

Histamine H1 receptor antagonists (promethazine, cyclizine, cinnarizine, doxylamine and dimenhydrinate) act on the vestibular nucleus and within the brainstem. Some antihistamines such as cyclizine and doxylamine have anticholinergic properties that inhibit muscarinic receptors at the same sites. Adverse effects include dizziness, drowsiness, dry mouth and fatigue. Antihistamines are used as first-line treatment for nausea and vomiting of pregnancy. Xonvea

is a delayed-release tablet containing doxylamine succinate (an antihistamine) and pyridoxine hydrochloride (vitamin B6) which is specifically licensed for the treatment of nausea and vomiting in pregnancy.

ANTI-INFLAMMATORY DRUGS

Non-Steroidal Anti-Inflammatory Drugs

Aspirin and NSAIDs do not produce structural defects. They readily cross the placenta and achieve higher concentrations in the fetus as they are albumin bound. Salicylates and NSAIDs may increase the risk of neonatal haemorrhage via inhibition of platelet function. NSAIDs may lead to oligohydramnios via effects on fetal kidney. If given in the third trimester, they can cause premature closure of ductus arteriosus and neonatal hypertension. Premature ductus closure and oligohydramnios are reversible. If used, they should be discontinued at 32 weeks. Low-dose aspirin is used in the prophylaxis of early-onset severe pre-eclampsia, migraine attacks and treatment of antiphospholipid syndrome. Aspirin in low doses inhibits thromboxane A_2 resulting in a decrease in vasoconstrictor prostaglandins.

Cyclooxygenase-2 Inhibitors. Cyclooxygenase (COX) enzymes are responsible for production of the prostaglandin series of bioactive compounds. Specifically COX converts arachidonic acid to prostaglandin H_2. There are three known COX isoforms, designated COX-1, COX-2 and COX-3. COX-1 and 2 are both expressed in tissues and have biological functions. COX-3 is a splice variant of COX-1. COX-1 is found in the gastric mucosa, kidney and platelets. COX-2 is an inducible form, although to some extent it is present constitutively in the CNS, juxtaglomerular apparatus of the kidney and placenta during late gestation. Recent development of selective COX-2 inhibitors is of major clinical interest as these have been related to lower incidence of gastrointestinal bleeding. Both COX-1 and -2 inhibitors can cause sodium retention and reduction of the GFR. Fetal COX-2 inhibition can be responsible for neonatal chronic renal failure and therefore maternal usage should be avoided until further studies confirm the safety of this group of drugs.

Colchicine. Colchicine reduces the inflammatory response to the deposition of monosodium urate crystals in joint tissue, in part by inhibiting neutrophil metabolism, mobility and chemotaxis. It also inhibits cell division in metaphase by binding tubulin and thereby interfering with mitosis. It is used to treat gouty arthritis and for prophylaxis of recurrent gout attacks. It is also used in familial Mediterranean fever, Behçet disease and amyloidosis. Colchicine given to either parent within 3 months of the time of conception may result in increased frequency of trisomy 21.

ANTIMICROBIALS

Antibiotics

Penicillin crosses the placenta and attains fetal concentrations equal to those found in the maternal circulation. It is considered safe in pregnancy and lactation. It does have the potential to modify the normal bacterial flora of the mother's genital and gastrointestinal tract.

Tetracyclines are derived from streptomyces species. They inhibit bacterial protein synthesis by binding to the bacterial ribosome and preventing access of transfer RNA (tRNA) to messenger RNA (mRNA) in ribosome complexes. It is a broad-spectrum antibiotic, crosses the placenta, chelates with calcium and is deposited in the developing teeth and bones of the fetus. The risk of tooth discoloration is highest from mid pregnancy up to 5 years postnatally. It also causes transient inhibition of bone growth if given in pregnancy. Maternal hepatoxicity can occur in the form of acute fatty liver. It is considered safe for breastfeeding by the American Academy of Pediatrics.

Quinolones act by targeting bacterial DNA gyrase and topoisomerase IV and inhibit DNA replication. In developing adolescents their use is associated with acute arthropathy of the weightbearing joints. Recent studies have shown no effect when used in the first trimester. They are not recommended when breastfeeding due to the risk of arthropathy and phototoxicity.

Aminoglycosides penetrate the cell wall and cytoplasmic membrane of susceptible microorganisms and act on the bacterial ribosome leading to cell death. Aminoglycosides are ototoxic in adults and streptomycin is definitely toxic to the fetal ear causing eighth nerve damage with auditory impairment. Gentamicin should not be withheld if indicated clinically. Single-dose gentamicin is safer for mother, but increased serum levels can cause renal and eighth nerve toxicity, hence divided doses are preferred. Gentamicin can interact with magnesium sulphate and cause rapid onset of respiratory arrest. Parenteral aminoglycosides carry a greater risk than oral aminoglycosides due to poor absorption of the latter into the systemic circulation. A small amount of the drug is excreted in the breast milk and therefore the risk to the neonate is low.

Chloramphenicol inhibits protein synthesis in bacteria and rickettsiae by preventing peptide bond synthesis in ribosomes. It also inhibits mitochondrial protein synthesis in mitochondrial ribosomes but not in cytoplasmic ribosomes in mammalian cells. Mammalian erythropoietic cells seem to be particularly sensitive and chloramphenicol can cause aplastic anaemia which limits its use to severe life-threatening conditions. It should be avoided in late pregnancy and during labour because of potential risk of grey baby syndrome which starts 2 to 9 days after the start of treatment. In the first 24 hours there can be vomiting, refusal to suck, irregular and rapid respiration, abdominal distension, periods of cyanosis and passage of loose, green stools. The baby then becomes flaccid, turns an ashen-grey colour and becomes hypothermic after the first 24 hours. This occurs due to a failure of the drug to be conjugated with glucuronic acid owing to inadequate enzyme in the liver or to inadequate renal excretion of the unconjugated drug. In a nursing infant it can also cause idiosyncratic bone marrow suppression.

Macrolides. Bacteriostatic antibiotics act at the same site as chloramphenicol. Erythromycin is safest. Erythromycin estolate can cause cholestatic hepatitis as a hypersensitivity reaction to the estolate ester. It has no adverse side effects in the nursing infant. It causes inhibition of cytochrome P450 and therefore can potentiate the actions of warfarin, anticonvulsants, digoxin and corticosteroids.

Clindamycin is a derivative of an amino acid. It binds to bacterial ribosomes and suppresses protein synthesis and is used in labour for patients who are sensitive to penicillin.

Sulphonamides are structural analogues and competitive antagonists of para-aminobenzoic acid and prevent utilisation of PABA (para-aminobenzoic acid) for synthesis of folic acid. They readily pass through the placenta and are sufficient to cause therapeutic and toxic effects. Sulphonamides should be avoided in the first trimester and during the latter part of pregnancy. If given to the mother near delivery they can cause haemolytic anaemia, hyperbilirubinaemia and kernicterus. They compete with bilirubin to bind with plasma albumin. Sulphonamides are excreted in low concentrations in breast milk and pose no risk for healthy, full-term infants. They are contraindicated if the infant is stressed, ill or premature, and in those with glucose-6-phosphate dehydrogenase (G6PD) deficiency or hyperbilirubinaemia.

Trimethoprim inhibits reduction of dihydrofolate to tetrahydrofolate and readily crosses the placenta. It is a highly selective inhibitor of the dihydrofolate reductase of unicellular organisms, and it has sufficient effect on human folate metabolism to cause megaloblastic anaemia and increase serum homocysteine concentrations. It causes neural tube defects if given in the first trimester.

Metronidazole is a prodrug that requires activation by susceptible organisms. Anaerobic bacteria contain ferredoxins that can donate electrons to metronidazole, unlike aerobic bacteria. This forms a highly reactive nitro radical anion that targets DNA and other vital biomolecules. Metronidazole is catalytically recycled and increasing levels of oxygen inhibit metronidazole-induced cytotoxicity. There is a possible association with oral clefts when it is used in early pregnancy, but a large meta-analysis (from Drug-Free America) has shown no effect. Its use in breastfeeding is controversial and lactation is withheld for 12 to 24 hours following a 2 g dose. It can cause diarrhoea and secondary lactose intolerance in breastfed infants.

Nitrofurantoin is reduced by bacteria into an active metabolite that causes DNA damage and is bacteriostatic at low concentrations and bactericidal at high concentrations. It is used for treatment and prophylaxis of urinary tract infection and is more potent in acidic urine. It can cause haemolytic anaemia in the newborn if given late in pregnancy. Nitrofurantoin is actively transported into human milk, achieving concentrations in milk greatly exceeding those in serum with an observed milk to serum ratio of 6.2 ± 2.7, and causes haemolytic anaemia in G6PD-deficient children.

Antiviral Agents

Acyclovir inhibits viral DNA synthesis. It is phosphorylated to acyclovir triphosphate by herpes simplex virus (HSV) thymidine kinase, which competes for endogenous deoxyguanosine triphosphate and acts as a chain terminator in the synthesis of viral DNA. Resistance to the drug is due to a mutation in the thymidine kinase enzyme. Acyclovir has poor oral bioavailability and the absorbed drug is reached in good concentrations in breast milk, amniotic fluid and the placenta. It is used in the treatment of HSV and varicella-zoster infection. It has been used in pregnancy and is believed to be safe. Common side effects include nausea, vomiting and headache and it occasionally causes renal insufficiency and neurotoxicity.

Interferons (INF) are potent cytokines secreted by virtually all cells in the body in response to viral infection. They possess antiviral, immunomodulatory and antiproliferative actions. Three major classes are recognised: α, β and γ. Clinically used INF-α are used in the treatment of chronic hepatitis B and C virus infections and in refractory condylomata acuminata (genital warts). Dose-limiting side effects are myelosuppression with granulocytopenia and thrombocytopenia. Febrile illness is more common after INF administration to which tolerance gradually develops.

Antifungals

Triazole antifungal drugs (e.g. fluconazole and itraconazole) inhibit sterol demethylase and thus impair the biosynthesis of ergosterol in the cytoplasmic membrane. Ketoconazole inhibits steroid biosynthesis by inhibition of cytochrome P450 and can cause menstrual irregularities, gynaecomastia and in high doses azoospermia. Itraconazole is less likely to cause hepatotoxicity and corticosteroid suppression. Triazole antifungals can cause anomalies similar to Antley–Bixler syndrome (an autosomal recessive disorder characterised by craniofacial and other skeletal abnormalities) if given in doses exceeding 400 mg in the first trimester. They are safe in breastfeeding.

Antithyroid Drugs

Thioamides (propylthiouracil, thiamazole and carbimazole) act principally by blocking the synthesis of T_4 by preventing iodination of tyrosine residues. Propylthiouracil also inhibits peripheral conversion of T_4 to T_3. Carbimazole is rapidly converted to thiamazole, the active metabolite. Thioamides cross the placenta, propylthiouracil less than carbimazole. Carbimazole exposure particularly in the first trimester is associated with birth defects such as aplasia cutis choanal atresia and tracheo-oesophageal fistula, therefore its use is not recommended in women of childbearing age unless they are using effective contraception. In high doses thioamides may cause fetal hypothyroidism and goitre. Thioamides can also cause agranulocytosis as a rare complication. The lowest possible dose to maintain the free thyroxine level within the normal range should be used. Block and replace regimens should not be used as thyroxine does not cross the placenta sufficiently to protect the fetus from hypothyroidism. Patients who are on maintenance carbimazole need to be switched to propylthiouracil prior to pregnancy. They are safe in breastfeeding, although neonatal thyroid function tests should be checked if high doses are used. Less propylthiouracil is excreted into breast milk as it is more protein bound.

BIOLOGIC AGENTS AND KINASE INHIBITORS

Biologic drugs are commonly used to treat a large number of immune-mediated conditions, such as rheumatic and inflammatory bowel diseases, idiopathic thrombocytopenic purpura, psoriasis and asthma.

Pharmacological agents act by inhibiting cytokines (tumour necrosis factor (TNF) or interleukin (IL)), inhibiting T-cell activation or depleting B cells.

Three approaches are used in order to downregulate or inhibit the functions of cytokines:

1. soluble receptor antagonists: bind to the cytokine in serum and inhibit its interaction with cell receptors.

2. monoclonal antibodies (mAb): homogenous preparations of antibodies (or fragments of antibodies) which binds to plasma protein (i.e. TNFα) and stops it from interacting with their normal targets.
3. cell surface receptor antagonist: compete with cytokines for binding in membrane receptor.

Tumour Necrosis Factor Inhibitors

Etanercept is a soluble receptor antagonist that consists in two TNF receptors bound to the Fc portion of immunoglobulin G. The medication is bivalent, which means that one etanercept molecule binds two TNF molecules.

Infliximab is a chimeric (human and murine) mAb directed against TNF.

Adalimumab is a recombinant human mAb and due to its humanised construction, it is associated with a lower risk of anti-drug antibody formation.

Certolizumab pegol is a humanised anti-TNF-α antibody Fab' fragment linked to polyethylene glycol (PEG). It lacks Fc portion and can't be actively transported by the placenta.

TNF inhibitors are not teratogenic but are actively transported through the placenta reaching a peak transfer after 28 weeks. Hence it is recommended that treatment is stopped, if possible, by the third trimester (Infliximab at 16 weeks due to its long half-life). If continued beyond the recommended gestational age, the neonate should not have any live vaccinations for the first 6 months of life due to the possibility of neonatal immunosuppression. The exception is Certolizumab which has a molecular structure that only allows slow diffusion across the placenta, therefore it can be safely used throughout pregnancy. All TNF inhibitors can be used during breastfeeding.

Interleukin Inhibitors

Anakinra is a IL-1 receptor antagonist. It should not be used in combination with other biologic agents due to increased risk of serious adverse events. Other examples of IL-1 inhibitors include canakinumab and rilonacept.

Tocilizumab and Sarilumab act by inhibiting IL-6, while Secukinumab and Ixekizumab inhibit IL-17.

Ustekinumab is a human monoclonal antibody that binds to the p40 subunit shared by IL-12 and IL-23, blocking those inflammatory cytokines.

There is insufficient evidence to support the use of IL inhibitors in pregnancy and breastfeeding, therefore they should be avoided.

T-Cell Activation Inhibitors

Abatacept prevents the suppression of T reg activity and prevents increased T effector cell activity. In view of insufficient evidence, its use should be avoided in pregnancy and breastfeeding.

B-Cell Inhibitors

Rituximab, a mAb, eliminates CD20-positive B cells, induces complement mediated cytotoxicity and stimulates apoptosis.

Belimumab is an anti-B lymphocyte stimulator (BLyS) mAb. It prevents stimulation of B cells.

There is insufficient evidence to support the use of B-cell depleting agents in pregnancy and breastfeeding, therefore they should be avoided.

Kinase Inhibitors

These agents are not biologics, but target pathways that mediate cell signalling, growth and division. Janus kinases (JAK) are cytoplasmic protein tyrosine kinases that are critical for signalling transduction to the nucleus from ILs 2, 4, 7, 9, 15 and 21. Tofacitinib and Baricitinib are examples of JAK inhibitors. An advantage of these agents is that they can be orally administered but should not be used in pregnancy or breastfeeding.

All biologic drugs supress the immune system and increase the risk of infection and reactivation of latent infections (i.e. tuberculosis). Once biologics are started, live vaccine is contraindicated, and chemoprophylaxis is required if latent tuberculosis is identified. Side effects include gastrointestinal (nausea, vomiting, diarrhoea, constipation), respiratory (coughing, dyspnoea), haematological (anaemia, leucopoenia, thrombocytopenia), neurological (musculoskeletal pain) and altered mood

CYTOTOXIC DRUGS

These drugs affect rapidly dividing cells. Methotrexate, chlorambucil and cyclophosphamide are all contraindicated in pregnancy. Cyclophosphamide may be used in life-threatening conditions like progressive proliferative glomerulonephritis because of its immunosuppressant actions.

Azathioprine is used commonly for conditions like systemic lupus erythematosus, inflammatory bowel disease and in transplant patients. It is a 6-mercaptopurine derivative which interferes with antibody production and halts proliferation of T cells. There is extensive experience of its use in pregnancy and current evidence suggests an increased risk of impaired fetal immunity, but that this is not sustained in the neonate. FGR has been reported, but it is hard to separate the effect of chronic maternal disease on fetal growth from the potential effect of azathioprine. Only a small proportion of azathioprine is transferred into breast milk.

Mycophenolate mofetil is a prodrug that is rapidly hydrolysed to mycophenolic acid (MPA), a selective, uncompetitive and reversible inhibitor of inosine monophosphate dehydrogenase. Since T and B lymphocytes are dependent on this pathway, it causes selective inhibition of antibody formation, cellular adhesion and migration. It is used primarily in prophylaxis of transplant rejection and is used in combination with glucocorticoids and a calcineurin inhibitor but not with azathioprine. Toxicity is mainly gastrointestinal and haematological. Its use is associated with an increased incidence of infections, especially sepsis associated with cytomegalovirus. It is excreted mainly by the kidney as an inactive phenolic glucuronide.

ALKYLATING AGENTS

Alkylating agents are derived from nitrogen mustard. They become strong electrophiles through formation of carbonium ion intermediates that react with various nucleophilic moieties, such as phosphate, amino, sulfhydryl, hydroxyl, carboxyl and imidazole groups forming covalent linkages and alkylating them.

Cyclophosphamide must be activated metabolically by microsomal enzymes of the cytochrome P450 system. The metabolites phosphoramide mustard and acrolein are thought to be the ultimate active cytotoxic moieties. Cyclophosphamide can be given either orally, intramuscularly or intravenously. It has a half-life of 4 to 8 hours in patients receiving it intravenously. It does not cross the blood–brain barrier and is eliminated primarily by the kidney. It is used to treat lymphoma,

myeloma, chronic leukaemia, breast cancer, small cell lung cancer and ovarian cancer, and may be used as an alternative to azathioprine in Wegener granulomatosis, childhood nephrosis and severe rheumatoid arthritis. Side effects include bone marrow suppression (affecting white cells more than platelets), alopecia, impaired function of both humoral and cellular immunity. Cystitis is relatively common due to renal excretion of the metabolite acrolein and this disappears after discontinuation of treatment.

Melphalan is an amino acid derivative of mechlorethamine, an alkylating agent. It is used for the treatment of multiple myeloma and cancer of the breast and ovary. It can cause relatively prolonged bone marrow suppression and affects both white cells and platelets but does not cause alopecia.

Ifosfamide is an analogue of cyclophosphamide. Its use is associated with relatively low levels of bone marrow suppression, but more bladder toxicity, and hence it is administered with mesna.

Chlorambucil is an aromatic nitrogen mustard and with an anti-tumour activity similar to melphalan. It is well absorbed orally and is used for palliative treatment of lymphomas, chronic lymphocytic leukaemia and myeloma. Bone marrow toxicity is relatively common.

Dacarbazine: the triazeno group of this alkylating agent causes methylation of DNA and RNA and inhibition of nucleic acid and protein synthesis. It is the most active agent in metastatic melanoma and is combined with doxorubicin for treatment of sarcomas and Hodgkin disease. Side effects include bone marrow depression, a flu-like syndrome and alopecia.

ANTIMETABOLITES

Methotrexate is an antimetabolite which competes for binding sites on dihydrofolate reductase and inhibits the binding of folic acid. Hence, the essential co-factor tetrahydrofolate for synthesis of thymidylate, purines, methionine and glycine is inhibited. Cells in the S phase of the cell cycle are very sensitive. Resistance can occur due to increase in intracellular dihydrofolate reductase levels or appearance of altered forms of dihydrofolate reductase. It is well absorbed orally and mainly excreted through the kidneys. Methotrexate is used in combination chemotherapy for acute lymphoblastic leukaemia, Burkitt lymphoma and trophoblastic choriocarcinoma and is used in low doses to cause immune suppression in non-malignant conditions like rheumatoid arthritis and psoriasis. The major dose-limiting toxic side effect is myelosuppression, and occasionally hepatitis and lung toxicity can occur due to a hypersensitivity reaction. High doses of methotrexate can also cause renal failure.

Purine analogues include thioguanine and mercaptopurine (which is converted to thioguanine). This is incorporated into DNA and prevents cell multiplication by inhibition of purine synthesis. These drugs are used in the treatment of leukaemia. Leukopenia and thrombocytopenia are common adverse effects.

5-Fluorouracil is a pyrimidine analogue that kills cells in the S phase of the cell cycle by competitively inhibiting DNA synthesis. It is metabolised largely in the liver and excreted in urine. Side effects include myelosuppression, skin rashes, nail discoloration and photosensitivity. 5-Fluorouracil is used in the treatment of breast cancer, gastrointestinal adenocarcinomas and carcinomas of the ovary, cervix and bladder.

Topical treatment has been useful in superficial basal cell carcinoma and treatment of premalignant keratoses of the skin.

ANTHRACYCLINE ANTIBIOTICS

Doxorubicin and daunorubicin are anthracycline antibiotics that have the ability to intercalate between base pairs and hinder DNA synthesis. Cells in the S phase are more sensitive. Drug resistance occurs due to enhanced active efflux of the drug. These drugs are not absorbed orally and cause necrosis if given intramuscularly or subcutaneously. Doxorubicin is used in the treatment of breast, ovary, endometrial, bladder and thyroid cancers. It can cause transient cardiac arrhythmias and depression of myocardial function. Myelosuppression occurs to a lesser extent and the drug may cause radiation recall reactions.

Bleomycin is a glycopeptide that binds to DNA and produces single- and double-strand scission and fragmentation of DNA. It is poorly absorbed orally and excreted mainly from the kidneys. Fatal lung toxicity can occur in 10% to 20% of cases. Skin toxicity may manifest as hyperpigmentation and erythematous rashes, and low-grade, transient fever is common. It is used in combination with platinum-based drugs to treat advanced testicular carcinomas and ovarian germ cell tumours.

PLATINUM-BASED DRUGS

α-Cisplatin

α-Cisplatin is a platinum coordination complex used in the treatment of epithelial malignancies. α-Cisplatin enters the cell by diffusion and reacts with water to yield a positively charged molecule. Platinum compounds react with DNA to form intrastrand and interstrand cross-links. The cross-linking is most pronounced during the S phase of the cell cycle. α-Cisplatin is used in the treatment of cancers of bladder, head and neck, endometrium and ovary. It is nephrotoxic and ototoxic. Nephrotoxicity can be abrogated by hydration and diuresis. Repeated cycles can cause neuropathy.

Carboplatin has a similar mechanism of action and clinical spectrum to cisplatin. Carboplatin is relatively well tolerated and there is less nausea, neurotoxicity, ototoxicity and nephrotoxicity than with cisplatin. A dose-limiting toxic side effect is myelosuppression, evident as thrombocytopenia. It is an alternative in patients with responsive tumours who cannot tolerate cisplatin clinically due to impaired renal function, refractory nausea, significant hearing impairment or neuropathy.

VINCA ALKALOIDS

Vincristine and vinblastine are plant alkaloids that bind avidly to tubulin and cause arrest in metaphase of cells. They act in the M phase of the cell cycle. Vinca alkaloids are used in the treatment of methotrexate-resistant choriocarcinoma, myelomas, Hodgkin and non-Hodgkin lymphomas, Ewing sarcoma and neuroblastoma. Vinblastine is more toxic to the bone marrow and vincristine is more neurotoxic.

TAXANES

Paclitaxel is a plant compound which binds to tubulin dimers and microtubulin filaments and prevents their depolymerisation. This causes disruption of mitosis and cytotoxicity. Major side effects include myelosuppression and peripheral neuropathy. It is used in treatment of breast, ovary, lung and head and neck carcinomas.

DIURETICS

Diuretics may cause a reduction in the intravascular volume and decrease placental perfusion. However, reviews of the use of diuretics in pregnancy have not shown any adverse fetal effects, although some diuretics can cause maternal electrolyte imbalances. Table 12.4 summarises the site and mode of action and the maternal and fetal side effects of commonly used diuretics.

DRUGS AFFECTING UTERINE ACTIVITY

Prostaglandins

Prostaglandins are eicosanoids derived from 20-carbon essential fatty acids of which arachidonic acid is the main precursor. Their role has been established in conception, menstruation and labour. Prostaglandin analogues are widely used for ripening of the cervix (PGE_2), treatment and prevention of postpartum haemorrhage ($PGF_{2\alpha}$ and PGE_1) and as an abortifacient.

Oxytocin

Oxytocin is a cyclic nonapeptide, synthesised in the paraventricular nuclei and secreted by the posterior pituitary. After intravenous infusion, oxytocin reaches a steady-state plasma concentration after 20 minutes, with a half-life of 3 minutes, and hence hyperstimulation resolves rapidly after stopping the infusion. It increases the frequency and force of uterine contractions. There is less response in the first trimester due to decreased numbers of oxytocin receptors, compared with a more marked response at term, as there is a 30-fold increase in oxytocin receptors. It acts on the breast and helps in milk ejection. Oxytocin acts through G-protein receptor and calcium–calmodulin complex. It is used in induction and augmentation of labour, and treatment and prevention of postpartum haemorrhage. Oxytocin infusion over a prolonged time can cause haemodilution and hyponatraemia due to vasopressin-like effects. High doses may provoke reflex hypotension and tachycardia. Carbetocin is a long-acting synthetic oxytocin analogue, 1-deamino-1-monocarbo-(2-O-methyltyrosine)-oxytocin. It has a greater biological effect and a longer half-life of 40 minutes (around 4 to 10 times longer than oxytocin) and uterine contractions occur in less than two minutes after intravenous administration.

Tocolytics

Tocolytics are drugs that inhibit uterine contractions. They have not been shown to improve perinatal morbidity or mortality and hence their use is restricted until after the administration of steroids or to facilitate *in utero* transfer.

β Agonists act through adenylate cyclase to increase cyclic adenosine monophosphate (cAMP), which inhibits myosin light chain kinase (MLCK) activity by direct phosphorylation and by reducing intracellular free calcium. They also interact with surface receptors on the trophoblast, leading to increased cAMP which increases

Table 12.4   Summary of the Site and Mode of Action, Maternal and Fetal Side Effects of Diuretics

	Site of Action	Mode of Action	Maternal Side Effects	Fetal Side Effects
Carbonic anhydrase inhibitors (acetazolamide)	Proximal tubular cells Inhibition of sodium bicarbonate absorption	Increase urinary pH Metabolic acidosis Bone marrow depression Skin toxicity Calcium phosphate stones	Open-angle glaucoma Acute mountain sickness Familial periodic paralysis	–
Loop diuretics (furosemide)	Thick ascending limb of loop of Henle Blockade of the Na–K symporter	Hyponatraemia Volume depletion Ototoxicity – tinnitus Hyperuricaemia Hyperglycaemia	Acute pulmonary oedema Congestive cardiac failure Hypertension Nephritic syndrome	Crosses the placenta and causes a diuretic effect on the fetus; changes in liquor volume not established
Thiazide diuretics	Distal convoluted tubule Inhibition of sodium transport	Hyperuricaemia Sexual dysfunction Fluid and electrolyte imbalance Hyponatraemia Hyperglycaemia	Congestive cardiac failure Cirrhosis Acute glomerulonephritis Reacts with quinidine to prolong QT interval leading to polymorphic ventricular tachycardia (torsade de pointes)	Not associated with malformation Adverse fetal effects are rare Neonatal thrombocytopenia Hyponatraemia and hypotonia have been reported
Potassium-sparing diuretics	Epithelial cells in the late distal tubule and collecting duct Competitive inhibition of binding of aldosterone to its receptor	Hyperkalaemia Metabolic acidosis in cirrhotic patients Gynaecomastia, impotence, decreased libido, hirsutism and menstrual irregularities, breast cancer on chronic administration	Co-administered with loop or thiazide diuretic in treatment of oedema and hypertension Primary hyperaldosteronism Diuretic of choice in patients with liver cirrhosis, hirsutism	Unlikely to cause abnormalities, limited data Consider use only if other treatments fail

progesterone production. Tachyphylaxis of the adrenergic receptor occurs throughout the body after prolonged exposure and occurs due to reduced receptor density and adenyl cyclase activity. Side effects include pulmonary oedema, myocardial ischaemia and cardiac dysrhythmia, hypotension, hyperglycaemia and hypokalaemia. They have been linked to increased risk of neonatal intraventricular haemorrhage, neonatal hypocalcaemia and hypoglycaemia.

Magnesium sulphate acts by competition with calcium either at the motor end plate, reducing excitation, or at the cell membrane, reducing calcium influx into the cell. It is used to prevent eclampsia in women with severe preeclampsia. Flushing, nausea, vomiting and headache are common side effects. It can cause respiratory depression in high doses, and this is treated by calcium gluconate intravenously.

Indomethacin inhibits COX and reduces synthesis of prostaglandins. Side effects include gastrointestinal bleeding, alterations in coagulation, thrombocytopenia and asthma in aspirin-sensitive patients. Contraindications include renal or hepatic disease, active peptic ulcer disease, poorly controlled hypertension, asthma and coagulation disorders. In neonates, indomethacin may cause constriction of the ductus arteriosus, oligohydramnios and neonatal pulmonary hypertension.

Oxytocin receptor antagonists: atosiban is a peptide analogue which inhibits uterine activity by interacting with oxytocin at its membrane receptor. It is a specific inhibitor of myometrial contractions and does not affect smooth muscles all over the body. It has limited transfer into the fetal circulation and does not have direct effects on the fetus. The disadvantage of atosiban is that administration is complex with different bolus and infusion rates and its use is not cost-effective compared with calcium channel blockers.

ERGOT ALKALOIDS

Ergot alkaloids are potent α-blockers that cause direct smooth muscle contraction. They are products of the fungus *Claviceps purpurea*. Only products of lysergic acid are of clinical importance. Ergotamine has a 100% first-pass metabolism and hence its derivatives, ergonovine and methyl ergonovine, are commonly used. They are used in the treatment of migraine and for prevention and treatment of postpartum haemorrhage. Side effects include nausea and vomiting. Also precordial distress and angina-like pain are known to occur after intravenous injection due to coronary spasm. In addition, there have been reports of gangrene of the limbs following repeated doses. Ergot alkaloids are contraindicated in patients with hypertension and cardiac disease.

Bromocriptine is 2-bromo-α-ergocryptine, which is used to control secretion of prolactin due to the dopamine agonist effect of the drug.

OPIOIDS

All centrally acting opioids cross the placenta. Pethidine is the most commonly used opioid. It reaches fetal blood within 2 minutes following intravenous administration and achieves steady-state concentration in the maternal blood within 6 minutes. Opioids have been used over many decades and are not known to cause any anomalies. Some important facts about specific opioids are outlined below:

- Morphine is not used as it causes more respiratory depression in the fetus and causes histamine release
- Methadone has the longest elimination half-life, that is, 23 hours in the fetus

- Pethidine is used as a sedative in labour to block the sympathetic response to pain. Respiratory depression in the neonate is common if delivered between 1 and 3 hours after intramuscular administration of the drug
- Fentanyl is an opioid used in epidural block and spinal anaesthesia to prolong and decrease the dose of local anaesthetics
- Codeine is widely used as an analgesic and is safe in pregnancy and lactation
- Meptazinol is an agonist–antagonist opioid analgesic believed to be unique in its selectivity for μ_1 (high affinity) receptors and its cholinergic activity. It is partially antagonised by naloxone and is used in the management of postoperative pain. It has recently been licensed for use as a labour analgesic. Meptazinol induces little respiratory depression and has low addictive potential.

Neither intravenous nor inhalational anaesthetics are good analgesics. Opioids are used to decrease the haemodynamic response to painful stimuli and to decrease the anaesthetic requirement. They are given during induction to decrease the pain response to intubation. Opioids act by agonist activity at μ receptors. Meperidine decreases shivering postoperatively due to its κ-receptor agonist activity. Side effects include hypotension and respiratory depression.

Naloxone is an opioid antagonist with no agonist properties. It is frequently used in neonates to treat respiratory depression secondary to opioids. It can cause severe withdrawal symptoms if given to a baby born to an addicted mother.

RETINOIDS

Acitretin and isotretinoin are synthetic vitamin A derivatives. They are used for severe resistant or complicated psoriasis and some congenital disorders of keratinisation. Vitamin A derivatives reduce sebum secretion and are used for the treatment of nodulocystic and conglobate acne and severe antibiotic-resistant acne. Teratogenic effects are seen in up to 25% of babies born to mothers who took retinoids. Isotretinoin is eliminated from the body within 4 weeks of stopping treatment but acitretin may take up to 2 years.

SELECTIVE β_2 AGONISTS

Inhalational β_2 agonists are a major breakthrough in treatment of asthma. They relax bronchial smooth muscle but also suppress release of leukotriene and histamine from mast cells, enhancing mucociliary action and inhibiting phospholipase A_2. They are mainly used in the treatment of asthma and chronic obstructive airway disease. Side effects include tremor, hyperglycaemia, tachycardia and pulmonary oedema with an increased risk in patients with cardiovascular decompensation. Selected drugs like salbutamol, terbutaline and ritodrine can be used for tocolysis.

Sulphonylureas

Sulphonylureas are oral hypoglycaemic agents that act by increasing insulin release from pancreatic β cells. They have varying half-lives ranging from approximately 5 hours (tolbutamide) to 36 hours (chlorpropamide). Some sulphonylureas are reported not to cross the placenta (glibenclamide), while others do (chlorpropamide). They have been reported to cause neonatal hypoglycaemia by exerting profound stimulatory effects on fetal pancreatic β cells thus enhancing the release of high levels of insulin.

VASODILATORS

α_2-Adrenergic Agonists

Clonidine activates α_2-adrenergic receptors in the cardiovascular control centres of the CNS and suppresses the outflow of sympathetic nervous system activity from the brain. It is 100% bioavailable with a half-life of 12 hours. Side effects include postural hypotension, dry mouth, sedation and sexual dysfunction. It is considered to be safe in pregnancy, although this is supported by fewer studies than methyldopa.

Methyldopa is a prodrug that is metabolised into α-methylnoradrenaline (norepinephrine) and acts centrally to decrease the adrenergic neuronal outflow from the brain stem. It readily crosses the placenta and achieves fetal concentrations similar to those found in the mother, although it does not affect the fetal vasculature. Methyldopa is used for the treatment of hypertension in pregnancy and 7.5 years of follow-up in children has not shown any adverse effects. Side effects are transient and include sedation, depression, decreased libido and hyperprolactinaemia. Rarely, hepatotoxicity, granulocytopenia, thrombocytopenia and haemolytic anaemia may occur.

Prazosin is a potent and selective α_1 antagonist with 1000 times more affinity to α_1 than α_2 receptors. It causes blockade of α_1 receptors in arterioles and veins and decreases peripheral vascular resistance leading to a decrease in the venous return to the heart, and hence an absence of reflex tachycardia. Its half-life is 2 to 3 hours and its duration of action is 7 to 10 hours. Profound postural hypotension with the first dose is a well-known side effect and hence it is always started at bedtime. Adverse fetal effects have not been observed as the fetal drug concentration is only 20% of the maternal concentration.

Hydralazine causes direct relaxation of the arteriolar smooth muscle. It causes a selective decrease in vascular resistance in the cerebral, coronary and renal circulations with a less marked effect on skin and muscle, and hence it does not cause postural hypotension. Side effects include reflex tachycardia and tachyphylaxis. It is used mainly in the acute control of blood pressure; intravenous administration may cause a rapid fall in blood pressure but does not affect placental vessels. Case reports of fatal maternal hypotension, a lupus-like syndrome in mother and offspring, neonatal thrombocytopenia and bleeding have been reported.

β-Adrenoceptor Antagonists

β-Blockers are used in a variety of conditions, including hypertension, angina, secondary prevention of myocardial infarction, cardiac arrhythmias, migraine, thyrotoxicosis, anxiety necrosis and glaucoma. Cardioselective β-blockers are those that act selectively on β_1 receptors and have effects only on the heart (e.g. atenolol, bisoprolol), while the majority act on both (e.g. labetalol, propranolol, oxprenolol and atenolol).

Labetalol is a competitive antagonist at both α_1 and β adrenergic receptors with partial agonist activity at β_2. α_1 receptor blockade leads to relaxation of arterial smooth muscle and vasodilatation. β_1 blockade contributes by decreasing the reflex sympathetic stimulation of the heart. It is used orally for control of chronic hypertension and intravenously for hypertensive emergencies.

Atenolol is a β_1-selective antagonist with no intrinsic sympathomimetic activity. Its half-life is 5 to 8 hours. It blocks release of renin from the juxtaglomerular apparatus. It has been used for treatment of hypertension and tachyarrhythmias. Its use in the first trimester has not been shown to be teratogenic but adverse perinatal effects have been reported. Intrauterine growth retardation was reported in association with the use of atenolol in some studies, although subsequent randomised trials have not confirmed this. When used in pregnancy atenolol can cause a decreased fetal heart rate and hyperglycaemia occurring shortly after birth.

Calcium Channel Blockers

Among the calcium channel blockers, the most commonly used is nifedipine. This is a dihydropyridine compound, which inhibits the influx of calcium (voltage-dependent fast channels) in the smooth muscle and causes vascular relaxation. It has no effect on the slow calcium channels, which control the sino-atrial node and hence can cause reflex tachycardia (this does not occur with diltiazem and verapamil). A single dose lasts for 6 hours. Although it can be used in the acute control of blood pressure it should not be given sublingually as it can affect the placental vessels with a rapid drop in blood pressure causing fetal distress. It is used to treat hypertension in pregnancy and to inhibit premature labour. The Cochrane review demonstrated that calcium channel blockers have superior effects for delaying delivery and a reduction in the risk of several neonatal morbidities. Side effects include flushing, headache and tachycardia. Evidence of exposure during the first trimester is limited and animal studies have shown embryotoxicity. Thus, their use should ideally be limited to the second and third trimester.

PSYCHOTROPIC DRUGS

LITHIUM

Lithium carbonate may rarely be indicated for treatment of the manic phase of bipolar disorder during pregnancy. The precise mechanism of action is unknown, but it is thought to be due to altered ion transport or inhibition of adenyl cyclase, influencing nerve excitation, synaptic transmission and neuronal metabolism in the CNS.

Lithium use is associated with an increased incidence of fetal abnormalities. Since the 1960s, an International Register of Lithium Babies has collected information about lithium-exposed children in the first trimester of pregnancy. It is estimated that 7.8% of lithium-exposed embryos develop abnormalities. Early data showed that the cardiovascular system is most affected, with mitral and tricuspid atresias, coarctation of the aorta and patent ductus arteriosus being reported. The disorder known as Ebstein anomaly (tricuspid valve distortion and displacement) occurs with particular frequency among lithium-exposed infants. There have also been reports suggesting an association between maternal lithium therapy and premature delivery.

ANTIDEPRESSANTS

Selective Serotonin Re-Uptake Inhibitors

Selective serotonin re-uptake inhibitors (SSRIs) inhibit the re-uptake of serotonin into pre-synaptic cells, thereby increasing extracellular levels of the neurotransmitter that are available to bind post-synaptic neurones. They have become the agents of first choice in the treatment of depression because of their safe side-effect profile. Several studies have evaluated the safety of SSRIs in pregnancy. The well powered studies have not shown any major teratogenic effect. Some have shown mildly increased risks of right ventricular outflow tract defects in particular, and also of omphalocele, septal defects and craniosynostosis. This is reported more commonly with paroxetine than other SSRIs. There is no evidence that SSRIs cause serious neonatal complications, but likewise there is no clear evidence that they are absolutely safe. The recommendation at present is that they should only be used if the benefit outweighs the potential harmful risks. There is variable transfer of SSRIs into breast milk, but overall transfer is low. Ideally nursing mothers should use SSRIs with a shorter half-life (e.g. sertraline or paroxetine).

Tricyclic Antidepressants

Tricyclic antidepressants are thought to act by inhibiting re-uptake of dopamine, serotonin and noradrenaline. There is considerable experience of their use in pregnancy and the older tricyclic antidepressants are not believed to be associated with risks of teratogenicity. They are found in breast milk at levels comparable with those demonstrated in the maternal plasma. Therefore it is recommended that they are used with caution in lactating women and, if they are used, tricyclic antidepressants with a short half-life are recommended.

ORAL CONTRACEPTIVES

Combined oral contraceptives are commonly used and contain oestrogen and progestogen.

Mechanism of Action of the Combined Pill

- Progestogen acts on the hypothalamus to inhibit gonadotrophin-releasing hormone (GnRH) pulses and on the pituitary to inhibit the oestrogen-induced luteinising hormone (LH) surge
- Oestrogen decreases the pituitary response to GnRH and in the follicular phase inhibits the follicle stimulating hormone (FSH) surge. Oestrogen and progestogen alter the transport of sperm, egg and fertilised ovum due to their effects on the fallopian tube
- Progestogen causes thickening of cervical mucus, thereby decreasing sperm penetration and inhibiting implantation.

MECHANISM OF ACTION OF THE PROGESTOGEN-ONLY PILL AND DEPOT INJECTIONS OF PROGESTOGEN

- 60% to 80% blockade of ovulation due to slowing of the GnRH pulse generator, which prevents the LH surge required for ovulation
- Thickening of cervical mucus and impairment of sperm penetration
- Alteration of the intrauterine environment and impairment of implantation.

Depot medroxyprogesterone injections inhibit ovulation in virtually all patients due to high plasma levels of progesterone.

METABOLIC EFFECTS OF THE COMBINED ORAL CONTRACEPTIVE PILL

The metabolic side effects of the combined pill are dose dependent and are uncommon with the introduction of low-dose preparations. The pill does not increase the risk of infarction/stroke in non-smokers, although it does alter coagulation by decreasing antithrombin III and plasminogen activator, thereby increasing platelet activation and the risk of venous thromboembolism. The magnitude of risk is small and is equated to half the risk in pregnancy. Hypertension is seen more often in patients on high-dose than low-dose preparations. The risk of venous thromboembolism decreases after stopping the pill. The low-dose preparations do not have any effect on HDL (high density lipoprotein) or LDL (low density lipoprotein) and cause a slight increase in triglycerides. Very long-term use has been shown to increase gall bladder disease and the high-dose pills increase insulin resistance.

THE COMBINED ORAL CONTRACEPTIVE PILL AND CANCER

The combined pill protects against endometrial cancer and ovarian cancer (due to the absence of gonadotropin stimulation of the ovaries). There is a slight increase in hepatic adenoma and hepatocellular carcinoma but no definite association has been proved. The relative risk of developing breast cancer is increased slightly and disappears 10 years after stopping the pill.

Drugs which induce microsomal enzymes (e.g. rifampicin, carbamazepine, phenytoin) decrease the efficacy of the pill. Theoretically, drugs that decrease the enterohepatic circulation (e.g. amoxicillin and other broad-spectrum antibiotics) may cause reduced plasma levels of oestrogens.

Drugs of Choice in Breastfeeding

The processes that govern the passage of a drug into milk are similar to the placenta. The maternal serum concentration is the main determinant. Maternal milk pH is slightly acidic in comparison to serum pH, so weak bases could become trapped in milk (ion trapping).

Conclusion

The use of drugs during pregnancy requires maintenance of a fine balance. Before prescribing a drug, consideration must be given to any potential harmful effects on the fetus. Equally, inadequately treating a disease can be associated with risk to mother and fetus. To minimise the fetal risks, the lowest possible effective dose should be used.

In addition to the dangers associated with fetal exposure to teratogenic drugs, there are risks associated with misinformation about the teratogenicity of drugs. This can lead to unnecessary termination of pregnancy or the avoidance

Table 12.5 Drugs That Involve Considerable Fetal Risks When Used in Pregnancy

Absolute	Relative
CYTOTOXIC DRUGS Busulfan, cyclophosphamide, methotrexate, MMF	**PSYCHOTROPIC DRUGS** Antipsychotic drugs – lithium
VITAMIN A ANALOGUES Etretinate, isotretinoin	**ANTICOAGULANTS** Warfarin, DOACs
ANTICONVULSANTS Sodium valproate	**ANTICONVULSANTS** Carbamazepine, phenytoin
THALIDOMIDE	**ENDOCRINE DRUGS** Carbimazole, propylthiouracil, chlorpropamide
CARDIOVASCULAR DRUGS Angiotensin-converting enzyme inhibitors, angiotensin II inhibitors, spironolactone	
ANTIFUNGAL DRUGS Griseofulvin, triazoles, itraconazole, terbinafine	**ANTIBIOTICS** Tetracycline, ciprofloxacin, aminoglycosides, chloramphenicol
	ANTI-INFLAMMATORY DRUGS Colchicine
ANTI-INFLAMMATORY DRUGS NSAIDs (third trimester), COX II inhibitors (limited data)	**OTHERS** Dapsone (third trimester)
ENDOCRINE DRUGS Radioactive iodine, sex hormones, octreotide	
ANTIHELMINTHIC DRUGS Mebendazole	
OTHERS Misoprostol, mefloquine, statins Bisphosphonates	

COX, Cyclooxygenase; *DOACs,* direct oral anticoagulants; *NSAIDs,* nonsteroidal anti-inflammatory drugs.

Table 12.6 Teratogen Information Services

UNITED KINGDOM
UK Teratology Information Service (UKTIS)
Web address: http://www.uktis.org/
(+44) 03448920909

UNITED STATES
Organization of Teratology Information Specialists (OTIS)
National toll-free number: (866) 626-OTIS, or (866) 626–6847 during normal business hours, Mountain Standard Time.
Web address: http://www.otispregnancy.org/

of essential treatment. Drug manufacturers and medical practitioners should make every effort possible to protect women and their unborn babies from both risks. Implicit in this statement is the need to counsel pregnant women about the safety as well as the associated risks of the use of certain drugs in pregnancy. Table 12.5 lists the drugs that are believed to involve the greatest risk to the fetus when used in pregnancy.

To receive up-to-date, evidence-based information on the safety of drugs during pregnancy, clinicians can consult a teratogen information service. Table 12.6 lists web addresses and telephone numbers of teratogen services.

13 Physics in Obstetrics and Gynaecology

SRDJAN SASO

Introduction

The application of the theories, principles and methods of physics to medicine and healthcare, in general, belongs to a branch of medicine called 'medical physics'. This chapter focuses on the use of medical physics in obstetrics and gynaecology, with a focus also on its surgical application.

Physics for Surgery

A trainee will encounter plenty of situations where the principles of physics are integral to the surgical learning experience. Summarised below are the most relevant, but, first, some basic physics and formulae.

Tissues are composed of cells, which are, in turn, composed of atoms. Electrons orbit the nucleus of an atom (composed of a neutron and proton) and bring about current flow when they move from one atom into an orbit of another atom. The flow is generated by a force that comes from a voltage which is, in turn, generated by a power generator.

Ohm's law, in simple terms, defines the current (electrons flowing through an electrical conductor, tissue or space during a period of time; *unit – ampere*) passing between two points as being directly proportional to the voltage (or the potential difference; work needed per unit of charge to move a test charge between two points; *unit – volt*) between the exact same two points. Resistance is the constant of that proportionality and the hindrance to the flow of current (*unit – ohm*).

The formula that binds all three together is: Current (I) = Voltage (V)/Resistance (R). In addition, Power (W) = Current $(I) \times$ Voltage (V).

ELECTROSURGERY

Electrosurgery (ES) is defined as the application of a high (radio) frequency electrical current during surgical operations on biological/human tissue. The concept was first initiated in the 20th century, by the father of neurosurgery, Harvey Cushing and a physicist, William Bovie. Four modes have been defined: *cutting, coagulation, desiccation* and *fulguration*.

All the modes rely on the application of an alternating electrical current, pioneered by the famous Serbian physicist, Nikola Tesla, onto tissue, which, in turn, generates heat. This basic principle has resulted in turning gynaecology into a full-blown surgical speciality. It involves improved, efficient procedures being performed to treat both benign and malignant conditions with less complications. Procedures include minimally invasive operations such as hysteroscopies and laparoscopies, open surgeries such as laparotomies (pelvic-focused and multivisceral resections), vulval/vaginal surgeries and treatments for cervical pathologies.

Equipment

In the operating room, the source of the voltage, electron flow, and, hence, electric current is the ES generator. The current then arrives to the instrument itself – in fact, the tip of the instrument –, which acts as the active electrode. The current subsequently returns to the generator via the patient and a different electrode, known as the patient return electrode. Therefore, the circuit consists of the following (in order): ES generator (or ES unit), active electrode, patient and patient return electrode.

Tissue acts as a conductor for the current, albeit a poor one, via interstitial fluid. During conduction, current meets resistance, resulting in generation of heat within the tissues, as the electrons overcome the resistance. To ensure that only required heat is produced, the generated voltage is modified by an ES generator. The modification usually depends on the variable tissue resistance.

An example is Faradic effect. Sixty kilohertz is the standard frequency at which an electric current alternates (examples include kitchen electrical appliances). An alternating current allows for modification of generated voltage and, hence, input frequencies to be increased to more than 400 kHz. This increase acts as a protection mechanism by reducing muscle and nerve stimulation. The stimulation is known as Faradic effect, occurring at frequencies below 100 kHz. Therefore, at much higher frequencies, electricity can pass through a patient with no risk of injury secondary to electrocution and minimal neuromuscular stimulation.

Modes

When we talk about heat, what do we actually mean? As explained above, the tissue radio frequency alternating current is the key. It is the radio frequency that causes molecules within cells to oscillate. This, in turn, increases the temperature within a cell, leading to heat generation.

At 60°C, the cell dies instantly. Between 60°C and 100°C, the tissue is completely dried out (dehydrated or desiccated) and simultaneously coagulated (non-liquid contents of the cell, i.e. protein). Above 100°C, intracellular contents turn to gas, the tissue expands in volume exponentially, and, consequently, it aggressively vaporises.

So, let us go through the four modes of ES (cut, coagulate, desiccate and fulgurate). At a high power, with a high frequency and constant waveform current, the water content of cells (and, therefore, tissue) is vapourised upon direct electrode contact. This allows for tissue to be cut (rapid increase to 100°C). Intermittent and, thus, lower power waveforms are used to coagulate tissue. Because of the lower power, the heat here is insufficient to bring about explosive vaporisation but, instead, results in occlusion of blood vessels and haemostasis. The area produced is known as a thermal coagulum.

Desiccation, like cutting, leads to vaporisation of the liquid cellular content. However, this cellular 'drying' here occurs with lower power and, hence, lower heat than required with cutting. Therefore, the exposed tissue on which the instrument electrode is placed dries out but only the surface and area directly underneath the surface. The damage caused to tissue with desiccation is significantly less than with cutting and coagulation.

In complete contrast to the above, fulguration occurs when the electrode is held away from the tissue in question. The result is similar to coagulation but in this case, only superficial. High voltage modulated waveforms bring about ionisation of the air gap between the electrode and the tissue. This results in an electric arc which superficially coagulates the tissue. This coagulation is superficial but spread to an area larger than the electrode tip.

It is worth highlighting that the above differs from electrocautery, which describes heat conduction by the application of an instrument heated via direct electric current to a high temperature onto tissue. This is what leads to cautery. Therefore, the current does not enter the patient's body. In ES, the current passes through the patient's tissue or body and, therefore, the patient becomes part of the current.

MONOPOLAR AND BIPOLAR DIATHERMY

Diathermy is an obvious and most common example of ES in the operating field. Diathermy relates to the instrument used. Two types exist: monopolar (single electrode) and bipolar (two electrodes); monopolar diathermy is the more common of the two.

The monopolar instrument itself acts as the 'active electrode' and is in the surgical site when galvanised. Therefore, the patient return electrode is on a different part of the patient's body. It acts as a 'dispersive electrode', which scatters the current that has passed through the patient. This closes the circuit but, importantly, prevents thermal injury to the underlying tissue.

An example of a bipolar diathermy instrument is forceps used to coagulate blood vessels. It includes two electrodes, both an active and a return electrode, whose functions are, therefore, carried out at the surgical site. This means that the only part of the patient that is included in the circuit is the tissue grasped between the electrodes. This is the main advantage of bipolar instruments: elimination of the risk of current diversion, a need for a patient return electrode and other risks. The main disadvantage is that it is difficult to vaporise or cut tissue with bipolar instruments.

The effect of heat on tissue when using either monopolar or bipolar diathermy will very much depend on the following variables: surface area, duration and proximity of instrument to tissue, as well as tissue conductivity. An increase in the latter three means more heat generated, but an increase in surface area results in a lower current concentration and less heat.

Thunderbeat, LigaSure and Harmonic

Integrated energy sources have vastly changed the landscape of minimally invasive surgery. They combine the ability to dissect tissues whilst simultaneously attaining haemostasis. Three are described here.

Thunderbeat (TB) is the only integrated form of surgical energy derived from a single instrument. It concurrently delivers ultrasonically generated frictional heat energy and electrically generated bipolar energy. It can realise 7-mm vessel sealing. Five variables determine the versatility of TB: haemostasis, histologic sealing, cutting, dissection and tissue manipulation.

LigaSure vessel sealing system (LVSS) is a bipolar device for sealing vascular tissue. It seals tissue by administration of high current and low voltage as compared to conventional ES. It provides a secure seal of blood vessels measuring up to 7 mm diameter.

Harmonic scalpel (HS) is a high-power system that works at a frequency of 55.5 kHz or 55,500 vibrations/s.

TB and HS apply ultrasonic dissection by applying ultracision. The handpiece contains a transducer 'comprised' of piezoelectric crystals sandwiched among metal cylinders. The ultrasound (US) generator transforms ultrasonic energy into mechanical energy. Ultimately, vessels are sealed because of denatured protein coagulum secondary to tamponade and coaptation.

TB differs in many ways from LVSS and HS. The versatile score of TB is higher than LVSS and HS. This is demonstrated in many ways. First, the dissection time with TB is shorter, ensuring a faster operation time, reliable 7 mm vessel sealing, accurate dissection with fine jaw design, inconsequential thermal spread and best visibility at time of surgery. Second, TB has higher bursting pressure and highly reduced thermal speed compared to LVSS and HS.

COMPLICATIONS

A quick word about potential complications from using ES in the context of laparoscopy. Injuries, in general, are similar to those during open surgery, for example, laparotomy, and can be attributed to inappropriate identification of anatomical structures, mechanical trauma or electrothermal injuries. Our focus here is on electrothermal injuries. They can be grouped into four areas: (1) direct application; (2) insulation failure, (3) direct and capacitive coupling of current; and (4) return electrode or alternative site burns.

Direct application causes injury either via unintentional activation or incorrect targeting. Both are commonly attributed to momentary lack of attention and increased speed of the procedure meaning more coagulation and thermal spread. Dwell time is also important as it determines the amount of tissue effect. Prolonged or unintended activation means increased involuntary dwell time, hence wider and deeper tissue damage.

Poor insulation means, in simple terms, a *stray current* escaping to injure bowel, bladder ureters or blood vessels. Attention to detail is paramount here, both pre- and postoperatively, to check the actual instruments for defective insulation. Frequent sterilisation, to ensure asepsis, leads to a weakening of insulation, as does repeated use of disposable equipment and a mismatch in size between an instrument and port size ('wear and tear').

Direct coupling occurs when the surgeon accidentally activates the active electrode when it is near to another metal instrument (e.g. laparoscope or metal grasper forceps). The metal instrument becomes energised, and, hence, the current will look to complete the circuit to the patient return electrode. Prevention of this involves visualising the active electrode and ensuring no contact with any other conductive instrument before its activation.

Coupling can be also *indirect* or *capacitive*. The process is as follows: electric current is transferred from the active electrode, that is, conductor, through its surrounding, unbroken insulation, into adjacent conductive tissue (e.g. bladder or bowel) without actual direct contact. Therefore, to prevent this, the surgeon must activate the active electrode only when it is in contact with target tissues. Additionally, ensuring appropriate and fail-proof insulation, shorter instrument length, and reduction in high-voltage peaks are beneficial.

The grounding (dispersive) pad offers the path of least resistance from the patient back to the generator and ensures an area of flow current density. If the return electrode is not able to disperse the current safely or is not completely in contact with the patient's skin, it results in the exiting current having a high enough density to produce an unintended burn. It is important to have good contact between the patient and a dispersive pad. A burn at an alternative site can occur if the dispersive (ground) pad is not well connected to the patient's skin. When the dispersive pad lacks in quantity or quality, or patient interface, the electrical circuit can be completed by a small grounded contact point, such as electrocardiogram leads and produce high current densities, causing a burn.

Laser

The effectiveness of Light Amplification by Stimulated Emission of Radiation (LASER) is derived from the production of a perfectly parallel beam, allowing extremely tight focusing. Concentrating energy into a very small area in a very brief pulse produces very high local temperatures, sufficient to vaporise tissue, surrounded very locally by a cauterising action, which seals the edges and reduces blood loss.

In the following description, the simplified Bohr model of the atom is used, modified where relevant by some of the constraints of wave mechanics. Neodymium-doped yttrium aluminium garnet (Nd-YAG) lasers are rod lasers that are pumped by a flash lamp, having a broad spectrum of light. A typical system is shown in Fig. 13.1. The flash excites electrons orbiting a nucleus to orbits of higher energy, from where they drop back and may emit a photon of light as they do. In suitable materials, some of these orbits are relatively stable, and electrons tend to dwell in them for a relatively long time. The rod has polished, squared off ends and is placed between mirrors with surfaces that are exactly parallel, so that any light emitted within the rod is reflected back and forth. Those electrons in unstable orbits soon drop back at random times and take no significant part in the true laser beam. Those in semi-stable orbits accumulate. When they drop back, they also emit a photon, although most are not parallel to the axis of the rod and mirrors. When a photon has a wavefront parallel to the mirrors, it is reflected exactly back to the other mirror, which sends it back to the first, etc. Because its wavelength is exactly the same as that represented by the energy difference in all the similar semi-stable electrons, they are stimulated to join in as the wave passes by, adding their energy to the beam in precisely the same direction and phase. The stronger the beam becomes, the more likely any remaining excited electrons are to join in, producing a sudden, very intense, flash of visible or infrared light. This is how lasers get their name: LASER.

Part of the light is allowed to escape through one of the mirrors, and it is described as 'coherent'. Coherent light is monochromatic and highly parallel, sharing the same spatial and temporal phase. Because it is so perfectly parallel, it can be focused onto much smaller spots than sunlight. Spots of 0.5 µm can be used to cut into single cells in vitro. Although the conversion efficiency from energy in the flash tubes to laser output is very small, typically less than 1/1000, this fine focusing produces very high local energy deposition, termed irradiance. For instance, a typical CO_2 laser might briefly produce an irradiance of up to 20 kW/cm² over a 0.3-mm diameter spot. The wavelength of the radiation (colour, if in the visible range) depends on the material doing the lasering. This has an important bearing on the effect on the tissue. CO_2 lasers produce infrared radiation at a 10.6 µm wavelength, which is strongly absorbed by water in the tissue. Tightly focused intensities of 100 W/cm² produce tissue vaporisation depths of 3 to

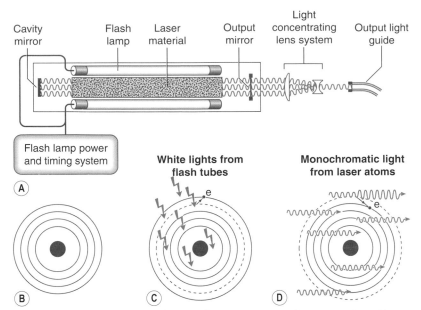

Fig. 13.1 Diagram of laser. (A) Flash lamp power and timing system; (B) electrons orbiting a nucleus; (C) electrons may emit a photon of light when orbiting a nucleus to orbits of higher energy; (D) monochromatic light from laser atoms.

4 mm, giving the effect of a laser knife. A laser knife has the further advantage that, at the edge of its beam, blood vessels become coagulated, sealing off the operative field as they cut. Cone excisions from the cervix may be produced by mechanical rotation of the beam. Spreading the beam by partial de-focusing is useful for surface ablation or thermocoagulation.

The physical properties of CO_2 lasers make them unsuitable for operating on thicker tissues, for example to ablate endometriosis. Here, the Nd-YAG laser is ideal because its wavelength is in the near infrared range (0.532 μm), at which water is transparent, but blood pigments readily absorb. The radiation is conducted to the site via a 0.4-mm diameter fibre light guide. This is a fine glass fibre whose outer surface is coated with a thin layer of another glass of a different refractive index. This ensures that any light not quite parallel to the axis of the fibre is totally reflected back into the fibre as if the fibre were surrounded by a perfect mirror. The fibre is flexible. It can then be passed down endoscopes and positioned using a pilot beam of normal light. When the desired position is attained, and the trigger button pressed, a shutter blocks the eyepiece, the flash lamp fires and the shutter re-opens. It is likely that a whole range of different laser beams will become available, each tailored to a specific surgical application.

Imaging

COMPUTED TOMOGRAPHY

Computed tomography (CT) represents an accurate and fast medical imaging technique. Whole body images are currently obtained using continuous, helical data acquisition instead of sequential and axial (transverse anatomical plane, which is perpendicular to the body). Hence, these images are taken by rotation around a fixed axis.

A single slice can be 1 to 5 mm thick and contains the attenuation of different tissues to ionising radiation. A mean value for a given volume of tissue is calculated and is known as a voxel. Furthermore, a voxel is represented in greyscale as a single point in the final 2D image. It is commonly referred to as a pixel. The greyscale of the image is measured using the Hounsfield scale, which is relative to the attenuation of water (water is 0 Hounsfield units). Air measures -1000 Hounsfield units and metal above a 1000. Common CT techniques include CT angiography, CT urography, perfusion CT and CT combined with positron emission tomography (PET).

With regards to the latter, it has become a key investigatory tool in oncology, both for diagnosis and follow-up. A gantry holds the CT and PET scanners together. The sequential images acquired from both devices are combined into a single superimposed image. PET images are functional, mapping glucose metabolism in the body. This is possible due to the uptake (by metabolically active tissues) of ^{18}F-fluorodeoxyglucose (FDG), a glucose analogue with a half-life of 2 hours. Its decay results in the release of a positron, whose positive electric charge, makes it seek an electron. It is this collision with an electron that brings about a release of high energy photons. They are subsequently detected by PET. In combination with CT images, one can see how the aforementioned activity correlates with anatomical imaging acquired by CT scanning. This allows for identification of hot spots, that is, primary carcinosis or metastases, where uptake of FDG is high.

MAGNETIC RESONANCE IMAGING

Magnetic Resonance Imaging (MRI) is a type of non-ionising radiation. It used to be called 'nuclear magnetic resonance', but that had negative associations in patients' minds. No beams of light or sound are produced; instead, the nuclei of certain atoms in the patient are induced to report their presence and condition by absorbing or sending out radio waves. Th SI for a magnetic field is a Tesla. A magnetic field of 0.5 to 3 T is produced by medical MRI magnetic equipment. This is a type of electromagnetic radiation that does not carry enough energy per quantum to ionise atoms or molecules. Images of body organs are generated by magnetic fields and their gradients and radio waves. The principle is based on fat and water (which, together, make up ~80% of the human body) containing a high number of hydrogen nuclei (unpaired protons).

These hydrogen nuclei have a positively charged spin that gives it magnetic polarity. When spinning within an external magnetic field, they are able to produce or absorb radio waves, manifested as radio frequency energy. Hence, the frequency is dependent on the electromagnetic field and the energy state of the radio waves. Moreover, the electromagnetic field aligns atomic (hydrogen) nuclei within the human body, an act that allows for the electromagnetic field to become rotating. Using resonant frequency, the radio frequency pulse flips nuclei away from their original alignment via an angle depending on the amount of energy they absorb. Upon cessation of the electromagnetic field, the radio frequency pulse stops, and the nuclei relax and flip back to their original alignment. An MRI machine will detect a photon, released as a difference in energy between the two states that the nuclei find themselves in. To get a picture of the internal abdominal contents, the difference in energy released is measured according to location.

The correct terminology for the greyscale seen on images is signal intensity. High signal is white and low signal is black. The time between the radio frequency pulses and the time between a radio frequency pulse and an ECHO determine weighting. Weighting is commonly divided into two groups for the purposes of MRI: T1-weighted (focus is on anatomy) and T2-weighted (focus is on pathology). T1 refers to spin-lattice relaxation time, which is the time taken for the nuclei to revert to their original energy state once the field is turned off (dissipating energy previously absorbed). In the images produced, fluid-containing tissues are dark and fat-containing tissues are bright. With the radiofrequency field off, the nuclei eventually lose their alignment, with a loss of synchronisation. As opposed to spin-lattice

relaxation time (T1), this is known as spin-spin relaxation time (T2). The opposite is the case here; water and fluid-containing tissues are bright and fat-containing tissues are dark.

Ionising Radiation

RADIATION DEFINED

First, we define radiation. The term 'radioactivity' refers to occurrences in the nuclei of atoms. The nucleus is the positively charged centre around which the negatively charged electrons of the atom circulate in orbits up to 10,000 times the nuclear diameter. There is continual exchange of energy between particles constituting the nucleus, and, in some atoms, it is possible for sufficient energy to be acquired by a particle to allow it to escape (Fig. 13.2).

Protons (carrying one positive charge) or neutrons (uncharged) may leave singly or in a two-plus-two group, which is then known as an α particle. Other particles are electrons (called β particles), electrons with positive charges (called positrons) and miscellaneous others, such as neutrinos and mesons, which are not yet of primary importance in medicine. Table 13.1 shows some of the radioactive substances that do have medical applications and the way in which energy is liberated.

The energy carried away from the nucleus by any particle is limited by wave mechanics to discrete values, and the nucleus may then be left with a surplus energy above its next lowest stable level. The surplus may then be carried away by a burst (quantum) of γ radiation. Since the energy of a γ quantum is proportional to its frequency, any quantity of energy can be carried by an appropriate frequency.

WHAT IS IONISATION?

Radiation can be divided into two groups: ionising and non-ionising. Ionisation, specifically, is the process by which an atom or molecule is converted into an ion subsequent to addition or removal of charged particles. An addition of an electron results in a negatively charged particle, and a

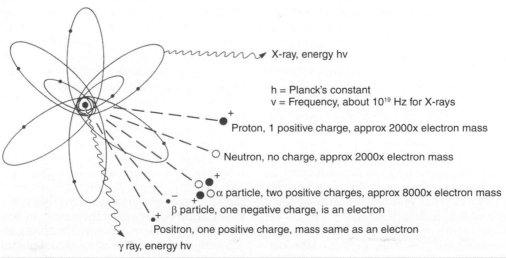

X-ray, energy hv

h = Planck's constant
v = Frequency, about 10^{19} Hz for X-rays

Proton, 1 positive charge, approx 2000x electron mass

Neutron, no charge, approx 2000x electron mass

α particle, two positive charges, approx 8000x electron mass

β particle, one negative charge, is an electron

Positron, one positive charge, mass same as an electron

γ ray, energy hv

Fig. 13.2 Principal ionising radiations.

Table 13.1   Principal Parameters of Some Isotopes Associated With Medicine

Name	Symbol	Half-Life	Radiation Energy (MeV)[a] Electromagnetic (γ- or X-rays)	Particle (β)
Caesium-137	^{137}Cs	30 years	0.662	0.51[b]
Carbon-14	^{14}C	5760 years		0.155
Cobalt-60	^{60}Co	5.26 years	1.17	0.31[b]
			1.33	0.96
Gold-198	^{198}Au	2.7 days	0.412	
Iodine-125	^{125}I	60 days	0.027	0.61
Iodine-131	^{131}I	8 days	0.36	1.71
Phosphorus-32	^{32}P	14 days		0.167
Sulphur-35	^{35}S	87 days		
Technetium-99m	$^{99}Tc^m$	6 h	0.14	0.018
Tritium (hydrogen-3)	^{3}H	12.3 years		

[a]1 MeV $= 1.6 \times 10^{-19}$ J.
[b]This form of radiation is not utilised for medical purposes.

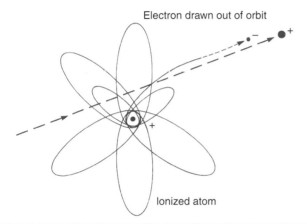

Fig. 13.3 Ion pair production: electron drawn out of orbit.

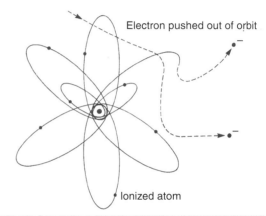

Fig. 13.4 Ion pair production: electron pushed out of orbit.

removal of an electron results in the opposite, that is, a positively charged particle.

Ionisation is usually considered the dominant effect, and, as it produces readily detected physical results, it is used as a marker or scalar of radiation activity. The ions referred to are those produced by each particle, not the particles themselves. An ejected proton, for instance, is travelling in a sea of electrons and exerting an attractive force on them as it passes through the orbital shells of various atoms. If the force is large enough and exerted for long enough, an electron may be dragged out of orbit round its parent nucleus (Fig. 13.3). This produces two new ions, positive and negative. It also slows the proton down slightly as it gives up energy to the electron, but only slightly because its mass is some 2000 times that of the electron. The proton will continue ploughing a trail of ion pairs as it goes. As it gradually loses energy, it spends longer in each atom through which it passes, thus having a greater effect on its electrons, increasing its ionisation efficiency. It eventually captures an electron and becomes a neutral hydrogen atom.

Such an unstable atomic nucleus spontaneously loses energy as it emits ionising particles. This process is commonly referred to as radioactive decay, a stochastic process defined by uncertainty and randomness involved in outcomes and predicting the atomic decay process. Radioactive decay that produces ionising radiation is grouped into three types: alpha (α) radiation, beta (β) radiation and gamma (γ) radiation.

Spontaneous radioactive decay favours the emission of a group of two protons and two neutrons as the heavy positive component (α particle). Having twice the charge/energy and four times the mass of a proton, it is highly efficient at ionisation. All nuclear particles have definite air path lengths, although it will be tortuous and, thus, effectively reduced in the case of the lighter and more easily deflected β and positron particles (Fig. 13.4). This means a low depth of penetration.

Two types of β-particles exist: β+ and β−. The former is a higher energy positron (electron-like particle with a positive charge), which is found following β+ decay of a neutron. The latter is an electron arising following β− decay of a neutron. γ-rays are high-frequency electromagnetic radiation that can also transfer energy to electrons in the material through which they pass, in ways that depend on the frequency of the ray. These mechanisms are pair production, Compton scattering and photoelectric absorption, in order of descending ray frequency and energy. The electrons subsequently escape from their parent atoms and cause the ionisation observed, like β particles. The γ-ray continues travelling, but its frequency is reduced, corresponding to the loss of energy. Furthermore, it is produced by radioactive decay, fusion or fission. Shielding from a γ-ray requires a large amount of mass (lead); α-particles only need a single sheet of paper.

X-rays are also electromagnetic radiation and differ from γ-rays in their origin and wavelength. They are generated by the circulating electrons of the atom, instead of its nucleus. Unlike the particles, X-ray velocity is unchanged, and the probability of interaction with another electron is largely unaltered. Therefore, it dies away exponentially with distance, rather than having a well-defined range.

MEASUREMENTS

What are the units for some of the terms described above?

X-Rays

A Roentgen measures an X-ray's ionising ability and, therefore, radiation exposure. It is defined as the electrostatic unit of charge of each polarity freed by the radiation in a specified volume of dry air (1 cm^3) divided by the mass of that air (coulomb per kilogram). Sievert units (Sv) measure the biological effect of radiation on the human body. One Sv is equal to 100 roentgen equivalent man (rem).

Finally, with regards to measuring absorbed dose of ionising radiation, one applies gray (Gy) and rad. One gray is defined as the absorption of one joule of radiation energy per kilogram of matter, hence, a unit of the radiation quantity absorbed dose, which calculates the energy deposited by ionising radiation in a unit mass of matter being irradiated. One gray and rad is equal to 100 rad, an old SI unit now replaced by Gy.

A chest X-ray is less than 0.01 mGy, and an abdominal X-ray is 4.2 mGy. The threshold dose for fetal malformation is 100 to 200 mGy and sterility is 3 to 6 Gy.

Radioactive Decay

Becquerel (Bq) is the SI unit of radioactive decay. It is defined as the activity of a radioactive material in which one nucleus decays per second. Any such measurement is only true at the moment it is made since the proportion left capable of transforming it is continually decreasing. A second parameter, half-life, defines the rate at which this is happening as the time required for half the initial quantity to have completed its transformation.

To determine these factors, it is only necessary to detect when transformations occur. To determine the effect these disintegrations are having requires measurement of the magnitude of the ionisation caused by the radiation emitted.

TREATMENT

Ionisation was the route by which radioactivity was discovered and by which it is usually measured. Excitations may be considered imperfect ionisations, in which sufficient energy is imparted to outer electrons of atoms to put them into orbits of higher energy than usual, but insufficient for them to escape from their parent nucleus.

Radiation also has a therapeutic function because the biological effects of radiation are due to both of the above phenomena described in the previous paragraph. Both lead to the production of new chemical species inside the cell, some of which lead, in turn, to further chains of damaging chemical reaction. DNA disruption is the most critical mode for cell killing, but other fatal or disabling reactions, such as impairment of membrane function, leading to osmotic changes, release of lysosome contents and mitochondrial damage, are also important.

It can be used to treat both malignant and non-malignant pathologies. The principle is simple: radiation is applied for the purpose of causing DNA damage. DNA damage is a consequence of direct or indirect ionisation of atoms that constitute the DNA chain. It, therefore, follows that both normal cells and cells that have undergone the 'carcinosis' process will be impaired.

To limit the extent of damage to normal cells and allow them time to recover, radiation is administered using a 'fractionation' method, that is, the radiation dose is given in fractions, rather than the whole dose in one administration. The gap between each fraction permits tumour cells found to be hypoxic to re-oxygenate and, hence, become more sensitive to the radiation prior to the next fraction, that is, dose. This is crucial as oxygen acts as a radiosensitiser, and, hence, hypoxic surroundings increase resistance of tumour cells to radiation. Solid tumours tend to find themselves in such environments if angiogenesis has not been beneficial.

The gap between each fraction also benefits the patient in that it allows those tumour cells found to be in a radiation-resistance phase of their cycle during the therapy to change to the next phase of the cell cycle. This is potentially more radiosensitive.

Nuclear Medicine

Imaging can be divided into two camps. Either external waves are passed through the patient to be picked up by a detector, or an internal source that has been introduced into a patient emits radiation that is measured. The latter is commonly referred to as nuclear medicine. As a spectrum of ionising radiation, it serves two purposes: diagnostic (PET scan) and therapeutic (iodine-131 in hyperthyroidism).

The introduction of an internal source can happen in three ways: injection, inhalation or ingestion. Molecules are labelled with radioactive isotopes and introduced into a patient. The radionuclides are atoms with an unstable nucleus that emit ionising radiation as part of their radioactive decay. The radiation is captured by a γ camera. Rather than providing information relevant to organ/tissue anatomy, the imaging in this scenario describes the physiological tissue or organ function. Examples include PET scans, ventilation/perfusion scans (V/Q scan), bone scintigraphy and nuclear imaging done to shed a light on thyroid disease, phaeochromocytoma, hyperparathyroidism and renal function.

STABLE ISOTOPES

Isotope (iso meaning same and topes meaning place) means occupying the same place in the periodic table, that is, they are atoms that happen to have the same number of protons in the nucleus and, hence, attract the same number of electrons, giving them the same chemical characteristics. The rest of their nuclei may be thought of as made up of neutrons of similar mass to protons but carrying no charge. Many of these combinations are unstable and break up to form daughter isotopes with different chemical characteristics, often producing radioactive effects. Some (Table 13.2), although relatively rare, are perfectly stable and can be incorporated into compounds as markers without disturbing chemical reactions. Most importantly, they can be detected and distinguished from the more commonly occurring isotopes, and do not emit ionising radiation.

Deuterium is an example. It is relatively cheap and easily incorporated but is also more easily accidentally 'lost' during processing. C-13 and N-14 are usually bonded more securely but are more expensive to obtain and incorporate. Since these markers are chemically identical to the majority of isotopes, physical methods have to be used to detect their presence by small differences in mass of the molecules into which they are incorporated. The primary tool for this is the mass electromagnetic spectrograph (Fig. 13.5).

Ultrasound

DIAGNOSTIC ULTRASOUND

US does not use electromagnetic radiation but, rather, longitudinal compression sound waves. Very high frequency sound is useful in diagnosis because it can be directed and will penetrate the body like X-rays, but it does not cause ionisation at the energy levels used. Hence, it is a safe and popular mode of imaging.

Frequencies are in the range of 2 to 15 MHz, the most common being around 3 MHz, about 200 times the highest frequency the average adult can hear. In our specialty, the frequency ranges 2 to 6 MHz for abdominal US and 7 to 9 MHz for transvaginal. Sound waves cause particles of the medium through which they are travelling to move a minute distance back and forth along the direction of their path. Such waves are called 'longitudinal' to indicate the direction of displacement of the particles supporting the wave.

The power to produce these waves is generated electrically. A US probe consists of two parts: a transducer and a receiver. The former is a device that transforms electric power into sound power. A common form of transducer uses a thin slice of piezoelectric ceramic or quartz. These materials alter their thickness according to the electric current or voltage (V) applied between their faces. The change in thickness is small, only a few micrometres in the highest-powered machines. It brings about a mechanical deformation, resulting in an electric charge or a voltage, leading to displacement of surrounding air and, ultimately, US waves.

Those waves allow for us to see an image as a result of the pulse echo principle. The produced US waves have displacements of about 1 nm, and the time for the reflected echo of those US waves to return is measured (travel through tissues at about 1540 m/s) (Fig. 13.6). In addition, a slice of the piezo material exposed to the returning ultrasonic echoes produces a corresponding electrical signal. This results in the formation of a grey-scale two-dimensional image on screen.

ULTRASOUND INTERACTION WITH TISSUE

US waves interact with tissue in five ways: *reflection*, *refraction*, *diffraction*, *absorption* and *scatter*. First, we define intensity: it describes how much energy is passing through a certain cross-sectional area, usually 1 cm^2, over a certain time period. It is usually defined in watts per square centimetre (W/cm^2).

Impedance, Reflection, Refraction and Scatter

The characteristic acoustic impedance of a material describes how it resists being moved in response to a given sound pressure wave. For soft tissues, it is roughly proportional to tissue density. When US encounters a boundary between tissues of different impedances, the mismatch of movements prevents a proportion of the sound energy from being transferred. The rest is reflected and produces the echoes used in diagnostic US (Fig. 13.7). Therefore, acoustic impedance decides what fraction of the original waves will be reflected. If the sound reaches the boundary at an angle, it will be reflected at the same angle, provided the reflecting surface is large compared with the sound wavelength.

Going back to acoustic impedance, the fraction of the wave that is not reflected can also be refracted, that is, it can pass through the medium it reaches. Again, the impedance

Table 13.2	Isotopes and Relative Abundance		
Isotope	Relative Abundance (%)	Isotope	Relative Abundance (%)
H-1	99.985	H-2 (D-2)	0.015
C-12	98.892	C-13	1.108
N-14	99.635	N-15	0.365
O-16	99.759	O-18	0.204
S-32	95.0	S-34	4.22
Cl-35	75.79	Cl-37	24.20
K-39	93.22	K-41	6.77

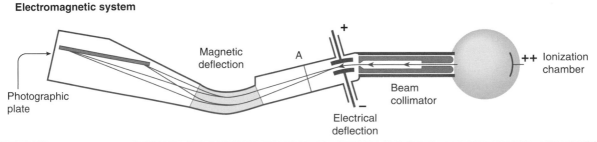

Electromagnetic system

Photographic plate

Magnetic deflection

A

Electrical deflection

Beam collimator

++ Ionization chamber

Fig. 13.5 Mass electromagnetic spectrograph.

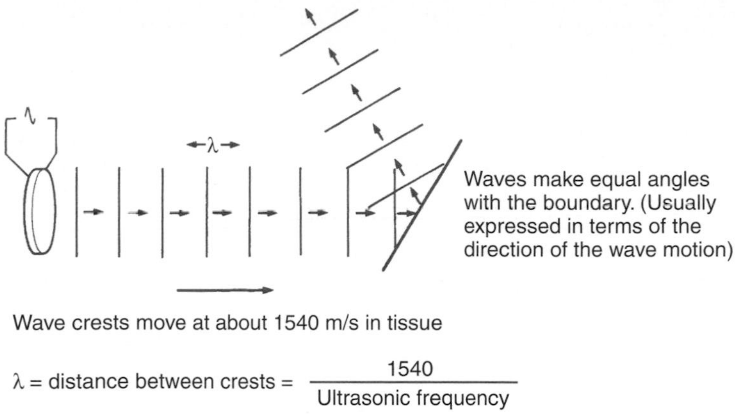

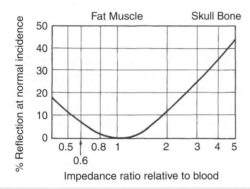

Waves make equal angles with the boundary. (Usually expressed in terms of the direction of the wave motion)

Wave crests move at about 1540 m/s in tissue

$$\lambda = \text{distance between crests} = \frac{1540}{\text{Ultrasonic frequency}}$$

Fig. 13.6 Ultrasound generation and reflection.

Fig. 13.7 Percentage reflection caused by interfaces of various impedance ratios.

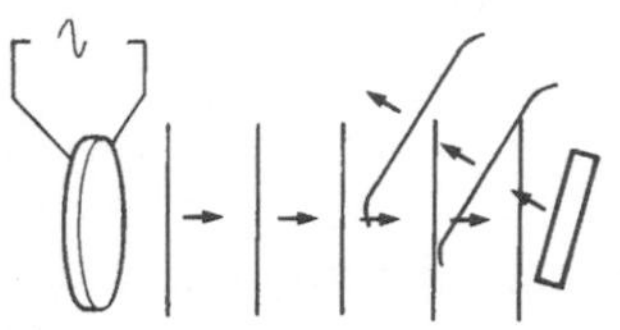

Fig. 13.8 Reflection.

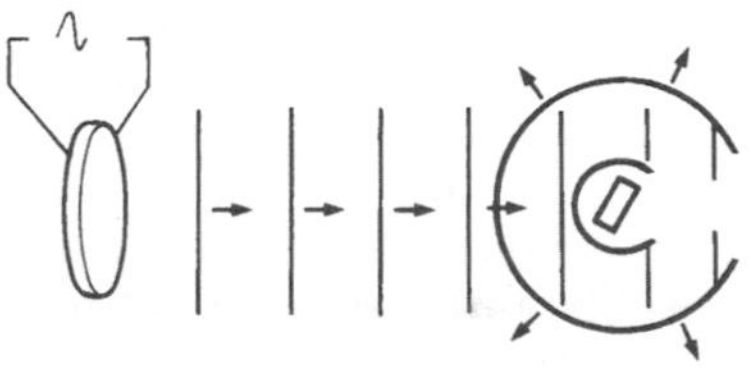

Fig. 13.9 Scattering.

of each medium determines the speed of the US wave in that medium. The greater the impedance difference, the greater the difference in speed between the media and, hence, the greater the change in angle and direction of the wave as it passes from one medium to the other.

Near the edge of the reflector, the local sound pressure pushes particles sideways, rounding off the edge of the reflected wave (Fig. 13.8) at the centre of the reflector local pressure balance. This is so that the reflected wave is flat. If the reflector is reduced in size, as it approaches half a wavelength, the flat portion disappears, and the reflection spreads in all directions, spherically (Fig. 13.9).

This form of reflection is known as scattering, since the direction of the reflected sound energy bears no relation to the direction of the incident wave, hence, a combination of irregular reflection, refraction and diffraction.

Absorption

US waves lose energy to the tissue by several mechanisms – viscous, relaxation and thermodynamic losses, for instance. Viscous losses are increased in non-homogeneous fluids, whose acoustic impedance varies on a microscopic scale. Relaxation mechanisms arise when, at one stage of the sound cycle, associated ions become separated and then require a certain specific minimum time to reassociate. Relaxation mechanisms have characteristic variations with frequency, which may depend on the chemical state

of the tissue. Thermodynamic losses occur because, as the tissue is compressed by the sonic pressure, its temperature rises slightly. Nearby, there is another region where the temperature has been reduced by decompression. Any thermal leakage between the two regions is energy lost to the sound wave. In soft tissues at diagnostic frequencies, thermodynamic losses are small compared with viscous and relaxation losses.

Diffraction

The ideal ultrasonic beam for diagnostic purposes would be needle thin to give the finest detail. Unfortunately, this is not possible because of diffraction. Diffraction is defined as a phenomenon arising when a wave confronts an impediment with a diameter equivalent to its wavelength. It commonly occurs when US waves bend around small obstacles and spread as they pass through small openings.

A point source transducer would produce spherical waves similar to a point scatterer. Wider transducer faces produce flatter wavefronts, but off-axis waves created at one part of the face may cancel or reinforce those from another. This results in sound being emitted at unwanted angles known as side lobes (Fig. 13.10). It is highly desirable to suppress side lobes and make the angle θ at which the first minima occur (defining the main lobe) as narrow as possible.

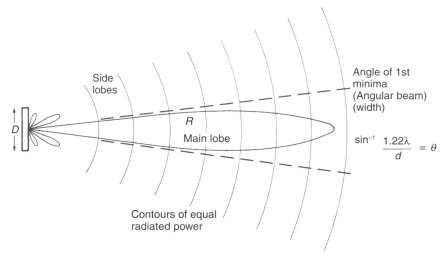

Fig. 13.10 Polar plot of radiated power vector *R* at angle d from a circular transducer of diameter *D*.

Focusing

It is possible to shape the transducer face, fit an acoustic lens or provide special electronic drive and, thus, generate a concave wave, directed to a point. Diffraction effects still limit the effectiveness of this technique. Nevertheless, in the region of this focal point, the beam is typically one-half to one-third of that from a flat transducer of the same dimensions, improving lateral resolution and raising the echo strength from the desired target (see Fig. 13.10).

Resolution deals with the ability to be able to distinguish two adjacent points from each other. Maximum resolution achieved by most US machines is 0.3 to 1 mm.

Doppler Effect

It is well known that, as a police car or fire engine passes, the note of its siren appears to drop. The same effect occurs if sound is reflected off a moving object. If the object is approaching, each sound wave has a shorter distance to travel than the one preceding it. A succession of such waves is received at a higher frequency than the frequency at which it was transmitted. This frequency shift is known as the Doppler shift. It is defined by a change in frequency of a wave following observation by an observer moving relative to the source of the wave. Therefore, the Doppler shift is the difference between transmitted and received frequencies.

If the reflector moves away from the transducer, the delay will increase, and the frequency will decrease. Mixing the transmitted signal and the echo can produce a new electrical signal at the difference frequency, representing the velocity of the reflector. Doppler systems, therefore, detect movement, rather than distance, and, since the difference frequencies are in the audible range, they may be fed directly to a loudspeaker for simple instruments, in particular, to detect and measure blood flow. Hence, the Doppler shift frequency depends on the angle between the direction of movement of blood and the sound beam, velocity of moving blood and the frequency of the insonating wave.

Three types of Doppler exist: pulse, power and colour.

Other Effects of Ultrasound

US is considered a safe modality, but it may still produce biological effects. Heating is self-explanatory. Micro-steaming is the establishment of minute, local fluid circulations found intracellularly or extracellularly. Finally, cavitation can also occur intracellularly or extracellularly. This process describes the formation, growth and oscillation of micro gas bubbles.

14 Statistics and Evidence-Based Healthcare

LOUISE C. BROWN, EMILY J. GREENLAY AND JENNIFER SUMMERS

Introduction

Many doctors often equate statistics with the numbers and equations seen in research papers, but the term 'statistics' does not mean 'numbers'; indeed, a competent statistical analysis of a paper should include non-numerical issues such as the nature of the sampling methods or the validity of a 'gold standard' diagnostic test. Furthermore, papers may be overflowing with numerical data but contain no statistics at all.

Statistics has been defined as the discipline concerned with:

- Data collection and presentation
- Inference from samples or experiments to the population at large
- Modelling and analysis of complex systems
- Broader issues to do with the application and interpretation of the above techniques in politics, management, the law, philosophy, ethics and the sciences.

One of the problems in getting to grips with statistics is that, in common with many other branches of medicine, it is becoming an increasingly sophisticated science, where standard textbooks appear to serve only those who are already members of its exclusive club. The analysis of large and complex datasets, and the techniques of mathematical modelling and statistical computer programming, are generally best left to the experts. However, the appraisal of many published articles relevant to the practicing obstetrician or gynaecologist can be greatly helped by an understanding of several basic principles, some of which are presented in this chapter.

Some Basic Statistical Principles

SAMPLING AND INFERENCE TO THE POPULATION AT LARGE

The most fundamental issue of statistics is that one is trying to relate data taken from a relatively small 'sample' to a

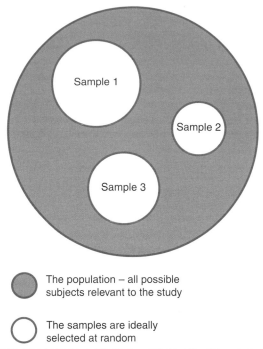

Sample 1

Sample 2

Sample 3

⬤ The population – all possible
   subjects relevant to the study

◯ The samples are ideally
   selected at random

Fig. 14.1 Representation of sample and population.

much larger group where it would be impractical to collect all the available data. In medical statistics, this large and rather nebulous group of subjects is known as 'the population' and it can often be hard to define. This may seem obvious but understanding the concept of sampling is crucial in the interpretation of results from studies. The application of statistics to research is an attempt to ensure that the results from your sample are in general agreement with the results that would have occurred if you had been able to conduct the experiment on all relevant members of the population in question. Fig. 14.1 demonstrates this simple relationship, and it is intuitive to see that, as the sample size increases, it moves closer to representing the population. In general, as the size of the sample increases, the bias in the study decreases; however, this is not always the case, and in some unusual statistical settings the bias will remain, but these are beyond the scope of this chapter (see Peacock and Peacock, 2011).

The most important 'take-home' message for you as an investigator is that, if you repeated your experiment, you would almost certainly get a different result. You may still draw the same conclusions from that result, but the numbers used in the statistical calculations would differ from sample to sample. On average, you would expect the results to be consistent, but when there is disagreement between sample and population, the following types of error (Type 1 and Type 2 errors) can occur and these should always be at the front of your mind when interpreting study results.

TYPE 1 ERROR

This occurs when 'the sample' used in your experiment generates a significant result for your hypothesis but there would not have been a significant result if you had performed the experiment on 'the population'; in other words,

it occurred by chance. When we set a 'significant' P value at .05, we are allowing a 5% chance of a type 1 error occurring for our study. To have zero chance of a type 1 error we would need to perform the experiment on 'the population' itself, and this is not possible as it implies recruiting an infinite number of subjects. The 5% level is entirely arbitrary and purely a convention that seems 'reasonable' in most research situations. Thus, P values should be interpreted cautiously, always bearing in mind the study design and the size of the difference observed between the comparative groups. P values are a continuum that runs from 0 to 1 and thresholds such as .05 are only used as a guide. On occasions, different levels are used, such as 1% (P value of .01) and 10% (P value of .10).

Another consideration when interpreting the results of a study is whether many comparisons have been made using the same sample. This is known as 'multiple testing' and it is a common flaw seen in a number of studies in the published literature (see Peacock and Peacock 2011 for further details on how to address this). By setting your P value for significance at .05, you are allowing a 5% chance of a type 1 error, that is, 1 in 20 statistical comparisons will produce a significant result by chance and thus, if a large number of variables in the dataset are tested for significance, there is a considerable risk of getting a type 1 error. Multiple testing often goes hand in hand with an unclear hypothesis and a poorly thought through study design. If you wish to test many outcomes and exposures using the same sample of patients, you need to account for this by setting yourself a more stringent P value for significance, for example, .01. In this case, you would need to make 100 comparisons in order for one of them to be significant by chance.

TYPE 2 ERROR

This occurs when 'the sample' used in your experiment fails to generate a significant result for your hypothesis but there would have been a significant result if you had performed the experiment on 'the population', that is, you have missed a real and possibly important effect. When we require a study to have 90% power, we are allowing a 10% chance that our sample will not detect a significant result that in truth exists in the population. This commonly occurs in small studies where there is insufficient power. Underpowered studies can be frustrating to interpret, particularly when there appears to be quite a large difference between the groups but the P value does not reach the magical threshold for acceptance as a significant result. Some statisticians argue that no under-powered studies should ever be undertaken as they cannot be interpreted and can raise ethical concerns in terms of unjustified patient research, and this would probably condense the world's research output to a fraction of its current amount. Most research funders now demand power calculations, but sometimes the assumptions on which power calculations are based are grossly optimistic. However, in many cases a balance can still be achieved between attaining sufficient power and setting a pragmatic target for the sample size.

THE NULL AND ACTIVE HYPOTHESES

It is always important to be able to define the null and active hypotheses for a study, and this means having clear definitions for both the outcome and the exposure or treatment. Under the null hypothesis, there is no difference between the groups that are being compared. This will tend to be the 'default' hypothesis unless the study sample accrues sufficient evidence to reject this null hypothesis and show that the active hypothesis is true.

BIAS AND GENERALISABILITY

When studies have been sampled in a non-random fashion, differences between the results from the sample and the true population can arise. Similarly, if treatments are allocated to patients non-randomly, estimates for differences between treatment groups can be biased. In other words, bias can arise if the sample is systematically unrepresentative of the population. However, bias and generalisability are not always the same thing. If one runs a well-powered randomised controlled trial (RCT), the results comparing randomised groups that are estimated from the sample are unlikely to be biased; however, they will only be generalisable to the subgroup of the population that met the inclusion criteria for the study. Thus, when interpreting the results from studies it is important to view them in relation to the study inclusion and exclusion criteria and the sampling methods that were employed when recruiting the subjects. There are many different types of bias and certain study designs are more prone to particular types of bias than others. This will be discussed in more depth in the section about types of study and experimental design (pp 10).

CONFIDENCE INTERVALS, ACCURACY AND PRECISION

When interpreting a result from a sample, it is useful to express the result with a range of possible values that it might have taken if other samples of the same size had been selected. This range of values is called a confidence interval (CI), and we can set the level of confidence as a percentage; 95% confidence is typically used. For example, if we measure the birth weight of 50 babies and calculate a point estimate for the mean weight of 3360 g and a 95% CI of 3200 to 3520 g, this means that we can be 95% confident that, given this sample size, the true mean birth weight for all babies in the population relevant to this study lies somewhere between 3200 and 3520 g. In general, as the sample size increases, the CI becomes narrower. The term precision is used to describe how wide the CI is around the point estimate, whereas accuracy gives an indication of how close the point estimate from the sample is to the true unmeasurable population value and is therefore more related to bias or generalisability. The calculation of CIs will be discussed in more detail on p. 7.

PRIMARY AND SECONDARY OUTCOMES

When designing a study, there will often be many research outcomes listed. In general, one or a few of these outcomes will be identified as the primary outcome(s). The primary outcome(s) is used to calculate the sample size for the overall study. A well-presented study will provide the P value along with the CI of the primary outcome(s) being measured, while the estimates of the secondary outcomes should be reported with CIs.

INDEPENDENCE AND MATCHED DATA

Many statistical tests make assumptions about the independence of the subjects analysed in the study. If data are not independent (e.g. the same mother can be included more than once in a study on childbirth) then account should be taken of this in the analysis. Many commonly used statistical tests assume that all observations are from separate individuals and, by including subjects more than once, you are making your sample less varied than it would be if subjects were only entered once. Similarly, if your study design selected cases and controls by matching them in terms of covariates such as age and ethnic group, then your analysis *must* account for this matching. In general, it is preferable not to match any subjects within a study as it is possible to adjust for potential differences between your groups at the analysis stage. Furthermore, in studies where subjects have been assessed before and after experiencing an exposure, they should be investigated in a 'paired' fashion by analysing the difference between the before and after measurements, as this accounts for the lack of independence between them. This also tends to improve the power of the study as within-patient differences tend to be less variable than absolute variation between patients.

Data Types, Distribution Assumptions and Parametric Tests

There are many different ways in which we can collate data on a subject of interest but, in general, data can be classified into the following types:

Quantitative or continuous – a continual spectrum of data measurements, for example, age, blood pressure, height or weight.

Ordinal – subjects are categorised into groups where there is some order to the categories, for example, mild, moderate or severe symptoms.

Categorical – subjects are categorised into groups but there is not necessarily any particular order to the categories, for example, ethnicity or country of birth.

Binary – this is a sub-group of ordinal and categorical data where there are just two possible categories, for example, pregnant or not pregnant, dead or alive.

Time-dependent data – where subjects have been followed up for different lengths of time, typically in cohort studies and RCTs when subjects have been recruited over an extended period of time. For example, the classification of a subject as pregnant or not pregnant may depend upon the length of their follow-up.

When analysing these data types, it is often necessary to make assumptions about how the data within our sample are likely to behave in relation to the population from which they came. In order to do this, it is helpful to assume a probability distribution which can be described by a mathematical equation, and this can then be used as a template to describe the sample data and make comparisons within it. There are many types of mathematical distribution used in statistics, but four of the most common ones are the binomial, Poisson, normal and chi-squared (χ^2) distributions:

The binomial distribution describes the probability distribution for binary data, and it relates to the common example of tossing a coin. For large sample sizes, the binomial distribution is very similar to the normal distribution and so the latter is often assumed in the statistical calculations.

The Poisson distribution can be assumed when investigating rates derived from time-to-event data, and it represents the idea that a certain event is occurring at a constant rate and thus, as we follow people through time, more events will occur. However, it should be noted that there are also more complex assumptions that are required when analysing time-to-event data, for example, Cox proportional hazards regression analysis is often used (see Peacock and Peacock, 2011).

The normal or Gaussian distribution is assumed when investigating measurements from continuous data, but it is also used as the basis for many aspects of medical statistics. More detail is provided for this distribution a little further on, as it is so important in understanding the application of statistics.

The chi-squared (χ^2) distribution is derived by squaring the normal distribution, and it has particular properties that make it useful for investigating proportions from categorical, ordinal or binary data.

THE NORMAL DISTRIBUTION

The normal distribution is one of the most important and widely used probability distributions in medical statistics. It can be described by a rather complex mathematical equation; however, if it is plotted in terms of probability, we can see that it generates the famous 'bell-shaped' curve shown in Fig. 14.2. The x-axis is standardised such that the mean corresponds to zero (the most probable value) with units of standard deviation (SD) falling above and below this value. It can be seen that 95% of the area under the curve lies between the points that fall 1.96 SDs on either side of the mean value, and this number is particularly important as we can use it to give

us an indicator of the range of values that would incorporate 95% of all possible values. In some cases, you may wish to know the range of values that incorporate 90% or even 99% of all values, and these ranges correspond to the 1.65 and 2.58 SDs on either side of the mean, respectively.

The beauty of the normal distribution is that this symmetrical property around the mean value holds whether we are plotting the actual data points from our sample or whether we are plotting the results of the study if we had repeated it over and over again. In this scenario, we would end up with the 'mean of the mean of the samples', and the range of mean values can be represented by the sampling distribution. The term standard error is essentially the SD of this sampling distribution and it is used throughout statistics to calculate CIs around point estimates. An example of how to calculate a CI for the mean is given on p. 7.

PARAMETRIC AND NON-PARAMETRIC TESTS

Parametric statistical tests are ones where assumptions are made about which mathematical distribution best represents the sample and the population from which it was taken. Non-parametric statistical tests are ones where no assumption has been made about the distribution of the data. See Table 14.1 'A guide to unifactorial statistical methods'. In general, parametric tests tend to be more powerful and sensitive than non-parametric tests and therefore tend to be preferred, as fewer observations are required to provide evidence in favour of the hypothesis if it is true. A typical example of a parametric test is the use of a Student's *t*-test to compare the mean values of a continuous variable between two groups. One of the test assumptions is that the continuous data measured in the sample can be assumed to follow the normal distribution. If this assumption is not valid, then the non-parametric Mann–Whitney *U* test can be used, which ranks the observations in order of size and compares the proportions that fall above and below the median value for each of the groups in question. Thus, the Mann–Whitney *U* test is less sensitive to large outlying values but also less informative as observations above or below the median are all treated in the same way.

Deciding Whether to Use Parametric or Non-Parametric Tests

For binary data, the assumption of a binomial distribution may be valid, as according to Peacock and Peacock, 2011, the normal distribution 'can be used as an approximation to the Binomial distribution when *n* is large. In precise this works if *np* and *n(1−p)* are both greater than 5 (where *np* and *n(1−p)* are number of successes and number of failures)'. When comparing proportions across binary, categorical or ordinal data, the chi-squared distribution is often assumed; however, if the numbers in the categories in a 2 × 2 table become very small (<5 in any one category) then it is often more appropriate to use Fisher's exact test, which is described in any standard statistical textbook.

Probably the most common example of deciding whether to use a parametric or non-parametric test is when you want to know whether the continuous data in your sample can be assumed to follow a normal distribution. In general, for small samples of less than about 15 observations, it is not safe to assume the data are normally distributed, and non-parametric methods should generally be employed.

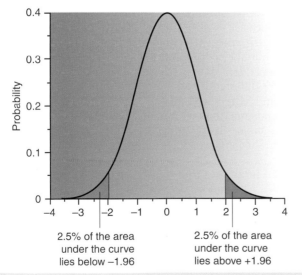

Fig. 14.2 Probability distribution function for the normal distribution. The horizontal axis has been standardised such that zero corresponds to the mean with units of standard deviation above and below the mean.

2.5% of the area under the curve lies below −1.96

2.5% of the area under the curve lies above +1.96

Table 14.1   A Guide to Unifactorial Statistical Methods

Design or Aim of Study	Type of Data/Assumptions	Statistical Method
COMPARE TWO INDEPENDENT SAMPLES		
Compare two means	Continuous, Normal distribution, same variance	t test for two independent means
Compare two proportions	Categorical, two categories, all expected values greater than 5	Chi-squared test
Compare two proportions	Categorical, two categories, some expected values less than 5	Fisher's exact test
Compare distributions	Ordinal	Wilcoxin two-sample signed rank test equivalent to Mann Whitney U test
Compare time to an event (e.g. survival) in two groups	Continuous	Logrank test
COMPARE SEVERAL INDEPENDENT SAMPLES		
Compare several means	Continuous, Normal distribution, same variance	One-way analysis of variance
Compare time to an event (e.g. survival) in several groups	Continuous	Logrank test
COMPARE DIFFERENCES IN A PAIRED SAMPLE		
Test mean difference	Continuous, Normal distribution for differences	t test for two paired (matched) means
Compare two paired proportions	Categorical, two categories (binary)	McNemar's test
Distribution of differences	Ordinal, symmetrical distribution	Wilcoxon matched pairs test
Distribution of differences	Ordinal	Sign test
RELATIONSHIPS BETWEEN TWO VARIABLES		
Test strength of linear relations between two variables	Continuous, at least one has Normal distribution	Pearson's correlation
Test strength of relationship between two variables	Ordinal	Spearman's rank correlation, Kendall's tau (if many ties)
Examine nature of linear relationship between two variables	Continuous, residuals from Normal distribution, constant variance	Simple linear regression
Test association between two categorical variables	Categorical, more than two categories for either or both variables, at least 80% of expected frequencies greater than 5	Chi-squared test
Test for trend in proportions	Categorical, one variable has two categories and the other has several categories which are ordered, sample greater than 30	Chi-squared test for trend

Reproduced from Peacock JL, Peacock PJ 2011 Oxford handbook of medical statistics, Oxford University Press, Oxford.

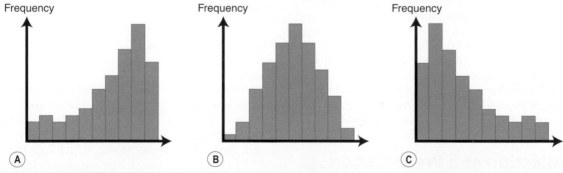

Fig. 14.3 Histograms representing skewness of data. (A) Negatively skewed (median > mean). (B) Normally distributed (median = mean = mode). (C) Positively skewed (median < mean).

However, it should be remembered that these tests are less powerful and the sample size is small, which will make the statistical results hard to interpret. If you have a reasonably large sample size, the first thing to do is to plot your data points on a scatter graph or group the data into bins and plot them on a histogram. Inspection of the graphs or histograms is the simplest way of assessing whether your distribution assumptions are valid. Deviations from the normal distribution can lead to significant skewness or kurtosis. Fig. 14.3 demonstrates histograms for data that follow a normal distribution or have a positively or negatively skewed distribution, and Fig. 14.4 shows how data can deviate from the classic 'bell-shaped' curve seen in the normal distribution and exhibit kurtosis. Kurtosis is concerned with the shape of the distribution and can have a considerable impact on the statistical analysis that you choose to perform on your data. When kurtosis is extreme, non-parametric tests should be used. It is worth noting that for data that are perfectly normally distributed, the mean, median and mode values are all the same, whereas for positively skewed data, the mean tends to be larger than the median and vice versa for negatively skewed data. When summarising skewed data

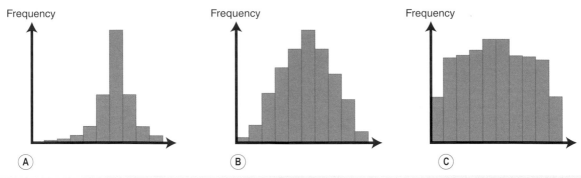

Fig. 14.4 Histograms representing kurtosis of data. (A) Lepto-kurtic (long-tailed). (B) Meso-kurtic (normally distributed). (C) Platy-kurtic (short-tailed).

Table 14.2   Typical Summary Statistics and Presentation Methods for Describing Data

Data Type	Summary Statistics	Presentation
Quantitative or continuous	Mean or average, standard deviation, variance, standard error, confidence intervals, mode, median, range, interquartile range	Scatter plots
		Line plots
		Box and whisker plots
		Histograms
Categorical, ordinal or binary	Mode	Histograms
	Percentage or risk	Pie charts
	Odds	Bar charts
Time-dependent event outcomes	Rate	Life table or
	Hazard (particular example for Cox modelling)	Kaplan–Meier curves

(and also reporting descriptive results from a non-parametric test), it is often better to quote the median and interquartile range rather than the mean and SD, which are generally used for summarising normally distributed data. The way to calculate these summary statistics is described in the next section. In some cases, it helps to convert skewed data into another variable that can be assumed to follow the normal distribution (this is called transformation). For example, data that are positively skewed can often be manipulated into a more normally distributed format by transforming them onto the log scale; the *t*-test can then be used on the log-transformed data. There are more formal ways of testing your assumptions about the normal distribution, such as normal plots and Shapiro–Francia or Shapiro–Wilk tests, but these should be used cautiously and, if there is doubt, you should revert to using non-parametric methods.

Data Collection and Presentation

There are numerous ways in which data can be summarised and presented, and the choice depends on the type of data. The previous section defined the different types of data and the distributions that are often assumed to analyse them. Table 14.2 shows some typical methods for summarising and presenting different data types. All statistical software packages will perform the analysis for summary statistics, but the following simple example shows how the basic ones can be calculated for a set of data.

For example, a study was conducted to investigate various aspects of pregnancy status, previous pregnancy, delivery type, birth weight and survival in a sample of 20 women recruited over 1 year and followed for 5 years.

MEAN

This is the sum of all the observations divided by the number of observations.

For example, mean systolic blood pressure at 20 weeks' gestation $= (105 + 107 + 107 + \cdots + 190 + 199)/20 = 144.35$ mmHg.

Similarly, the mean age $= 32.05$ years.

VARIANCE

This is an indication of the variability of the observations. Each observation is subtracted from the mean, squared, added up and divided by the number of observations, minus 1.

For example, variance of systolic blood pressure at 20 weeks' gestation $= [(105 - 144.35)^2 + (107 - 144.35)^2 + \cdots + (190 - 144.35)^2 + (199 - 144.35)^2]/(20 - 1) = 804.66$ mmHg.

Similarly, the variance of age $= 71.94$ years.

STANDARD DEVIATION

This is also an indication of the variability of the observations as it is the square root of the variance.

For example, SD of systolic blood pressure at 20 weeks' gestation $= \sqrt{804.66} = 28.37$ mmHg.

Similarly, the SD of age $= 8.48$ years.

STANDARD ERROR OF THE MEAN

The standard error is used to indicate how well the sample mean measurement represents the true population mean value. Standard errors are used to calculate CIs (see next section).

For example, standard error of the mean (SEM) systolic blood pressure at 20 weeks' gestation = SD divided by the square root of the number of observations = $28.37/\sqrt{20}$ = 6.34 mmHg.

Similarly, the standard error for the mean age is 1.90 years.

CONFIDENCE INTERVAL FOR THE MEAN

Earlier in the chapter, the characteristics of the normal distribution were discussed, and these properties are central to the construction of CIs. The most common CI is set at 95%, as this corresponds to a P value of .05. Once the standard error has been calculated, the 95% CI for the mean blood pressure can be constructed using the 1.96 multiplier described on page 4. Thus, the point estimate with the 95% CI for the mean blood pressure is $144.35 \pm (1.96 \times 6.34)$ = 131.9 to 156.8 mmHg.

Similarly, the 95% CI around the mean age is 28.3 to 35.8 years.

If you wish to be more stringent with your data, you can set your P value threshold for statistical significance at .01, rather than .05, as this corresponds to a 99% CI. In this case, the 1.96 number increases to 2.58. Alternatively, a less stringent threshold would be a P value of .1 where the 1.96 value is decreased to 1.65 to generate a 90% CI.

MODE

This is the most common value in the dataset. It is typically used with categorical and ordinal data but can also be used for continuous data. The mode can become a more complicated parameter when the distribution of data has more than one most common value, for example, bi-modal, but this will not be discussed further here.

For example, the mode for ethnic group is white and the mode for delivery type is home delivery.

MEDIAN

The median is the midpoint of all the observations, indicating that 50% of the observations lie above and 50% lie below the median. Sometimes it is more appropriate to quote the median rather than the mean as it is less sensitive to large outlying values. Similarly, when data are skewed, it is generally better to quote the median rather than the mean.

For example, the median for blood pressure at 20 weeks' gestation is midway between the 10th and 11th observation when arranged in rank order, that is, 146 mmHg.

Similarly, the median age is 32 years.

RANGE

This is the total range of values between the largest and the smallest observation. It indicates how widely varied the data are and is often quoted with the median.

For example, the range for blood pressure at 20 weeks' gestation is 105 to 199 mmHg.

Similarly, the range for age is 20 to 49 years.

INTERQUARTILE RANGE

This is similar to the median, although the lower value indicates that 25% of the observations lie below it and the upper value indicates that 25% of the observations lie above it. Thus, it represents the central 50% range of values and is usually quoted with the median and often used to summarise skewed data.

For example, the The interquartile range for blood pressure at 20 weeks' gestation is 118.5 to 163.5 mmHg.

Similarly, the interquartile range for age is 24.5 to 37 years.

PROPORTION AND RISK

Table 14.3 is a 2 × 2 table that shows the results of delivery type by previous full-term pregnancy. The percentages can be used to represent the proportion of previous full-term pregnancies within hospital or home birth deliveries, that is, 3 of 7 hospital deliveries occurred in women who had a previous full-term pregnancy (42.9%) compared with 5 of 13 home deliveries (38.5%). Risks and percentages cannot be used for time-dependent data unless subjects have all been followed for the same length of time.

ODDS

The odds are calculated as the ratio of the number of subjects classified in one category (usually an exposure, e.g. smoking while pregnant) to the number of subjects classified in another category (usually a disease status or case, e.g. miscarriage). Again, using Table 14.3, the odds of previous full-term pregnancy within delivery types are 3 of 4 = 0.75 for hospital delivery and 5 of 8 = 0.63 for home delivery. Odds should not be used for time-dependent data unless all subjects have been followed for the same length of time. The reasons for using odds rather than risk are to do with mathematical restrictions which make it more appropriate in certain analysis situations.

RATE

In many situations, subjects are followed for a certain period of time to see if a certain event occurs, for example, death, surgical intervention, subsequent pregnancy, etc. If these events occur at a steady rate over time, the number of events that occurred divided by the amount of time subjects have been followed will generate a rate of events. As such, rates are ratios between two related quantities and are usually expressed as 'per' unit of the denominator. A common type of rate would be per unit time, such as heart

TABLE 14.3 Results of Hospital/Home Delivery and Previous Full-Term Pregnancy

	Previous Full-Term Pregnancy	No Full-Term Pregnancy	Total
Hospital	3	4	7
Home	5	8	13
Total	8	12	20

rate, which is expressed as 'beats per minute'. Another type is birth rate, which is often used to compare population growth. For example, it is conventional to report number of live births per 1000 in a year. For a given population, this might be 10.6. This can be interpreted as meaning that, if you follow 1000 subjects for 1 year, 10.6 births will occur, but this is a very crude summary as it assumes that births occur at a constant rate across years, and this may not be the case. Calculation of crude rates in this way makes many assumptions about the frequency of the events over time, and alternative methods are often used, such as Kaplan–Meier curves for presentation and Cox modelling for generating hazard ratios, as a measure of outcome between groups. It is also worth noting that rates should always be used when subjects have been followed for different lengths of time, otherwise risks can be overestimated.

Measures of Outcome, Exposure and Effect

When investigating the relationships between cause and treatment of diseases, it is useful to talk in terms of the exposures (the factors that are thought to relate to the presence or progression of the disease or the treatment that is thought to cure or slow the development of the disease) and the outcome (the variable that describes whether the disease is present or how severe the disease is in terms of some defined symptom or event). At this point, it is worth formally defining the difference between the prevalence and incidence of a disease, as these are commonly used as outcome measures in epidemiology.

PREVALENCE

This refers to the number of individuals with the disease at one point in time as a proportion of the total number of individuals in the population of interest at the same point in time. Thus, the prevalence represents a 'snap-shot' of the proportion of people with the outcome of interest at a given point in time and is therefore dimensionless in terms of time. It therefore relates to the risk of the outcome.

INCIDENCE

This is defined as the number of new cases of a disease that develop in a group of individuals who are at risk during a specified period of time. Thus, as time passes the cumulative incidence of disease will increase, and this is dependent on the length of the study and relates to the rate of disease.

Earlier in this chapter, risk, odds and rates were defined, and these are commonly used as measures of outcome. Ratios and differences for these outcomes can be used as measures of effect between exposed and unexposed groups. These measures of effect should always be quoted with their CIs, and all statistical software packages will calculate these for you, but the methodology describing how to do this is too detailed to provide here. However, interpretation of these types of outcomes can be illustrated using the data such as in Table 14.4, by investigating the relationships between various exposures and outcomes.

Question – Is There Any Difference in Previous Full-Term Pregnancy Between Delivery Type?

This can be investigated by calculating either the risk or the odds ratio (OR).

Table 14.4 Summary of Dataset to Investigate Various Aspects of Patient Status Following Pregnancy Which Reached at Least 20 Weeks Gestation

Age at Start of Pregnancy (Years)	Hospital or Home Birth (Delivery Type)	Ethnic Group	Systolic Blood Pressure of Patient at 20 Weeks' Gestation (mmHg)	Previous Full-Term Pregnancy	Birth Weight (kg)
22	Hospital	White	105	Yes	3.6
45	Home	Afro-Caribbean	107	No	3.1
34	Hospital	White	107	Yes	3.5
21	Home	White	109	No	3.6
36	Home	White	115	Yes	2.4
24	Home	Asian	122	No	2.2
22	Home	White	132	No	4.0
33	Home	Asian	133	No	2.3
33	Home	White	136	Yes	1.9
42	Hospital	White	144	No	2.5
25	Hospital	Afro-Caribbean	148	Yes	4.6
31	Hospital	White	155	No	3.8
49	Hospital	White	155	No	3.5
29	Home	White	156	Yes	2.4
38	Home	Asian	160	Yes	1.8
20	Home	White	167	No	2.6
43	Home	Afro-Caribbean	167	Yes	2.4
36	Hospital	White	180	No	1.9
27	Home	White	190	No	2.0
31	Home	Afro-Caribbean	199	No	3.9

The risk ratio (RR) for previous full-term pregnancy between delivery type = 38.5%/42.9% = 0.90 [95% CI 0.30 to 2.69].

Thus, the point estimate suggests that women having a home birth are 10% less likely to have had a previous full-term pregnancy than women having a hospital birth, but given the size of our sample, we are 95% confident that the true RR for the population lies somewhere between 0.30 and 2.69. As our 95% CI includes the RR that corresponds to the null hypothesis value of 1.0, we do not have sufficient evidence to reject the null hypothesis and conclude that women having a home birth are significantly more or less likely to have had a previous full-term pregnancy.

The OR for previous full-term pregnancy between delivery type = 0.63/0.75 = 0.83 [95% CI 0.14 to 4.88]. Thus, the odds of having had a previous full-term pregnancy is nearly a fifth less for women having a home birth, but once again the CI includes the null hypothesis value of 1.0 so there is insufficient evidence to suggest a difference.

It is also possible to calculate differences in outcomes rather than ratios, but these tend to be used more in the realms of public health where absolute numbers tend to be more relevant.

Risk difference (attributable risk) for previous full-term pregnancy by delivery type = 38.5% − 42.9% = −4.4% [95% CI −5.0% to 4.1%].

As before, the 95% CI includes the null hypothesis value of zero, and therefore would correspond to *P* values >.05.

CONFOUNDING AND INTERACTION

If one is trying to investigate whether a particular exposure or behaviour is affecting a group of subjects when compared with an unexposed control group, how can one be certain that the difference observed between the groups is attributable to the exposure? If the treated and the control group are different in ways other than the exposure of interest, for example if there are more older mothers in the control group, it is very difficult to tease out how much of the difference between the two groups is due to the exposure and how much is due to the younger age of the exposed group. In this case, age is a confounder, and it is a classic example as there are very few diseases that do not show some association with age. In order to be a confounder, the variable must be associated with *both* the outcome and the exposure of interest. Fig. 14.5 demonstrates two classic examples where confounding is likely and unlikely to be occurring. Intuitively, it is tempting to think that because obesity (body mass index (BMI) > 30) and smoking are both risk factors during pregnancy, one must always adjust for each of these variables when investigating the effects of the other. However, although this is advisable for studies investigating the effects of obesity and smoking on pre-eclampsia, it is not necessarily required when studying the effects of obesity and smoking on gestational diabetes mellitus (GDM). There is evidence to suggest both a protective effect of smoking and a damaging effect of smoking on the incidence of pre-eclampsia, as well as a strong link between obesity and the development of pre-eclampsia. It is also known that smoking and obesity can be related and are both ill-advised for pregnant women; therefore, all three sides of the confounding triangle show significant association. Conversely, in

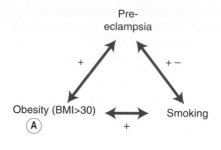

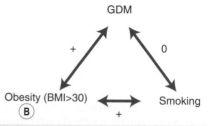

Fig. 14.5 Confounding relationship between obesity and smoking when investigating risk factors for pre-eclampsia and gestational diabetes mellitus. (A) Confounding. (B) No confounding.

studies investigating the effect of obesity on GDM one does not need to adjust for smoking status as there is little or no evidence to suggest that smoking is associated with an increased risk of GDM. Thus, smoking is a confounder in Fig. 14.5A but not a confounder in Fig. 14.5B.

In the real world, there are probably many variables having a confounding effect on our results and many of them will not be obvious to us, which is why RCTs are so valuable. By randomly assigning your subjects to either the treatment or the control group, you are minimising the chance that there are any associations between all the potential confounding variables and the decision to be in the treatment or control group. Thus, one side of the triangular relationship that is required for confounding to occur no longer exists. However, there are often times when randomisation is not possible as people cannot randomly be assigned to develop a disease, and other studies are required to investigate these situations. Thus, in non-randomised comparisons, the tendency for confounding can be high and this often makes interpretation of results very difficult. Adjustment for potential confounders is one way in which the presence of confounding can be assessed. In the pre-eclampsia example in Fig. 14.5, if you find there is a twofold increase in the incidence of pre-eclampsia between obese and not obese mothers but this risk decreases to 1.5 when adjusted for smoking, it might be interpreted that half of the increase in risk of developing pre-eclampsia is attributable to smoking and the other half to obesity; providing all other factors are equal. This example raises another issue that often requires investigation, and this is called interaction.

Interaction occurs when two risk factors do not combine to produce the expected effect in outcome when they are both present in an individual. For example, if being obese and not smoking you have a threefold increase in the risk of developing pre-eclampsia, and by smoking but not being obese, you have a twofold increase in the risk of developing pre-eclampsia, then one might expect individuals who both smoke and are obese to have a sixfold increase in the risk of developing pre-eclampsia compared with individuals who neither smoke nor are obese. If you tested this hypothesis in an experiment and found that there was a 10-fold increase in the risk of pre-eclampsia rather than the expected six fold, then there might be evidence to suggest that obesity and smoking are interacting in some way that exacerbates the risk of pre-eclampsia. Often, investigators are tempted to analyse treatment effects in subgroups, for example, hospital versus home delivery, but this is not advisable as it is an unpowerful and inefficient use of data, and tests for interaction are recommended. There are formal ways of testing for interaction, but these will not be discussed here; the description is merely included as an alert to the reader that these types of issue should be considered when interpreting results from studies.

TYPES OF STUDY AND EXPERIMENTAL DESIGN

Epidemiology is essentially concerned with the investigation of health and illness across and within populations of people, and numerous study design methods have been developed for the analysis of this often complex subject. Fig. 14.6 summarises the most common types of epidemiological study and shows that the main division occurs between experimental and non-experimental studies. Non-experimental studies are principally concerned with the causation and progression of disease, while experimental studies are generally concerned with the treatment or prevention of disease.

There are also other types of study concerned with diagnosis and testing for disease and each study type is a major subject in its own right. The next section will summarise some of the most common study designs and discuss the pros and cons of each in relation to the research topic in question, and in particular discuss some of the issues relating to bias. There are many different types of bias but some of the most common types are discussed below, and the impact that they can have on the different study types is given in Table 14.5. It is also worth stressing that, for all studies, a *consecutive series* should be obtained whenever possible, and if exclusions occur, they should be documented with reasons for exclusion so that the generalisability of the results can be considered.

TYPES OF BIAS

Collectively, most types of bias seen in epidemiological studies can be embraced by the term *measurement bias*, as they relate to the incorrect classification of a patient or the inaccurate measurement of some parameter such as blood pressure. Two common types to consider when designing and interpreting studies are selection bias and responder/observer bias.

Selection Bias

When a sample has not been selected at random from the population, selection bias can occur. For example, if you choose to investigate factors associated with blood pressure

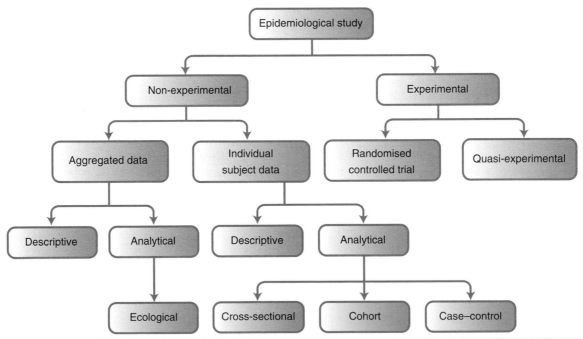

Fig. 14.6 The common types of epidemiological study.

Table 14.5 Impact of Study Design on Bias and Confounding

Probability of:	Ecological	Cross-Sectional	Cohort	Case–Control	Randomised Trial
Selection bias	N/A	Medium	Low	High	Low
Responder or observer bias	N/A	Medium	Low	High	Low (in blinded trials)
Recall bias	N/A	High	Low	High	Low
Confounding	High	Medium	Low (with adjustment)	Medium	Very low
Loss to follow-up	N/A	N/A	High	Low	Medium

and you select your subjects from hospital clinics rather than the general public, selection bias may occur in two separate ways. First, blood pressure may be higher for people in hospital clinics than when they are outside of the hospital and, second, patients tend to be in hospital because they are ill, and you do not know whether their condition relates to blood pressure or interacts with any of the factors that you are investigating. Similarly, if you are using hospital records retrospectively to investigate survival following a particular operation, you should bear in mind that hospital records for patients who have died are often archived differently from those of patients who are alive, and thus the availability of patients' notes is not random, as it relates to the outcome of interest and considerable bias may creep into your study.

When investigating the impact of treatment on disease, RCTs are the best way of reducing the effects of selection bias, particularly in trials where subjects and clinicians are blinded to the allocated treatment. The main benefit of randomisation is 'concealment', which means that when the decision is made to enter a subject into a trial, nobody knows what the treatment allocation will be. Thus, quasi-randomised trials, where the treatment is decided according to some freely available factor, like month of birth or alternate allocation to treatment or control, are not adequate at reducing levels of selection bias as a clinician may chose not to enter a subject into the trial because he knows what the allocation will be.

Responder or Observer Bias

Observer bias occurs when the investigator is aware of the disease status, treatment group or outcome of the subject, and their ability to interview the subject, collect or analyse the data in an unbiased manner is compromised. Similarly, the subject (responder) may respond differently to questions relating to their levels of exposure if they have been classified as a subject with or without the disease under investigation. A classic example of the latter is also known as *recall bias*, and it can be very problematic in cross-sectional and case-control studies, particularly when using self-report outcomes. For example, pregnant mothers may be untruthful about their alcohol intake or smoking status due to social desirability or perceived stigma; or they may find it difficult to remember specific amounts, such as how many years they have had a pre-existing condition for, or when they last went to their doctor.

TYPES OF STUDY

Ecological Studies

These tend to be hypothesis-generating studies rather than providing any strong causal evidence. They are concerned with observations made on large groups of the population (e.g. one might postulate that the increase in the incidence of multiple births over the last 20 years is due to women choosing to have children later on in life). However, this is entirely speculative and would require a far more detailed study to investigate such a hypothesis. Thus, the tendency for confounding is extremely high in ecological studies, as countless other factors may be responsible and, unless data are collected on these as part of a fuller investigation, reliable conclusions cannot be drawn. Nevertheless, these types of studies can act as important pointers towards areas of public health that might be worthy of further investigation.

Cross-Sectional Studies

Cross-sectional studies are often chosen because they tend to be fairly easy to perform and are thus relatively inexpensive. Data are collected from a sample of subjects at a given point in time and comparisons are made between the variables to investigate the extent of the disease of interest or to assess which exposures may be linked with the disease. Thus, these studies represent a 'snap-shot' in time, and therefore the prevalence is generally the main outcome measure, as no information is obtained on the incidence of the disease over time. Surveys are a typical example of a cross-sectional study, and the main problem is that they do not provide good information on the chronology of events, as data for both exposure and disease are being measured simultaneously. Thus, it is difficult to assess any temporal relationship between the exposure and the disease, as the former should always precede the latter for there to be any evidence of a causal link between the two. Selection bias can also be problematic as people who chose not to complete survey questionnaires can often be the people with the greatest extent of exposure or disease, and they end up being excluded from any analysis. Responder bias can also occur as many surveys ask the subjects to give details on various aspects of their life, and people are not always accurate when estimating these types of data (e.g. most smokers tend to underestimate the amount that they smoke). In particular, if you ask people to give details on their retrospective history of smoking when they are aware that the study is investigating the effects of smoking, considerable recall bias may creep into the results, and this should be considered when designing the study and inspecting the results.

Cohort Studies

Subjects are recruited into a cohort study and followed over time to assess the incidence of a particular disease or the progression of a disease if they have already been diagnosed. A full baseline assessment of data is collected on potential risk factors and other exposures and then follow-up commences to monitor the progress of the subjects. Thus, these studies are far more informative than cross-sectional studies as they provide information on incidence of events and allow temporal assessments to be made on whether the exposures preceded the outcomes of interest. They are particularly useful for investigating the effects of relatively rare exposures, as the classification of being exposed or not occurs at baseline, and they can also be used to investigate a wide range of disease outcomes potentially linked with the exposure of interest. Conversely, cohort studies are not very good at investigating rare diseases as many people will need to be recruited in order to accrue enough cases for analysis. Thus, cohorts tend to be used when the disease is common and the effects of various exposures are not very well understood, and they are particularly beneficial because data can be collected on many potential confounding variables and these can be used for adjustment in the final analyses at the end of the follow-up period. The main disadvantage is that cohorts are costly in both time and resources and usually require large sample sizes to attain sufficient power for the analyses of interest. There can also be considerable loss to follow-up as it is often hard to keep people involved with the study for many years.

Case–Control Studies

As discussed in the previous section, cohort studies are not very useful at investigating rare diseases, so case–control studies are often performed in this situation. The cohort can be seen as a prospective study following subjects forward through time, whereas the case–control study is retrospective in that it recruits cases (subjects with the disease) and then finds a concurrent group of controls (subjects without the disease) and looks back through time to compare their exposures to see if any appear to relate to the development of the disease. Case–control studies tend to be relatively quick and cheap to perform and can be used to investigate a number of different exposures simultaneously. The difficulties often lie in the selection of the control group, and this is generally harder than it may first appear; hence, case–control studies can often experience considerable selection bias problems. They are also particularly prone to recall bias as subjects are being asked about past exposures with the knowledge that they are a case or a control and this may influence their ability to remember the extent of their exposure. This is also the case for the investigator, and considerable observer bias can occur. Case-control studies also differ from cohorts in that they are not good at investigating rare exposures, as a large number of subjects need to be recruited to attain enough evidence of the exposure. They cannot be used to make estimates for the incidence of a disease and are not very helpful in trying to investigate the sequence of events leading to the diagnosis of a disease. Confounding can also be problematic in case–control studies and, in some cases, investigators choose to match cases and controls for variables that are thought to be potential confounders, such as age and ethnicity. This should be done very cautiously as it is possible to 'over-match' the two groups such that variables of importance are 'matched' out of the analysis and valuable results can be missed. Most importantly, if cases and controls are matched in any way, it is extremely important that the statistical analysis of the data accounts for this matching because the study has forced the cases and controls to be more similar than they would be in the population and, thus, the precision of the estimates will be incorrect. A simpler method is not to match the cases and controls, but to collect data on potential confounders and adjust for any differences at the analysis stage.

Randomised Controlled Trials

These are used to investigate the effects of therapies and interventions in a particular treatment situation. Subjects with a particular condition who meet certain trial entry criteria are randomly allocated to either receive the treatment of interest or some form of control (generally no treatment, a placebo or the current 'gold standard' treatment). The randomisation is usually performed by a computer program and should be based separately from the participating centres, usually with an online/email service to request the randomisation procedure. Where

possible, it is preferable for the subjects and the investigators to be blinded to their randomised allocation and for the control group to be provided with some form of placebo. The groups are then exposed to their allocation and the outcome of interest is measured to see if one group experiences any benefit over the other. There are various types of randomised study – for example, cross-over trials, factorial design or cluster randomised trials – and they do not have to be limited to just two comparative groups. The main benefits of randomised trials are the concealment of the treatment allocation and thus minimisation of selection bias, as well as the low chance of confounding (providing the study is of adequate size and power). However, the disadvantages to RCTs are similar to those seen for cohort studies in that they tend to be time consuming and expensive, and there can be appreciable loss to follow-up if the infrastructure is not in place to ensure good data collection.

The Intention-to-Treat Principle

Once you have gone to all the effort of conducting an RCT, it is very important that primary analysis keeps the subjects in their randomised group regardless of the treatment that they actually received. By not doing this, you will negate most of the benefits of having randomised your subjects and run the risk of selection bias and confounding occurring. It is very rare that 100% of subjects will comply fully with their randomised allocation, and investigators often feel justified in performing a 'per protocol' or 'treatment received' analysis, which excludes subjects who did not receive their intended treatment or who crossed over to the other randomised group. This is generally not advisable and, in the cases where it may be justified, it should be performed with caution and as a secondary analysis to the primary intention-to-treat analysis. The decision to do this additional analysis should also be made in an *a priori* fashion before any of the data are seen.

Diagnostic Testing Studies

It is often important to assess how well a particular diagnostic test detects people with a particular condition. Table 14.6 shows the standard terms used for describing the usefulness of a diagnostic or screening test, which can be derived from a cross-sectional study of the test against a known 'gold standard'. As shown in Table 14.6, a *sensitive* test has a low false-negative rate (i.e. it successfully identifies most or all of the people with the condition), and a *specific* test has a low false-positive rate (i.e. it successfully excludes most or all of those without the condition). Screening tests, such as the Guthrie test for phenylketonuria in neonates, tend to have high sensitivity in order to not miss any cases at the first hurdle; a definitive (and more expensive) *diagnostic* test with high *specificity* can be carried out on all those who test positive on the screening test.

The effectiveness of a particular diagnostic test to confirm or exclude a particular diagnosis is known as the *likelihood ratio* of that test; as Table 14.6 shows, it is calculated from the formula *sensitivity/(1 − specificity)*. The likelihood ratio can be thought of as an index of the usefulness of a diagnostic test. The higher the likelihood ratio, the more a positive test result should influence decisions.

Table 14.6   Features of a Diagnostic Test Which Can be Calculated by Comparing It With a 'Gold Standard' in a Validation Study

		Disease Status (Result Of 'Gold Standard' Test)		
		Disease – Positive	Disease – Negative	Total
Test Results	Test – Positive	A (True Positive)	B (False Positive)	A + B
	Test – Negative	C (False Negative)	D (True Negative)	C + D
	Total	A + C	B + D	N

Sensitivity = A / (A + C) (proportion of true positives)
Specificity = D / (B + D) (proportion of true negatives)
Positive Predictive Value (PPV) = A / (A + B) (probability that following a positive test result the individual truly has the specific disease)
Negative Predictive Value (NPV) = D / (C + D) (probability that following a negative test result the individual truly does not have the specific disease)
Likelihood ratio of positive test = Sensitivity / (1 - Specificity)

A likelihood ratio of 1.0 means that the patient is no more or less likely to have the condition than before the test was performed.

Studies in the United States suggest that any woman of childbearing age attending the emergency department has a 6% chance of being pregnant, and that those who think they are pregnant have a 40% to 60% chance of being right. Helpful questions to 'rule in' pregnancy include morning sickness (likelihood ratio: 2.7), breast engorgement (likelihood ratio: 2.7) and uterine size on vaginal examination (likelihood ratio: 3.7). A story of delayed menstrual period is fairly unhelpful (likelihood ratio: 1.56) compared with uterine artery pulsation (likelihood ratio: 11).

These numerical estimates confirm the value of vaginal examination by a competent gynaecologist in the diagnosis of early pregnancy. The world would be a simpler place if all clinical and laboratory tests were safe, readily reproducible by junior staff, and had high likelihood ratios. Unfortunately, clinical signs are often equivocal, definitive investigations impractical or contraindicated, and results of next-best tests incomplete or inconclusive. This is the 'grey area' seen frequently in primary care and the casualty department.

Equations for Basic Power Calculations

For Continuous Outcomes

$$n \text{ per group} = 2 \times (Z_{\text{alpha}/2} + Z_{\text{beta}})^2 \times \sigma^2/\delta^2$$

where σ = SD (standard deviation) and δ = d (clinically meaningful difference).

This formula consists of four parts. For a continuous variable, δ is the clinically meaningful difference in mean value (e.g. blood pressure). σ is the estimate of variability; specifically, it is the SD of the blood pressure.

The other two elements, $Z_{\text{alpha}/2}$ and Z_{beta}, refer to the type I and type II error rates. The letter Z that precedes alpha and beta in the formula refers to numbers derived from the normal distribution. It is usual practice to require a power of 80% or 90%, and a significance level of 5%. Thus, alpha = 5% and this gives $Z_{\text{alpha}/2} = 1.96$. If beta = 10% (for a power of 90%), then $Z_{\text{beta}} = 1.28$. These values may be taken as constants in the formula.

Suppose the object of appraisal was a study involving a treatment for hypertension during pregnancy which might reasonably be expected to make a difference of 5 mmHg of diastolic blood pressure (DBP) compared with a placebo. This could be taken as the clinically meaningful difference to be detected (δ). In the population of interest, the SD of DBP might be 10 mmHg – this will be the σ. The aim is to show this difference as statistically significant at the 5% level with 90% power. Thus:

$$n \text{ per group} = 2 \times (1.96 + 1.28)^2 \times 10^2/5^2 = 84.$$

The total sample size required is 168 (84+84); therefore, if it was noted that the authors of the study had included only 20 patients per group, we would know that the study was underpowered.

For Categorical Outcomes

The above formula needs to be modified a little if the outcome of interest is an event. The percentage of subjects who would experience the event in the control group (π_1) must first be estimated, as well as the percentage for the group receiving the new treatment (π_2). The δ would now represent the difference in these two percentages, = $\pi_1 - \pi_2$.

However, the notion of an SD is less intuitive for a variable representing an event. In fact, instead of σ^2, it is $[\pi_1 \times (1 - \pi_1)] + \pi_2 \times (1 - \pi_2)]$.

Thus, the whole formula for a power calculation when the outcome is an event becomes:

$$n \text{ per group} = (Z_{\text{alpha}/2} + Z_{\text{beta}})^2 \times$$

$$[\pi_1 \times (1 - \pi_1) + \pi_2 \times (1 - \pi_2)]/\delta^2$$

By using the blood pressure example again, if you expected 50% of the treated group to have their DBP reduced by 5 mmHg, but only 30% of the control group to experience this drop, the equation indicates that 121 subjects would be required per group (242 in total).

$$\boldsymbol{n \text{ per group}} = (1.96 + 1.28)^2$$
$$\times [0.5(1 - 0.5) + 0.3(1 - 0.3)]$$
$$/(0.5 - 0.3)^2 = 121$$

It is worth noting here that choosing a dichotomised continuous outcome at design stage generally requires a larger sample than using a mean. If you are planning a research study yourself, make a point of consulting this text or, preferably, a statistician before deciding how many subjects to recruit. It is also recommended to apply inflation factors to your target recruitment to allow for patients 'crossing over' between groups and for loss to follow-up.

Acknowledgement

The sections on diagnostic testing and power calculations were provided previously by Trisha Greenhalgh.

Recommended Statistics Texts

Altman DG 1990 Practical statistics for medical research. Chapman & Hall, London.

Bland M 2000. An introduction to medical statistics, 3rd edn. Oxford University Press, Oxford.

Greenhalgh T 2006 How to read a paper: The basics of evidence-based medicine, 3rd edn. Wiley–Blackwell, Chichester.

Kirkwood B Sterne J 2003 Essential medical statistics, 2nd edn. Wiley–Blackwell, Chichester.

Peacock JL, Peacock PJ 2011 Oxford handbook of medical statistics, 1st edn. Oxford University Press, Oxford.

Peacock JL, Kerry SM, Balise RR, 2017. Presenting medical statistics from proposal to publication, 2nd edn. Oxford University Press, Oxford.

15 *Clinical Research Methodology*

ANDREW SHENNAN AND ANNETTE BRILEY

Introduction

Research is an organised, systematic and rigorous process of enquiry to develop concepts and theories and describe phenomena. It aims to add to a scientific body of knowledge. A fundamental understanding of how to approach clinical research is now a basic requirement for any specialist. In recent years, regulation around research governance has resulted in many mandatory requirements to set up, monitor and execute research in a clinical arena. This chapter will outline the approach required to manage any clinical research, but specific details pertinent to the UK and Europe will be included.

Types of Clinical Investigation

Evidence that informs knowledge ranges from personal experience of an individual case through to meta-analysis of several randomised controlled trials. The quality of research is improved by limiting confounding factors and ensuring the study is large enough to answer the research question. However, best evidence regarding management of a rare disease may be a simple case report. The study design will depend on previous evidence, the rarity of the clinical situation being investigated, and the feasibility and resources available to investigate the question.

Studies that have a control population will help eliminate chance findings unrelated to the research question.

TYPES OF STUDY

A case–control study is a retrospective study (collection of data from past events) investigating the relationship between a risk factor and one or more outcomes. People with a pre-defined risk factor or outcome are selected (cases) and compared with people who do not have these factors (controls). A case–control study primarily aims to investigate cause and effect. Generally speaking, prospective studies will reduce bias, as the research question is predefined, and then evaluated.

A cohort study is a prospective, observational study looking at a specific effect of a treatment or risk factor over a period of time.

Systematic research is the process whereby a project is based on an agreed set of rules and processes (protocol) and these are rigorously adhered to. It is against this protocol that the research is evaluated. This will reduce bias, as pre-defined rules are adhered to, and selecting significant findings of interest from numerous variables that could occur by chance is avoided.

Qualitative research is research undertaken in the field (natural settings) and usually analysed by non-statistical methods.

Quantitative research involves measurements and analysis of observations using statistical methods.

Surveys are based on a representative sample of a population being questioned at one time point.

Randomised controlled trials (RCTs) are viewed as the 'gold standard' for evaluating health services effectiveness and interventions in relation to specific conditions. Participants are randomly allocated to two or more groups, and direct comparisons can be made between the groups. The only difference between the groups should be the investigation intervention. Therefore, any differences found between the groups should be attributable only to the intervention, and a causal relationship is far more likely (rather than association).

Cluster randomised trials (CRTs) differ from RCTs in that the unit of randomisation is not the individual participant but something else, for example a ward, a department or a service provider. CRTs are particularly useful when testing differences in a method or approach to patient care or evaluating a new standard of care or other practice-wide, hospital-wide or system-wide change that impacts patient outcomes. Randomising at the cluster level as opposed to individual patients reduces the potential for contamination because all patients within the cluster are highly likely to receive the same treatment or care, and thereby have similar outcomes. Thereby, this is an effective method to test an intervention by some clusters randomised to using it in practice and others not using it at all. The number of clusters will be dependent on cluster size and outcomes, but typically a minimum of eight clusters is required.

Stepped wedge cluster randomised trial is a pragmatic study design increasingly popular for evaluating service delivery type interventions. In a stepped wedge study design, more clusters are exposed to the intervention towards the end of the study than at the start. In the initial study phase, none of the clusters are exposed to the intervention. At regular intervals (steps) one cluster (or group of clusters) is randomised to introduce the intervention, until all clusters are using it; there is then a period when all clusters are exposed to the intervention. Continuous data collection throughout the study period means all clusters contribute to both the control and intervention phases.

WHAT IS AUDIT?

Audit is not research. The differences are outlined in Table 15.1. Clinical audit is a quality improvement process that seeks to improve patient care and outcome. This is achieved through systematic review of care against explicit criteria and the implementation of change. Aspects of the structure, processes and outcomes of care are selected and systematically evaluated against explicit criteria (Fig. 15.1). Where indicated, changes are implemented at an individual, team or service level and further monitoring is used to confirm improvement in healthcare delivery (*definition endorsed by the National Institute for Clinical Excellence*, NICE, 2002). In short, audit is the process used by health professionals to assess, evaluate and improve care of patients in a systematic way in order to enhance their health and quality of life (NICE, 2021).

Audit does not require ethical committee review or approval, nor is it under the same regulatory requirements as research. Most hospital trusts will have a robust infra-structure that deals with clinical audit, including registration of projects, which has become an integral part of clinical practice.

Table 15.1 The Differences Between Audit and Research

Research	Audit
Discovers and defines the 'right' thing to do	Determines whether the right thing is being done
Each project 'stands alone'	A cyclical series of reviews
Collects complex and unique data	Collects routine data
Often possible to generalise findings (aims for this to be possible)	Reports individual situation, therefore never possible to generalise findings

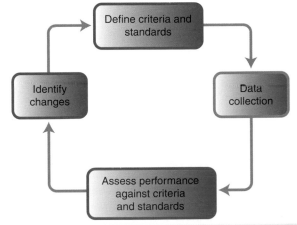

Fig. 15.1 The audit cycle.

The Clinical Research Process

Once a research question is established, a funding source must be identified, an appropriate literature review performed, study design chosen and the protocol written. There are also mandatory requirements to be undertaken before the project can begin. These will depend partly on the study design and the intervention being investigated. Generally, any research involving human subjects (including analysis of data or samples derived from a human source) requires ethical and, in the UK, research and development (R&D) approval.

INTEGRATED RESEARCH APPLICATION SYSTEM

The European Union (EU) Directive says 'Member States shall take the measures necessary for the establishment and operation of Ethics Committees'. The responsibilities of the ethics committee are to safeguard the rights and wellbeing of trial subjects, and to ensure proposals meet the requisite standards. It is unlikely that this EU Directive changes for studies in the UK in light of Brexit.

It is stipulated that there must be at least seven members of an ethics committee, including scientific/expert and lay representatives. Research ethics committees (REC) can be either Main or Local (MREC/LREC), depending on their size and the experience of their members. All clinical trials of a medicinal product and multicentre studies need to be ethically reviewed and approved by a Main REC, following which, Local REC approval is granted for Site Specific Information (SSI). Every study should have a chief investigator (CI) and each site must have a local principal investigator (PI), who has overall local responsibility for the trial or study. The ethics committee assesses the suitability of the local PI and support staff in addition to the appropriateness of the local research environment.

An electronic application form (www.myresearchproject.org.uk) must be used for applications in the UK. This consists of three parts: part A gives general details of the research project, part B involves information on specialised topics, including the use of existing or newly obtained biological specimens and part C is SSI (local assessor). A separate (duplicate) application form can be accessed on the Integrated Research Application System (IRAS) website for R&D approval (see below). Once completed, with the requisite signatures, both forms can be processed through the R&D department for the participating Trust or PCT.

Once logged in, the form can be edited any number of times by the individual with the pass code and can be electronically transferred to collaborators for comments and editing.

When complete, details of how to make your booking for ethical review can be found on the 'e-submission' tab of the form you wish to submit. This provides step-by-step instructions and a direct link to the booking portal. When you book make sure you have your application available as you will need to answer questions to determine which RECs are suitable to review your study. This is dependent on the study type and population, for example some committees focus on patient groups, paediatrics for example. The form can then be locked and submitted online and one paper copy, with requisite signatures accompanied by the study protocol, including patient information and informed consent forms, should be delivered to the ethics committee administrator. The administrator will check all the paperwork is present and then send confirmation of receipt of the application. For single-centre studies, parts A and B of the form need to be completed. If the study is undertaken in more than one institution/hospital, SSI will need to be sought in all additional centres. The letter of receipt gives details as to how to ensure this process happens concurrently with MREC consideration.

RECs meet frequently, and the date when the application will be discussed will be notified to the applicant. Each committee will only review a certain number of proposals at each meeting, and an applicant can choose an appropriate committee, according to their commitments and time schedule. A local committee will not therefore always review research from its own institution. A multicentre study (three or more centres) will require a Main REC. Attendance by applicants is not mandatory, but applicants can be invited to attend to clarify any ambiguous or difficult ethical issues. The REC can ask for alteration or clarification of the application on one occasion – at this point the clock stops, and any delay is entirely the responsibility of the applicant. Apart from this delay, a decision will be given within 60 days.

RESEARCH AND DEVELOPMENT APPROVAL

All projects involving NHS patients, staff or services require approval from the local research and development committee. The form is available online and interconnects with the ethics forms. This needs to be completed at every participating centre, including single-centre sites and academic projects. Most research and development committees expect an early application. Advice is available from your local Research and Development or Research and Development Support Unit (RDSU).

INTERNATIONAL CONFERENCE ON HARMONISATION GUIDELINE ON GOOD CLINICAL PRACTICE

This document sets out an internationally agreed quality standard for designing, conducting, recording and reporting trials involving human participants. This ensures unified standards of research in the EU, but also covers Japan and the United States. Good clinical practice guidelines from Australia, Canada, the Nordic countries and the World Health Organization (WHO) were also considered in the preparation of these guidelines. The principles of the International Conference on Harmonisation Guideline on Good Clinical Practice (ICH GCP) originate from the Declaration of Helsinki (1964) last updated in 2000. Accordance gives assurance to the public that the rights and wellbeing of the subjects is protected, and that trial data are credible. Information can be found at www.ich.org.

THE EUROPEAN UNION CLINICAL TRIALS DIRECTIVE

The EU Clinical Trials Directive (2001/20/EC) is the legislative framework that implements ICH GCP in the EU and also in Iceland, Norway and Liechtenstein, which form the

European Economic Area (EEA). The aims of this Directive are three-fold:

1. To protect the rights, safety and wellbeing of trial participants
2. To establish transparent procedures that will harmonise trial conduct in the EU and ensure the credibility of results
3. To simplify and harmonise administrative provisions governing clinical trials.

The original clinical trials regulations were superseded by the Clinical Trial Regulation (Regulation (EU) No 536/2014). The aim of this Regulation is harmonisation in the assessment and supervision processes for clinical trials throughout the EU, via the Clinical Trials Information System (CTIS). This will provide a centralised EU portal and database for all clinical trials under the jurisdiction of the Regulation. Although the Clinical Trials Regulation was adopted and came into force in 2014, the timing of its application is reliant on confirmation of the full functionality of the CTIS, which will involve an independent audit. This was scheduled for December 2020 but has been postponed due to the global COVID-19 pandemic. Updates are available on the European Medicines Agency website (www.ema.europa.eu).

Key benefits of the updated Regulation are to create a favourable environment to undertake clinical trials, in the EU developing and maintaining high safety standards for participants and transparency of trial information, thereby necessitating consistent rules for conducting clinical trials throughout the EU and publicly available information regarding the authorisation, conduct and results of each clinical trial undertaken in the UK. The key benefits of the Regulation include:

- Harmonised electronic submission and assessment processes for clinical trials conducted in multiple Member States
- Improved collaboration, information-sharing and decision making between and within Member States
- Increased transparency of information on clinical trials
- Highest standards of safety for all participants in EU clinical trials (EMA, 2018).

The UK Government has confirmed it is committed to implementing the EU Clinical Trials Regulation 534/2014 into UK law post-Brexit and this is referred to in the MHRA Five Year Plan 2018–2023 (MHRA, 2021).

INVESTIGATIONAL MEDICINAL PRODUCTS

The regulations cover all clinical research on 'investigational medicinal products (IMPs) for human use' (excluding non-interventional trials, see below). The Regulation (EU) No 536/2014 Article 2(5) defines an IMP as 'a medicinal product which is being tested or used as a reference, including as a placebo, in a clinical trial'. This includes products already with a marketing authorisation but which are used or assembled differently from the authorised form, or to gain further information regarding an authorised form. The regulations are required when the trial is designed to support a medical claim, and when the IMP will influence (treat or prevent) a disease process.

AUXILLARY MEDICINAL PRODUCTS

This is defined as 'a medicinal product used for the needs of a clinical trial as described in the protocol, but not as an investigational medicinal product'. So, an Auxillary Medicinal Product (AMP) would be required when a protocol requires the use of a medicinal product as a challenge agent, a rescue medication or background treatment. Note that AMPs are defined as medicinal products, therefore not all products need to be recorded as such. Additionally, concomitant medications do not fall into this category.

MEDICAL DEVICES

A medical device is not recognised as an IMP, that is, this is when the principal intended action of an intervention in a trial is fulfilled by physical means (device), not pharmacological, immunological or metabolic means (medicinal product). However, medicinal devices may be assisted in their function by a medicinal product (e.g. intrauterine contraceptive (device) with progestogen (medicinal product)), and under these circumstances will require conformity to these regulations.

Although there is no legislative requirement to follow the exact requirements of ICH GCP when an IMP is not investigated (e.g. in a trial of a surgical procedure), it remains good practice to follow the same basic principles, although reporting requirements to the MHRA may not be mandatory (see below).

A practical implementation of the ICH GCP guidelines can be found in Table 15.2.

RESPONSIBILITIES OF AN INVESTIGATOR

The chief investigator (CI) must adhere to the 13 principles of GCP (see Table 15.2). In addition, according to ICH CGP the investigator must, by education, training and experience be qualified to fulfil this role, as evidenced through an up-to-date CV or other documentation. They must facilitate monitoring and auditing of the study by the sponsor and inspection by the regulatory authorities. They must maintain a list of the individuals to whom significant trial-related duties have been delegated, demonstrating appropriate qualifications for their relevant tasks.

The investigator must show that recruitment in the agreed timeframe is realistic. They are responsible for ensuring that there is sufficient time to undertake the project, and there is adequate staffing to execute the study. This includes guaranteeing that all staff employed will be adequately trained to undertake the responsibilities expected of them during the study. They also should examine the reason a subject withdraws from a trial prematurely and communicate all significant matters with the ethics committee. They must ensure compliance with the trial protocol. They should be knowledgeable about all aspects of the investigational project and have responsibility for it. This includes responsibility for randomisation procedures and unblinding policies where necessary, as well as for obtaining informed consent from all trial participants. All trial-related medical decisions are the responsibility of a qualified medical practitioner. Attending clinicians should be aware of a participant's involvement in a trial.

Table 15.2   Practical Implementation of the 13 Principles of International Conference on Harmonisation

1	Clinical trials should be conducted in accordance with the ethical principles that have their origin in the Declaration of Helsinki and are consistent with good clinical practice (GCP) and the applicable regulatory requirements.
2	Before a trial is initiated, foreseeable risks and inconveniences should be weighed against the anticipated benefit for the individual trial participant and society. A trial should be initiated and continued only if the anticipated benefits justify the risks.
3	The rights, safety and wellbeing of the trial participant are of utmost importance and should prevail over the interests of science and society.
4	The available non-clinical and clinical information on an investigational product should be adequate to support the proposed clinical trial.
5	Clinical trials should be scientifically sound and described in a clear detailed protocol.
6	A trial should be conducted in compliance with the protocol that has received prior independent ethics committee approval.
7	The medical care given to, and the medical decisions made on behalf of, the participants should always be the responsibility of a qualified physician.
8	Each individual involved in conducting the trial should be qualified by education, training and experience to perform appropriate tasks.
9	Freely given informed consent should be obtained from each subject prior to participation in any clinical trial.
10	All clinical trial information should be recorded, handled and stored to facilitate accurate reporting, interpretation and verification. 'If it's not documented, it did not happen'.
11	The confidentiality of records that could identify subjects should be protected, respecting the privacy and confidentiality rules in accordance with regulatory requirements (Data Protection Act, 1998).
12	Investigational products should be manufactured, handled and stored in accordance with Good Manufacturing Practice (GMP), and used as per an approved protocol.
13	Systems with procedures that assure the quality of every aspect of the trial should be implemented.

The investigator also has responsibilities regarding records and reports. They have overall responsibility for the accuracy, completeness and timeliness of the data. This includes consistency between data recorded in the case report form (CRF) (study records) and the source documents (medical records). They must be able to explain any discrepancies. Alteration to the CRF should be initialled and dated and should not obscure the original entry. All computer records should be made using programs employing audit trails. Safe storage of the trial records and documentation (including electronically stored data) is necessary during, and after closure of, the trial for the requisite time period (dependent on trial type). This can be up to 25 years for maternity records. The CI is responsible for ongoing mandatory reports during the course and at the end of the trial. This includes progress reports, annually to the medicines and healthcare products regulatory agency (MHRA), funding bodies, etc.; safety reporting of serious unexpected adverse events (SUAES) and suspected unexpected serious adverse events/reactions (SUSARs) (see below); premature suspension of the trial, for example safety reasons; and final reports to the MHRA, M/LREC, sponsor and funding bodies.

WHEN ARE STUDIES NOT COVERED BY THE EUROPEAN UNION DIRECTIVE?

When a medicinal product is used in the manner within the terms of its marketing authorisation, or patient allocation is not dictated by protocol but falls within the remit of current practice, the regulations governed by the EU Directive are not required. This also includes when the decision to prescribe the IMP is independent from the decision to include the patient in the trial. This includes mechanistic trials which are not part of clinical research into the efficacy and/ or safety of an IMP. Psychotherapy and surgery trials with no IMP comparator, and diet trials with no IMP, are also not covered by these laws. This regulation is also not relevant when a patient undergoes diagnostic or monitoring procedures that are part of normal clinical practice, or when data are analysed using epidemiological methods.

THE MEDICINES AND HEALTHCARE PRODUCTS REGULATORY AGENCY

The MHRA is the government agency responsible for ensuring the safety of medicines and medical devices in the UK. It considers no product to be 'risk-free' but applies robust and fact-based judgements to ensure that benefits to patients and the general public justify the risks. The MHRA monitors medicines and devices and ensures, when necessary, that prompt action is taken to protect the public. Within the remit of the MHRA greater access to products and the timely innovation of treatments benefits patients and the public.

The MHRA has produced an algorithm to enable researchers to clarify whether their research question falls within the scope of the EU Clinical Trials Directive. The MHRA will also advise on an individual basis (www.mhra.gov.uk).

All trials falling into the remit of the EU Directive legally require *Clinical Trials Authorisation* (CTA) from the MHRA (Fig. 15.2). If the trial is international, similar approval will be required from any competent authority in each member state. The MHRA must make a decision within 60 days of application. An Investigator Brochure must be kept for all clinical trials, which is a compilation of all the relevant clinical and non-clinical data available regarding the investigational product in human subjects.

Registration of Trials

EudraCT

This has now been superseded by the latest Regulation and the CTIS register.

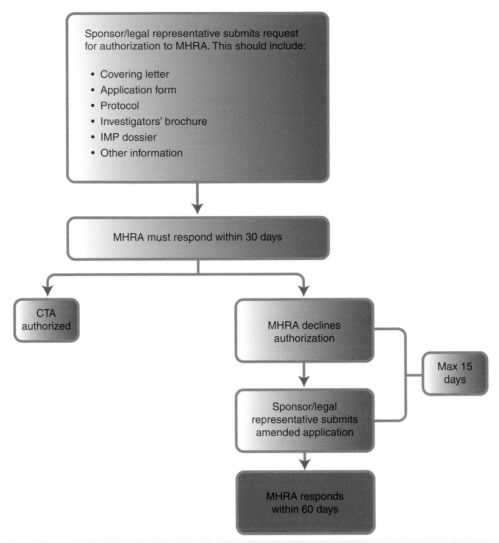

Fig. 15.2 Application process to the Medicines and Healthcare Products Regulatory Agency *(MHRA)* for Clinical Trials Authorisation *(CTA)*.

INTERNATIONAL STANDARD RANDOMISED CONTROLLED TRIAL NUMBER

In June 2005, the International Committee of Medical Journal Editors (De Angelis et al., 2005) issued a statement that, after 1 July 2005, all trials must be registered prior to recruiting the first subject as a prerequisite to publication, thus ensuring a comprehensive, publicly available database of clinical trials. Randomised controlled trials and other studies designed to assess the efficacy of healthcare interventions should all be registered. The International Standard Randomised Controlled Trial Number (ISRCTN) Register is owned by the ISRCTN, a 'not for profit' organisation, and the scheme is administered on their behalf by Current Controlled Trials Ltd.

Application for an ISRCTN is the responsibility of the sponsor or CI and is undertaken online at: www.isrctn.com. The form is divided into five sections:

1. Applicant details – the contact details of the person making the application. This should be the person who will deal with any queries regarding the application.

2. Sponsor details – the organisation taking primary responsibility for ensuring the study design meets the standards of GCP and that measures are in place to ensure appropriate conduct and reporting.
3. Chief investigator (lead principal investigator) – contact details for the individual with legal and scientific responsibility for the trial (also required for multicentre trials) (Fig. 15.3).
4. Details of the trial – from the protocol.
5. Additional information – general information about where you found out about the ISRCTN scheme.

Receipt of the online application will be acknowledged by e-mail, and after the administrators have checked the eligibility of the application, an administrative charge will be made. The 2021 rate is currently GB£226 + tax per entry. This may be reduced or waived for trials in developing countries. There is also a reduced rate for organisations registering more than 100 trials. Once payment is received, the ISRCTN Editorial Office informs the applicant and the CI of the ISRCTN assigned to the trial, and the record will

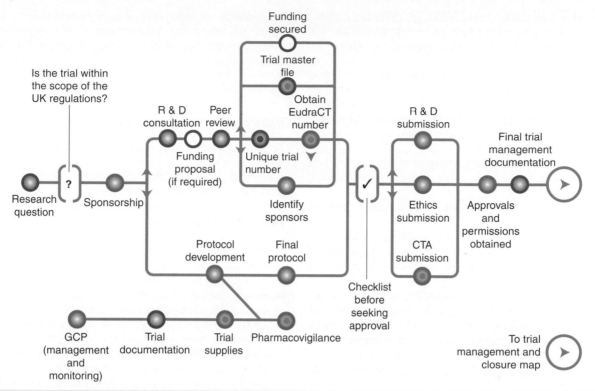

Fig. 15.3 What a researcher needs to set up a multicentre clinical trial. (From Department of Health/MRC, the Clinical Trials Tool Kit 2006.)

appear in the register. This number should then be used on trial documentation.

*meta*REGISTER OF CONTROLLED TRIALS

The metaRegister of Controlled Trials (*m*RCT) was initiated in the UK in July 1998 as a result of an initiative involving the UK Medical Research Council, the National Health Service Executive, medical charities, pharmaceutical companies, the UK Cochrane Centre and journal representatives (i.e. *BMJ* and *Lancet*). This is an international searchable database of current ongoing randomised controlled trials in all areas of healthcare. All trial entries are currently in English, although there is an introduction in French, German, Spanish and Italian, with other languages to be added at a later date.

The *m*RCT has been formed by combining registers held by trial sponsors from the public, charitable and commercial sectors. It is a free service which aims to:

- Facilitate those wanting to be confident they are aware of all trial evidence available relevant to a particular question (clinicians and scientists)
- Assist research funding bodies who want to make funding decisions in the light of information about ongoing relevant research, thus avoiding duplication and facilitating collaboration
- Inform potential participants regarding ongoing trials they may wish to consider.

Although not compulsory, it would be prudent to register any clinical investigation involving an intervention into all three registers.

Data

The UK General Data Protection Regulation (UK GDPR) 2018 sits alongside the Data Protection Act 2018 to form the primary data protection legislation in the UK. Whilst the principles remain the same, and in practice there is little difference in the principles, rights and obligations in EU GDPR, which will apply if you are collaborating with researchers in Europe.

Regulation around GDPR is undertaken by the Information Commissioner's Office (ICO). This relates to data in all sectors and is not research specific. Advice and guidance are available on their website (www.ico.org.uk).

GDPR affords research certain privileges. Recognising that data is useful for research and that research can be a long-term activity, the ICO state data can be stored indefinitely, as long as the data controller can justify indefinite retention. Thus, research data are exempt from the purpose and storage limitations set out in the Act, as long as other data protection principles and specific safeguards are in place.

DATA PROCESSING MUST BE LAWFUL, FAIR AND TRANSPARENT

The greatest changes to the previous Data Protection Act 1988 are around implementing transparency requirements and meeting the safeguards necessary, where these are not already reflected in good clinical practice. In clinical research, these are often already evidenced through university or National Health Service governance systems, for example, ethical and local R&D approvals are in place.

Data processing must adhere to all relevant legal requirements, for example, the common law of confidentiality, and specify the lawful basis for these activities. There are six lawful bases for data processing (set out in Article 6 of the UK GDPR, 2018), and at least one must apply (ICO, 2018).

(a) Consent: the individual has given clear consent for you to process their personal data for a specific purpose.
(b) Contract: the processing is necessary for a contract you have with the individual, or because they have asked you to take specific steps before entering into a contract.
(c) Legal obligation: the processing is necessary for you to comply with the law (not including contractual obligations).
(d) Vital interests: the processing is necessary to protect someone's life.
(e) Public task: the processing is necessary for you to perform a task in the public interest or for your official functions, and the task or function has a clear basis in law.
(f) Legitimate interests: the processing is necessary for your legitimate interests or the legitimate interests of a third party, unless there is a good reason to protect the individual's personal data which overrides those legitimate interests. (This cannot apply if you are a public authority processing data to perform your official tasks.)

More detailed information about each of these can be found on the ICO website (www.ico.org).

It should be remembered that consent as a legal basis for legally processing personal data is *not* the same as consent obtained from individuals to participate in a clinical trial. Consent discussions prior to gaining consent from someone to take part in a clinical trial must include details of all that is entailed, including risk and benefits, and include information about sharing confidential information and data processing. But the definition of consent within GDPR means it is not likely to be the legal basis for processing personal data in a research context.

BEING FAIR AND TRANSPARENT

Respecting participants' rights and ensuring their personal data is used in line with their expectations means that transparency and fairness are intrinsically linked, and ultimately gives participants greater awareness as to how their data is used and therefore increases their autonomy and control.

Transparency information should be concise and easy to understand. Clear statements in patient information sheets and consent forms are required. Transparency is best addressed at organisational and research study levels. Seek advice from your data protection officers regarding your local implemented strategies to address this.

It is important that people notice transparency information, and how this is achieved will be dependent on level and frequency of contact with participants. For example, if you have direct contact with participants, regular updates or newsletters could be used. Where there is no direct contact, posters and fliers in clinical areas or social media announcements might ensure participants are updated.

Where research methodology dictates information is not collected from individuals but other sources there are exemptions to the transparency requirements. In cases where providing this information is 'impossible' or would take a 'disproportionate effort' the minimum GDPR requirements are that the transparency information must be publicly available. If this applies to your research project, discuss with your data protection officer.

WHAT IS 'PERSONAL DATA'?

Personal data comprises information about living people who can be directly or indirectly identified from the data, or combinations of the data, which the person in charge of the data has, or may have in the future.

It is worth noting that: anonymising data is considered processing personal data for the purposes of GDPR.

- *Pseudoanonymised data:* identifiers have been separated, but this may still be personal data, depending on how difficult it is to reconnect the identifiers with the dataset
- *Anonymised data:* no individual can be identified from these data, although it was generated from personal data
- *Linked anonymised data:* these data are anonymous to the researchers (who hold the information) but contain codes or other information that would enable others to identify people from them. For example, study ID on sample (for researcher) links to hospital number and date of birth (for clinicians)
- *Unlinked anonymised data:* there is no information that could identify an individual to anyone. For example, a multiple-choice survey containing no demographic data
- *Coded data:* all information that could identify a participant is concealed in a code, and can be decoded by the researchers
- *Confidential information:* all information obtained on the understanding that it will not be disclosed to others or gathered in circumstances when it is expected that such information will not be disclosed. The law assumes that whenever personal information is imparted to healthcare professionals it is confidential for as long as anyone is identifiable.

Data protection law does not apply to data that has been anonymised in such a way that the data subject cannot be identified at all.

Complete anonymisation of personal data is possible and is useful in servicing society's information needs whilst maintaining privacy.

DATA SECURITY

Ensuring data are maintained securely is a legal obligation under the Data Protection Act. Documented procedures to ensure data security must form part of the Standard Operating Procedures (SOP) of each research project. These procedures require regular review; this is especially relevant with IT systems and data transfers.

Procedures should be in place for:

- Overall management and control of data
- Expedient response and reactions to breaches of security
- Back-up policies and recovery procedures
- Minimising the number of duplicate files in existence

- Limiting access rights, including reacting promptly to staff changes
- Immediate access to chief investigator regarding issues of data security.

Consent, Information and Sponsors

Informed consent is a process by which a trial subject voluntarily confirms his or her willingness to participate after having been informed of all aspects of the trial that are relevant to the subject's decision to take part. It is the investigator's responsibility to ensure the subject (or his or her legal representative) is informed regarding all pertinent aspects of the trial, in language he or she understands. This includes any new information that comes to light during the duration of the study.

PATIENT INFORMATION SHEET

All clinical studies should have a patient information leaflet (PIL). This describes the research in lay-person's terms. Many institutions have explicit information to be included in all their patient information leaflets. The UK Research and Innovation (UKRI) publication, Consent and Participant Information Guidance (UKRI, 2020), provides advice and templates for research projects (www.hra-decisiontools.org.uk/consent/docs/PIS-Template_version2.pdf).

Whilst there is flexibility in the format of a PIL, all should contain:

- The purpose and background of the research and invitation to take part (explanation).
- The nature and purpose of the research.
- What is already known and how your study will add to existing knowledge?
- What interventions are extra to standard care, being clear about what potential participants are being asked to consider agreeing to?
- Is this research educational, for example, part of a higher degree? This is totally reasonable but needs to be outlined clearly in the PIL.
- Is this a therapeutic study? In which case you will need to explain the condition and alternative treatment options
- How many people will be in the study?
- Re-iterate the invitation to participate and explain why this person has been approached.

What does taking part involve?

Potential participants need to know exactly what taking part entails, and what is different from routine care. This could include:

How long their participation in the research will be?
How long the research will take to complete?
Frequency of research visits: How often they will need to see the researcher/attend clinic or general practitioner?
What will happen at each visit, for example, sample collection, questionnaire, interview, etc. (in addition to those required for standard care)?

Will the participants be asked sensitive information? Knowing what would be sensitive demands understanding of your study population but being warned this is going to happen often means participants are better prepared for this.
How will being part of the research study work with their clinical care?
Are there long-term monitoring or follow up plans?
Does the study use audio/video recording or photography? Note specific consent is required if published materials identify participants.
Potential recruits need to know that if they agree to participate you will be collecting data about their health and/or treatment. You must explain.
Types of data you will be collecting.
Who will have access to these?
The name of the Data Controller.
Your plan to optimise use of the data in the future. Data storage, re-use of data after completion of primary project, potential sharing of anonymous data or identifiable information with other researchers. Potential participants should be made aware of the importance of data sharing.

Their rights in relation to their data, and any rights that may be restricted in order to ensure the integrity of the research (in line with data protection legislation).

The Potential Benefits of Participation

It is usually not possible to identify any direct benefits of participation, even though some participants may derive benefit.
Potential participants should be aware that the researcher is unaware of what the outcome will be, that is the reason for the research.
Consultation with service users and community groups may aid identification of indirect benefits of taking part in this research. These could include: empowering individuals to learn more about their condition, being seen more frequently or feeling more supported as a consequence of enrolling in the research.
The most likely benefit will be to others with the same condition in the future, rather than personal benefit for participants

What are the disadvantages of taking part?

The PIL must contain an honest and complete evaluation of the consequences of the research, including significant benefits and harms with likelihood ratios.
Potential participants must be given an honest assessment of the likelihood that something could go wrong, and the level of harm that might ensue.
Risk assessment is subjective based on what is already known about the intervention.
Consultation with service users and lay representatives may help determine what is likely to be considered a significant risk, and how to present this risk to potential participants.
The precise risk of the research is often unknown.
Each study has its own inherent risks determined by the interventions involved, the participant population and the assessment tools and many other things.

You need to ensure potential recruits can distinguish the risks of having a specific condition, the risk associated with routine care and the risks inherent in the research.

Risk of physical harm: explain the likelihood of harm and likely impact, for example:

1 in 10 people are likely to suffer from a minor stomach upset or

1 in 10 people are likely to suffer from severe diarrhoea or

1 in 1000 people are likely to suffer from severe diarrhoea or

1 in 1000 people are likely to suffer from a mild stomach upset.

Risk to confidentiality also needs to be covered.

Psychological risk: some research may pose specific psychological risk; therefore participants should be made aware of this potential and informed of support available to them should this occur.

The PIL can also include information on the following:

- Collaborations between universities (and other organisations) and the National Health Service (NHS), and transfer of information between these institutions
- The funding source for the research
- That the research is independently reviewed
- That research staff have the same duty of confidence as the health professionals caring for them
- That there is no obligation to take part in the research and the volunteer is free to withdraw at any time without giving a reason, and that current or future healthcare will not be affected by this decision
- Who to contact for further information about the project
- Who to contact if they have any cause for complaint.

When writing a patient information sheet, it is advisable to keep language simple; the Literacy Trust recommends equivalence to a reading age of 11 years. Avoid jargon and medical terminology and keep sentences short and concise. By piloting the leaflet on family and friends, many of the pitfalls can be addressed before submission to an ethics committee.

INFORMED CONSENT FORM

An Informed Consent Form (ICF) is a form which records that informed consent was given (by the subject) and must include who explained the study and obtained the consent and when. Most institutions insist all trial participants sign a generic consent form, where only the name of the study and very specific lines are altered. General consent to participation and for the researchers to examine medical notes are mandatory. The consent form must be submitted to ethics committee for approval before use, and at each revision. Informed consent guidelines are available on the IRAS website (www.myresearchproject.org.uk).

SPONSORSHIP

Sponsorship is now a legal requirement in all trials that use NHS resources and are under the EU Directive. The responsibilities of the sponsor are listed in Table 15.3.

Table 15.3 The Sponsor's Responsibilities

Quality assurance and quality control
Contract Research Organization (CRO)
Medical expertise
Trial design
Trial management, data handling and record keeping
Financing
Notification/submission to regulatory authorities
Confirmation of review by institutional review board (IRB)/independent ethics committee (IEC)
Information on investigational product(s)
Manufacturing packaging, labelling and coding of investigational products
Supplying and handling investigational product(s)
Record access
Safety information
Adverse drug reaction reporting
Monitoring
Audit
Non-compliance
Premature termination or suspension of a trial
Clinical trial study reports
Multicentre trials

Trial Steering Committees and Data Monitoring and Ethics Committees

All trials should have a committee to oversee the organisation and running of the study. The committee includes investigators and other individuals with expertise in the area, usually including appropriate lay representation. A separate data monitoring (and ethics committee) will report to the steering group, but final decisions remain with the TSC. The Data Monitoring and Ethics Committee (DMEC) will view safety data, including unblinding when necessary at predefined points, although stopping rules should also be predefined and be appropriately robust.

Review of the Literature

In order to develop the aims and objectives of any research question, the first step is to review the existing literature around the topic. Electronic databases have facilitated comprehensive literature reviews, but hand searching remains valuable, as some articles will not be coded as expected. Grey literature is unpublished non-significant data that tend to remain in internal reports. Therefore it is accessed through 'networking' with experts interested in the area but is an essential part of developing cutting-edge research.

Amendments and Reports

During the course of the trial it may be necessary to make amendments. This may be the result of protocol change, due to new information becoming available (from other trials or scientific discovery) or because an extension to the trial is required.

SUBSTANTIAL AMENDMENTS

A notice of substantial amendment needs to be made when a significant alteration to the initial protocol (or any other supporting documentation) is made. This includes aspects that affect the safety or physical or mental integrity of the subjects, impacts on the scientific value of the trial, influences the conduct or management of the trial or affects the quality or safety of any IMP used in the trial. Substantial amendment should be submitted to the REC that gave the favourable opinion. In clinical trials of investigational medicinal products (CTIMPs) use the 'notification of amendment' form from the EudraCT website (see Useful Sources of Information).

For all other research, use the 'Notice of substantial amendment' form on the IRAS website: www.myresearchproject.org.uk. This form will need to be completed and signed by the CI. It is then necessary to forward this with altered documentation, with changes tracked, to the ethics committee that originally approved the study. Substantial amendments normally require favourable ethical approval before implementation, the only exceptions being:

- Where urgent safety measures are required
- Where substantial amendments require authorisation from the competent authority (MHRA) but are submitted to the main REC for information only.

The MHRA should also be notified of substantial amendments.

Further guidance can be found at www.gov.uk/clinical-triolas-for-medicines-manage-your-authorisation-report-safety-issues.

NON-SUBSTANTIAL AMENDMENTS

Non-substantial amendments do not have to be notified to the MHRA, but should be recorded centrally, with all the relevant information available for inspection purposes.

REPORTING ADVERSE REACTIONS

When reporting any event, adherence to UK GDPR and DPA 2018 is mandatory in all written reports, that is, retaining the participant's anonymity by using unique code numbers. Within the context of any clinical trial there will be some adverse reactions or events. Many of these will be outlined in the study protocol or investigator brochure, that is, are known. These are expected adverse events because they are predefined. All other adverse events are usually unexpected, that is, are not consistent with the information about the medicinal product being investigated or the condition.

When adverse expected events or reactions occur, that is, those that are outlined in the protocol, they need to be listed and reported in the annual safety report to the MHRA, ethics committee and the sponsor. The exception to this is any adverse event that is identified in the protocol as essential in the safety evaluation of the trial, and these will need to be reported to the sponsor, within the timeframe specified in the protocol.

SERIOUS ADVERSE EVENTS AND SERIOUS UNEXPECTED ADVERSE EVENTS

Adverse reactions are 'serious' if they result in death; are life-threatening; require hospitalisation or prolong existing admission; result in persistent or significant incapacity or disability; or result in a congenital anomaly or birth defect. Both serious adverse events (SAEs) and SUAEs must be reported. The timing will depend on whether they are mentioned in the protocol. If not in the protocol, it must be within 7 days (if they are listed in the protocol they must be included in the Annual Report).

Related and unexpected SAEs must be reported to the REC within 15 days of the CI being aware of it, using the IRAS 'Report of a serious adverse event' form, downloaded from the IRAS website (www.myresearchproject.org.uk). These forms need to be completed in typescript and signed by the CI. In double-blinded trials, SAE reports should be unblinded. The REC administrator acknowledges receipt of these reports within 30 days.

SUSARs are defined as an 'adverse reaction' and is 'any untoward and unintended response in a subject to an investigational medicinal product which is related to any dose administered to that subject'. The Medicines for Human Use (Clinical Trials) Regulations 2004 (MHRA, 2004).

For those SUSARs that are life-threatening or result in death, the sponsor needs to be informed within 7 days. There will be an agreement between the CI and the sponsor as to who will inform the MHRA. Using forms supplied by the local R&D office, the MHRA must be notified within 7 days following the sponsor being informed and will require a follow-up report within 8 days. For those SUSARs which are not fatal or life-threatening, the sponsor should be informed as soon as possible, and the MHRA needs to be informed within 15 days of the sponsor knowing.

All adverse events reports and follow-up forms should be sent to the R&D office, and the ethics committee should also be informed. Any reaction should be recorded in the participant's CRF and documented in their medical records.

THE END OF THE TRIAL

The definition of the end of the trial is usually the date the last patient is seen, or reaches the defined endpoint (i.e. date of delivery); this is usually specified in the protocol. The MHRA must be notified within 90 days of the end date, using the 'Declaration of the End of a Clinical Trial'. If the trial ends early, the MHRA must be notified within 15 days, with a clear explanation of the early termination. In addition to the end of trial declaration to the MHRA, a final report must be sent to the ethics committee (use the 'Declaration of the End of a Clinical Trial' form as used for the MHRA), the R&D Department and the funding body.

Promoting and Maintaining a Trial

Regular meetings with investigators and management team are an essential part of a successful trial. Regular, realistic targets should be set. Review recruitment, staff issues and outcome data collection regularly, and deal with problems/potential problems as they arise. Keep others informed of progress of the trial and thank those who help. It is wise to have obvious trial identification, including logos, newsletters and labels to identify participants' notes. Outcome data are as important as recruitment rates – ensure strategies are in place to optimise opportunities to get outcome data.

Common Statistical Terms Used in Clinical Trials

Power

The power of a study is the probability that it will detect a statistically significant difference. Therefore, if the anticipated effect is large, a small study is required, but if the effect is smaller a larger sample size is required.

Incidence

The number of new cases (of a condition) in a given timeframe.

Intention to Treat

This is an analysis that includes all the participants randomised to a group, even if they are subsequently withdrawn and do not receive the allocated intervention.

Likelihood Ratio

This is the likelihood that a test result would be expected in patients with a condition, divided by the likelihood of the same result occurring in patients without that condition.

Sensitivity

This is the number of patients with a condition testing positive for that condition. It describes the effectiveness of a test at picking up a condition.

Specificity

This describes the proportion of people without a condition who test negative – the rate of elimination of a disease by a test.

Positive Predictive Value

When a person tests positive for a condition the positive predictive value (PPV) is the chance that they actually have that condition.

Negative Predictive Value

In the presence of a negative test, this is the chance that the person does not have the condition.

Numbers Needed to Treat

The number of patients who need to be treated, for one to gain benefit.

Numbers Needed to Harm

The number of patients who need to be treated, for one to be harmed by the treatment.

Relative Risk Reduction

The proportion by which the intervention reduced the event rate.

Odds Ratio

This is a relative measure of effect, allowing comparison of the intervention group relative to the control (placebo) group.

$$\frac{\text{The numerator is the odds in the intervention arm}}{\text{The denominator is the odds in the control (placebo) arm}} = \text{Odds ration (OR)}$$

Consequently, an OR of 1 shows no difference in risk between groups. OR >1 the control is better than the intervention, <1 the intervention is better than the control (Hicks, 2013).

Risk

Risk is the probability of an event happening and is calculated by dividing the number of events by the number of people at risk.

Risk Ratio (Can Be Referred to As Relative Risk)

Risk ratio is calculated by dividing risk in a treated (or exposed) group by the risk in a control (or unexposed) group (Harris & Taylor, 2004). Risk ratio is the ratio of the probability of an outcome in an exposed group to the probability of an outcome in an unexposed group. Together with risk difference and odds ratio, relative risk measures the association between exposure and outcome (Sistrom & Garvan, 2004).

P Values

The probability of any observed difference happening by chance is expressed as a P value. A P value of .5 means that the probability of any difference happening by chance is .5 in 1, therefore 50:50. The lower the P value, the less likely a difference has occurred by chance; $P = .01$ means a difference will only happen by chance 1 in 100 times and therefore is considered significant. Similarly, $P = .001$ means a difference will only happen due to chance 1 in 1000 times and is therefore considered very highly significant.

Type I and Type II Errors

- Type I errors occur when a correct hypothesis is rejected.
- Type II errors occur when an incorrect hypothesis is accepted.

References

De Angelis C, Drazon JM, Frizelle, FA, et al. 2005 Is this clinical trial fully registered? – a statement from the International Committee of Medical Journal Editors. New England Journal of Medicine 352, 2436–2438.

Department of Health/MRC 2006 Clinical Trials Tool Kit – planning a new trial. Online. www.ct-toolkit.ac.uk. Accessed 30 March 2006.

European Medicines Agency (EMA). Human regulatory. EMA 2018. www.ema.europa.eu/en/human-regulatory/research-development/clinical-trials/clinical-trial-regulation. Accessed 17 April 2021.

Harris M, Taylor G 2004 Medical statistics made easy. Taylor & Francis, London.

Hicks T. A beginner's guide to interpreting odds ratios, confidence intervals and p-values Students 4 best Evidence 2013. www.s4be.cochrane.org. Accessed 19 April 2021.

Information Commissioner's Office (ICO), 2018. Data Protection Act 2018. www.ico.org.uk/about-the-ico/what-we-do/legislation-we-cover/data-protection-act-2018. Accessed 1 July 2022.

Medicines and Healthcare products Regulatory Authority. MHRA Corporate Plan 2018–2023. www.gov.uk/government/publications/mhra-corporate-plan-2018-2023. Accessed 17 April 2021.

MHRA 2004 Description of the Medicines for Human Use (Clinical Trials) Regulations.

NICE 2002 Principles for best practice in clinical audit (supported by NHS, NICE, CHI).

NICE 2021 Audit and service improvement 2021. www.nice.org.uk/about/what-we-do/into-practoce/audit-and-service-improvement. Accessed 1 July 2022.

Sistrom CL, Garvan CW 2004 Proportions, odds, and risk. Radiology 230 (1), 12–19.

UKRI: Consent and Participation Information Guidance NHS Health Research Authority 2020. www.Hra-decisiontools.org.uk/consent. Accessed 19 April 2021.

Useful Sources of Information

Integrated Research Application System (IRAS): www.myresearchproject.org.uk

Medical Research Council (MRC): www.mrc.ac.uk
Tel: +44 (0)20 7636 5422, Fax: +44 (0)20 7436 6179

MHRA:
https://www.gov.uk/government/organisations/medicines-and-healthcare-products-regulatory-agency

16 | *Self-Assessment*

CHARITY KHOO AND ERNA BAYAR

Chapter 1: Structure and Function of the Genome

QUESTIONS

1. How many pairs of autosome chromosomes does each adult possess?
   A. 11
   B. 22
   C. 23
   D. 44
   E. 46

2. What is the most common process used for identifying chromosomes in the lab?
   A. Geisma stain
   B. PCR
   C. FISH
   D. Leishman stain
   E. Q banding

3. How many possible combinations of DNA are there?
   A. 22
   B. 46
   C. 64
   D. 82
   E. 108

4. Which of the following is a base pair in DNA?
   A. Cytosine and thymine
   B. Adenine and guanine
   C. Adenine and cytosine
   D. Thymine and guanine
   E. Cytosine and guanine

5. Which of the following is not a prerequisite for DNA replication?
   A. DNA template
   B. Oxygen
   C. Free DNA nucleotides
   D. DNA polymerase
   E. Primer

6. Which form of cell division results in haploid cells?
   A. Mitosis
   B. Meiosis
   C. Splicing
   D. Translocation
   E. Transcription

7. What is one of the roles of mitochondrial DNA?
   A. Confirming identity
   B. Confirming maternal origins
   C. Confirming paternal origins
   D. Predicting familial bowel cancer
   E. Predicting familial pancreatic cancer

8. Who first proposed the laws of disease inheritance patterns?
   A. Mendal
   B. Crick
   C. Watson
   D. Franklin
   E. Sanger

9. What procedure occurs by amplifying an RNA sequence to generate enough copies to visualise or manipulate?
   A. FISH
   B. PCR
   C. Southern blot
   D. Western Blot
   E. RT PCR

10. What is the basic principle of DNA electrophoresis?
    A. DNA molecules are slightly negatively charged and hence, under the right conditions, will migrate towards a buffer.
    B. DNA molecules are slightly negatively charged and hence, under UV conditions, will migrate towards a positive charge.
    C. DNA molecules are slightly negatively charged and hence, under the right conditions, will migrate towards a positive charge.
    D. DNA molecules are slightly positively charged and hence, under the right conditions, will migrate towards a negative charge.
    E. DNA molecules are slightly positively charged and hence, under UV conditions, will migrate towards a negative charge.

11. Which type of blot is used for protein analysis?
    A. Western
    B. Eastern
    C. Southern
    D. Northern
    E. Hybrid

Chapter 2: Clinical Genetics

QUESTIONS

1. Patau's syndrome is a trisomy of which chromosome?
   A. 18
   B. 13
   C. 20
   D. 21
   E. 15

2. Which trisomy will not survive to birth?
   A. 18
   B. 13
   C. 20
   D. 21
   E. X

3. Which of the following syndromes is an example of monosomy?
   A. Edwards'
   B. Patau's
   C. Down's
   D. Turner
   E. Jenner

4. Following up a patient after her surgical management of miscarriage, the histopathology describes a partial hydatidiform molar pregnancy. What type of numerical disorder of the chromosomes is this?
   A. Aneuploidy
   B. Polyploidy
   C. Monosomy
   D. Trisomy
   E. Mixoploidy

5. Which of the following is NOT a characteristic of DiGeorge syndrome (microdeletion 22q)?
   A. Cleft palate
   B. Autism
   C. Congenital heart problems
   D. Moon face
   E. Hypoparathyroidism

6. Which of the following characterise ring chromosome disorders?
   A. Intellectual disability, normal life expectancy
   B. Seizures, cleft palate
   C. Intellectual disability, cleft palate
   D. Seizures, normal life expectancy
   E. Intellectual disability, seizures

7. Which of the following is NOT an example of a single gene mutation at DNA level?
   A. Substitution
   B. Duplication
   C. Inversion
   D. Insertion
   E. Deletion

8. What type of mutation is described as mutation 'occurring when single base pair substitutions cause the generation of a premature stop codon'?
   A. Nonsense
   B. Silent
   C. Mistake
   D. Missense
   E. Frameshift

9. Which of the following is not an autosomal dominant disease?
   A. Huntington's
   B. Cystic fibrosis
   C. Marfan
   D. Tuberose sclerosis
   E. Osteogenesis imperfecta

10. A couple are both known to be carriers for an autosomal recessive condition. When planning their pregnancy, which of the following statements is correct?
    A. 75% risk of having an affected child
    B. 100% chance the child is a carrier
    C. 75% chance the child is not a carrier
    D. 66% chance unaffected sibling of an affected child will be a carrier
    E. 100% chance child will be affected

11. Which of the following is not an autosomal recessive disease?
    A. Phenylketonuria
    B. Cystic fibrosis
    C. Congenital adrenal hyperplasia
    D. Neurofibromatosis type 1
    E. Usher syndrome

Chapter 3: Embryology

QUESTIONS

1. Which of the following best describes the loss of ovarian follicles that occurs after birth?
   A. Apoptosis
   B. Necrosis
   C. Hypoplasia
   D. Atresia
   E. Aplasia

2. A 37-year-old woman asks what dose of folic acid she should be taking antenatally to prevent neural tube defects. Which of the following is not an indication for 5 mg folic acid?
   A. BMI >30
   B. Age >35
   C. Use of anti-epileptic medication
   D. Thalassaemia
   E. Diabetes mellitus

3. Where does the majority of fertilisation take place?
   A. Fimbria
   B. Infundibulum
   C. Ampulla
   D. Isthmus
   E. Fundus of the uterus

4. Compaction is defined as a change in the embryo shape that leads to the formation of:...
   A. The morula
   B. The blastocoele
   C. The trophoblast
   D. The cytotrophoblast
   E. The syncytiotrophoblast

5. Sertoli cells release
   A. Progesterone
   B. Oestrogen
   C. Testosterone
   D. Anti-müllerian hormone
   E. Follicular stimulating hormone

6. The ligamentum venosum is a remnant of
   A. Umbilical vein
   B. Umbilical artery
   C. Ductus venosus
   D. Ductus arteriosus
   E. Ligamentum teres

7. Which of the pharyngeal arches is associated with the glossopharyngeal nerve?
   A. 1st arch
   B. 2nd arch
   C. 3rd arch
   D. 4th arch
   E. 6th arch

8. A 41-year-old pregnant woman receives her combined screening result as high risk for trisomy 21. She is offered amniocentesis. Which cells obtained from the amniotic fluid are typically cultured for karyotyping?
   A. Epithelial cells
   B. Amniotic cells
   C. Glial cells
   D. Fibroblasts
   E. Red blood cells

9. Regarding the development of the urogenital system, the bladder and urethra are derived from:
   A. The primitive streak
   B. The ureteric bud
   C. The genital tubercle
   D. The mesonephric ducts
   E. The primate urogenital sinus

10. Regarding the development of the alimentary system, the hindgut is supplied by
    A. The superior mesenteric artery
    B. The inferior mesenteric artery
    C. The coeliac trunk
    D. The splenic artery
    E. The carotid artery

11. The mesoderm gives rise to all of the following except
    A. Muscles
    B. Connective tissue
    C. Reproductive system
    D. Blood vessels
    E. Nervous system

Chapter 4: Fetal and Placental Physiology

QUESTIONS

1. Following delivery, umbilical arteries constrict under the influence of:
   A. Serotonin and thromboxane A_2
   B. Serotonin and prostaglandins
   C. Dopamine and thromboxane A_2
   D. Serotonin and nitric oxide
   E. Progesterone and prostaglandins

2. Following delivery, the umbilical vein degenerates to become the:
   A. Ligamentum arteriosum
   B. Ligamentum flavum
   C. Ligamentum teres hepatis
   D. Ligamentum teres
   E. Ligamentum venosum

3. In the context of congenital heart disease, patency of the ductus arteriosus can be maintained with:
   A. Bradykinins
   B. Endothelin
   C. Acetylcholine
   D. Prostaglandin-E
   E. Oxygen

4. At what gestation do diaphragmatic breathing movements begin in the fetus?
   A. From 3 to 4 weeks
   B. From 5 to 16 weeks
   C. From 16 to 25 weeks
   D. From 26 weeks
   E. From 32 weeks

5. After birth, the GFR reaches adult levels by:
   A. Age 1
   B. Age 2
   C. Age 5
   D. Age 12
   E. Age 16

6. Fetal heart rate variability is best described as:
   A. Fluctuations in the fetal heart-rate baseline
   B. Transient increases in the fetal heart rate
   C. Transient decreases in the fetal heart rate
   D. A drop in the fetal heart rate to below 100 beats/min
   E. A rise in the fetal heart rate to above 160 beats/min

7. A 32-year-old woman is 24 weeks pregnant and presents with a gush of fluid. On examination, she is found to be 3 cm dilated. Which of the following should be administered within 24 hours of delivery to reduce the risk of cerebral palsy?
   A. Corticosteroids
   B. Progesterone
   C. Nifedipine
   D. Magnesium sulphate
   E. Surfactant

8. A patient experiencing tocophobia from a previous traumatic birth asks you what proportion of cerebral palsy cases are attributed to intrapartum fetal hypoxia:
   A. 10%
   B. 20%
   C. 30%
   D. 50%
   E. 60%

9. In utero, fetal temperature is regulated by the:
   A. Fetal liver
   B. Keratinised fetal skin
   C. Amniotic fluid
   D. Fetal gut
   E. Placenta

10. Hypoxic-ischaemic encephalopathy is defined as:
    A. Central nervous system dysfunction secondary to prolonged hypoxia.
    B. Bleeding inside or around the ventricles of the brain.
    C. A softening of white brain tissue near the ventricles.
    D. A group of disorders that involve a motor disability.
    E. Weakness or paralysis of muscles that can occur with injury to the brachial plexus.

11. A woman is 34 weeks pregnant and presents with increased leg swelling, headaches and visual symptoms. Her blood pressure is 150/95, and she is diagnosed with pre-eclampsia. By what gestational age is remodelling of the spiral arteries completed?
    A. 6 weeks
    B. 10 weeks
    C. 14 weeks
    D. 24 weeks
    E. 34 weeks

Chapter 5: Applied Anatomy

QUESTIONS

1. Which of the following is NOT a characteristic of a somatic nerve?
   A. The afferent pathways transmit sensor information.
   B. The efferent pathways innervate skeletal muscles.
   C. They cross the midline.
   D. The sensory cells are derived from the neural crest.

2. Which of the following is NOT a sympathetic effect?
   A. Increase in heart rate
   B. Constriction of detrusor muscle
   C. Dilation of bronchial tree
   D. Relaxation of the ciliary muscle
   E. Dilation of coronary arteries

3. What structures make up the brain stem?
   A. Cerebral hemispheres, lateral ventricle, midbrain
   B. Aqueduct of Sylvius, forebrain, pons
   C. Pons, medulla, forebrain
   D. Pons, medulla, midbrain
   E. Cerebral hemispheres, pons, medulla

4. Pituitary tumours usually grow upwards to cause which symptom?
   A. Temporal hemianopia
   B. Dysphagia
   C. Expressive dysphasia
   D. Hemiplegia
   E. Diplopia

5. Which of the following statements about the lymphatics vessels is incorrect?
   A. The function of the lymphatics is to remove fluid and debris from the extracellular system.
   B. This fluid is returned to the venous circulation.
   C. The lymphatics in the limbs are superficial.
   D. The thoracic duct drains lymph from the upper half of the body.
   E. The right thoracic duct drains the right thorax, upper limb, head and neck.

6. What tissues do the deep inguinal lymph nodes drain?
   A. Vulva, clitoris
   B. Superficial inguinal nodes, deep part of leg
   C. Clitoris, superficial inguinal nodes, vulva
   D. Superficial inguinal nodes, vulva, deep part of leg
   E. Deep part of leg, superficial inguinal nodes, clitoris

7. At which point does the aorta divide into the common iliac arteries?
   A. L3
   B. L4
   C. T12
   D. L2
   E. L5

8. Which of these is NOT a paired arterial branch of the aorta?
   A. Phrenic arteries
   B. Splenic arteries
   C. Lumbar segmental arteries
   D. Renal arteries
   E. Gonadal arteries

9. Which of the following does not drain into the IVC?
   A. Hepatic veins
   B. Left renal vein
   C. Left gonadal vein
   D. Right renal vein
   E. Right gonadal vein

10. The pelvis is made up of the sacrum, ischium, pubis and which other bone?
   A. Coccyx
   B. Ilium
   C. L5 vertebrae
   D. L4 vertebrae
   E. Femoral head

11. What is the name of this diagrammatic representation of a pelvic shape (see Fig. 5.8)?
   A. Android
   B. Gynaecoid
   C. Anthropoid
   D. Platypoid
   E. Rachitic

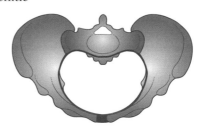

12. Which pelvic ligament runs from the lower aspect of the sacrum to the ischial spine?
   A. Sacrospinous
   B. Sacroilious
   C. Iliolumbar
   D. Sacrotuberous
   E. Lumbosacral

13. What is the average diameter of the fetal skull at vertex presentation?
   A. 9.5 cm
   B. 10 cm
   C. 10.5 cm
   D. 11 cm
   E. 11.5 cm

14. 'Submentobregmatic' refers to which fetal presentation?
   A. Occipital
   B. Face
   C. Brow
   D. Vertex
   E. Shoulder

15. Which fetal bone is highlighted in Fig. 5.10?
   A. Parietal bone
   B. Occipital bone
   C. Frontal bone
   D. Mandible

16. Which structure does not lie in the transpyloric plane?
   A. Duodenojejunal flexure
   B. Renal hila
   C. Neck of pancreas
   D. Fundus of gallbladder
   E. Liver edge

17. Which important landmark lies at the plane of the iliac crests?
   A. Pylorus of stomach
   B. Bifurcation of the abdominal aorta
   C. McBurney's point
   D. Termination of the spinal cord
   E. Origin of the inferior mesenteric artery

Chapter 6: Pathology

QUESTIONS

1. Which of the following is a feature of apoptosis?
   A. Cell swelling
   B. Inflammation
   C. Release of proinflammatory cytokines
   D. Absence of tissue destruction
   E. Disruption of normal tissue architecture

2. Hyperplasia is defined as
   A. Cytological changes associated with malignancy
   B. Reversible increase in cell size
   C. An increase in the number of cells in a tissue or organ
   D. A reduction in the cell number within an organ or tissue
   E. The process of new growth of cells

3. Which of the following is an example of hypertrophy?
   A. Postmenopausal changes to the endometrium
   B. Changes to the uterus during pregnancy
   C. Changes in the transformation zone of the cervix from columnar to squamous cells
   D. Changes to breast glands during pregnancy and lactation
   E. Cellular changes detected during a cervical smear test

4. Which of the following is not a cytological feature of malignancy?
   A. Abnormal nuclear shape
   B. Abnormal mitosis
   C. Cytological heterogeneity
   D. Increased nuclear to cytoplasmic ratio
   E. Abnormal differentiation

5. Cervical intraepithelial neoplasia precedes cervical carcinoma by approximately how many years?
   A. 1 year
   B. 5 years
   C. 10 years
   D. 20 years
   E. 30 years

6. A 29-year-old woman is seen in clinic with a 4-week history of postcoital bleeding. Which of the following is not a risk factor for cervical cancer?
   A. HIV infection
   B. Smoking
   C. Number of sexual partners
   D. Family history
   E. Prolonged use of oral contraceptives

7. The most carcinogenic sub-type of human papilloma virus (HPV) is:
   A. HPV-16
   B. HPV-18
   C. HPV-31
   D. HPV-33
   E. HPV-35

8. Which of the following dermatological conditions is most associated with vulval malignancy?
   A. Lichen sclerosus
   B. Lichen planus
   C. Psoriasis
   D. Candida infection
   E. Lichen simplex

9. Miscarriage occurs in what proportion of clinical pregnancies?
   A. 5%
   B. 15%
   C. 30%
   D. 50%
   E. 75%

10. A woman is 18 weeks pregnant and presents with spotting and abdominal cramping. What is the commonest cause of late second-trimester spontaneous miscarriage?
    A. Chromosomal abnormalities
    B. Ascending genital tract infection
    C. Urinary tract infection
    D. Alcohol consumption
    E. Antiphospholipid syndrome

11. What percentage of partial hydatidiform pregnancies progress into choriocarcinoma?
    A. 0.5%
    B. 5%
    C. 15%
    D. 25%
    E. 50%

Chapter 7: Microbiology and Virology

QUESTIONS

1. Regarding gram-positive bacteria, which statement is false?
   A. Gram-positive bacteria have a thick peptidoglycan layer.
   B. Gram-positive bacteria stain blue or black.
   C. Gram-positive bacteria have a complex outer membrane of lipoprotein and lipopolysaccharides.
   D. Group B streptococcus is gram positive.
   E. Gram-positive bacteria have teichoic acids present in their cell walls.

2. Which of the following components within the structure of gram-positive bacteria can contribute to the development of toxic shock?
   A. Exotoxins
   B. Teichoic acids
   C. Peptidoglycans
   D. Phospholipids
   E. Flagellin

3. A woman is 34 weeks pregnant and presents with vomiting, diarrhoea and flu-like symptoms. *Listeria monocytogenes* is seen as:
   A. Gram-positive rods

B. Gram-negative rods
C. Gram-positive cocci
D. Gram-negative cocci
E. Gram-positive spirillum

4. A 22-year-old woman reports a change in her vaginal discharge and superficial dyspareunia following unprotected sex with a new partner 3 weeks ago. Which of the following is correct regarding *Neisseria gonorrhoea?*
   A. *N. gonorrhoea* is gram positive.
   B. *N. gonorrhoea* is a commensal of the genital tract.
   C. Infection is asymptomatic in 10% of women.
   D. *N. gonorrhoea* is an anaerobic organism.
   E. It is a gram-negative diplococci bacteria.

5. Which of the following viruses does not have oncogenic ability?
   A. Human immunodeficiency virus
   B. Human T-cell lymphotrophic virus type 1
   C. Varicella zoster virus
   D. Human papilloma viruses
   E. Epstein–Barr virus

6. Infection with which virus can lead to T-cell leukaemia?
   A. Human immunodeficiency virus
   B. Human T-cell lymphotrophic virus type 1
   C. Varicella zoster virus
   D. Human papilloma virus
   E. Epstein-Barr virus

7. Which of the following is a DNA virus?
   A. Hepatitis A
   B. Human immunodeficiency virus
   C. Japanese B virus
   D. Cytomegalovirus
   E. Rubella

8. The SARS-CoV-2 genome is:
   A. Double-stranded DNA
   B. Single-stranded DNA
   C. Double-stranded RNA
   D. Single-stranded RNA
   E. Approximately 200,000 base pairs long

9. A 27-year-old woman presents with an increase in thin grey-coloured vaginal discharge with an offensive fishy odour. Microscopy demonstrates clue cells. What is the most likely causative organism?
   A. *Staphylococcus aureus*
   B. *Trichomonas vaginalis*
   C. *Neisseria gonorrhoea*
   D. *Candida albicans*
   E. *Gardnerella vaginalis*

10. Which of the following is not routinely screened for as part-antenatal booking bloods?
    A. Syphilis
    B. Hepatitis B
    C. Varicella zoster virus
    D. Human immunodeficiency virus
    E. Sickle cell disease

11. Which of the following HPV subtypes can cause genital warts?
    A. 6 and 11
    B. 16 and 18
    C. 6 and 16
    D. 11 and 18
    E. 18 and 31

Chapter 8: Immunology

QUESTIONS

1. A 32-year-old woman presents with an acute asthma attack. Which immunoglobulin type binds to mast cells and basophils leading to release of histamine?
   A. IgA
   B. IgG
   C. IgM
   D. IgD
   E. IgE

2. A 37-week pregnant woman asks about the benefits of breastfeeding. Which immunoglobulin is found in mucosal secretions, such as breast milk?
   A. IgA
   B. IgG
   C. IgM
   D. IgD
   E. IgE

3. Which of the following immune cells stimulate naïve T cells?
   A. Natural killer cells
   B. Macrophages
   C. Mast cells
   D. Dendritic cells
   E. Cytotoxic T cells

4. In which part of the immunoglobulin structure is the antigen binding region found?
   A. Variable light chain
   B. Variable heavy chain
   C. Variable light chain and heavy chain
   D. Hinge region
   E. Constant domain

5. Which of the following immune cells destroy virally infected cells?
   A. B cells
   B. T cells
   C. T-helper cells
   D. Cytotoxic T cells
   E. Mast cells

6. Which of the following statement about the adaptive immune system is false? The adaptive immune system:
   A. Is slow
   B. Relies on memory
   C. Is activated with re-exposure

D. Consists of B- and T-cell lymphocytes
E. Produces antibodies

7. Haemolytic disease of the newborn occurs when...
    A. Maternal Rhesus positive, fetus Rhesus positive
    B. Maternal Rhesus positive, fetus Rhesus negative
    C. Maternal Rhesus negative, fetus Rhesus positive
    D. Maternal Rhesus negative, fetus Rhesus negative
    E. All of the above

8. Which of the following immunoglobulin subtypes can cross the placenta?
    A. IgA
    B. IgG
    C. IgM
    D. IgD
    E. IgE

9. Which of the following steps is in common in all of the complement pathways?
    A. Binding of lectin to mannose on pathogens
    B. Activation of C1 by antigen-antibody complexes
    C. Cleavage of C3 into C3a and C3b
    D. Binding of C3b directly with a microbe
    E. Activation of C2

10. Which of the following immune cells destroy neoplastically transformed cells?
    A. B cells
    B. T cells
    C. T-helper cells
    D. Cytotoxic T cells
    E. Mast cells

11. Which of the following is not a main function of antibodies?
    A. To act as the B-cell receptor for antigens
    B. To bind directly to toxins, viruses and other molecules, blocking their ability to bind to target cells
    C. To recruit effector mechanisms to the target cell
    D. To activate the complement system
    E. To destroy viral infected cells

Chapter 9: Biochemistry

QUESTIONS

1. Which of the following statements about the cell nucleus is false?
    A. The cells nucleus contains cytoplasm.
    B. The cells nucleus contains the chromosomes.
    C. The nucleus walls are made up of a lipid bilayer.
    D. The nucleus may contain more than one nucleolus.
    E. RNA is transported out of the nucleus.

2. What is the function of ribosomes?
    A. Oxidative phosphorylation
    B. mRNA generation
    C. Splicing of genomes
    D. Catalysis and synthesis of proteins

E. Release of energy

3. What type of collagen is predominantly found in the fetus?
    A. Type 0
    B. Type I
    C. Type II
    D. Type III
    E. Type IV

4. Where in the adult is albumin synthesised?
    A. Liver
    B. Kidneys
    C. Adrenal glands
    D. Lungs
    E. Duodenum

5. Which of the following amino acids cannot be synthesised in vivo?
    A. Alanine
    B. Aspartic acid
    C. Asparagine
    D. Cysteine
    E. Arginine

6. Glycolytic enzymes are found in which part of a cell?
    A. Nucleus
    B. Cell membrane
    C. Cytoplasm
    D. Mitochondria
    E. Golgi apparatus

7. Where does the citric acid cycle take place?
    A. Golgi apparatus
    B. Mitochondrian
    C. Filament
    D. Centriole
    E. Endoplasmic reticulum

8. Where are erythrocytes degraded?
    A. Liver
    B. Spleen
    C. Adrenal glands
    D. Bone marrow
    E. Pancreas

9. At which temperature are most enzymes destroyed?
    A. 100°C
    B. 80°C
    C. 60°C
    D. 40°C
    E. 20°C

10. What is missing from the above equation describing a single substrate reaction?

Enzyme + Substrate
→ Enzyme – Substratecomplex
→ Enzyme +

    A. Complex
    B. Amino acid

C. Gas
D. Product
E. ATP

11. In competitive enzyme inhibition, what happens to the V_{max} when the Michaelis constant is increased?
A. It increases.
B. It remains constant.
C. It is doubled.
D. It is halved.
E. It is reduced.

Chapter 10: Physiology

QUESTIONS

1. Which of the following situations does not cause an increase in the anion gap?
A. Myeloma
B. Ketoacidosis
C. Lactic acidosis
D. Salicylate poisoning
E. Hypoalbuminaemia

2. Which of the following shortens the QT interval?
A. Hypocalcaemia
B. Hypokalaemia
C. Rheumatic carditis
D. Digoxin
E. Citalopram

3. What is the normal resting cardiac output in females?
A. 3.5 L/min
B. 4 L/min
C. 4.5 L/min
D. 5 L/min
E. 5.5 L/min

4. Which of the following regarding cardiac function in pregnancy is false?
A. Plasma volume increases.
B. Red cell mass increases.
C. Haematocrit increases.
D. Cardiac output increases.
E. Stroke volume increases.

5. What is the maximum healthy blood pressure at term?
A. 110/70 mmHg
B. 120/80 mmHg
C. 130/90 mmHg
D. 145/95 mmHg
E. 150/95 mmHg

6. Which of the following acts as a vasodilator?
A. Endothelin
B. Angiotensin
C. Thromboxane
D. Nitric oxide
E. Oxytocin

7. Levels of which clotting factors fall in pregnancy?
A. Fibrinogen and protein S
B. Fibrinogen and factor V
C. Factor V and factor VIII
D. Factor VIII and endogenous anticoagulant
E. Endogenous anticoagulant and protein S

8. A 25-year-old woman who uses the combined oral contraceptive pill presents with shortness of breath and pleuritic chest pain. Which of the following would be consistent with a pulmonary embolism?
A. Respiratory acidosis
B. Respiratory alkalosis
C. Metabolic acidosis
D. Metabolic alkalosis
E. Normal acid-base balance

9. How is cardiac output calculated?
A. Cardiac output = stroke volume × heart rate
B. Cardiac output = stroke volume × systolic blood pressure
C. Cardiac output = heart rate × systolic blood pressure
D. Cardiac output = systolic blood pressure − diastolic blood pressure
E. Cardiac output = stroke volume × diastolic blood pressure

10. During pregnancy,
A. Ventilation decreases.
B. Tidal volume increases.
C. FEV_1 increases.
D. Peak flow rate increases.
E. Peak flow rate decreases.

11. During pregnancy, bronchoconstriction is caused by:
A. Nitric oxide
B. Progesterone
C. Oxytocin
D. Prostaglandin E_2
E. Prostaglandin F_2

Chapter 11: Endocrinology

QUESTIONS

1. Steroid hormones are synthesised from:
A. Prostaglandins
B. Arachidonic acid
C. Cholesterol
D. Leukotrienes
E. Catecholamines

2. Aldosterone secretion occurs in the:
A. Outer zona glomerulosa of the adrenal cortex
B. Middle zona fasciculata of the adrenal cortex
C. Inner zona reticularis of the adrenal cortex
D. Anterior pituitary
E. Posterior pituitary

3. Arachidonic acid is a precursor molecule for:
   A. Guanylyl cyclase
   B. Prostaglandins
   C. Nitric oxide
   D. Cholesterol
   E. Testosterone

4. The pineal gland plays a role in producing the following hormone, which is involved in the regulation of the 'body clock' and puberty:
   A. GnRH-associated peptide
   B. Melatonin
   C. Kisspeptin
   D. Leptin
   E. Dihydroepiandrostenedione

5. The adenohypophysis secretes all of those below except for:
   A. Luteinising hormone
   B. Follicle-stimulating hormone
   C. Thyroid-stimulating hormone
   D. Oxytocin
   E. Prolactin

6. In females, what proportion of circulating testosterone is produced in the ovary?
   A. <1%
   B. 5%
   C. 25%
   D. 50%
   E. 75%

7. Leptin expression is increased by all the below except for:
   A. Insulin
   B. Food
   C. Noradrenaline
   D. Glucocorticoids
   E. Oestrogen

8. What is the average age of menarche in the United Kingdom?
   A. 11
   B. 12
   C. 13
   D. 14
   E. 15

9. What is the average age of menopause in the United Kingdom?
   A. 48
   B. 49
   C. 50
   D. 51
   E. 52

10. A 37-year-old woman presents with amenorrhoea for 1 year, accompanied with hot flushes and reduced libido. Which of the following blood tests, if taken on two occasions 4 to 6 weeks apart, can assist in the diagnosis?
    A. Anti-müllerian hormone
    B. FSH
    C. Progesterone

D. Inhibin A
E. Inhibin B

11. Which of the following statements about growth hormone is false?
    A. Growth hormone is a 191 amino acid peptide.
    B. Growth hormone is released from the anterior pituitary gland.
    C. Growth hormone promotes fat lipolysis.
    D. Growth hormone levels are increased by somatostatin.
    E. Exercise stimulates growth hormone release.

Chapter 12: Drugs and Drug Therapy

QUESTIONS

1. What is the Henderson-Hasselbalch equation used to calculate?
   A. The volume of plasma cleared of the drug in unit time
   B. The rate at which a drug leaves its site of administration
   C. The pH at which half the drug is in its ionised form
   D. The ratio of ionised to non-ionised drug at each pH
   E. The fractional extent to which a dose of drug reaches its site of action

2. At what gestation is the risk of teratogenicity highest?
   A. 7–10 weeks
   B. 0–11 weeks
   C. 3–7 weeks
   D. 4–16 weeks
   E. 9–12 weeks

3. What type of drug transport is described as the diffusion of the drug through the cell membrane along a concentration gradient by virtue of its lipid solubility?
   A. Active
   B. Passive
   C. Transcellular
   D. Transcapillary
   E. Facilitated diffusion

4. A patient is on $MgSO_4$ following an eclamptic seizure. She is noted to have respiratory depression, and $MgSO_4$ levels are high. What is the key contributory factor to this?
   A. Oliguria
   B. Pulmonary oedema
   C. Tachycardia
   D. Sedation
   E. Anaemia

5. Which of the following physiological changes of pregnancy does NOT affect drug metabolism?
   A. Hyperemesis
   B. Delayed gastric emptying
   C. Increased $\alpha 1$-acid glycoprotein levels
   D. Increased GFR
   E. Decreased albumin concentrations

6. A patient is taking 30 mg prednisolone. She wishes to breastfeed. What is the best advice to give her?
   A. Do not breastfeed.
   B. Breastfeed, but wait 2 hours until after the dose to feed the infant.
   C. Breastfeed, but wait 4 hours until after the dose to feed the infant.
   D. Breastfeed, but wait 6 hours until after the dose to feed the infant (use expressed milk in meantime).
   E. Breastfeed, but wait 12 hours until after the dose to feed the infant (use expressed milk in meantime).

7. A patient presents in threatened preterm labour. She is offered steroids. What % of the maternal dose of β-methasone will cross the placenta?
   A. 20
   B. 40
   C. 60
   D. 80
   E. 100

8. Which of the following antiepileptic drugs is NOT teratogenic?
   A. Sodium valproate
   B. Carbamazepine
   C. Phenobarbital
   D. Lamotrigine
   E. Phenytoin

9. You are seeing a 25-year-old epileptic patient in clinic. She is 18 weeks pregnant and taking 100 mg lamotrigine/day. She has been fit free for 1 year and is feeling well. What advice will you give her regarding her medicine?
   A. It will need stepwise increments as her pregnancy increases.
   B. Levels do not need to be checked.
   C. Her levels will need checking regularly during the pregnancy.
   D. Stop taking the medicine as she has been fit-free for 1 year.
   E. She will need dose reduced due to impaired clearance during pregnancy.

10. You are in the early pregnancy unit scanning a patient who presented following referral from her GP with PV bleeding at 11 weeks. The scan shows a viable intrauterine pregnancy. In the consultation, she brings up that she has been struggling with hyperemesis, and taking a variety of antiemetics. She is suffering from a dry mouth, blurred vision and constipation. Which antiemetic is likely to be the cause of this?
    A. Ondansetron
    B. Domperidone
    C. Cyclizine
    D. Promethazine
    E. None of the above

11. Which antibiotic causes 'grey baby syndrome' and thus should be avoided in labour and the third trimester?
    A. Streptomycin
    B. Chloramphenicol
    C. Tazocin

D. Nitrofurantoin
E. Gentamicin

Chapter 13: Physics in Obstetrics and Gynaecology

QUESTIONS

For each of the questions below, please select the single most appropriate answer from the five options listed.

1. What are the four defined modes of electrosurgery?
   A. Cutting, diathermy, coagulation, cauterisation
   B. Desiccation, cutting, coagulation, cauterisation
   C. Coagulation, desiccation, cutting, fulguration
   D. Faridation, coagulation, desiccation, cutting
   E. Diathermy, cutting, coagulation, desiccation

2. A surgeon applies diathermy forceps to an artery clip holding a 6 mm bleeding vessel. What is this an example of?
   A. Direct coupling
   B. Indirect coupling
   C. Capacitive coupling
   D. Direct application
   E. Poor insulation

3. What does LASER stand for?
   A. Long Amplification by Stimulated Emission of Radiation
   B. Low Amplification by Simulated Emission of Radiation
   C. Light Amplification by Simulated Emission of Radiation
   D. Light Amplification by Stimulated Emission of Radiation
   E. Low Amplification by Stimulated Emission of Radiation

4. Which of the below would show up as white on a T2-weighted MRI scan?
   A. Fat- and water-containing tissues
   B. Fluid-containing tissues
   C. Fat-containing tissues
   D. Water-containing tissues
   E. Fluid- and water-containing tissues

5. What is the absorbed dose of ionising radiation for a chest x-ray in a pregnant patient?
   A. 1 mGy
   B. 0.1 mGy
   C. 0.01 mGy
   D. 10 mGy
   E. 100 mGy

6. Known side-effect(s) of ultrasound scans is/are...
   A. Doppler Shift
   B. Cavitation, heating, microsteaming
   C. Cavitation, microsteaming, heating, cellular destruction
   D. Cavitation, microsteaming
   E. Cavitation, heating

7. Listening to the fetal heartbeat is feasible due to which effect?
   A. Sonic auscultation
   B. Power velocity
   C. Pulse reflection
   D. Doppler shift
   E. Colour flow

8. Which best describes the ways that an ultrasound wave will react with tissues?
   A. Reflection, diffraction, absorption, Doppler and scatter
   B. Reflection, refraction, diffraction, absorption and scatter
   C. Reflection, refraction, absorption and scatter
   D. Reflection, refraction, diffraction and absorption
   E. Reflection, refraction, diffraction, absorption and scatter

9. A 16 weeks pregnant woman with a history of preterm birth attends an appointment for transvaginal ultrasound assessment of her cervical length. What is the frequency range for transvaginal ultrasounds?
   A. 2–6 MHz
   B. 7–9 MHz
   C. 20–60 MHz
   D. 70–90 MHz
   E. 2–15 MHz

10. A 14 weeks pregnant woman has experienced abdominal pain and PV spotting. What is the frequency range for transabdominal ultrasounds?
    A. 2–6 MHz
    B. 7–9 MHz
    C. 20–60 MHz
    D. 70–90 MHz
    E. 2–15 MHz

11. Acoustic impedance is best described as:
    A. An estimate of mean velocity of flow within a vessel
    B. The bending of waves around the corners of an obstacle
    C. The ultrasound behaviour within a tissue
    D. A phenomenon arising when a wave confronts an impediment with a diameter equivalent to its wavelength
    E. The difference between transmitted and received frequency

Chapter 14: Statistics and Evidence-Based Health Care

QUESTIONS

1. A study is looking at whether all women in the population have regular periods. 34 women aged 18 to 24 were questioned, and it was found that all of them had periods at intervals of 26 to 42 days. The study therefore surmised that all women in the population had periods at 26 to 42 days. This is an example of:
   A. Under-powered study
   B. Type 1 error
   C. Type 2 error
   D. Unclear hypothesis
   E. Multiple influence

2. What is the definition of a type 2 error?
   A. When 'the sample' used in your experiment fails to generate a significant result for your hypothesis, but there would not have been a significant result if you had performed the experiment on 'the population'
   B. When 'the sample' used in your experiment generates a significant result for your hypothesis, but there would have been a significant result if you had performed the experiment on 'the population'
   C. When 'the sample' used in your experiment generates a significant result for your hypothesis, but there would not have been a significant result if you had performed the experiment on 'the population'
   D. When 'the sample' used in your experiment fails to generate a significant result for your hypothesis, but there would have been a significant result if you had performed the experiment on 'the population'
   E. When studies have been sampled in a non-random fashion, differences between the results from the sample and the true population can arise

3. A patient is asking about her scan review. The fetal growth falls on the 30th centile. She is concerned that it is not sitting on the black dot in the centre and is therefore undergrown. What is the best explanation of this?
   A. Using confidence intervals within a population, we can estimate that 95% of all babies will fall outside the lines, and thus, your baby falls within the remits of normal.
   B. Using confidence intervals within a sample, we can estimate that 95% of all babies will fall between the lines, and thus, your baby falls within the confidence intervals of normal.
   C. Using type 2 errors within a population, we can estimate that 95% of all babies will fall between the lines, and thus, your baby falls within the confidence intervals of normal.
   D. Using confidence intervals within a population, we can estimate that 95% of all babies will fall between the lines, and thus, your baby falls within the confidence intervals of normal.
   E. Using confidence intervals within a sample, we can estimate that 95% of all babies will fall outside the lines, and thus, your baby falls within the confidence intervals of normal.

4. In a study looking at menorrhagia, the data is sorted into three groups – mild bleeding, moderate bleeding and severe bleeding. What type of data is this?
   A. Ordinal
   B. Categorised
   C. Qualitative
   D. Binary
   E. Continuous

5. Which of the following is NOT a type of mathematical distribution used in statistics?
   A. Binomial
   B. Poisson
   C. Binary
   D. Normal
   E. Chi-squared

6. Which presentation method is not appropriate for qualitative data?
   A. Scatter plots
   B. Line plots
   C. Box plots
   D. Bar charts
   E. Histograms

7. In an audit looking at the age of women presenting at the early pregnancy clinic on a certain day the following ages were recorded:
   29, 30, 22, 45, 31, 22, 17, 38 and 36.

   What is the median?
   A. 22
   B. 29
   C. 30
   D. 36
   E. 39

8. The below table looks at the outcome of early pregnancy scans in smokers for early embryonic demise and the management plans.

MANAGEMENT OF MISCARRIAGE	SMOKER	NON-SMOKER	TOTAL
Surgical	3	6	9
Conservative	4	3	7
Total	7	9	16

   What are the odds of having a surgical management of pregnancy in a smoker?
   A. 3/6 – 50%
   B. 3/4 – 75%
   C. 7/9 – 78%
   D. 6/3 – 200%
   E. 3/16 – 19%

9. A new variant of a respiratory infection is noted to be in the UK, and 36,000 people have this new respiratory infection. What is this?
   A. Incidence
   B. Prevalence
   C. Rate
   D. Risk
   E. Proportion

10. What is the odds ratio?
   A. Measure of association between exposure and outcome
   B. Measure of association between time and outcome
   C. Ratio of the probabilities of risk in one group compared to the possibilities of an occurrence of risk in another group
   D. Ratio of time and exposure
   E. Likelihood of one event happening in place of another

11. A patient comes to the day assessment unit at 36 weeks with possible rupture of membranes. You perform a test for rupture of membranes. She wants to know what the 95% accuracy rate of the tests means.
   A. How good is this test at correctly excluding people without the condition?
   B. How good is this test at picking up people who have the condition?
   C. What proportion of all tests have given the correct result?
   D. If a person tests positive, what is the probability that they have the condition?
   E. If a person tests negative, what is the probability that they do not have the condition?

Chapter 15: Clinical Research Methodology

QUESTIONS

1. A study is set up to look at vaping in pregnancy. The notes are reviewed of women who vape in pregnancy compared with those who continued to smoke. The outcomes of their pregnancy were looked into, including birthweight, mode of delivery and gestation at delivery.
   What type of clinical research is this?
   A. Case control study
   B. Randomised control trial
   C. Qualitative research
   D. Quantitative research
   E. Cohort study
   F. Systematic research

2. What trial is considered the gold standard for NHS care?
   A. Case control study
   B. Randomised control trial
   C. Qualitative research
   D. Quantitative research
   E. Cohort study
   F. Systematic research

3. A hospital wants to look at the effect of different shift patterns of nursing staff on patient satisfaction. It selects its eight medical wards and introduces differing shift patterns to each, with two remaining on the old pattern. The outcomes are evaluated using patient and nursing feedback. This is an example of what type of trial?
   A. Audit
   B. Cluster randomised trial
   C. Cohort study
   D. Case control study
   E. Stepped wedge cluster randomised trial

4. You are conducting a clinical trial to assess whether a new drug can improve success rates of in vitro

fertilisation. During your study, a serious, unexpected adverse event that was not mentioned in the protocol occurs. How soon should this be reported?
A. Within 24 hours
B. Within 48 hours
C. Within 7 days
D. Within 28 days
E. In the annual report

5. In which year was the Data Protection Act updated alongside the UK GDPR act to form the primary data protection legislation in the UK?
A. 2015
B. 2016
C. 2017
D. 2018
E. 2019

6. In RCTs, the only difference between the two groups should be:
A. Intervention
B. Time for study
C. Risk factors
D. Age
E. Place of trial

7. What are the responsibilities of the ethics committee?
A. Ensuring proposals meet the requisite standards
B. Safeguarding the rights and wellbeing of trial subjects
C. Ensuring proposals meet the requisite standards and protecting the rights and wellbeing of trial subjects
D. Ensuring proposals meet the international ethics standards and safeguarding the rights and wellbeing of trial subjects
E. Ensuring proposals meet the requisite ethics standards and protecting the rights of the trial subjects

8. Which of the following is NOT an aim of the European Union Clinical Trials Directive?
A. To protect the rights, safety and wellbeing of trial participants
B. To establish transparent procedures that will harmonise trial conduct in the EU
C. To establish transparent procedures to ensure the credibility of results
D. To simplify and harmonise administrative provisions governing clinical trials.
E. To protect the rights of the principal investigator

9. Which of the following is NOT a key benefit of updated Clinical Trials Regulation?
A. Harmonised electronic submission and assessment processes for clinical trials conducted in multiple member states
B. No requirement for each site to submit to the Clinical Trials Directive
C. Improved collaboration, information-sharing and decision-making between and within member states
D. Increased transparency of information on clinical trials
E. Highest standards of safety for all participants in EU clinical trials

10. How many days does the MHRA have to make its decision with regard to an application for investigation?
A. 10
B. 21
C. 32
D. 45
E. 60

11. Which of these is not a lawful basis for data processing (GDPR)?
A. Consent
B. Contract
C. Legal obligation
D. Vital interests
E. Personal task

Mock Exam Papers

MOCK EXAM PAPER 1

1. A mother has suffered a stillbirth at 36 weeks. When discussing the postmortem she asks about extraction of DNA from the baby. Which of these methods will not yield DNA?
A. Bone extraction
B. Formaldehyde fixed tissue blocks
C. Fetal blood
D. Fetal saliva
E. Fetal urine

2. What are single-base DNA mutations called?
A. Point mutations
B. Germ-line mutations
C. Somatic mutations
D. Genomic mutations
E. Polymerised mutations

3. What are the mutations found in cancerous tumours known as?
A. Point mutations
B. Germ-line mutations
C. Somatic mutations
D. Genomic mutations
E. Polymerised mutations

4. Which of the following is NOT tested for in the heel prick test on the fifth day of life?
A. Phenylketonuria
B. Congenital adrenal hyperplasia
C. Homocystinuria
D. Cystic fibrosis
E. Sickle cell disease

5. Sickle cell disease is the result of which single amino acid change?
A. Glutamine to valine
B. Valine to glutamine
C. Alanine to glutamine
D. Alanine to valine
E. Glutamine to alanine

6. Which of the following is NOT an X-linked recessive condition?
   A. Turner syndrome
   B. Duchenne muscular dystrophy
   C. Haemophilia A
   D. G6PD deficiency
   E. Haemophilia B

7. The thick glycoprotein layer surrounding the secondary oocyte is known as the
   A. Corpus luteum
   B. Zona pellucida
   C. Antrum
   D. Corona radiata
   E. Trophectoderm

8. At which stage of meiosis does the primary oocyte arrest?
   A. Prophase I
   B. Prophase II
   C. Metaphase I
   D. Metaphase II
   E. Interphase

9. Which of the following hormones drives spermatogenesis?
   A. ACTH
   B. AMH
   C. FSH + LH
   D. Progesterone + oestrogen
   E. FSH + AMH

10. Which of the following does not cause low birth weight?
    A. Smoking
    B. Anorexia nervosa (<500 kcal/day)
    C. Chronic maternal inflammatory disease
    D. Pre-eclampsia
    E. Alcohol (in the absence of fetal alcohol syndrome)

11. In the absence of fetal alcohol syndrome, alcohol consumption in pregnancy can lead to...
    A. Abnormal spiral artery remodelling
    B. Reduced placental weight
    C. Fetal growth restriction
    D. Maternal hypertension
    E. Macrosomia

12. Which of the following hormones is not produced by the placenta?
    A. Oestrogen
    B. Progesterone
    C. Luteinising hormone
    D. Human chorionic gonadotrophin
    E. Pregnancy-associated plasma protein A

13. A complete molar pregnancy is caused by:
    A. A single sperm fusing with an anucleate oocyte
    B. Two sperm fusing with a normal oocyte
    C. Splitting of a blastocyst into two embryos
    D. Two sperm fusing with two sperm
    E. A Robertsonian translocation

14. What genotype occurs in a partial molar pregnancy?
    A. 46XX
    B. 46XY
    C. 69XXY
    D. 45X0
    E. 44XXY

15. In pregnancy, ascending genital infection can lead to all except for:
    A. Chorioamnionitis
    B. Preterm prelabour rupture of membranes
    C. Late second-trimester loss
    D. Preterm birth
    E. Maternal hypertension

16. Which of the following viral infections can lead to the development of Kaposi sarcoma?
    A. Hepatitis B
    B. Hepatitis C
    C. Varicella zoster virus
    D. Human immunodeficiency virus
    E. Cytomegalovirus

17. In the UK, what is the incidence of HIV-1 infection among pregnant women in inner city regions?
    A. 0.05%
    B. 0.5%
    C. 5%
    D. 15%
    E. 25%

18. To what extent does the use of antiretroviral therapy reduce transmission of HIV-1 from an infected mother to the fetus?
    A. From 20% to 2%
    B. From 20% to 5%
    C. From 15% to 2%
    D. From 15% to 5%
    E. From 30% to 2%

19. Where do T cells mature?
    A. Peripheral circulation
    B. Thymus
    C. Bone marrow
    D. Liver
    E. Thyroid

20. MHC II molecules mostly interact with which type of immune cells?
    A. Mast cells
    B. Macrophages
    C. B cell lymphocytes
    D. CD4 T cells
    E. CD8 T cells

21. The alternate pathway of the complement system is activated by:
    A. Lectin binding to mannose on pathogens
    B. Antigens bound to MHC molecules
    C. Microorganisms
    D. Antigen-antibody complexes
    E. Membrane attack complexes

22. A patient in clinic tells you that she has had a letter from her GP stating that she is deficient in thiamine. Which vitamin do you tell her to buy from the pharmacy for supplementation?
   A. Vitamin B12
   B. Vitamin B7
   C. Vitamin B6
   D. Vitamin B3
   E. Vitamin B1

23. Which of the following is NOT a fat-soluble vitamin?
   A. A
   B. C
   C. D
   D. E
   E. K

24. Regarding the digestion of protein, which of the following statements is correct?
   A. Digestion of protein begins in the pancreas. The 'chief' cells secrete pepsinogen. The parietal (oxyntic) cells secrete hydrochloric acid, and the resulting low pH causes the hydrolysis of pepsinogen into pepsin, which is a proteolytic enzyme.
   B. Digestion of protein begins in the stomach. The oxyntic cells secrete pepsinogen. The parietal cells secrete hydrochloric acid, and the resulting low pH causes the hydrolysis of pepsinogen into pepsin, which is a proteolytic enzyme.
   C. Digestion of protein begins in the stomach. The parietal cells secrete pepsinogen. The chief cells secrete hydrochloric acid, and the resulting low pH causes the hydrolysis of pepsinogen into pepsin, which is a proteolytic enzyme.
   D. Digestion of protein begins in the stomach. The 'chief' cells secrete pepsinogen. The parietal (oxyntic) cells secrete hydrochloric acid, and the resulting high pH causes the hydrolysis of pepsinogen into pepsin, which is a proteolytic enzyme.
   E. Digestion of protein begins in the stomach. The 'chief' cells secrete pepsinogen. The parietal (oxyntic) cells secrete hydrochloric acid, and the resulting low pH causes the hydrolysis of pepsinogen into pepsin, which is a proteolytic enzyme

25. Carbon monoxide:
   A. Shifts the haemoglobin dissociation curve to the to the right
   B. Has a lower affinity for haemoglobin than oxygen
   C. Toxicity causes immediate cyanosis
   D. Prevents peripheral liberation of oxygen that is combined with haemoglobin
   E. Reduces the oxygen capacity of haemoglobin by 80%

26. A 25-year-old woman is 32 weeks pregnant and has been admitted with urosepsis. Which of the following is normal in pregnancy?
   A. Dilatation of the right pelvicalyceal system
   B. Protein (mg):creatinine (mmol) ratio greater than 0.30
   C. Raised heart-rate of 140 beats/min

D. Reduced secretion of antidiuretic hormone
E. Raised creatinine greater than 77 µmol/L

27. A woman is at 30-weeks' gestation with twins, and her most recent bloods show haemoglobin of 93 g/L. The most likely cause of anaemia in pregnancy is...
   A. Reduced absorption of dietary iron
   B. Haemodilution
   C. Increased urinary excretion of iron
   D. Reduced rate of erythropoiesis
   E. Reduced life cycle of the erythrocyte

28. Which of the following regarding vitamin D is false?
   A. Vitamin D is synthesised from cholesterol.
   B. Vitamin D is mostly acquired from UV light.
   C. 10% of vitamin D is acquired from diet.
   D. Parathyroid hormone levels control vitamin D levels.
   E. 25-hydroxylation occurs in the kidneys.

29. In pregnancy,
   A. Circulating levels of thyroid binding hormones are decreased.
   B. The total circulating levels of thyroid hormones decrease.
   C. hCG has a thyrotrophic effect.
   D. Hyperemesis gravidarum can markedly elevate TSH levels.
   E. Thyroid function should routinely be assessed every 4 to 6 weeks.

30. Development of the external male genitalia is promoted by the action of:
   A. Anti-müllerian hormone
   B. Oestrogen
   C. Dihydrotestosterone
   D. Dihydroepiandrostenedione
   E. Growth hormone

31. Which of these is not attributable to carbimazole use during the first trimester?
   A. Choanal atresia
   B. Fetal aplastic anaemia
   C. Fetal goitre
   D. Fetal hypothyroidism
   E. Tracho-oesophageal fistula

32. Doxorubicin is used in the treatment of breast, ovarian, endometrial, bladder and thyroid cancers. Which cancer is not treated with Doxorubicin?
   A. Breast
   B. Bladder
   C. Ovarian
   D. Endometrial
   E. Bowel

33. Which diuretic acts by inhibiting sodium transport in the distal convoluted tubule of the nephron?
   A. Frusemide
   B. Spironolactone
   C. Bendroflumethiazide
   D. Acetazolamide
   E. Amiloride

34. Which of the following imaging modalities involves the use of ionising radiation?
    A. Magnetic resonance imaging
    B. Ultrasound imaging
    C. Diathermy
    D. X-ray
    E. Electrocautery

35. Which of the following statements about magnetic resonance imaging (MRI) is false?
    A. MRI uses non-ionising radiation.
    B. The international system unit used to determine magnetic field strength is the Tesla.
    C. In T2-weighted MRI images, fat and bone appear dark.
    D. In T1-weighted MRI images, water and fluid appear bright.
    E. MRI relies on the movement of protons within tissues to produce an image.

36. The process by which an unstable atomic nucleus loses energy by radiation is known as:
    A. Attenuation
    B. Decay
    C. Doppler shift
    D. Diffraction
    E. Absorption

37. In performing an audit into presentations to gynaecology clinic, there is difficulty in attaining notes, and thus only notes from telephone clinics are used as they are available on the computer system. What type of bias is this?
    A. Measurement bias
    B. Selection bias
    C. Responder bias
    D. Observer bias
    E. Recall bias

38. In a focus group on the postnatal ward, recently delivered mothers are invited to give their opinion on their birth experience and asked specifically about how long it took for them to be offered analgesia postdelivery. The mothers discuss this and give estimates of time between 2 and 6 hours. A check of the maternal notes suggests that this length of time does not correlate with the drug charts or midwifery notes. What type of bias does this demonstrate?
    A. Measurement bias
    B. Selection bias
    C. Responder bias
    D. Observer bias
    E. Recall bias

39. An SHO is asked to look into all the women who have had a perineal repair in the last week, and how many of those were given the antibiotic prophylaxis. This is an example of what type of study?
    A. Cohort study
    B. Cross sectional study
    C. Ecological study
    D. Case control study
    E. Randomised controlled trial

40. In GDPR, what lawful basis can be described as 'the processing is necessary for your legitimate interests or the legitimate interests of a third party unless there is a good reason to protect the individual's personal data which overrides those legitimate interests'.
    A. Legitimate interests
    B. Contract
    C. Legal obligation
    D. Vital interests
    E. Personal task

41. Researchers in a clinical trial give each participant a code number. Only the researchers can identify the participants from the code. What type of data is this?
    A. Pseudo-anonymised data
    B. Anonymised data
    C. Coded data
    D. Pseudo-coded data
    E. Unlinked coded data

42. A researcher is talking to a patient about using part of their placenta for a research study. All the data will be anonymised. Which of the following does the researcher not have to give to the patient?
    A. Patient information leaflet
    B. Types of data you will be collecting
    C. The name of the data controller
    D. The fact that the data will be stored
    E. Type of anonymisation

43. Which of the following is NOT contained within the rectus sheath?
    A. Pyramidalis muscle
    B. Inferior epigastric artery
    C. Superior epigastric artery
    D. Rectus abdominis muscle
    E. Internal oblique muscle

44. At which point does the external iliac artery become the femoral artery?
    A. The midpoint of the inguinal ligament
    B. Halfway between the anterior superior iliac spine and pubic tubercule
    C. Two thirds laterally along a line from the umbilicus and anterior superior iliac spine
    D. 1 cm lateral to the pubic tubercle
    E. Halfway between the anterior superior iliac spine and symphysis pubis

45. The round ligament passes through which canal or foramen?
    A. Inguinal canal
    B. Deep inguinal ring
    C. Superficial inguinal ring
    D. Femoral ring
    E. Inguinal triangle of Hesselbach

46. Which of these is not a border of the femoral ring?
    A. Pectineus muscle
    B. Pubic tubercle
    C. Lacunar ligament
    D. Femoral vein
    E. Inguinal ligament

47. Where should the surgical incision for appendicectomy be in pregnancy?
    A. Over McBurney's point
    B. 2 cm superior to McBurney's point
    C. Over point of maximal tenderness
    D. 2 cm lateral from point of maximal tenderness
    E. Two thirds laterally along a line from the umbilicus and anterior superior iliac spine

48. Which hormones do chromaffin cells secrete?
    A. Oestrogen
    B. Adrenocortical hormones
    C. Catecholamines
    D. Luteinising hormone
    E. Follicular stimulating hormone

MOCK EXAM PAPER 2

1. Polymerase chain reaction is a laboratory technique:
   A. Where a sequence of DNA is amplified millions of times to generate enough copies to visualise
   B. That allows DNA, RNA or protein molecules to be separated according to their charge
   C. That transfers molecules from a gel onto a blotting membrane
   D. That locates a specific DNA sequence on a chromosome by attaching a small DNA sequence with a fluorescent probe
   E. That determines the number and size of cells using a flow cytometer

2. Which of the following statements about DNA polymerase is true:
   A. DNA polymerase synthesises DNA in the 3′ to 5′ direction.
   B. DNA polymerase synthesises DNA in the 5′ to 3′ direction.
   C. DNA polymerase synthesises RNA in the 3′ to 5′ direction.
   D. DNA polymerase synthesises RNA in the 5′ to 3′ direction.
   E. DNA polymerase synthesises DNA and RNA in the 3′ to 5′ direction.

3. Which of the following base pairs does RNA not contain?
   A. Adenine
   B. Cytosine
   C. Uracil
   D. Guanine
   E. Thymine

4. Deficiency of which factor is responsible for haemophilia A?
   A. VII
   B. IX
   C. X
   D. XI
   E. XII

5. In fragile X syndrome, there is expansion of the DNA segment of the promotor region in which gene?
   A. CHD2
   B. FGHFR3
   C. FMR1
   D. SCN5A
   E. FGHFR2

6. You see a couple in clinic who are known to carry the cystic fibrosis gene. Which of the following gene sequencing methods is best for detecting cystic fibrosis?
   A. FISH
   B. Karyotype
   C. QF-PCR
   D. Chromosomal microarray
   E. DNA Sequencing

7. Nuclear material is stored in which part of the sperm?
   A. Sperm head
   B. Sperm neck
   C. Sperm midpiece
   D. Sperm principal piece
   E. Sperm endpiece

8. A couple present to clinic with primary subfertility. What is the normal sperm count in an average ejaculate?
   A. 6×106 / mL
   B. 60×106 / mL
   C. 600×106 / mL
   D. 6000×106 / mL
   E. $60,000 \times 106$ / mL

9. The endoderm gives rise to:
   A. The nervous system and skin
   B. Muscles and bone
   C. Endocrine glands and blood vessels
   D. The gastrointestinal tract and endocrine glands
   E. The respiratory tract and connective tissue

10. Which of the following statements about fetal haemoglobin (HbF) is correct?
    A. Adult haemoglobin (HbA) has a greater affinity for oxygen than HbF.
    B. Fetal haematocrit is higher than in adult life.
    C. HbA has a higher saturation of oxygen at a lower partial pressure than HbF.
    D. HbF forms 10% of adult haemoglobin.
    E. The fetal oxygen content of the blood is inadequate to meet its needs in normal circumstances.

11. Prematurity increases the risk of all the below except for:
    A. Exomphalos
    B. Necrotising enterocolitis
    C. Respiratory distress syndrome
    D. Hirschsprung's
    E. Hypoxic-ischaemic encephalopathy

12. Which cells synthesise surfactant?
    A. Bronchial endothelial cells
    B. Type I pneumocytes

C. Bronchial epithelial cells
D. Type II pneumocytes
E. Fetal erythrocytes

13. Which of the following is not considered a risk factor for ectopic pregnancy?
    A. Smoking
    B. Pelvic inflammatory disease
    C. Human papilloma virus
    D. In vitro fertilisation
    E. Intrauterine device in situ

14. The most common site of an ectopic pregnancy is:
    A. Tubal
    B. Cervical
    C. Ovarian
    D. Caesarean section scar
    E. Abdominal

15. During pregnancy, a bicornuate uterus may increase the risk of:
    A. Intrauterine death
    B. Fetal sepsis
    C. Breech presentation
    D. Subchorionic haematoma
    E. Hydatidiform mole

16. A 20-week pregnant woman is diagnosed with Parvovirus B19 infection. Which of the following fetal complications is not associated with Parvovirus B19 infection?
    A. Fetal anaemia
    B. Developmental defects
    C. Viral myocarditis
    D. Fetal hydrops fetalis
    E. Spontaneous abortion

17. Which of the following viral infections can lead to fetal birth defects?
    A. HIV-1
    B. Coxsackie B virus
    C. Hepatitis C
    D. Parvovirus B19
    E. Varicella zoster virus

18. How is culture medium sterilised?
    A. Disinfectant
    B. Boiling
    C. Autoclaving
    D. Hot air oven
    E. Ionising radiation

19. Helper T cells are usually:
    A. CD4 +
    B. CD8 +
    C. CD95+
    D. CD4+ and CD8+
    E. CD3+

20. Which complement components directly form the membrane attack complex?
    A. C1, C4, C2, C3a, C3b
    B. C1, C4, C2, C3b, C5b

C. C3a, C3b, C5a, C5b
D. C3b, C5b, C7, C8, C9
E. C5b, C6, C7, C8, C9

21. Which of the following immune cell types produce IgE?
    A. Eosinophils
    B. Mast cells
    C. Basophils
    D. Plasma cells
    E. Neutrophils

22. Which of the following statements regarding aspirin is NOT true?
    A. A low dose of aspirin works in the hepatic portal system.
    B. Aspirin permanently inhibits platelet thromboxane synthesis.
    C. Most aspirin is inactivated within the liver.
    D. Small volumes of aspirin enter the general circulation.
    E. Aspirin promotes prostacyclin synthesis within the hepatic portal system.

23. Where is ANP secreted?
    A. Atriums of the heart
    B. Adrenal glands
    C. Stomach
    D. Pancreas
    E. Spleen

24. Which of the following is NOT a function of insulin?
    A. Glucose uptake and glycogen synthesis in skeletal muscle
    B. Produces glycogen from glucose
    C. Promotes liver uptake of glucose
    D. Stimulates adipocytes to make glycerol
    E. Activates potassium influx into many cell types

25. A woman experiences a massive obstetric haemorrhage secondary to atony. Blood tests indicate disseminated intravascular coagulation (DIC). Which of the following is seen in DIC?
    A. Thrombocytopenia
    B. Raised fibrinogen
    C. Increased factor VII
    D. Reduced activated partial thromboplastin time
    E. Low D-dimer

26. Which antibody type is involved in causing haemolytic disease of the newborn?
    A. IgA
    B. IgD
    C. IgE
    D. IgG
    E. IgM

27. The first sensation of bladder filling occurs at what bladder volume?
    A. 10 mL
    B. 50 mL
    C. 150–200 mL
    D. 220–320 mL
    E. 320–420 mL

28. In a 28-day cycle, when do circulating oestrogen levels rise?
    A. Day 0–5
    B. Day 5–8
    C. Day 8–10
    D. Day 12–14
    E. Day 15–20

29. During the menstrual cycle, progesterone levels are highest during:
    A. The luteal phase
    B. The follicular phase
    C. Menstruation
    D. Ovulation
    E. Throughout

30. In pregnancy, the hCG levels peak at
    A. 10 days after ovulation
    B. 4–6 weeks' gestation
    C. 8–10 weeks' gestation
    D. 10–12 weeks' gestation
    E. From 16 weeks' gestation

31. Which of the following is NOT a use of prostaglandin agonists?
    A. Ripening of the cervix
    B. Induction of labour
    C. Abortifacient
    D. Treatment of menorrhagia
    E. Treatment of PPH

32. A 32-year-old multip is due to start oxytocin for prolonged SROM. She has been told of the risk of tachysystole and hyperstimulation. She is asking what the half-life of oxytocin is. What do you tell her?
    A. 1 minute
    B. 3 minutes
    C. 5 minutes
    D. 10 minutes
    E. 20 minutes

33. Which of the following statements about β agonist tocolytics is true?
    A. They act by reducing progesterone production.
    B. They improve perinatal mortality rates.
    C. Pulmonary oedema is a known side effect.
    D. They decrease the risk of neonatal microhaemorrhages.
    E. They can be used to extend gestation even when steroids have been administered.

34. Which of the following influences the speed of ultrasound?
    A. Wavelength
    B. Amplitude
    C. Impedance
    D. Decay
    E. Scatter

35. Ultrasound waves can lose energy to the tissue through...
    A. Viscous, relaxation and thermodynamic losses
    B. Decay, relaxation and thermodynamic losses
    C. Decay and thermodynamic losses
    D. Scatter, decay and thermodynamic losses
    E. Scatter, viscous and thermodynamic losses

36. Which of the following imaging modalities allows for functional imaging and can measure changes in metabolic processes?
    A. Magnetic resonance imaging
    B. Positron emission imaging
    C. X-ray imaging
    D. Ultrasound
    E. Computerised tomography

37. Standard deviation is:
    A. The square root of the variance
    B. Used to indicate how well the sample mean measurement represents the true population mean value
    C. The most common value in the dataset
    D. The midpoint of all the observations
    E. The total range of values between the largest and smallest observation

38. A research team wants to explore whether a new medication reduces the risk of preterm birth. Participants are randomly allocated to receive the new medication or a placebo. What kind of study is this?
    A. Case-control study
    B. Observational study
    C. Cohort study
    D. Randomised control trial
    E. Cross-sectional study

39. Which of the following regarding screening tests is false?
    A. Screening tests should be cheap.
    B. Screening tests should be widely available.
    C. Screening tests should have a high specificity.
    D. Screening tests should identify rare conditions.
    E. Screening tests should only be used for treatable conditions.

40. What literacy age is recommended when writing a patient information sheet?
    A. 10 years
    B. 11 years
    C. 12 years
    D. 14 years
    E. 16 years

41. In a research trial involving a new hay fever vaccine, one of the participants is hospitalised with a life-threatening serious side effect. The chief investigator is informed. Within how many days does the CI have to tell the REC?
    A. 7
    B. 10
    C. 15
    D. 21
    E. 30

42. In the same trial above, the CI also has to inform the sponsor after how many days?
    A. 7
    B. 10
    C. 15
    D. 21
    E. 30

43. Which of the following crosses the left ovarian artery?
    A. Middle colic vessels
    B. Ileocolic vein
    C. Descending colon
    D. Terminal ileal vein
    E. IVC

44. Which vein do the superficial external pudendal veins drain directly into?
    A. Femoral vein
    B. Great saphenous vein
    C. Deep external pudendal vein
    D. IVC
    E. External iliac vein

45. Which muscle does the femoral nerve supply?
    A. Piriformis muscle
    B. Quadriceps muscle
    C. Obturator internus
    D. Psoas muscle
    E. Gluteus medius

46. Which nerve on the posterior division of the sacral plexus goes through the sacrotuberous ligament?
    A. Superior gluteal
    B. Common peroneal part of sciatic
    C. Posterior cutaneous nerve of thigh
    D. Perforating cutaneous nerve
    E. Inferior gluteal

47. Which of the following is not found in the deep perineal pouch?
    A. External urethral sphincter
    B. Ischiocavernosus muscles
    C. Deep transverse perineal muscle
    D. Glands of Cowper
    E. Areolar tissue

48. The blood supply to the upper two thirds of the vagina is from which arteries?
    A. Perineal artery
    B. Dorsal artery
    C. Internal iliac arteries
    D. Pudendal artery
    E. Uterine artery

MOCK EXAM PAPER 3

1. Complementary base pairs are joined by:
    A. Peptide bonds
    B. Hydrogen bonds
    C. Phosphodiester bonds
    D. Histone proteins
    E. Molecular bonding

2. What technique was used to identify the double helix structure of DNA?
    A. Electrophoresis
    B. Flow cytometry
    C. X-ray crystallography
    D. Polymerase chain reaction
    E. Western blotting

3. Which of the following laboratory methods is used for the analysis of compositional properties of DNA?
    A. Northern blotting
    B. Southern blotting
    C. Western blotting
    D. PCR
    E. Flow cytometry

4. Which karyotype gives the clinical picture of a female infant with low birthweight, small chin, narrow palpebral fissures, overlapping fingers, rocker bottom feet, congenital heart defects and death, usually within few weeks of birth?
    A. 47, XX + 18
    B. 47, XY + 18
    C. 47, XX + 13
    D. 47, XY + 13
    E. 47, XX + 21

5. Which of the following is QF PCR NOT the first line test for detecting?
    A. Angelman
    B. Klinefelter
    C. Edwards'
    D. Patau's
    E. Prader-Willi

6. Which cytogenetics test allows the rapid simultaneous analysis of multiple regions of DNA in a single reaction?
    A. FISH
    B. MLPA
    C. QF-PCR
    D. Chromosomal microarray
    E. DNA sequencing

7. In females, the genital tubercle develops into the
    A. Labia minora
    B. Labia majora
    C. Clitoris
    D. Bladder
    E. Urethra

8. Which of the following is not true regarding amniotic fluid?
    A. Amniotic fluid has a lower partial pressure of oxygen than maternal arterial blood.
    B. Amniotic fluid is more alkaline than maternal blood.
    C. Amniotic fluid contains lipids, carbohydrates and protein.
    D. Amniotic fluid has antibacterial properties.
    E. The amino acid concentration in amniotic fluid is similar to that of maternal plasma.

9. In males, the genital tubercle develops into the...
   A. Prostate
   B. Penis
   C. Scrotum
   D. Urethra
   E. Bladder

10. Surfactant synthesis is promoted by:
    A. Thyroid hormones
    B. Glucocorticoids
    C. Epidermal growth factor
    D. All of the above
    E. None of the above

11. Prematurity can lead to the following complications, except:
    A. Retinopathy
    B. Periventricular leukomalacia
    C. Respiratory distress
    D. Hyaline membrane disease
    E. Haemolytic disease

12. Transfer of IgG across the placenta occurs by:
    A. Active transport
    B. Vesicular transport
    C. Simple diffusion
    D. Glucose transporters
    E. Exchanger transporters

13. In the case of a hydatidiform, surveillance to detect persistent disease should involve:
    A. Maternal progesterone levels
    B. Maternal βHCG serum levels
    C. Transvaginal ultrasound scanning
    D. Urine βHCG levels
    E. No surveillance needed

14. Which of the following is not true of ovarian tumours?
    A. 90% of malignant ovarian tumours are derived from surface epithelium.
    B. Ovarian adenocarcinoma usually affects adolescents.
    C. Germ cell tumours typically occur in younger patients.
    D. Teratomas are the commonest ovarian neoplasms.
    E. Sex cord stromal tumours are usually hormone producing.

15. Abnormal placentation, which can occur secondary to the presence of a caesarean-section scar, can lead to:
    A. First trimester miscarriage
    B. Chorioamnionitis
    C. Placenta accreta
    D. Choriocarcinoma
    E. Hydatidiform mole

16. A 24 weeks pregnant woman has recently completed a course of cefalexin for a urinary tract infection. She now presents with thick, white and itchy vaginal discharge. What is the first-line management?
    A. Repeat course of cefalexin
    B. Metronidazole
    C. Clindamycin
    D. Clotrimazole
    E. Amoxicillin

17. A 34-year-old woman presents with frothy, offensive vaginal discharge. On speculum examination, findings are in keeping with a strawberry cervix. Which of the following is identified by flagella movements in wet preparations?
    A. *Trichomonas vaginalis*
    B. *Toxoplasmagondii*
    C. *Neisseria gonorrhoea*
    D. *Gardnerella vaginalis*
    E. *Streptococcus agalactiae*

18. Which of the following is a gram-negative bacterium?
    A. *Streptococcus* spp.
    B. *Enterococcus* spp.
    C. *Lactobacillus* spp.
    D. *Neisseria* spp.
    E. *Staphylococcus* spp.

19. In anti-phospholipid syndrome, circulating antibodies against which molecules exist?
    A. C3b
    B. C5b
    C. Cardiolipin
    D. Rhesus blood group antigen
    E. Thyroid peroxidase

20. What is the main function of the complement system?
    A. Hypersensitivity
    B. Opsonisation
    C. Conferring fetal immunity
    D. Avoiding autoimmunity
    E. Destruction of neoplastically transformed cells

21. A 35-year-old woman is 12 weeks pregnant and reports exposure to chicken pox. Which of the following blood results indicate previous exposure to chicken pox?
    A. Varicella zoster IgG positive
    B. Varicella zoster IgM positive
    C. Cytomegalus virus IgG positive
    D. Cytomegalus virus IgM positive
    E. Epstein-Barr virus IgM positive

22. What is the Warburg effect?
    A. Cancer cells have less oxidative phosphorylation activity and more glycolytic activity than normal cells, even in the presence of sufficient oxygen.
    B. Cancer cells have more oxidative phosphorylation activity and more glycolytic activity than normal cells, even in the presence of sufficient oxygen.
    C. Cancer cells have less oxidative phosphorylation activity and less glycolytic activity than normal cells, even in the presence of sufficient oxygen.
    D. Cancer cells have more oxidative phosphorylation activity and less glycolytic activity than normal cells, even in the presence of sufficient oxygen.
    E. Cancer cells have less oxidative phosphorylation activity and more glycolytic activity than normal cells, even in the presence of sufficient oxygen.

23. What is the name of the process that causes a reduction in the oxygen affinity of RBCs in response to raised CO_2 in the blood?
    A. Bohr effect
    B. Krebs cycle
    C. Gluconeogenesis
    D. Eicosanoid synthesis
    E. Hypercapnea oxyreduction acidosis

24. Which of the following statements about Bilirubin is true?
    A. Haem is broken down in the spleen into microhaem
    B. The microhaem binds with serum albumin and produces bilirubin.
    C. The bilirubin is moved to the liver to produce glucose.
    D. The glucose produces bile for storage in the small intestine.
    E. Bile in the small intestine helps to break down fats.

25. In which obstetric condition are bile salts raised?
    A. Pre-eclampsia
    B. HELLP syndrome
    C. Obstetric cholestasis
    D. Gestational diabetes
    E. Cholelithiasis

26. Which of the following liver enzymes increases in pregnancy?
    A. ALP
    B. AST
    C. GGT
    D. ALT
    E. Bilirubin

27. Where is renin mostly produced?
    A. Pulmonary endothelial cells
    B. Capillaries of the glomerulus
    C. Kupffer cells
    D. Juxtaglomerular apparatus of the kidney
    E. Vascular endothelial cells

28. Prolactin...
    A. Is released from the posterior pituitary
    B. Is stimulated by dopamine
    C. Is inhibited by TRH
    D. Controls the milk-ejection reflex
    E. Release is continued in response to suckling

29. Hormones synthesised by the hypothalamus include:
    A. Gonadotrophin-releasing hormone, growth hormone-releasing hormone and prolactin.
    B. Gonadotrophin-releasing hormone, growth hormone-releasing hormone and corticotrophin-releasing hormone.
    C. Prolactin, FSH and TSH.
    D. Somatostatin, prolactin and corticotrophin-releasing hormone.
    E. Gonadotrophin-releasing hormone, corticotrophin-releasing hormone and prolactin.

30. The posterior pituitary gland secretes:
    A. Vasopressin
    B. Prolactin
    C. Growth hormone
    D. ACTH
    E. LH

31. A patient is about to commence magnesium sulphate for severe pre-eclampsia. Her midwife is orientating, but the unit is very busy, so she is the only midwife looking after the patient. She asks for warning signs for toxicity to look out for on the MEOWS. What do you tell her to look for?
    A. High pulse rate, low respiratory rate, high blood pressure
    B. High pulse rate, low respiratory rate, low saturations, high blood pressure
    C. Low pulse rate, low respiratory rate, low blood pressure
    D. Low pulse rate, low saturations, high respiratory rate, low blood pressure
    E. High pulse rate, low respiratory rate, low saturations, low blood pressure

32. A patient on $MgSO_4$ is on the labour ward. She is awaiting a caesarean delivery of her 28-week-old preterm breech baby for abnormal Dopplers on scan today. She is very anxious, and you are asked to see her to consent her for the delivery. On arrival in the room, she is feeling very sleepy and has vomited. She has a BP 70/30, her pulse rate is 90, her resp. rate is 4. What are the most appropriate next steps for you to take?
    A. A, B C management, fast bleep anaesthetist
    B. A, B C management, stop MgSO4, call 2222
    C. Stop MgSo4
    D. A, B C management, stop MgSO4, call 2222, administer 1% calcium gluconate
    E. A, B C management, call 2222, administer 1% calcium gluconate

33. Which of the following drugs is a relative contraindication for use in pregnancy?
    A. Griseofulvin
    B. Sodium valproate
    C. Lithium
    D. Methotrexate
    E. Atorvastatin

34. Electrons with positive charge are known as:
    A. Protons
    B. Neutrons
    C. α particles
    D. Positrons
    E. Measons

35. The biological effect of radiation on the human body is measured as:
    A. Sieverts (Sv)
    B. Becquerel (Bq)
    C. Megahertz (MHz)

D. Ohms
E. Volts

36. When using diathermy, the effect of heat on tissue will depend on all the below except for:
    A. Surface area
    B. Duration
    C. Proximity of instrument to tissue
    D. Tissue conductivity
    E. Body mass index of patient

37. In a sample of 100 women, the mean age of menarche is 14 years old, and shows a normal distribution. The standard deviation is 1 year. The standard error of the mean is therefore:
    A. 0.01
    B. 0.1
    C. 0.02
    D. 0.2
    E. 0.5

38. An obstetric unit looks at the fetal fibronectin result for women who end up delivering before 37 weeks' gestation. Data from 500 women is obtained and shows a normal distribution. The mean fetal fibronectin result is 225 and the variance is 9. What is the standard deviation for this data set?
    A. 3
    B. 5
    C. 10
    D. 15
    E. 81

39. Which of the following is true regarding the P value?
    A. The P value indicates the likelihood of a type 1 error.
    B. The P value assumes the null hypothesis is false.
    C. A P value of $>.05$ suggests a significant difference.
    D. The P value is the probability of detecting a significant finding if the null hypothesis is true.
    E. The standard P value used in most statistical analyses is 0.01.

40. What does the following describe?
    'This is the number of patients with a condition testing positive for that condition. It describes the effectiveness of a test at picking up a condition'.
    A. Specificity
    B. Sensitivity
    C. Positive predictive value
    D. Likelihood ratio
    E. Incidence

41. Hospital workers are asked to take a flow test for a highly contagious infection, and only attend work if they are negative. The have a negative predictive value of 90%. What does this mean?
    A. If the test is negative, they are 90% likely not to have the infection.
    B. If the test is positive, they are 10% likely to have the infection.
    C. If the test in negative, they are 10 % likely to have the infection.
    D. If the test is positive, they are 90% likely to have the infection.
    E. If they take 10 tests in 1 day, 9 tests will be negative.

42. What is the P valuc?
    A. Probability threshold for statistical significance
    B. Estimation of variance among groups
    C. Likelihood of observed outcome happening by chance
    D. Difference between the observed outcome and the expected outcome
    E. Number of standard deviations away from the mean

43. The vagina is lined by what type of epithelium?
    A. Simple squamous
    B. Stratified squamous
    C. Simple cuboidal
    D. Stratified cuboidal
    E. Stratified transitional

44. Lymphatic drainage of the rectum is to which nodes?
    A. Pararectal and external iliac nodes
    B. Internal and external iliac nodes
    C. Pararectal and internal iliac nodes
    D. Superficial inguinal nodes and pararectal nodes
    E. Superficial inguinal nodes and internal iliac nodes

45. What is the normal capacity of the bladder?
    A. 350 mL
    B. 400 mL
    C. 500 mL
    D. 550 mL
    E. 600 mL

46. What is the blood supply to the urethra?
    A. Inferior vesical artery
    B. Inferior pudendal artery
    C. Superior vesical artery
    D. Inferior vesical artery and inferior pudendal artery
    E. Superior vesical artery and inferior pudendal artery

47. Alveolar development of the breast is due to which hormone?
    A. Progesterone
    B. Oestrogen
    C. Growth hormone
    D. Parathyroid hormone
    E. Insulin

48. The base of the breast is in the midclavicular line over which ribs?
    A. Second to fourth
    B. Second to fifth
    C. Second to sixth
    D. Third to fifth
    E. Third to sixth

Answers

CHAPTER 1: STRUCTURE AND FUNCTION OF THE GENOME

1. B
2. A
3. C
4. E
5. B
6. B
7. B
8. A
9. E
10. C
11. A

CHAPTER 2: CLINICAL GENETICS

1. B
2. C
3. D
4. B
5. D
6. E
7. C
8. A
9. B
10. D
11. D

CHAPTER 3: EMBRYOLOGY

1. D
2. B
3. C
4. A
5. D
6. C
7. C
8. D
9. E
10. B
11. E

CHAPTER 4: FETAL AND PLACENTAL PHYSIOLOGY

1. A
2. C
3. D
4. D
5. B
6. A
7. D
8. B
9. C
10. A
11. D

CHAPTER 5: APPLIED ANATOMY

1. C
2. B
3. D
4. A
5. D
6. D
7. B
8. C
9. C
10. B
11. B
12. A
13. E
14. B
15. B
16. E
17. B

CHAPTER 6: PATHOLOGY

1. D
2. C
3. B
4. C
5. D
6. D
7. A
8. A
9. B
10. B
11. A

CHAPTER 7: MICROBIOLOGY AND VIROLOGY

1. C
2. A
3. A
4. E
5. C
6. B
7. D
8. D
9. E
10. C
11. A

CHAPTER 8: IMMUNOLOGY

1. E
2. A
3. D
4. C
5. D
6. A
7. C
8. B
9. C
10. D
11. E

CHAPTER 9: BIOCHEMISTRY

1. A
2. D
3. D
4. A
5. E
6. C
7. B
8. B
9. C
10. D
11. B

CHAPTER 10: PHYSIOLOGY

1. A
2. D
3. C
4. C
5. D
6. D
7. E
8. B
9. A
10. B
11. E

CHAPTER 11: ENDOCRINOLOGY

1. C
2. A
3. B
4. B
5. D
6. C
7. E
8. C
9. C
10. B
11. D

CHAPTER 12: DRUGS AND DRUG THERAPY

1. D
2. A
3. B
4. A
5. C
6. C
7. D
8. D
9. C
10. C
11. B

CHAPTER 13: PHYSICS IN OBSTETRICS AND GYNAECOLOGY

1. C
2. A
3. C
4. E

5. C
6. B
7. D
8. E
9. B
10. A
11. C

CHAPTER 14: STATISTICS AND EVIDENCE-BASED HEALTH CARE

1. B
2. D
3. D
4. A
5. C
6. D
7. C
8. B
9. B
10. A
11. C

CHAPTER 15: CLINICAL RESEARCH METHODOLOGY

1. A
2. B
3. E
4. C
5. D
6. A
7. C
8. E
9. B
10. E
11. E

MOCK EXAM PAPER 1

1. E
2. A
3. C
4. B
5. B
6. A
7. B
8. A
9. C
10. E
11. B
12. C
13. A
14. C
15. E
16. D
17. B
18. C
19. B
20. D
21. C
22. D
23. B

24. D
25. D
26. A
27. B
28. E
29. C
30. C
31. B
32. E
33. C
34. D
35. D
36. B
37. B
38. E
39. B
40. A
41. C
42. E
43. E
44. E
45. A
46. B
47. C
48. C

MOCK EXAM PAPER 2

1. A
2. B
3. E
4. A
5. C
6. E
7. A
8. B
9. D
10. B
11. D
12. D
13. C
14. A
15. C
16. B
17. E
18. C
19. A
20. E
21. D
22. D
23. A
24. C
25. A
26. D
27. C
28. D
29. A
30. D
31. D
32. B
33. C
34. C
35. A

36. B
37. A
38. D
39. D
40. B
41. C
42. A
43. C
44. B
45. B
46. D
47. B
48. C

MOCK EXAM PAPER 3

1. B
2. C
3. B
4. A
5. B
6. A
7. C
8. B
9. B
10. D
11. E
12. B
13. B
14. B
15. C
16. D
17. A
18. D
19. C
20. B
21. A
22. E
23. A
24. E
25. C
26. A
27. D
28. E
29. B
30. A
31. E
32. E
33. C
34. D
35. A
36. E
37. B
38. A
39. D
40. B
41. A
42. C
43. B
44. C
45. C
46. D
47. A
48. C

Index